Acupuncture and Acupressure

Acupuncture and Acupressure

Edited by Patrick Lampard

SYRAWOOD
PUBLISHING HOUSE

New York

Published by Syrawood Publishing House,
750 Third Avenue, 9th Floor,
New York, NY 10017, USA
www.syrawoodpublishinghouse.com

Acupuncture and Acupressure
Edited by Patrick Lampard

International Standard Book Number: 978-1-68286-488-3 (Hardback)

Cataloging-in-Publication Data

Acupuncture and acupressure / edited by Patrick Lampard.
    p. cm.
Includes bibliographical references and index.
ISBN 978-1-68286-488-3
1. Acupuncture. 2. Acupressure. 3. Alternative medicine. 4. Traditional medicine. I. Lampard, Patrick.
RM184 .A28 2017
615.892--dc23

Printed in the United States of America.

TABLE OF CONTENTS

PREFACE

It is often said that books are a boon to mankind. They document every progress and pass on the knowledge from one generation to the other. They play a crucial role in our lives. Thus I was both excited and nervous while editing this book. I was pleased by the thought of being able to make a mark but I was also nervous to do it right because the future of students depends upon it. Hence, I took a few months to research further into the discipline, revise my knowledge and also explore some more aspects. Post this process, I began with the editing of this book.

Acupuncture and acupressure are both widely practiced forms of alternative medicine. Acupuncture is a part of traditional Chinese medicine that requires the insertion of needles to pre-determined pressure points. Acupuncture and acupressure methods operate on muscles and muscle clusters to relieve tension and pain. Diagnosis of pain is made according to its acuteness and the response of the body to the same. In this book, using case studies and examples, constant effort has been made to make the understanding of the difficult concepts of acupuncture and acupressure as easy and informative as possible, for the readers. This book will be useful for students and researchers in the fields of alternative medicine, physiotherapy and pain management.

I thank my publisher with all my heart for considering me worthy of this unparalleled opportunity and for showing unwavering faith in my skills. I would also like to thank the editorial team who worked closely with me at every step and contributed immensely towards the successful completion of this book. Last but not the least, I wish to thank my friends and colleagues for their support.

Editor

Modulatory Effect of Acupuncture at Waiguan (TE5) on the Functional Connectivity of the Central Nervous System of Patients with Ischemic Stroke in the Left Basal Ganglia

Junqi Chen[1][¶], Jizhou Wang[2][¶], Yong Huang[3]*, Xinsheng Lai[4]*, Chunzhi Tang[4], Junjun Yang[4], Junxian Wu[5], Tongjun Zeng[6], Shanshan Qu[3]

1 Department of Rehabilitation, The Third Affiliated Hospital of Southern Medical University, Guangzhou, China, 2 The First Clinical Medical School, Southern Medical University, Guangzhou, China, 3 School of Traditional Chinese Medicine, Southern Medical University, Guangzhou, China, 4 School of Acupuncture and Rehabilitation, Guangzhou University of Traditional Chinese Medicine, Guangzhou, China, 5 Department of Acupuncture and Moxibustion, Shantou Central Hospital, Shantou, China, 6 The First People's Hospital of Shunde, Foshan, China

Abstract

Objective: To study the influence of acupuncture at Waiguan (TE5) on the functional connectivity of the central nervous system of patients with ischemic stroke.

Methods: Twenty-four patients with ischemic stroke in the left basal ganglia were randomized based on gender to receive TE5 acupuncture (n = 12) or nonacupoint acupuncture (n = 12). Each group underwent sham acupuncture and then verum acupuncture while being scanned with functional magnetic resonance imaging. Six regions of interest (ROI) were defined, including bilateral motor, somatosensory, and bilateral basal ganglia areas. The functional connectivity between these ROIs and all voxels of the brain was analyzed in Analysis of Functional NeuroImages(AFNI) to explore the differences between verum acupuncture and sham acupuncture at TE5 and between TE5 acupuncture and nonacupoint acupuncture. The participants were blinded to the allocation.

Result: The effect of acupuncture on six seed-associated networks was explored. The result demonstrated that acupuncture at Waiguan (TE5) can regulate the sensorimotor network of the ipsilesional hemisphere, stimulate the contralesional sensorimotor network, increase cooperation of bilateral sensorimotor networks, and change the synchronization between the cerebellum and cerebrum. Furthermore, a lot of differences of effect existed between verum acupuncture and sham acupuncture at TE5, but there was little difference between TE5 acupuncture and nonacupoint acupuncture.

Conclusion: The modulation of synchronizations between different regions within different brain networks might be the mechanism of acupuncture at Waiguan (TE5). Stimulation of the contralesional sensorimotor network and increase of cooperation of bilateral hemispheres imply a compensatory effect of the intact hemisphere, whereas changes in synchronization might influence the sensorimotor function of the affected side of the body.

Trial Registration: Chinese Clinical Trial Registry ChiCTR-ONRC-08000255

Editor: Cornelis Jan Stam, VU University Medical Center, Netherlands

Funding: This study was supported by National 973 Program of China (no.: 2006CB504505), National 973 Program of China (no.: 2012CB518504) and Third Key Subject of the '211 Project' of Guangdong Province. The funders had no role in study design, data collection and analysis, decision to publish, or preparation of the manuscript.

Competing Interests: The authors have declared that no competing interests exist.

* E-mail: nfhy@fimmu.com (YH); lai1023@163.com (XSL)

¶ These authors contributed equally to this work.

¶ These authors joint senior authors on this work.

Introduction

Acupuncture is one of the most widely used alternative treatments whose curative effect has been recognized and approved by the World Health Organization [1]. In traditional Chinese medicine, it is believed that acupuncture can affect the energy flow through the body which in turn modulates functions of the whole body system. However, the mechanism of its effect has not been well characterized to date. Clinical and experimental studies suggest that the modulatory effect of acupuncture might be mediated via the central and peripheral nervous systems [2,3].

Functional magnetic resonance imaging (fMRI) is an efficient, noninvasive method of studying the mechanism by which acupuncture affects the central nervous system (CNS). Many fMRI studies indicated that acupuncture can activate or deactivate certain areas of the brain related to a corresponding disease or function [4–12]. Meanwhile, its effect seems to be relevant to the regulation of brain networks, such as the default mode network, sensorimotor network, amygdala-associated network, and vision network [6,13–15]. Distinct from the conventional fMRI, functional connectivity MRI (fcMRI) can be used to detect the temporal correlation of the blood oxygen level–dependent (BOLD) signals of spatially remote brain regions. The connectivity of two areas, including functional connectivity and effective connectivity, depicts the cooperation pattern of these areas. Functional connectivity is the pattern of statistical dependency resulting from the nonlinear dynamics of neurons and neuronal populations within the neuroanatomical substrate [16], which reflects the existence and the strength of the connectivity between remote brain regions.

Patients with stroke in the basal ganglia have significant deficiency in the sensorimotor function of the contralesional side of their body. To date, researchers have found several relevant changes in the CNS of these patients, such as changes in the effective connectivity of core motor areas [17]. Recovery seems to be related to the extent of connectivity between the ipsilesional primary motor area and contralesional postcentral gyrus, change in the topological structure, centrality of the ipsilesional primary sensorimotor area, recruitment of bilateral somatosensory association areas and contralesional SII, and activation of the contralesional cerebellum [18,19]. Similarly, the abnormal function of many regions of the brain is also crucial in the deficiency in somatosensory function [20–22]. The sensorimotor function is regulated by complex functional networks formed by the neuronal populations of the cortex and subcortex [23]. Thus, ischemic stroke lesions may affect the functional network architecture in both hemispheres [24–28] and break the balance of the network, which in turn causes the deficiency in sensorimotor function.

Acupuncture is one of the most important treatments for stroke rehabilitation. Several studies demonstrated that acupuncture not only regulates the functional state and connectivity of sensorimotor areas of normal people [9,14,29] but also affects the functional state of the bilateral sensorimotor cortex of stroke patients [30,31].

TE5 is an important traditional acupuncture point common in the treatment of stroke-related motor, neurological and autonomic nerve problems in clinical practice [32]. We hypothesize that acupuncture at TE5 has a specific influence on the functional networks, including sensorimotor areas, of the CNS to improve the sensorimotor function of the body [33].

Twenty-four patients with ischemic stroke in the left basal ganglia were recruited to investigate this hypothesis. Data extracted from fMRI were assessed with seed-based analysis to discover the differences between TE5 verum acupuncture and nonacupoint acupuncture and between TE5 verum acupuncture and TE5 sham acupuncture. Results of this study elucidate the specific influence of acupuncture at TE5 on sensorimotor networks.

Methods

Subject

The study was carried out during October 2008 and August 2010 in the Imaging Center of Nanfang Hospital, Guangzhou, China. Twenty-four patients admitted to the First Affiliated Hospital of Guangzhou University of Chinese Medicine and matching the diagnostic criteria of ischemic stroke in ICD-9 434 and ICD-8 433 [34] were screened based on the following inclusion criteria: ischemic stroke in the left basal ganglia that occurred more than a month ago but less than a year, significant right hemiplegia (the score of the muscle strength of the upper limb and the lower limb ≤4), stable condition and receiving usual treatment (including antiplatelet medicine like aspirin and clopidogrel, and lipid-lowering drugs like statins et al.), right handedness, naive to acupuncture or not being treated by acupuncture for at least 4 weeks, no severe aphasia, no previous neurological or psychiatric disease, and no coagulation or other severe diseases. The experimental protocol was approved by the Ethical Committee of the First Affiliated Hospital of Guangzhou University of Chinese Medicine. This study was registered on the Chinese Clinical Trial Registry (http://www.chictr.org, ChiCTR-ONRC-08000255). All patients signed a written informed consent.

The participants were randomly (using random number table) divided into two groups of 12: Waiguan (TE5) group and nonacupoint group. Each group underwent sham acupuncture and then verum acupuncture.

Experiment Design

The fMRI brain scan was conducted on a 3.0-T whole-body scanner (GE Signa) with a standard head coil. The participants were prevented from experiencing auditory and visual activities via earplugs and eyeshades, respectively. The scanning procedure (Fig. 1) began after the participants rested on the bed for 5 min. The participants in each group were given sham acupuncture stimulus and then verum acupuncture while being simultaneously scanned. Each stimulus lasted for 6 min and 30 s. The two stimuli had an interval lasting for 6 min and 2 s, which was considered sufficient for restoring the sensitivity of cutaneous sensory receptor. The participants were blinded as to which stimulus was given to them; they were only aware of receiving acupuncture. The experiment operator, data analyst, and researcher were strictly separated from each other.

Verum Acupuncture Stimulation

TE5 is located on the dorsal aspect of the forearm at midpoint of the interosseous space between the radius and the ulna, 2 cun proximal to the dorsal wrist crease, whereas the nonacupoint is medial to TE5 at midpoint between the two meridians, i.e. triple energizer meridian and small intestine meridian (Fig. 2). During stimulation, a sterile silver needle 0.30 mm in diameter and 40 mm in length (tube purchased from Dongbang AcuPrime Co. and needle from Zhongyan Taihe Co., Beijing, China) was inserted vertically into the skin at a depth of 15±2 mm. The needle was twisted for ±180° evenly at a frequency of 60 circles per min after the needling sensation (de qi), i.e., the feeling of increased resistance to further insertion, was assured by the acupuncturist.

Sham Acupuncture Stimulation

In this study, sham acupuncture served as the tactile control. Tactile stimulation has been widely used as a noninvasive control for acupuncture neuroimaging studies. The procedure involved pushing the end of the needle with its tip out of the tube within 1 mm and touching the skin.

Acupuncture was conducted manually by an experienced acupuncturist. During experimental stimulation, the subjects were required to keep quiet and remain calm without speaking.

fMRI Scan

After the patients rested on the bed for 5 min, 3D anatomy images were collected with a T1-weighted 3D gradient echo-pulse

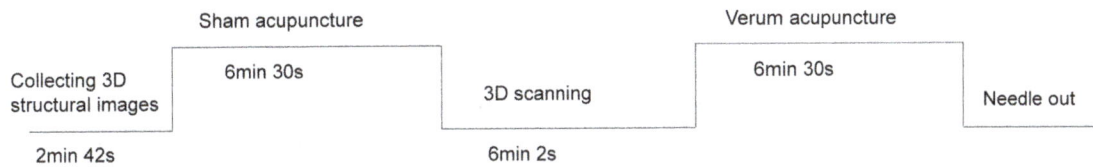

Figure 1. Stimulation and scanning pattern.

fast spin sequence, with axial view T1 fluid-attenuated-inversion-recovery scan. The exact scanning parameters were as follows: TR = 2.3 s, TE = 21 ms, TI = 920 ms, slice thickness = 6.0 mm, gap = 1.0 mm, 20 layers for a total of 2 min and 45 s, field of view (FOV) = 240×180 mm^2, matrix = 320×256, number of excitations (NEX) = 2, echo train length = 9, and band width = 50. During the acupuncture stimulation, BOLD functional images were collected with a T2-weighted single-shot, gradient-recalled echo-planar imaging sequence. The exact scanning parameters were as follows: TR = 3 s, TE = 20 ms, flip angle = 90°, FOV = 240×240 mm^2, slice thickness = 6.0 mm, slice gap = 1.0 mm, matrix = 96×96, NEX = 1, phase per location = 130, and 2600 phases per 6 min and 30s.

Data Analysis

The preprocessing steps were implemented in AFNI (Cox, 1996; http://afni.nimh.nih.gov/afni). The functional images from each run were aligned, slice timing corrected, temporally standardized, space smoothed (6 mm full width at half maximum Gaussian kernel), and transformed into Talairach space (Talairach and Tournoux, 1988).

For each subject, we analyzed the functional connectivity using the average activity of a seed region defined by the anatomical template in AFNI to find other voxels in the brain that behaved similarly. The ROIs (seeds) selected were areas related to motor ability [Brodmann area (BA) 4 and BA6], sensations (BA1, BA2, BA3, BA5, and BA7), and basal ganglia area. The objective was to

find the changes in correlations between these regions and other parts of the brain, which might affect the function of motor ability and sensations. The low-frequency BOLD correlations (0.01 Hz to 0.1 Hz) or functional connectivity between the time series of a given seed and that of all voxels in the brain was partially correlated by Pearson correlation analysis with covariance of head motion and time series from white matter and cerebrospinal fluid. Individual correlation coefficient maps for both the acupuncture and tactile conditions were generated and transformed to Fisher's z-distribution for group-level analysis. All the resultant t-maps were set to the threshold level of P<0.05. Multiple-comparison error was corrected with Monte Carlo simulation.

Results

Baseline Data

Two participants from the Waiguan (TE5) group and one participant from the nonacupoint group were excluded for significant movement during the scan, and three participants from the nonacupoint group were excluded for spoiled data (Fig. 3). No significant difference was found in the baseline data of the remaining 18 participants (Table 1).

Functional Connectivity

The different effects of TE5 verum acupuncture, TE5 sham acupuncture, and nonacupoint acupuncture on six seed-associated networks were observed through seed-based analysis (Table 2 and Fig. 4).

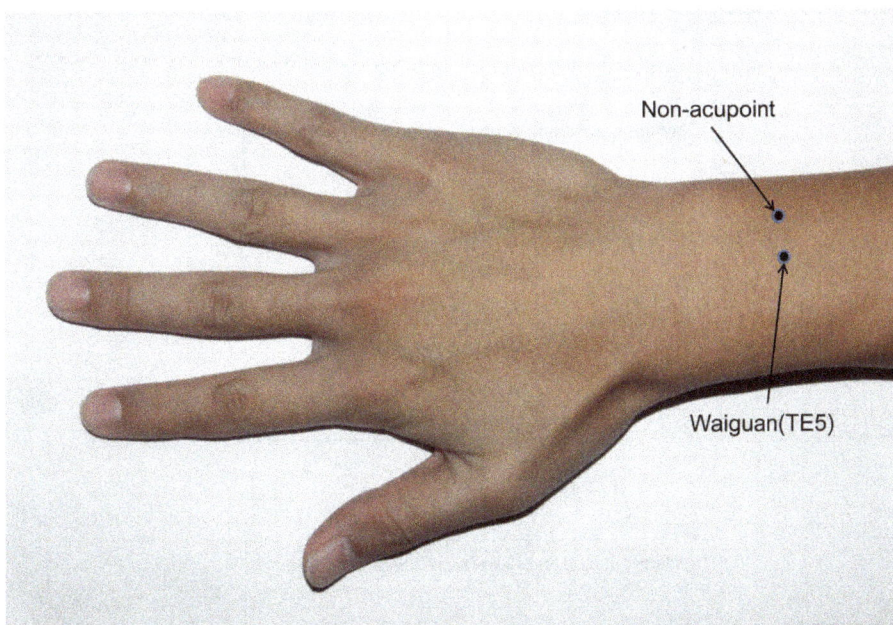

Figure 2. *Waiguan* and nonacupoint on the right forearm.

Table 1. Baseline data.

Items	Waiguan (TE5) (n = 10)	Nonacupoint (n = 8)	Statistics	P
Gender (M/F, n)	9/1	7/1		1*
Age	56.10±5.53	58.50±7.05	t = −0.811	0.429
Duration, months	5.30±3.71	3.38±3.29	t = 1.148	0.268
CSS score	18.20±4.02	17.13±4.76	t = 0.520	0.611
Hypertension (Yes/No, n)	9/1	6/2		0.559*
Diabetes mellitus (Yes/No, n)	2/8	1/7		1*

The P values with "*"were obtained using Fisher's Exact Test, whereas the rest were the result of independent samples t-test.

The correlation between the left precuneus and the left motor area was stronger under acupuncture than under the tactile control. Greater correlation was found between the left precuneus and the left somatosensory area, the latter being the seed. Stronger correlation was found between the left basal ganglia area and the right middle frontal gyrus, with the former being the seed.

The three seed-associated networks of the ROIs in the right hemisphere were more complicated than that in the left hemisphere. The correlation between the right motor area and the left postcentral gyrus, right middle frontal gyrus, and left thalamus was stronger under acupuncture than under the tactile control. Meanwhile, the correlation between the right somatosensory area and the bilateral postcentral gyrus and left putamen was stronger under acupuncture than under the tactile control. The right cerebellum and cerebellar culmen had greater connectivity with the right basal ganglia, whereas the left cerebellum had weaker correlation with the right motor and somatosensory areas.

Unlike the many differences demonstrated in the comparison of TE5 verum acupuncture and TE5 sham acupuncture stated before, only the left thalamus and left cuneus showed greater connectivity with the right motor area and right basal ganglia, respectively, when TE5 verum acupuncture was compared with nonacupoint acupuncture. Interestingly, stronger connectivity between left thalamus and right motor area was also aroused by verum acupuncture relative to sham acupuncture.

Discussion

Specific Effects of TE5 Acupuncture Compared with TE5 Sham Acupuncture

First, the left precuneus showed stronger connectivity with both the left motor area and left somatosensory area. Anatomical connectivity exists between the precuneus and the sensorimotor cortex and subcortex [35]. A clinical study indicated that

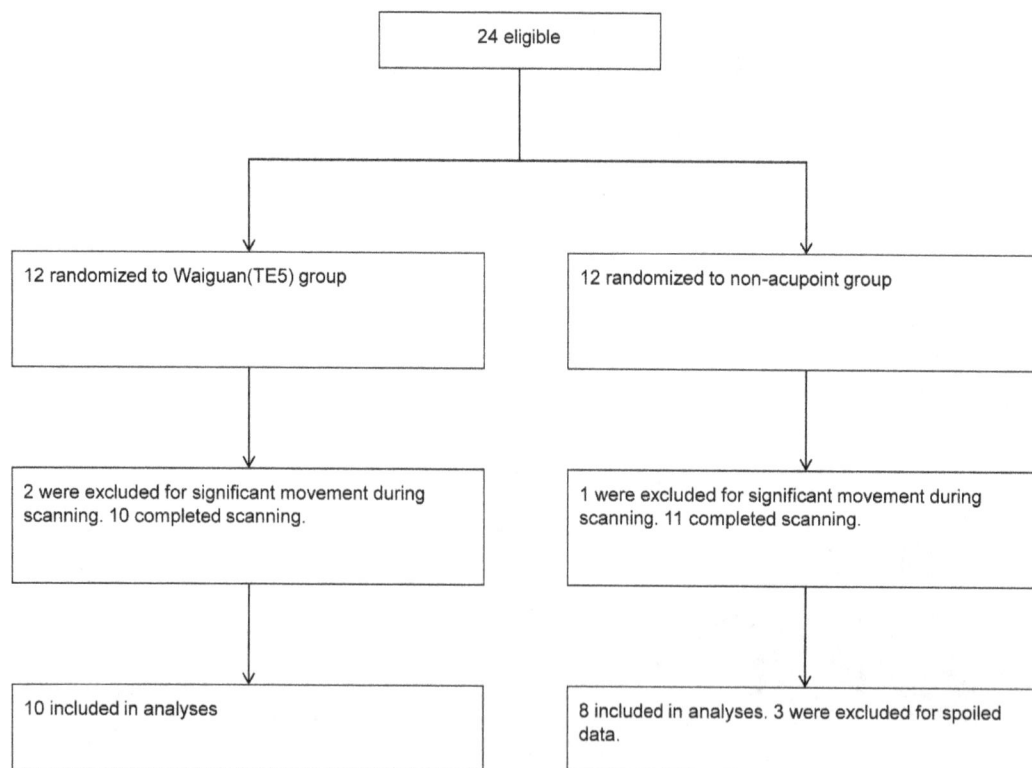

Figure 3. Consort flow diagram.

Table 2. Localization of the acupuncture specific effects by comparing TE5 verum acupuncture (Group A) vs. TE5 sham acupuncture (Group B) and TE5 verum acupuncture (Group A) vs. nonacupoint acupuncture (Group C).

ROI	Group A vs. Group B							Group A vs. Group C						
	Anatomical structures	BA	X	Y	Z	vox	t	Anatomical structures	BA	X	Y	Z	vox	t
Left motor area	Left precuneus	7	−10	−40	47	69	3.5							
Left somatosensory area	Left precuneus	5,7	−1	−37	47	48	5.2							
	Right paracentral lobule	4*	23	−37	50	33	3.5							
Left basal ganglia area	Right middle frontal gyrus	6	32	5	50	53	4.2							
Right motor area	Left postcentral gyrus	3	−25	−31	50	133	4.2	Left thalamus	N/A	−16	−22	5	31	3.8
	Left thalamus	N/A	−16	−25	8	66	4							
	Right middle frontal gyrus	6	32	−7	47	40	5.8							
	Left cerebellar	N/A	−19	−79	−34	38	−4.4							
Right somatosensory area	Right postcentral gyrus	3	20	−31	50	121	4.4							
	Left postcentral gyrus	3	−28	−31	50	69	3.5							
	Left putamen	N/A	−31	−16	8	50	4							
	Left cerebellar	N/A	−19	−79	−34	44	−7.2							
Right basal ganglia area	Right cerebellar	N/A	5	−55	−25	113	4.9	Left cuneus	18	−10	−85	17	41	5.2
	Cerebellar culmen	N/A	2	−34	−1	47	5.2							
	Left lingual gyrus	18	−25	−79	−4	44	−3.1							

Abbreviation: BA, Brodmann area; Vox, voxel (represents the number of voxels); N/A, not available (means that the peak voxel was out of the BA zone). The BA area marked by "*"was corrected by a neurological physician.

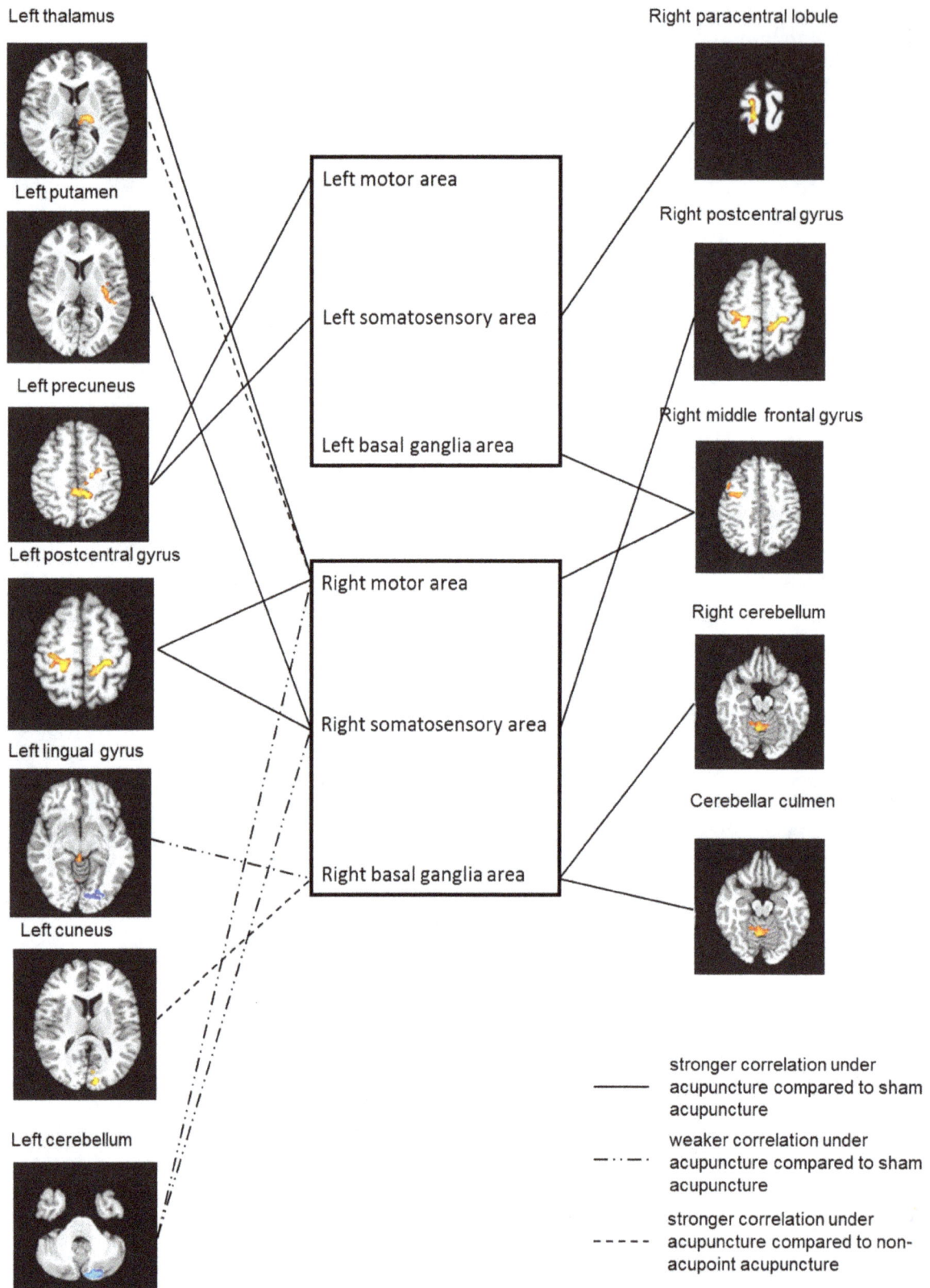

Figure 4. Differences of seed associated networks between ROIs from the left hemisphere and the right hemisphere. Full line represents stronger correlation under acupuncture compared with sham acupuncture, whereas the "dash–dot–dot" line represents weaker correlation. Dash line stands for weaker correlation compared with nonacupoint acupuncture (P<0.05, multiple comparison error corrected using Monte Carlo simulation). Regions of the left hemisphere and right hemisphere that had significant differences in correlation with seeds are placed on left side and right side, respectively, and ROIs in the same box are from the same hemisphere.

acupuncture can activate regions of ipsilesional hemisphere, which is correlated with the extent of rehabilitation [31]. Taking the anatomical connectivity and this clinical study into account, we hypothesize that acupuncture at TE5 can change the functional connectivity among ipsilesional neuronal populations of sensorimotor cortexes and subcortexes, leading to the modulation of the sensorimotor network, which might have a positive effect on the recovery of the affected side of the body. In addition, the precuneus was also found to have strong correlation with other brain regions [11], implying that the precuneus affects the efficiency of acupuncture.

Second, the correlation between the right sensorimotor areas and the left somatosensory area (left postcentral gyrus), right somatosensory area (right postcentral gyrus), right motor area [right middle frontal gyrus (BA6, premotor area)], and left basal ganglia area (left thalamus, left putamen) was stronger under acupuncture than under sham acupuncture. Meanwhile, a clinical study suggested that the regions activated or deactivated by acupuncture at TE5 of the affected forearm are mainly the components of the contralesional hemisphere [30]. Hence, the modulatory effects of acupuncture at TE5 might be attributed to the enhancement of compensatory process by the redistribution of functions to the sensorimotor areas of the contralesional hemisphere and to the increase in the cooperation of functioning between the bilateral sensorimotor areas. Our results were similar to those of Johansen-Berg [36,37] and Grefkes [17], who indicated that the sensorimotor areas of the contralesional hemisphere might have a role in modulating the function of the affected side of the body. Moreover, Grefkes et al. also found that the contralesional M1 of patients with stroke in the left basal ganglia was not only significantly activated while moving the affected limb but also exerted a negative influence on the ipsilesional M1. This result was not observed in healthy people. According to these studies, the negative influence can be attributed to the abnormal coupling between bilateral M1 caused by the damage of basal ganglia. Our analysis methods are different from theirs. Hence, ensuring whether or not the change in connectivity between the bilateral sensorimotor areas implies a modulatory effect on the coupling of these areas warrants further study.

Moreover, the connectivity between the left cerebellar cortex and the right motor area was weaker. The left cerebellum and the right motor area cooperate to control the left limb. Therefore, the result might reflect a decrease in the modulation of the sensorimotor function of the left limb. Meanwhile, the cerebella medial zone and the right cerebellar intermediate zone, which regulate the tension and cooperation of the body and proximal limb muscles and modulate the motor function of the right distal limb muscle, respectively, were more correlated with the right basal ganglia under acupuncture than under the tactile control. This result implies that the cooperation possibly aroused by the acupuncture between the right basal ganglia area and the right cerebellum might have a modulatory effect on the sensorimotor function of the right side (affected side) of the body. Moreover, the correlation between the right basal ganglia and the cerebellar culmen might regulate the sensorimotor function of both sides. Similar to our study, some clinical studies found that the functional recovery of patients improves with more activity in the contralesional cerebellum and with weaker centrality of the ipsilesional cerebellum [18,38]. Nevertheless, the reasons behind why the correlations between the cerebellum and other sensorimotor areas did not show significant differences need further study. In general, acupuncture at the right TE5 of stroke patients attenuates the cooperation of the right hemisphere and the left cerebellum responsible in modulating the sensorimotor function of the

unaffected limb while enhancing the cooperation of the right hemisphere and the right cerebellar to promote the regulation of the sensorimotor function of the right side (affected side) body.

Finally, a difference in correlation was also found between the visual cortex and the ROI, apart from the one between the sensorimotor function-associated areas and ROIs. Lingual gyrus is a part of the visual cortex, which also has functions in word comprehension and in the regulation of emotion and motor ability. Hence, the weaker correlation between these areas implies an attenuated cooperation on these functions with the use of acupuncture. However, a clinical study reported that acupuncture at TE5 can activate the bilateral occipital lobe compared with the baseline; however, the activation is not significant relative to that of tactile stimulation [30]. One reason that could account for this result is the different stimulation patterns of the verum and sham acupuncture on the visual cortex, such that distinction was found in its connectivity with the right basal ganglia, but not in activity. However, further studies are needed to investigate the exact benefit of this difference for the rehabilitation of stroke patients.

Specific Effects of TE5 Acupuncture Compared with Nonacupoint Acupuncture

Only the left thalamus and the left cuneus exhibited greater connectivity with the right motor area and the right basal ganglia, respectively, when TE5 acupuncture was compared with nonacupoint acupuncture. The stronger correlation between the left thalamus and the right motor areas implies an enhancement in the compensatory effect of the right intact sensorimotor areas. Interestingly, stronger connectivity between the left thalamus and the right motor area was also observed when TE5 acupuncture was compared with sham acupuncture. Thus, it can be a relatively specific effect of acupuncture at TE5. As stated above, the difference in the correlation between the left cuneus and the right basal ganglia might have resulted from the distinct stimulation pattern on the visual cortex and the augmented correlation under acupuncture when compared with nonacupoint acupuncture. When referring to the comparison between acupuncture and sham acupuncture, the correlation between the left visual cortex and the right basal ganglia was attenuated by acupuncture. This seemingly conflict needs to be clarified in further study with more exact data.

We propose the fact that little difference was found between the two groups might be related to the location of the nonacupoint. Locating the acupoint and the nonacupoint is rather arbitrary, and the surface area and spatial structure of an acupoint vary with the acupoint [39–41]. Thus, stimulating the nonacupoint and TE5 might have similar effects since these two points were close to each other, and the small difference in location might contribute to the differences in functional connectivity. Another possibility is that the nonacupoint is a new acupoint that might have a similar effect because it is situated close to TE5. Moreover, the fact that little difference was found might proceed from the analysis of acupuncture's instant effects. Acupuncture's long lasting effects have been demonstrated by many researchers. Hence more difference might be found if these effects were measured [42]. Although nonacupoint is commonly used as a control, investigating how to design a nonacupoint to reflect the actual effect of acupuncture is necessary to avoid the influence of nervous tissue, connective tissue, and other anatomic structures.

Characteristics of Connectivity Difference

Differences in connectivity were observed in several pairs of brain regions when TE5 acupuncture was compared with TE5 sham acupuncture and nonacupoint acupuncture (Table 2 and

Fig. 4). A pair of brain regions consisted of an ROI and another brain region. Most of the ROIs within these pairs were from the right hemisphere, whereas the other parts of the pairs were mainly areas of the left hemisphere and the left cerebellum. This type of distribution pattern implies that the main effect of acupuncture at TE5 of stroke patients might be the enhancement of the association between the two hemispheres, which cooperate to modulate the sensorimotor function of the affected side. Moreover, it could also be a sign of increasing the compensatory effect of the unaffected side of the brain.

Limitations

The sample size of our study was relatively small, and all participants were diagnosed of ischemic stroke in the left basal ganglia. We were unable to distinguish the exact regions of stroke. Therefore, our results only gave a preview on the mechanism of the effect of acupuncture on the CNS of patients with left basal ganglia ischemic stroke. In addition, the functional connectivity only refers to the correlation of the BOLD signal of two distinct brain regions, which indirectly reflects the correlation or cooperation of the neuronal activities. However, the correlation cannot indicate the effect passage of the neural function. Hence, further studies on the topic should use effective connectivity or graph theory, which is effective in revealing the direction of neural function, to enhance our understanding of the effect of acupuncture at TE5. We only focused on the connectivity between ROIs and all the voxels of the brain. Thus, the connectivity between the voxels that showed significant change in correlation with ROIs and the connectivity between regions other than the chosen ROIs and all voxels of the whole brain were not studied. Acupuncture is known to have a long lasting effect [13,15,43], and this characteristic was not investigated in this study. Further studies are warranted to explore the sustained effects of acupuncture on functional connectivity and its correlation with function recovery.

The commonly used TE5 sham acupuncture and nonacupoint acupuncture served as controls. However, previous research indicated that sham acupuncture and nonacupoint acupuncture have certain curative effects [44,45]. Therefore, the present study also neglected the connectivity, which did not show significant difference between groups that might influence the effect of acupuncture. A more suitable control needs to be adopted to reflect the exact effects of acupuncture.

Conclusion

The present study found that acupuncture helps regulate the functional connectivity between the sensorimotor areas of intra-hemisphere and inter-hemispheres as well as between the cerebellum and cerebrum. Results indicate that the compensatory effect of the intact sensorimotor network of contralesional hemisphere might be enhanced. The cooperation of the sensorimotor network of the ipsilesional hemisphere might be augmented. The impact on the functional connectivity between the cerebellum and cerebrum might also be important for the acupuncture's effects. The modulation of synchronizations between different regions within different brain networks might be the mechanism of acupuncture at Waiguan (TE5). A number of limitations were discussed.

Supporting Information

Checklist S1 Stricta checklist.
(DOCX)

Protocol S1 Trial protocol.
(DOC)

Acknowledgments

We would like to give our sincere appreciation to all the participants and their families, and to Prof. Yanping Chen and Dr. Shanshan Tang for the technical support from the Imaging Center of Nanfang Hospital, China.

Patient consent: Obtained.

Ethical approval: The Ethical Committee of the First Affiliated Hospital of Guangzhou University of Chinese Medicine.

Author Contributions

Conceived and designed the experiments: YH XSL. Performed the experiments: JQC. Analyzed the data: SSQ. Wrote the paper: JQC JZW. Enrolled subjects: CZT JJY. Integrated all experiment data: TJZ JXW.

References

1. (1998) NIH Consensus Conference. Acupuncture. JAMA 280: 1518–1524.
2. Cheng XN (2000) Chinese Acupuncture and Moxibustion. Beijing: People's Medical Publishing House.
3. Han JS (2003) Acupuncture: neuropeptide release produced by electrical stimulation of different frequencies. Trends Neurosci 26: 17–22.
4. Liu P, Qin W, Zhang Y, Tian J, Bai L, et al. (2009) Combining spatial and temporal information to explore function-guide action of acupuncture using fMRI. J Magn Reson Imaging 30: 41–46.
5. Claunch JD, Chan ST, Nixon EE, Qiu WQ, Sporko T, et al. (2012) Commonality and specificity of acupuncture action at three acupoints as evidenced by FMRI. Am J Chin Med 40: 695–712.
6. Zhang Y, Liang J, Qin W, Liu P, von Deneen KM, et al. (2009) Comparison of visual cortical activations induced by electro-acupuncture at vision and nonvision-related acupoints. Neurosci Lett 458: 6–10.
7. Hui KK, Napadow V, Liu J, Li M, Marina O, et al. (2010) Monitoring acupuncture effects on human brain by FMRI. J Vis Exp.
8. Huang W, Pach D, Napadow V, Park K, Long X, et al. (2012) Characterizing acupuncture stimuli using brain imaging with FMRI–a systematic review and meta-analysis of the literature. PLoS One 7: e32960.
9. Liu J, Qin W, Guo Q, Sun J, Yuan K, et al. (2011) Divergent neural processes specific to the acute and sustained phases of verum and SHAM acupuncture. J Magn Reson Imaging 33: 33–40.
10. Feng Y, Bai L, Ren Y, Chen S, Wang H, et al. (2012) FMRI connectivity analysis of acupuncture effects on the whole brain network in mild cognitive impairment patients. Magn Reson Imaging 30: 672–682.
11. Liu P, Zhang Y, Zhou G, Yuan K, Qin W, et al. (2009) Partial correlation investigation on the default mode network involved in acupuncture: an fMRI study. Neurosci Lett 462: 183–187.
12. Hsu SF, Chen CY, Ke MD, Huang CH, Sun YT, et al. (2011) Variations of brain activities of acupuncture to TE5 of left hand in normal subjects. Am J Chin Med 39: 673–686.
13. Qin W, Tian J, Bai L, Pan X, Yang L, et al. (2008) FMRI connectivity analysis of acupuncture effects on an amygdala-associated brain network. Mol Pain 4: 55.
14. Hui KK, Marina O, Claunch JD, Nixon EE, Fang J, et al. (2009) Acupuncture mobilizes the brain's default mode and its anti-correlated network in healthy subjects. Brain Res 1287: 84–103.
15. Dhond RP, Yeh C, Park K, Kettner N, Napadow V (2008) Acupuncture modulates resting state connectivity in default and sensorimotor brain networks. Pain 136: 407–418.
16. Sporns O, Chialvo DR, Kaiser M, Hilgetag CC (2004) Organization, development and function of complex brain networks. Trends Cogn Sci 8: 418–425.
17. Grefkes C, Nowak DA, Eickhoff SB, Dafotakis M, Kust J, et al. (2008) Cortical connectivity after subcortical stroke assessed with functional magnetic resonance imaging. Ann Neurol 63: 236–246.
18. Wang L, Yu C, Chen H, Qin W, He Y, et al. (2010) Dynamic functional reorganization of the motor execution network after stroke. Brain 133: 1224–1238.
19. Askim T, Indredavik B, Vangberg T, Haberg A (2009) Motor network changes associated with successful motor skill relearning after acute ischemic stroke: a longitudinal functional magnetic resonance imaging study. Neurorehabil Neural Repair 23: 295–304.
20. Dinomais M, Groeschel S, Staudt M, Krageloh-Mann I, Wilke M (2012) Relationship between functional connectivity and sensory impairment: red flag or red herring? Hum Brain Mapp 33: 628–638.

21. Gao JH, Parsons LM, Bower JM, Xiong J, Li J, et al. (1996) Cerebellum implicated in sensory acquisition and discrimination rather than motor control. Science 272: 545–547.
22. O'Reilly JX, Beckmann CF, Tomassini V, Ramnani N, Johansen-Berg H (2010) Distinct and overlapping functional zones in the cerebellum defined by resting state functional connectivity. Cereb Cortex 20: 953–965.
23. Breakspear M, Terry JR, Friston KJ (2003) Modulation of excitatory synaptic coupling facilitates synchronization and complex dynamics in a biophysical model of neuronal dynamics. Network 14: 703–732.
24. Grefkes C, Fink GR (2011) Reorganization of cerebral networks after stroke: new insights from neuroimaging with connectivity approaches. Brain 134: 1264–1276.
25. Hummel F, Celnik P, Giraux P, Floel A, Wu WH, et al. (2005) Effects of non-invasive cortical stimulation on skilled motor function in chronic stroke. Brain 128: 490–499.
26. Murase N, Duque J, Mazzocchio R, Cohen LG (2004) Influence of interhemispheric interactions on motor function in chronic stroke. Ann Neurol 55: 400–409.
27. He BJ, Snyder AZ, Vincent JL, Epstein A, Shulman GL, et al. (2007) Breakdown of functional connectivity in frontoparietal networks underlies behavioral deficits in spatial neglect. Neuron 53: 905–918.
28. Nomura EM, Gratton C, Visser RM, Kayser A, Perez F, et al. (2010) Double dissociation of two cognitive control networks in patients with focal brain lesions. Proc Natl Acad Sci U S A 107: 12017–12022.
29. Fang J, Jin Z, Wang Y, Li K, Kong J, et al. (2009) The salient characteristics of the central effects of acupuncture needling: limbic-paralimbic-neocortical network modulation. Hum Brain Mapp 30: 1196–1206.
30. Huang Y, Chen JQ, Lai XS, Tang CZ, Yang JJ, et al. (2013) Lateralisation of cerebral response to active acupuncture in patients with unilateral ischaemic stroke: an fMRI study. Acupunct Med.
31. Schaechter JD, Connell BD, Stason WB, Kaptchuk TJ, Krebs DE, et al. (2007) Correlated change in upper limb function and motor cortex activation after verum and sham acupuncture in patients with chronic stroke. J Altern Complement Med 13: 527–532.
32. Maciocia G (1994) The practice of Chinese medicine: the treatment of diseases with acupuncture and Chinese herbs. Edinburgh, UK: Churchill Livingstone. 342–385 p.
33. Liu B, Liu X, Chen J, Long Y, Chen ZG, et al. (2009) Study on the effects of acupuncture at acupoint and non-acupoint on functional connectivity of different brain regions with functional magnetic resonance imaging. Zhongguo Zhen Jiu 29: 981–985.
34. (1999) MONICA Manual.
35. Cavanna AE, Trimble MR (2006) The precuneus: a review of its functional anatomy and behavioural correlates. Brain 129: 564–583.
36. Johansen-Berg H, Dawes H, Guy C, Smith SM, Wade DT, et al. (2002) Correlation between motor improvements and altered fMRI activity after rehabilitative therapy. Brain 125: 2731–2742.
37. Johansen-Berg H, Rushworth MF, Bogdanovic MD, Kischka U, Wimalaratna S, et al. (2002) The role of ipsilateral premotor cortex in hand movement after stroke. Proc Natl Acad Sci U S A 99: 14518–14523.
38. Small SL, Hlustik P, Noll DC, Genovese C, Solodkin A (2002) Cerebellar hemispheric activation ipsilateral to the paretic hand correlates with functional recovery after stroke. Brain 125: 1544–1557.
39. Leibing E, Leonhardt U, Koster G, Goerlitz A, Rosenfeldt JA, et al. (2002) Acupuncture treatment of chronic low-back pain – a randomized, blinded, placebo-controlled trial with 9-month follow-up. Pain 96: 189–196.
40. Fink MG, Kunsebeck HW, Wippermann B (2000) Effect of needle acupuncture on pain perception and functional impairment of patients with coxarthrosis. Z Rheumatol 59: 191–199.
41. Molsberger AF, Manickavasagan J, Abholz HH, Maixner WB, Endres HG (2012) Acupuncture points are large fields: the fuzziness of acupuncture point localization by doctors in practice. Eur J Pain 16: 1264–1270.
42. Li Y, Liang F, Yang X, Tian X, Yan J, et al. (2009) Acupuncture for treating acute attacks of migraine: a randomized controlled trial. Headache 49: 805–816.
43. Zhong C, Bai L, Dai R, Xue T, Wang H, et al. (2012) Modulatory effects of acupuncture on resting-state networks: a functional MRI study combining independent component analysis and multivariate Granger causality analysis. J Magn Reson Imaging 35: 572–581.
44. Moffet HH (2009) Sham acupuncture may be as efficacious as true acupuncture: a systematic review of clinical trials. J Altern Complement Med 15: 213–216.
45. Wang JJ, Wu ZC (2009) [Thinking about the conclusion of no difference between the acupuncture and sham-acupuncture in the clinically therapeutic effects on migraine abroad]. Zhongguo Zhen Jiu 29: 315–319.

2

How Current Clinical Practice Guidelines for Low Back Pain Reflect Traditional Medicine in East Asian Countries: A Systematic Review of Clinical Practice Guidelines and Systematic Reviews

Hyun-Woo Cho[1], Eui-Hyoung Hwang[1,2], Byungmook Lim[3], Kwang-Ho Heo[1], Jian-Ping Liu[4], Kiichiro Tsutani[5], Myeong Soo Lee[6], Byung-Cheul Shin[1,2]*

1 Department of Rehabilitation Medicine of Korean Medicine, Spine and Joint Center, Pusan National University Korean Medicine Hospital, Yangsan, Republic of Korea, 2 Division of Clinical Medicine, School of Korean Medicine, Pusan National University, Yangsan, Republic of Korea, 3 Division of Humanities and Social Medicine, School of Korean Medicine, Pusan National University, Yangsan, Republic of Korea, 4 Center for Evidence-Based Chinese Medicine, Beijing University of Chinese Medicine, Beijing, China, 5 Department of Drug Policy and Management, Graduate School of Pharmaceutical Sciences, The University of Tokyo, Tokyo, Japan, 6 Brain Disease Research Center, Korea Institute of Oriental Medicine, Daejeon, Republic of Korea

Abstract

Objectives: The aims of this study were to investigate whether there is a gap between evidence of traditional medicine (TM) interventions in East-Asian countries from the current Clinical Practice Guidelines (CPGs) and evidence from current systematic reviews and meta-analyses (SR-MAs) and to analyze the impact of this gap on present CPGs.

Methods: We examined 5 representative TM interventions in the health care systems of East-Asian countries. We searched seven relevant databases for CPGs to identify whether core CPGs included evidence of TM interventions, and we searched 11 databases for SR-MAs to re-evaluate current evidence on TM interventions. We then compared the gap between the evidence from CPGs and SR-MAs.

Results: Thirteen CPGs and 22 SR-MAs met our inclusion criteria. Of the 13 CPGs, 7 CPGs (54%) mentioned TM interventions, and all were for acupuncture (only one was for both acupuncture and acupressure). However, the CPGs did not recommend acupuncture (or acupressure). Of 22 SR-MAs, 16 were for acupuncture, 5 for manual therapy, 1 for cupping, and none for moxibustion and herbal medicine. Comparing the evidence from CPGs and SR-MAs, an underestimation or omission of evidence for acupuncture, cupping, and manual therapy in current CPGs was detected. Thus, applying the results from the SR-MAs, we moderately recommend acupuncture for chronic LBP, but we inconclusively recommend acupuncture for (sub)acute LBP due to the limited current evidence. Furthermore, we weakly recommend cupping and manual therapy for both (sub)acute and chronic LBP. We cannot provide recommendations for moxibustion and herbal medicine due to a lack of evidence.

Conclusions: The current CPGs did not fully reflect the evidence for TM interventions. As relevant studies such as SR-MAs are conducted and evidence increases, the current evidence on acupuncture, cupping, and manual therapy should be rigorously considered in the process of developing or updating the CPG system.

Editor: Sonia Brucki, University Of São Paulo, Brazil

Funding: The authors have no support or funding to report.

Competing Interests: The authors have declared that no competing interests exist.

* E-mail: drshinbc@gmail.com

Introduction

Low back pain (LBP) is a common condition that affects a significant proportion of the population, with an estimated prevalence of 70%–85% [1]. Current Clinical Practice Guidelines (CPGs) recommend various LBP treatments, such as pharmaco-therapy, physical therapy, manual therapy, educational therapy, psychological therapy, and invasive therapy [2,3].

Traditional medicine (TM) is defined as indigenous medicine used to maintain health and to prevent, diagnose, and treat physical and mental illnesses and is distinct from allopathic medicine based on theories, beliefs, and experiences [4]. In East-Asian countries, especially China, Korea, and Japan, the main therapeutic methods of TM consist of acupuncture, moxibustion, cupping therapy, herbal medicines, and manual therapies (called Tuina in China, Chuna in Korea, and Shiatsu in Japan) [5]. In East-Asian countries, 80% of the population depends on TM for primary health care, and 70% to 80% of the population in many developed countries has used some form of alternative or complementary medicine (e.g., acupuncture) [4]. Although studies on the use of TM are increasing [6,7], differences in medical circumstances, culture, or poor evidence in support of TM seem to complicate the inclusion of TM in CPGs.

CPGs are systematically developed to assist practitioners and patients in making decisions about appropriate healthcare in specific clinical circumstances [8]. In contrast with previous approaches that were often based on tradition or authority, modern CPGs are based on an examination of current evidence within the paradigm of evidence-based medicine [9]. SR-MAs are literature reviews focused on a research question that attempts to identify, appraise, select, and synthesize all high-quality research evidence relevant to that question. SR-MAs of high-quality randomized controlled trials (RCTs) are crucial for evidence-based medicine [10]. Although it seems easy to write an SR-MA, good SR-MAs take time, and they frequently encounter delays but do not update the literature review. The additional typical delays for peer review and publishing add extra time, and SR-MAs may be printed two to four years after the end of the information retrieval. Finally, most SR-MAs are published worldwide without an accompanying CPG [11].

The purpose of this review was to investigate whether there is a gap between evidence of traditional medicine (TM) interventions in East-Asian countries from the current Clinical Practice guideline (CPGs) and evidence from current systematic reviews and meta-analyses (SR-MAs) and to analyze the impact of this gap on present CPGs.

Methods

Data Sources and Searches

Two types of databases were searched according to their database content. The first database was a CPG-related database for LBP that was used to understand the current status of LBP management. The other database included systematic reviews or meta- analyses (SR-MAs) and was used to compare the current evidence to current CPGs. Following the core, standard, ideal search (CoSI) model [12], we searched the following electronic databases from database inception to December 2012.

Our CPG database searches were the core searches because representative databases were more highly recommended than ideal searches. The CPG databases included the National Guideline Clearinghouse (NGC), Guidelines International Network (G-I-N), National Institute for Health and Clinical Excellence (NICE), and Scottish Intercollegiate Guidelines Network (SIGN). Additionally, we searched 3 representative East-Asian countries' databases: the Chinese National Knowledge Infrastructure (CNKI) for China, the Korean Medical Guideline Information (KoMGI) for Korea, and the Medical Information Network Distribution Service (MINDS) for Japan.

For SR-MAs, we conducted an ideal search because all relevant SR-MAs of LBP were needed for the TM area. We found TM in the following databases: The Cochrane Database of Systematic Review (CDSR), PubMed, MEDLINE, EMBASE, DH-DATA, AMED, Chinese databases (China Knowledge Resource Integrated Database, Wanfang database, and Chinese VIP information), a Korean database (Oriental Medicine Advanced Searching Integrated System), and a Japanese database (Japan Medical Abstracts Society).

Each East-Asian country's CPG and SR-MA databases were searched by authors from their own county.

The search keywords for CPG were (back pain OR low back pain OR lumbago) in each CPG database mentioned above. The search keywords for SR-MAs were (acupuncture OR acup*) for acupuncture, (moxa OR moxibustion) for moxibustion, (cupping) for cupping therapy, (herbal medicine OR traditional Chinese medicine OR Chinese herbal medicine) for herbal medicine, (manual therapy OR manipulation OR massage OR Chinese massage OR Tuina OR Chuna OR Shiatsu) for manual therapy, (low back pain OR back pain OR lumbago) for LBP, and (systematic review OR meta analysis OR meta analyze) for SR-MAs in each language. These search terms were combined in the form of [(LBP) AND (TM interventions) AND (SR-MA)]. This search strategy was adjusted for each database.

In addition, the bibliographies of relevant CPGs and SR-MAs were manually searched. Gray literature, consisting of theses, dissertations, letters, government documents, research reports, conference proceedings, and abstracts, was searched to avoid publication bias. The reference section for each study was searched. Personal contacts were made with the original authors of the searched studies to identify any data that were potentially missing from the publications.

The title and abstract of searched articles were read by a single primary researcher (H-WC), who conducted the screening process. Articles that were not written in English were translated into Korean or English prior to screening. The articles for potential inclusion in our review were checked by 2 independent reviewers (H-WC, E-HH). After screening the titles and abstracts retrieved in our search, we excluded all articles that did not meet our pre-defined inclusion/exclusion criteria. Then, the full text of the articles for inclusion was carefully read. The final inclusion was determined by two independent reviewers (H-WC, E-HH), who used the matching method.

Study Selection

Types of CPG and SR-MA. Current CPGs regarding the treatment of non-specific LBP, which were used universally and considered the standard, were evaluated. When we conducted the preliminary search, there were few CPGs not written in English, and they were from the Netherlands, Spain, Germany, France, Finland, and Brazil. The CPGs' development dates were relatively older than the English versions, and the relevance of their content was low. Thus, we concluded that they would have no effect on the analysis. Because we wanted to show the current state of TM through the representative CPGs, the authors reached a consensus to limit the language of the CPGs to English.

Non-specific LBP was searched and evaluated to understand the current evidence from SR-MAs research studies on the effectiveness of 5 major TM interventions (acupuncture, moxibustion, cupping therapy, manual therapy, and herbal medicine). Language was not restricted during the selection of SR and MA.

Types of participants in CPG and SR-MA. LBP was defined as pain localized to the area between the costal margin or the 12th rib to the inferior gluteal fold. Non-specific LBP indicated the lack of a detectable specific cause, such as infection, neoplasm, metastasis, osteoporosis, rheumatoid arthritis, fracture, or inflammatory process [13].

The CPGs and SR-MAs in our review included all stages of non-specific LBP with or without radiating pain, such as acute (lasting up to six weeks), sub-acute (lasting six to 12 weeks), or chronic (lasting longer than 12 weeks) non-specific LBP [14].

Types of interventions in SR and MA. We analyze the TM of the primary therapeutic interventions, including acupuncture, moxibustion, cupping therapy, herbal medicines, and manual therapies, found in East-Asian countries. We selected these 5 types of interventions because they were medical insurance reimbursement items in East-Asian countries [15].

Table 1. Comparison of Clinical Practice Guidelines for Low Back Pain.

Database	Guideline & Year	Target population	Interventions and practices considered	Presence of Traditional Medicine Interventions	Recommendation	AGREE II Overall Assessment
NGC (USA)	NGC-8959/2012 [21]	(Sub)acute/Non-specific LBP with or without radiculopathy/ including pregnant women	1, 2, 3, 5	None	NA	6/Y
	NGC-8744/2011 [24]	(Sub)acute/Non-specific LBP with or without back-related leg symptoms	1, 2, 3	None	NA	5/YWM
	NGC-8517/2011 [28]	(Sub)acute & chronic/ Non- specific LBP	1, 2, 3, 5, 6	Yes (acupuncture/ Acupressure)	Acupuncture/Acupressure considered, but are not recommended	6/Y
	NGC-8193/2010 [22]	(Sub)acute & chronic/ Non- specific LBP with or without radiculopathy	1,2,3,4	None	NA	3/YWM
	NGC-8009/2010 [26]	(Sub)acute/Non-specific LBP	1,2,3,6	None	NA	3/YWM
	NGC-7704/2009 [25]	(Sub)acute & chronic/ Non-specific LBP	(sub)acute LBP : 1, 2, 3, 5, 6/ Chronic LBP : 1, 2, 5, 6	Yes (acupuncture)	1. (Sub)acute: acupuncture - Do Not Know/2. Chronic: acupuncture - Do	3/YWM
	NGC-7510/2009 [27]	Work-related injuries or illnesses related to the low back, elbow, shoulder, forearm, wrist, or hand	2, 3, 4	None	NA	3/YWM
	NGC-7428/2009 [2]	Chronic/Non-specific LBP	6	None	NA	4/YWM
	NGC-6456/2007 [23]	Work-related low back disorders with radiculopath	1, 2, 3, 5, 6	Yes (acupuncture)	1.(Sub)acute LBP:acupuncture - Not recommended (Insufficient)/ 2.Chronic LBP: acupuncture for select use during a limited course with a clear objective and functional goals –Recommended (C-weak)/acupuncture - Notrecommended (Insufficient)	4/YWM
	NGC-5968/2007 [20]	(Sub)acute & chronic/ Non- specific LBP	1, 2, 3, 4, 5, 6	Yes (acupuncture)	Moderate quality evidence, Weak recommendation	3/YWM
NICE (UK)	CG-88/2009* [29]	(Sub)acute & chronic/ Non-specific LBP	1, 2, 3, 4, 5, 6	Yes (acupuncture)	Consider offering a course of acupuncture needling comprising up to a maximum of 10 sessions over a period of up to 12 weeks.	5/YWM
G-I-N (International)	Prodigy(UK) Back pain - low (without radiculopathy) /2009 [3]	(Sub)acute & chronic/ Non-specific LBP without radiculopathy(sciatica) (including sprains and strains)	1, 2, 3, 4, 5, 6	Yes (acupuncture)	The course should have up to 10 sessions given over a period of up to 12 weeks	3/YWM
MINDS (Japan)	Clinical Practice guideline for the management of LBP/2012 [30]	(Sub)acute & chronic/ Non-specific LBP	1, 2, 3, 4, 5, 6	Yes (acupuncture)	(Sub)acute – Do not know/ Chronic- It is hard to say acupuncture is better than other conservative therapies.	4/YWM

Abbreviations: LBP, low back pain; AT, acupuncture; NA, Not applicable YMA, yes with modification; Y, yes.
Items of Interventions and practices: 1 = pharmacological therapy, 2 = physical therapy, 3 = education, 4 = psychological therapy, 5 = manual therapy, 6 = invasive therapy; Items of outcomes considered: 1 = pain, 2 = Global measure, 3 = functional status, 4 = Quality of Life, 5 = Safety, 6 = Cost effectiveness, 7 = Other outcomes.; All AGREE II items are rated with the following 7-point scale: Score of 1 (Strongly Disagree) = There is no information relevant to the AGREE II item or very poor reporting of the concept.; Score of 7 (Strongly Agree) = quality of reporting is exceptional and the full criteria and considerations articulated in the User's Manual have been met.; Scores between 2 and 6 = The reporting of the AGREE II item does not meet the full criteria or considerations. A score is assigned depending on the completeness and quality of reporting. Scores increase as more criteria are met and considerations are addressed. We classified scores of 1 or 2 as low quality, scores of 3, 4 or 5 were moderate quality and 6 or 7 were high quality.; Domain scores are calculated by summing all the scores of the individual items in a domain and by scaling the total as a percentage of the maximum possible score for that domain. The scaled domain score will be: (Obtained score – Minimum possible) score/(Maximum possible score – Minimum possible score)*100.
*: NGC-7269 was originated from CG88 and it was summary of CG-88; thus, it was excluded.

Table 2. Systematic Reviews of Low Back Pain.

Type of Traditional Medicine	Stage of LBP	First Author & Year	Intervention	Outcome measurement	Direction of Outcome (Number of RCTs)	Level of Evidence/ Recommendation (SIGN)	Total AMSTA R score
Acupuncture							
	(Sub)acute						
		McIntosh 2008 [45]	Acupuncture	1, 2, 3, 7	P+(3)	1−/A	5
	Chronic						
		Hutchinson 2012 [44]	Acupuncture	1, 3, 4, 6, 7	P+ (7)	1+/A	4
		Trigkilidas 2010 [40]	Acupuncture	1, 3, 4, 6	I (4)	Not applicable	2
		Rubinstein 2010 [42]	Acupuncture	1, 3	P+ (18)	1+/A	10
		Yuan 2009 [39]	Acupuncture	1, 3, 4	Chronic LBP: P+ (23)	1+/A	7
		Ammendolia 2008 [37]	Acupuncture	1, 3, 4, 5, 7	I (19)	1+/A	4
		McIntosh 2008 [38]	Acupuncture	1, 2, 3, 7	P+ (32)	1−/A	4
		Henderson 2002 [34]	Acupuncture	Not reported	I (5)	2+/C	2
	Mixed						
		Furlan 2012 [41]	Acupuncture	1, 3, 5, 6	(Sub)acute LBP : I/chronic LBP : P+ (33)	1−/B	9
		Lu 2011 [43]	Acupuncture	1, 3, 4, 6, 7	P+ (5)	1+/A	8
		Furlan 2005 [35]	Acupuncture	1, 2, 3, 4, 5, 7	(Sub)acute LBP : I (3)/chronic LBP : P+ (32)	1+/A	3
		Maurits 2005 [46]	Acupuncture	1, 3, 7	acute LBP : I (2)/chronic LBP : P+ (13)	1+/A	9
		Manheimer 2005 [36]	Acupuncture	1, 2, 3, 7	P+ (33)	1+/B	8
		Ernst 2002 [33]	Acupuncture	1, 3	I (12)	1−/A	10
		Smith 2000 [32]	Acupuncture	1, 2, 7	(sub)acute LBP : N+ (2)/chronic LBP : N+ (8)	1+/A	7
		Tulder 1999 [31]	Acupuncture	1, 3, 7	I (11)	1−/A	8
Cupping Therapy							
	Mixed						
		Kim 2011 [52]	Dry/Wet cupping	1, 5	(sub)acute & chronic LBP : P+ (2)	1−/B	8
Manual Therapy							
	Chronic						
		Kim 2012 [50]	Acupressure	1, 3, 7	P++ (3)	1−/B	10
		Imamura 2008 [47]	Acupuncture massage, Acupressure	1, 2, 3, 4, 5, 6, 7	P+ (4)	1+/A	5
	Mixed						
		Moon 2012 [51]	Chuna	1	P+ (2)	1−/B	6
		Robinson 2011 [49]	Shiatsu, Acupressure	1, 3	Shiatsu: I (1)/Acupressure : P+ (3)	1−/B	6
		Furlan 2009 [48]	Acupuncture massage, Acupressure	1, 2, 3, 4, 5, 6, 7	P++ (5)	1+/A	10

Abbreviations: LBP, low back pain; I, insufficient; P, positive; N, negative;
+ = weak; ++ = moderate; +++ = strong.
Items of outcomes measurement: 1 = pain; 2 = Global measure; 3 = functional status; 4 = Quality of Life; 5 = Safety; 6 = Cost effectiveness; 7 = Other outcomes.
The total AMSTAR score was calculated by adding the average scores for all 11 items. We averaged item scores across guidelines. Item scores were classified such that 0–3 indicated low quality, 4–7 indicated moderate quality and 8–11 indicated high quality.

1. Acupuncture: only included needle acupuncture with or without electrical stimulation. Acupuncture without needling, such as laser or TENS on acupoints, was excluded.

2. Moxibustion: included when acupoints were heated with moxibustion.

3. Cupping therapy: included both dry and wet cupping.

4. Manual therapy: included Tuina in China or Chuna in Korea. Massage techniques were included, such as Chinese massage, acupressure, acupuncture massage, or Shiatsu when applied to acupoints or meridians.

5. Herbal medicine: included herbal medicine according to the TM diagnosis.

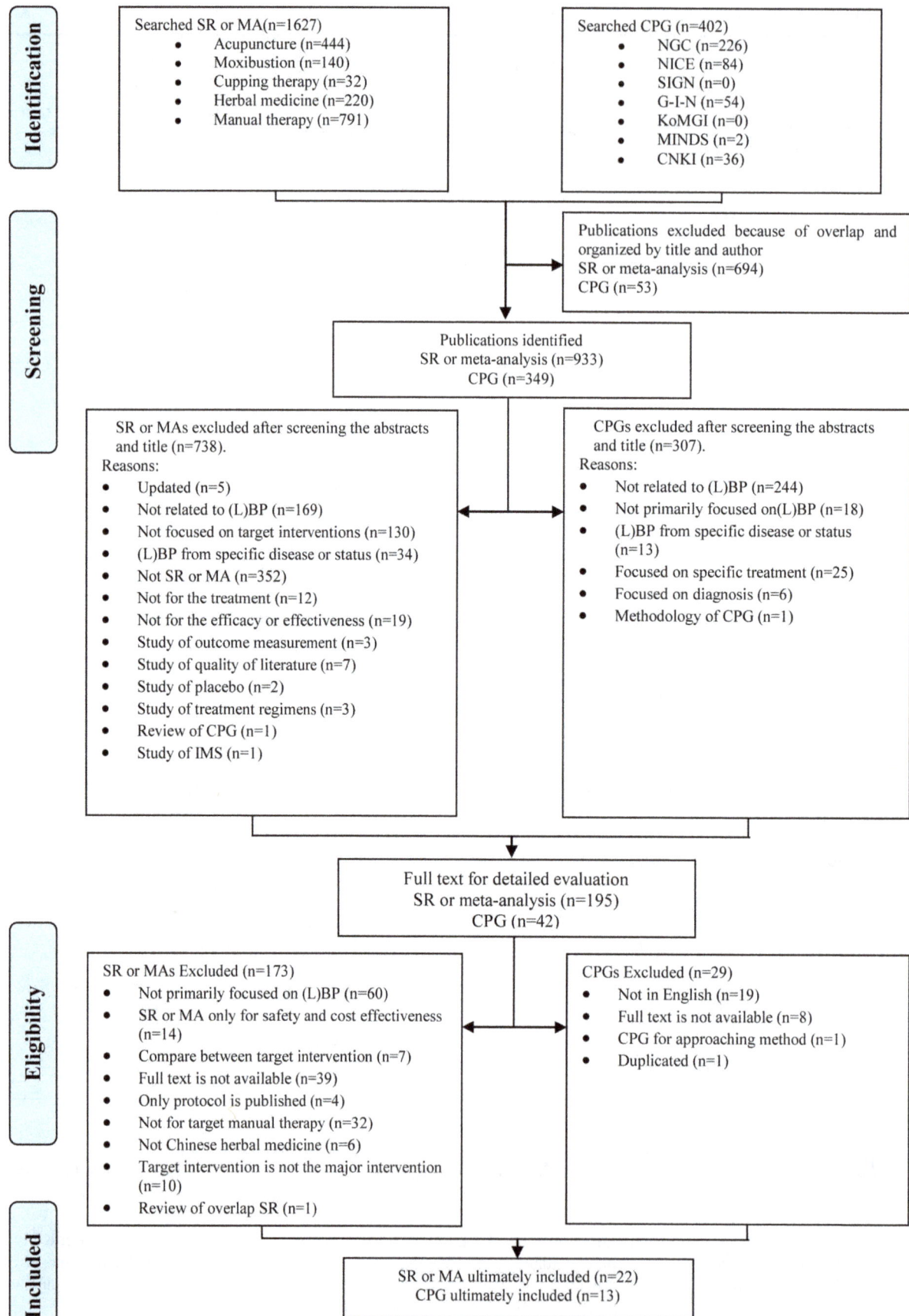

Identification

Searched SR or MA(n=1627)
- Acupuncture (n=444)
- Moxibustion (n=140)
- Cupping therapy (n=32)
- Herbal medicine (n=220)
- Manual therapy (n=791)

Searched CPG (n=402)
- NGC (n=226)
- NICE (n=84)
- SIGN (n=0)
- G-I-N (n=54)
- KoMGI (n=0)
- MINDS (n=2)
- CNKI (n=36)

Screening

Publications excluded because of overlap and organized by title and author
SR or meta-analysis (n=694)
CPG (n=53)

Publications identified
SR or meta-analysis (n=933)
CPG (n=349)

SR or MAs excluded after screening the abstracts and title (n=738).
Reasons:
- Updated (n=5)
- Not related to (L)BP (n=169)
- Not focused on target interventions (n=130)
- (L)BP from specific disease or status (n=34)
- Not SR or MA (n=352)
- Not for the treatment (n=12)
- Not for the efficacy or effectiveness (n=19)
- Study of outcome measurement (n=3)
- Study of quality of literature (n=7)
- Study of placebo (n=2)
- Study of treatment regimens (n=3)
- Review of CPG (n=1)
- Study of IMS (n=1)

CPGs excluded after screening the abstracts and title (n=307).
Reasons:
- Not related to (L)BP (n=244)
- Not primarily focused on(L)BP (n=18)
- (L)BP from specific disease or status (n=13)
- Focused on specific treatment (n=25)
- Focused on diagnosis (n=6)
- Methodology of CPG (n=1)

Full text for detailed evaluation
SR or meta-analysis (n=195)
CPG (n=42)

Eligibility

SR or MAs Excluded (n=173)
- Not primarily focused on (L)BP (n=60)
- SR or MA only for safety and cost effectiveness (n=14)
- Compare between target intervention (n=7)
- Full text is not available (n=39)
- Only protocol is published (n=4)
- Not for target manual therapy (n=32)
- Not Chinese herbal medicine (n=6)
- Target intervention is not the major intervention (n=10)
- Review of overlap SR (n=1)

CPGs Excluded (n=29)
- Not in English (n=19)
- Full text is not available (n=8)
- CPG for approaching method (n=1)
- Duplicated (n=1)

Included

SR or MA ultimately included (n=22)
CPG ultimately included (n=13)

Figure 1. Flow chart of the study selection process. SR = systematic review; MA = meta-analysis; CPG = clinical practice guideline; (L)BP = (low) back pain; IMS = Intra Muscular Stimulation.

When studies addressed various symptoms or interventions in one acupuncture SR, we limited the inclusion criteria if the majority (>50%) of the participants and the intervention were acceptable for predefined criteria because there were numerous acupuncture SR-MAs. However, there were few available SR-MAs of moxibustion, cupping, manual therapy, and herbal medicine. Therefore, we included the SR-MAs when the RCTs of those interventions were greater than 10% of all RCTs when the data could be separately extracted.

When it was difficult to evaluate the independent effectiveness of TM intervention, such as comparing the same interventions or mixed treatments, the SR-MAs were excluded.

Data Extraction and Quality Assessment

Two reviewers (H-WC, E-HH) independently extracted the data based on predefined characteristics to describe each study (refer to Tables 1, 2). In CPG, we extracted the type of interventions, the presence of TM, and the recommendation. In SR-MAs, we extracted outcome measures and their directions of outcome for each intervention and condition of LBP.

Outcome measures. The outcome measures that we considered are described below. SR-MAs that used at least one outcome measure related to pain were included. The other outcome measures were considered, and their inclusion may be important for the study of LBP.

1. Primary outcome: Pain intensity
2. Secondary outcome: Global measure of improvement or recovery/Back-specific functional status/Quality of life/Safety/Cost-effectiveness/Other outcomes

Level of Evidence and Recommendation

We reassessed the evidence level and recommendations of the SR-MAs using the SIGN grading system [16]. All disagreements were resolved through discussion and consensus or by the first author (H-WC).

Quality Assessment of CPGs and SR-MAs

The SR-MAs of 24 different appraisal tools and some studies have shown that the Appraisal of Guidelines for Research & Evaluation (AGREE) instrument is an acceptable standard for guideline evaluation. Therefore, the AGREE Instrument for reporting the quality of CPGs was used [17,18], and the Assessment of Multiple Systematic Reviews (AMSTAR) checklist for reporting the quality of SR-MAs was used to evaluate the methodological quality of the included publications. The AMSTAR instrument has recently been used in another study [19].

Four reviewers (H-WC, E-HH, K-HH, and B-CS) were fully trained in the quality assessment and data extraction methodology.

Data Synthesis and Analysis

We identified the directions for future CPG of LBP through deep discussion and expert consensus among authors. All authors were CPG-related experts from East-Asian countries (China, Korea, and Japan). The authors discussed and reached consensus through e-mail contact. In cases of disagreement, the final recommendation was made by consensus. Per the authors' recommendations, we recommend studies based on the results in Table 1 and Table 2.

Results

Study Description

A total of 402 CPGs and 1627 SR-MAs were identified. After manually removing the duplicates and screening the titles and abstracts, 42 CPGs and 195 SR-MAs were identified as potentially relevant. After a detailed evaluation of the full text, 29 CPGs and 173 SR-MAs were excluded. Finally, 13 CPGs and 22 SR-MAs met our inclusion criteria. The literature search process is summarized in Figure 1, following the Preferred Reporting Items for Systematic Reviews and Meta-Analysis (PRISMA) flow diagram. The key data are summarized in Table 1.

Current Clinical Practice Guidelines

Of the 13 CPGs, 10 originated in the USA [2,20–28], 2 were from the UK [3,29], and 1 was from Japan [30]. There were no CPGs from any East-Asian country. There were 7 CPGs for both (sub)acute and chronic LBP [3,20,22,25,28–30], 1 for chronic LBP [2], 3 for (sub)acute LBP [21,24,26], and 2 for work-related LBP [23,27]. The CPGs addressed various interventions, such as pharmacological therapy, physical therapy, education, psychological therapy, manual therapy, and invasive therapy. However, TM interventions were only included in 7 CPGs [3,20,23,25,28–30]. All TM interventions were for acupuncture, and only 1 CPG [28] mentioned both acupuncture and acupressure.

Of 7 CPGs, 6 recommended acupuncture, but all of these CPGs had weak recommendation strength or made the recommendation with session limitations [3,20,23,25,29,30]. However, 3 CPGs did not recommend acupuncture for (sub)acute LBP [23,25,28]. Only 1 CPG [28], which analyzed acupressure, did not recommend the treatment (Table 1).

Quality Assessment of Clinical Practice Guidelines

The overall assessment mean of the included CPGs was 4±1 (range: 3–6), indicating that CPGs have moderate quality. There were 2 high-quality CPGs [21,28], 11 moderate-quality CPGs [2,3,20,22–27,29,30], and no low-quality CPGs. We assessed 2 CPGs [21,28] as "recommend without modification" due to high quality and 11 other CPGs as "recommend with modifications" (Table 1). In each domain, the CPGs showed comparatively more than moderate quality (Table S1).

Evidence of Systematic Review and Meta-analysis

Of 22 SR-MAs, 16 were for acupuncture [31–46], 5 were for manual therapy (Chuna, acupressure, acupuncture massage, shiatsu) [47–51], and 1 was for cupping therapy [52]. For chronic LBP, 1 SR reported a moderately negative conclusion [32], 5 SR-MAs reported an insufficient conclusion [31,33,34,37,40], and 9 SR-MAs reported weakly positive effects of acupuncture [35,36,38,39,41–44,46]. For (sub)acute LBP, 1 SR reported a moderate negative conclusion [32], 5 SR-MAs reported insufficient conclusions [31,33,35,41,46], and 3 SR-MAs reported weakly positive effects of acupuncture [36,38,43]. The evidence level and recommendation strength were reassessed using the SIGN grading system. For the level of evidence, 5 SR-MAs were assessed 1− [31,33,38,41,45], 9 SR-MAs were 1+ [32,35–37,39,42–44,46], 1 SR was 2+ [34], and 1 SR was not applicable [40]. For recommendation strength, 12 SR-MAs were assessed as grade A [31–33,35,37–39,42–46], 2 SR-MAs were grade B [36,41], 1 was grade C [34], and 1 was not applicable [40].

Table 3. Directions for future Clinical Practice Guideline of Low Back Pain.

Database	Guideline & Year	Acupuncture		Moxibustion		Cupping Therapy		Manual Therapy		Herbal Medicine	
		Level of Evidence	Grade of Recommendation	Level of Evidence	Grade of Recommendation	Level of Evidence	Grade of Recommendation	Level of Evidence	Grade of Recommendation	Level of Evidence	Grade of Recommendation
Current											
NGC (USA)	NGC-8959 2012	–		–		–		–		–	
	NGC-8744 2011	–		–		–		–		–	
	NGC-8517 2011	U		–		–		U		–	
	NGC-8193 2010	–		–		–		–		–	
	NGC-8009 2010	–		–		–		–		–	
	NGC-7704 2009	E		–		–		–		–	
	NGC-7510 2009	–		–		–		–		–	
	NGC-7428 2009	–		–		–		–		–	
	NGC-6456 2007	U		–		–		–		–	
	NGC-5968 2007	U		–		–		–		–	
NICE (UK)	CG-88 2009	U		–		–		–		–	
G-I-N (International)	Prodigy (UK) 2009	U		–		–		–		–	
MINDS (Japan)	CPG for the management of LBP 2012	E		–		–		–		–	
Future											
Authors Recommendation	Condition of LBP										
	(Sub)acute	1–	B	–	–	1–	B	1–	B	–	–
	Chronic	1+	A	–	–	1–	B	1–	B	–	–
Recommendation		Moderate recommendation for chronic LBP/Inconclusive for (Sub)acute LBP		Do not know		Weak recommendation for both (Sub)acute and chronic LBP		Weak recommendation for both (Sub)acute and chronic LBP		Do not know	

Abbreviations: U, underestimated; E, enough.
–: There were no available data, and assessments were not applicable.

Only 1 SR-MA on cupping for pain, including 2 RCTs for both (sub)acute and chronic LBP, reported weakly positive conclusions. The study partially considered pain and safety (adverse effect). The evidence level was assessed to be 1−, and the recommendation strength received a grade of B [52].

Of 5 SR-MAs of manual therapy, 1 considered Chuna [51], and 4 considered acupressure (including acupuncture massage and Shiatsu) [47–50]. All of these SR-MAs were compared with other interventions and reported positive conclusions, except for an inconclusive conclusion reported in 1 study of Shiatsu [49]. The study evidence level was assessed to be 1−, and the recommendation strength received a grade of B [51]. In 4 studies of acupressure, 2 were on chronic LBP alone [47,50], and the other 2 included both (sub)acute LBP and chronic LBP [48,49]. The evidence level was assessed to be 1− in 2 studies [49,50] and 1+ in the other 2 studies [47,48]. The recommendation strength received a grade of A in 2 studies [47,48] and B in the other 2 studies [49,50] (Table 2).

Quality Assessment of Systematic Reviews

The mean (± standard deviation) score of total quality assessment of the SR-MAs was 6.59±2.65 (range: 2–10) (Table S2). A total of 10 SR-MAs (47.6%) were assessed to be high quality [31,33,36,41–43,46,48,50,52], 9 SR-MAs (38.1%) were moderate quality [32,37–39,44,45,47,49,51], and 3 SR-MAs (14.3%) were low quality [34,35,40](Table 2).

Directions for Future CPG of LBP

Of the 7 CPGs that included acupuncture, 2 showed a similar recommendation compared with current research on SR-MAs [25,30], but 5 CPGs were underestimated [3,20,23,28,29]. Only 1 CPG included manual therapy and showed effectiveness underestimation [28]. Similar to moxibustion, cupping therapy and herbal medicine were not discussed in current CPGs and thus could not be compared.

We moderately recommended acupuncture for chronic LBP with a 1+/A evidence level and recommendation grade. However, we inconclusively recommended acupuncture for (sub)acute LBP due to the current SR-MA evidence. We weakly recommended cupping therapy for both (sub)acute and chronic LBP with a 1−/B evidence level and recommendation grade. We weakly recommend manual therapy for both (sub)acute and chronic LBP with a 1−/B evidence level and recommendation grade. Moxibustion and herbal medicine were not applicable due to the lack of data available at this time (Table 3).

Discussion

The main aim of our review was to analyze TMs in East-Asian countries (China, Korea, and Japan) in the current CPGs for LBP. The results showed that TMs in East-Asian countries were not sufficiently included in current CPGs.

Notably, moxibustion, cupping therapy, and herbal medicine are not mentioned in current CPGs. The lack of eligible RCTs and the aggregation of SR of moxibustion for LBP might be the primary causes of this lack of inclusion. This omission leads to a lack of evidence for the CPG. The use of moxibustion has become more common; 67% of Korean Oriental medical doctors have used moxibustion [53]. Additionally, 40% of health care in China is currently based on traditional Chinese medicinal approaches that include moxibustion [54]. The adverse effects and difficulties of placebo moxibustion that are reported in the literature [55] may have emerged due to the limited moxibustion studies.

The relevant studies on cupping therapy were of poor quality [56], which might lead to a lack of inclusion in current CPGs. However, the only SR showed a positive effect for both sub(acute) and chronic LBP.

The heterogeneity of herbal medicine products may be a considerable problem. The various types of preparation and the amount of chemical constituents per dose influence the pharmacokinetics and relative efficacy of the herbal medicine [57]. These differences may make it difficult to conduct a high-quality study.

Some acupuncture recommendations had both favorable and unfavorable conclusions. Of all of the studies, 7 CPGs (54%) mentioned acupuncture, but only 1 study recommended acupuncture for chronic LBP without use limitations. The other studies recommended acupuncture for limited treatment sessions or did not recommend acupuncture. These results demonstrate a gap with the results of current SR-MAs. Negative or insufficient effects in SR-MAs were dominant for (sub)acute LBP [31–33,35,41]. However, the positive effects were dominant for chronic LBP [35,36,38,39,41–44]. Similar results were reported for the evidence-based medicine approach to LBP [58]. Therefore, we conclude that the recommendations for (sub)acute LBP seem appropriate, and the recommendations for chronic LBP are underestimated.

Regarding manual therapy, 1 CPG mentioned acupressure but did not recommend acupressure for both (sub)acute and chronic LBP. However, we found some gaps in SR-MAs. There were 5 SR-MAs with a positive result [47–51] (1 on Chuna [51] and 4 on acupressure or acupuncture massage [47–50]) and 1 insufficient SR on Shiatsu [49]. Additionally, 1 related SR-MA that was not included in this study supported the possibility of Tuina-integrated treatment t for LBP [59]. Thus, we find that the current CPGs underestimate the effectiveness of TM manual therapy for LBP.

The overall evidence available was usually published in the US and European countries, Thus, a lack of familiarity with East-Asian TM may influence the lack of interventions. These problems may explain the underpowered evidence for TM.

One important thing to consider is the need for more objective methods in TM practice. In contradistinction to classical approaches in Eastern medicine, where the methodology is much more concrete, TM is mainly considered an "art". This understanding complicates an objective study of the results.

We also conducted a quality assessment that included CPGs and SR-MAs. The AGREE assessment showed that the quality of included CPGs was acceptable. The average scores of 5 domains (with the exception of 1 domain) were greater than 60%, and the mean score in the overall assessment was 4±1 [range: 3–6], indicating a moderate quality of CPG (Table 1). The domains of applicability obtained the lowest score, suggesting that more attention should be paid to quality enhancement during CPG development (Table S1).

The SR-MAs were assessed using the AMSTAR instrument [19]. Although the item "Was a priori design provided?" received the lowest score, the overall scores were quite high. The total mean score showed moderate quality of 6.59 [range: 2–10] for included SR-MAs (Table S2). Therefore, future authors should conduct an a priori design to ensure better study quality.

The strength of our study is its successful completion of the first review of TM in current CPGs for LBP. Previous CPGs of Traditional Chinese Medicine [60] did not focus on specific diseases or make further suggestions to address the lack of evidence. To prevent this bias, we attempted to determine whether current TM interventions were adequately included in current, rigorous CPGs of LBP. Thus, we searched current available CPGs and SR-MAs with systematic search methods and assessed CPG and SR-MA quality. In this study, we reanalyzed the evidence level and grade of recommendation of SR-MAs and aimed to identify directions for future research via a CPG-related expert consensus.

Several study limitations should be considered. Despite our best efforts to retrieve all CPGs and SR-MAs on this subject, we are not convinced that our search was inclusive. Notably, the definition of manual therapy categories in Oriental medicine is a considerable problem. Because we selected the subjects for TM in East-Asian countries, there is a potential question regarding whether the 5 types of intervention represent all TM interventions. To address this problem, we selected the interventions that consider the use of traditional Chinese medicine [61]. Although we suggested recommendation reassessments, we did not follow the entire procedure involved in crafting CPGs [62]. Instead, we made decisions via the expert consensus method. Therefore, biased conclusions are possible.

To address these weaknesses, we suggest important recommendations for future research in this area. First, high-quality RCTs were not conducted despite the use of TM, and there is a remarkable lack of studies on moxibustion, cupping therapy, Tuina (or Chuna), and herbal medicine, which deserve increased interest and further study. Second, a broader scope of TM interventions should be searched in further studies, and accurate recommendations for TM interventions should be drawn via proper procedures by larger organizations or teams. The increasing TM evidence should be included in the process of updating CPGs, and TM interventions based on LBP CPGs should be developed in collaboration with TM experts.

Conclusion

Although interest in and use of TM is increasing, the CPGs identified did not fully reflect the TM interventions in East-Asian countries. In particular, acupuncture, cupping therapy, and manual therapy were underestimated or not mentioned despite their current evidence. The current evidence on acupuncture for chronic LBP and evidence on cupping and manual therapy for both (sub)acute and chronic LBP should be rigorously considered in the process of developing or updating the CPG system. However, a lack of evidence on moxibustion and herbal medicine prevented us from providing recommendations in these areas.

Supporting Information

Table S1 Assessment of Clinical Practice Guidelines (CPG) by AGREEII.
(DOCX)

Table S2 Assessment of Systematic Reviews by AM-STAR.
(DOCX)

Checklist S1 PRISMA checklist.
(DOCX)

Author Contributions

Conceived and designed the experiments: H-WC E-HH K-HH B-CS. Performed the experiments: H-WC E-HH. Analyzed the data: H-WC BML B-CS. Wrote the paper: H-WC. Contributed to assess the level of evidence, grade of recommendation and methodological quality of the CPGs and SR-MAs: H-WC J-PL KT. Contributed to search the CPGs and SRs from each countries: H-WC E-HH K-HH B-CS. Contributed to the consensus of recommendation of future CPGs: H-WC E-HH B-CS BML K-HH J-PL KT MS-L.

References

1. Andersson GB (1999) Epidemiological features of chronic low-back pain. Lancet 354: 581–585.
2. Manchikanti L, Boswell MV, Singh V, Benyamin RM, Fellows B, et al. (2009) Comprehensive evidence-based guidelines for interventional techniques in the management of chronic spinal pain. Pain Physician 12: 699–802.
3. SCHIN - Sowerby Centre for Health Informatics at Newcastle (2009) Back pain - low (without radiculopathy) (Prodigy).
4. World Health Organization Media Centre (2012) "Traditional medicine,". World Health Organization Media Centre.
5. Cheung F (2011) TCM: Made in China. Nature 480: S82–S83.
6. Frass M, Strassl RP, Friehs H, Mullner M, Kundi M, et al. (2012) Use and acceptance of complementary and alternative medicine among the general population and medical personnel: a systematic review. Ochsner J 12: 45–56.
7. Ernst E, Schmidt K, Wider B (2005) CAM research in Britain: the last 10 years. Complement Ther Clin Pract 11: 17–20.
8. Field MJ, Lohr KN (1990) Committee to Advise the Public Health Service on Clinical Practice Guidelines IoM. Clinical practice guidelines: directions for a new program. Washington: National Academy Press.
9. Graham R, Mancher M, Wolman DM, Greenfield S, Steinberg E (2011) Committee on Standards for Developing Trustworthy Clinical Practice Guidelines Institute of Medicine. Clinical Practice Guidelines We Can Trust: The National Academies Press.
10. Sackett DL, Rosenberg WM, Gray JA, Haynes RB, Richardson WS (1996) Evidence based medicine: what it is and what it isn't. BMJ 312: 71–72.
11. Dijkers M (2013) Want your systematic review to be used by practitioners? Try this! KT Update 1: Available from http://www.ktdrr.org/products/update/v1n4.
12. Bidwell S, Jensen MF (2004) Chapter 3: Using a search protocol to identify sources of information: the COSI model. In: Topfer L-A, Auston I, editors. Etext on Health Technology Assessment (HTA) Information Resources. Bethesda, MD: National Information Center on Health Services Research and Health Care Technology (NICHSR).
13. Waddell G (1996) Low back pain: a twentieth century health care enigma. Spine (Phila Pa 1976) 21: 2820–2825.
14. Koes BW, van Tulder M, Lin CW, Macedo LG, McAuley J, et al. (2010) An updated overview of clinical guidelines for the management of non-specific low back pain in primary care. Eur Spine J 19: 2075–2094.
15. Park HL, Lee HS, Shin BC, Liu JP, Shang Q, et al. (2012) Traditional medicine in china, Korea, and Japan: a brief introduction and comparison. Evid Based Complement Alternat Med 2012: 429103.
16. Harbour R, Miller J (2001) A new system for grading recommendations in evidence based guidelines. BMJ 323: 334–336.
17. AGREE Collaboration (2003) Development and validation of an international appraisal instrument for assessing the quality of clinical practice guidelines: the AGREE project. Qual Saf Health Care 12: 18–23.
18. MacDermid JC, Brooks D, Solway S, Switzer-McIntyre S, Brosseau L, et al. (2005) Reliability and validity of the AGREE instrument used by physical therapists in assessment of clinical practice guidelines. BMC Health Serv Res 5: 18.
19. Shea BJ, Grimshaw JM, Wells GA, Boers M, Andersson N, et al. (2007) Development of AMSTAR: a measurement tool to assess the methodological quality of systematic reviews. BMC Med Res Methodol 7: 10.
20. Chou R, Qaseem A, Snow V, Casey D, Cross JT, Jr., et al. (2007) Diagnosis and treatment of low back pain: a joint clinical practice guideline from the American College of Physicians and the American Pain Society. Ann Intern Med 147: 478–491.
21. Goertz M, Thorson D, Bonsell J, Bonte B, Campbell R, et al. (2012 Jan) Institute for Clinical Systems Improvement (ICSI). Adult acute and subacute low back pain. Bloomington (MN): Institute for Clinical Systems Improvement (ICSI).
22. Goertz M, Thorson D, Bonsell J, Bonte B, Campbell R, et al. (2010 Nov) Institute for Clinical Systems Improvement (ICSI). Adult low back pain. Bloomington (MN): Institute for Clinical Systems Improvement (ICSI).
23. Hegmann K (2007) Low back disorders. Occupational medicine practice guidelines: evaluation and management of common health problems and functional recovery in workers. 2nd ed. Elk Grove Village (IL): American College of Occupational and Environmental Medicine (ACOEM).
24. Michigan Quality Improvement Consortium (2011 Sep) Management of acute low back pain. Southfield (MI): Michigan Quality Improvement Consortium.

25. Toward Optimized Practice (2009 Mar 2) Guideline for the evidence-informed primary care management of low back pain. Edmonton(AB): Toward Optimized Practice. 21 p.
26. University of Michigan Health System (2010 Jan) Acute low back pain. Ann Arbor (MI): University of Michigan Health System.
27. National Guideline Clearinghouse (2009) Occupational therapy practice guidelines for individuals with work-related injuries and illnesses. Rockville MD: Agency for Healthcare Research and Quality (AHRQ).
28. National Guideline Clearinghouse (2011) Low back - lumbar & thoracic (acute & chronic). Rockville MD: Agency for Healthcare Research and Quality (AHRQ).
29. National Collaborating Centre for Primary Care (2009 May) Low back pain. Early management of persistent non-specific low back pain. London (UK): National Institute for Health and Clinical Excellence (NICE). pp. 25.
30. Japanese Orthopaedic Association (2012) Clinical Practice Guideline for the Management of Low Back Pain. Tokyo: Nankodo Co., Ltd.
31. van Tulder MW, Cherkin DC, Berman B, Lao L, Koes BW (1999) The effectiveness of acupuncture in the management of acute and chronic low back pain. A systematic review within the framework of the Cochrane Collaboration Back Review Group. Spine (Phila Pa 1976) 24: 1113–1123.
32. Smith LA, Oldman AD, McQuay HJ, Moore RA (2000) Teasing apart quality and validity in systematic reviews: an example from acupuncture trials in chronic neck and back pain. Pain 86: 119–132.
33. Ernst E, White AR, Wider B (2002) Acupuncture for back pain: Meta-analysis of randomised controlled trials and an update with data from the most recent studies. Schmerz 16: 129–139.
34. Henderson H (2002) Acupuncture: evidence for its use in chronic low back pain. Br J Nurs 11: 1395–1403.
35. Furlan AD, van Tulder M, Cherkin D, Tsukayama H, Lao L, et al. (2005) Acupuncture and Dry-Needling for Low Back Pain: An Updated Systematic Review Within the Framework of the Cochrane Collaboration. Spine (Phila Pa 1976) 30: 944–963.
36. Manheimer E, White A, Berman B, Forys K, Ernst E (2005) Meta-analysis: acupuncture for low back pain. Ann Intern Med 142: 651–663.
37. Ammendolia C, Furlan AD, Imamura M, Irvin E, van Tulder M (2008) Evidence-informed management of chronic low back pain with needle acupuncture. Spine J 8: 160–172.
38. Hall H, McIntosh G (2008) Low back pain (chronic). Clin Evid (Online) 2008.
39. Yuan J, Purepong N, Kerr DP (2009) Effectiveness of acupuncture for low back pain: A systematic review (Spine (2008) 33, (E887–E900)). Spine (Phila Pa 1976) 34: 1630.
40. Trigkilidas D (2010) Acupuncture therapy for chronic lower back pain: a systematic review. Ann R Coll Surg Engl 92: 595–598.
41. Furlan AD, Yazdi F, Tsertsvadze A, Gross A, Van Tulder M, et al. (2012) A systematic review and meta-analysis of efficacy, cost-effectiveness, and safety of selected complementary and alternative medicine for neck and low-back pain. Evid Based Complement Alternat Med 2012: 953139.
42. Rubinstein SM, van Middelkoop M, Kuijpers T, Ostelo R, Verhagen AP, et al. (2010) A systematic review on the effectiveness of complementary and alternative medicine for chronic non-specific low-back pain. Eur Spine J 19: 1213–1228.
43. Lu SC, Zheng Z, Xue CC (2011) Does acupuncture improve quality of life for patients with pain associated with the spine? A systematic review. Evid Based Complement Alternat Med 2011: 301767.
44. Hutchinson AJ, Ball S, Andrews JC, Jones GG (2012) The effectiveness of acupuncture in treating chronic non-specific low back pain: a systematic review of the literature. J Orthop Surg Res 7: 36.
45. Hall H, McIntosh G (2008) Low back pain (acute). Clin Evid (Online) 2008.
46. van Tulder MW, Furlan AD, Gagnier JJ (2005) Complementary and alternative therapies for low back pain. Best Pract Res Clin Rheumatol 19: 639–654.
47. Imamura M, Furlan AD, Dryden T, Irvin E (2008) Evidence-informed management of chronic low back pain with massage. Spine J 8: 121–133.
48. Furlan AD, Imamura M, Dryden T, Irvin E (2009) Massage for low back pain: an updated systematic review within the framework of the Cochrane Back Review Group. Spine (Phila Pa 1976) 34: 1669–1684.
49. Robinson N, Lorenc A, Liao X (2011) The evidence for Shiatsu: a systematic review of Shiatsu and acupressure. BMC Complement Altern Med 11: 88.
50. Kim YC, Lee MS, Park E-S, Lew J-H, Lee B-J (2012) Acupressure for the Treatment of Musculoskeletal Pain Conditions: A Systematic Review. J Musculoskelet Pain 20: 116–121.
51. Moon TW, Choi TY, Park TY, Lee MS (2012) Chuna therapy for musculoskeletal pain: A systematic review of randomized clinical trials in Korean literature. Chin J Integr Med 19: 228–232.
52. Kim JI, Lee MS, Lee DH, Boddy K, Ernst E (2011) Cupping for treating pain: a systematic review. Evid Based Complement Alternat Med 2011: 467014.
53. Han CH, Shin MS, Shin SH, Kang KW, Park SH, et al. (2007) Telephone survey for grasping clinical actual state of moxibustion therapeutics in Korea. J Meridian Acupoint 24: 17–31.
54. Hesketh T, Zhu WX (1997) Health in China. Traditional Chinese medicine: one country, two systems. BMJ 315: 115–117.
55. Park JE, Lee SS, Lee MS, Choi SM, Ernst E (2010) Adverse events of moxibustion: a systematic review. Complement Ther Med 18: 215–223.
56. Cao H, Li X, Liu J (2012) An updated review of the efficacy of cupping therapy. PLoS ONE 7: e31793.
57. Gagnier JJ, van Tulder M, Berman B, Bombardier C (2006) Herbal medicine for low back pain. Cochrane Database Syst Rev: CD004504.
58. Dagenais S, Haldeman S (2011) Evidence-Based management of low back pain: Elsevier Health Sciences.
59. Kong LJ, Fang M, Zhan HS, Yuan WA, Pu JH, et al. (2012) Tuina-focused integrative chinese medical therapies for inpatients with low back pain: a systematic review and meta-analysis. Evidence-based complementary and alternative medicine : eCAM 2012: 578305–578305.
60. Yu WY, Xu JL, Shi NN, Wang LY, Han XJ, et al. (2011) Assessing the quality of the first batch of evidence-based clinical practice guidelines in traditional Chinese medicine. J Tradit Chin Med 31: 376–381.
61. Xu J, Yang Y (2009) Traditional Chinese medicine in the Chinese health care system. Health Policy 90: 133–139.
62. Moret L, Lefort C, Terrien N (2012) [How to write, how to implement and how to evaluate a practice guideline in order to improve quality of care?]. Transfus Clin Biol 19: 174–177.

3

Assessing the Quality of Reports about Randomized Controlled Trials of Acupuncture Treatment on Mild Cognitive Impairment

Xiao Lu[1,2], Shang Hongcai[1,2]*, Wang Jiaying[1,3], Hu Jing[4], Xiong Jun[5]

1 Tianjin University of Traditional Chinese Medicine, Tianjin, China, 2 MOE Virtual Research Center of Evidence-Based Medicine, Chengdu, China, 3 Evidence Based Medicine Center in Tianjin, Tianjin, China, 4 Peking University, Beijing, China, 5 Department of Acupuncture, Jiang Xi Hospital of Traditional Chinese Medicine, Jiangxi Province, China

Abstract

Objective: To evaluate the reports' qualities which are about randomized controlled trials (RCTs) of acupuncture treatment on Mild Cognitive Impairment (MIC).

Methods: Nine databases including the Cochrane Central Register of Controlled Trials (CENTRAL,2010), PUBMED (1984-5/2010), EMbase (1984-5/2010), MEDLINE (1984-5/2010), CINAL (1984-5/2010), China National Knowledge Infrastructure (CNKI, 1980-5/2010), China Biomedicine Database disc (CBMdisc, 1980-5/2010), VIP (a full text issues database of China, 1989-5/2010) were searched systematically. Hand search for further references was conducted. Language was limited to Chinese and English. We identified 14 RCTs that used acupuncture as an intervention and assessed the quality of these reports against the Consolidated Standards for Reporting of Trials (CONSORT) statement and Standards for Reporting Interventions in Controlled Trials of Acupuncture (STRICTA).

Results: In regard to the items in the CONSORT statement, 13(92.86%) RCTs described baseline demographic and clinical characteristics in each group. 7 (50.0%) mentioned the method of generating the random sequence, only 2 (14.3%) RCTs had adequate allocation concealment. No RCTs used blinding. RCTs reported the sample size calculation. In regard to the items in STRICTA, 10 (71.43%) mentioned the depths of insertion, 6 (42.86%) reported acupuncture response, 11 (78.57%) mentioned the technique of acupuncture, 12 (85.71%) recorded the time, and only 3 (21.43%) RCTs reported the numbers of needles inserted. No RCTs reported the background of the acupuncture practitioners and professional title of practitioners.

Conclusion: The reporting quality of RCTs of acupuncture for mild cognitive impairment was moderate to low. The CONSORT statement and STRICTA should be used to standardize the reporting of RCTs of acupuncture in future.

Editor: Joseph Ross, Yale University School of Medicine, United States of America

Funding: New Century Excellent Talent Project Grant (No 2009613). The funders had no role in study design, data collection and analysis, decision to publish, or preparation of the manuscript.

Competing Interests: The authors have declared that no competing interests exist.

* E-mail: shanghongcai@foxmail.com

Introduction

Mild Cognitive Impairment (mild cognitive disorder) is a clinical state with disease characteristics between normal aging and mild dementia. Most clinical researches show that 44% of the patients diagnosed as cognitive impairment turn into Alzheimer's transit (AD) within 3 years in follow-up studies at an annual average rate of 15% [1]. Recognizing cognitive impairment and identifying individuals at high risk of dementia have become a hot issue in dementia studies in recent years. Lacking in effective drugs and rehabilitation treatment, many patients with mild cognitive impairment begin to try alternative and complementary medicine therapies which include acupuncture treatment. However, despite the publication of a number of case-based research papers the effectiveness of acupuncture on mild cognitive impairment is to be tested and to do so a reliable scientific method is needed. Some

research teams decide to adopt the randomized controlled trials (RCTs). RCTs, also known as randomized clinical trials, is a prospective study to test the efficacy and effectiveness of certain treatment or protective measures after comparing the results of the treatment group with those of the control group, thus the subjects involved in the study being randomized divided into two groups [2]. At present, randomized controlled trials (RCTs) is generally considered as the best design plan to verify the efficacy of intervention measures for it boasts rigorous design and scientific methods. It contributes to ensure high-quality systematic reviews, health technology assessment reports, and a variety of other reports for decision analysis, which meets the top requirements of evidence-based medical research [3]Therefore, we have adopted the internationally recognized standards for trial reporting (the CONSORT statement) [4] and the international standards for clinical trials of acupuncture interventions (STRICTA) [5] to evaluate the quality of reports of randomized controlled trials of acupuncture treatment for mild cognitive impairment in order to shed light on its further improvement.

Methods

Search strategy

The nine databases we have searched include Cochrane Central Register of Controlled Trials(CENTRAL,2010), PUBMED(1984-5/2010), EMbase(1984-5/2010), MEDLINE(1984-5/2010), CI-NAL(1984-5/2010), China National Knowledge Infrastructure (CNKI, 1980-5/2010), China Biomedicine Database disc (CBMdisc, 1980-5/2010), and VIP(a full text issues database of China,1989-5/2010). The work was done comprehensively and systematically and further references were searched by hand. Our search is featured by a wide coverage of reports and prospective studies in this field to provide enough information for research.

However, our search confined itself to reports written or published either in Chinese or in English. For one thing, it is because a majority of journal papers on acupuncture are published in these two languages and it is apparently impossible for reports written in Chinese to be included in non-Chinese databases. Besides, our team members were unable to read reports in languages other than Chinese and English. It may constitute to a limitation of this study.

We did not limit our search to a specific publication date range at the beginning of this study because we wanted to find as many reports as possible concerning mild cognitive impairment in the above databases. However, the databases themselves have such limitations.

Eligibility of the study

We included original reports in Chinese or English that described acupuncture as an intervention, stated the method, and provided specific data in this study and excluded commercials, speeches, letters and meeting reports.

Selection of reports to be studied

At first, one researcher (XL) picked out duplications of these reports using NoteExpress, and scanned the title and abstract of the citation retrieved by the selection search engine (first scanning). Another researcher (WJY) then viewed the full text of all potentially eligible reports obtained. After that, similar reports were marked "suspicious duplications" and compared. If the similarity rate of these articles was beyond 80% (including 80%), the one with the fullest information was included while the others were omitted. Disagreements between the two researchers were discussed by the whole team and were solved at last. (Figure 1)

Data abstraction

Two researchers (XL and WJY) compiled a table to list the general information of the final included reports. Items of the table include report title, journal name, year of publication, type of control, number of participants and country of publication. Any missed information was coded as "not reported" and disagreements were resolved after getting more information from related references before finalizing the table. Two reviewers scanned the full text of all 14 reports and filled the table.

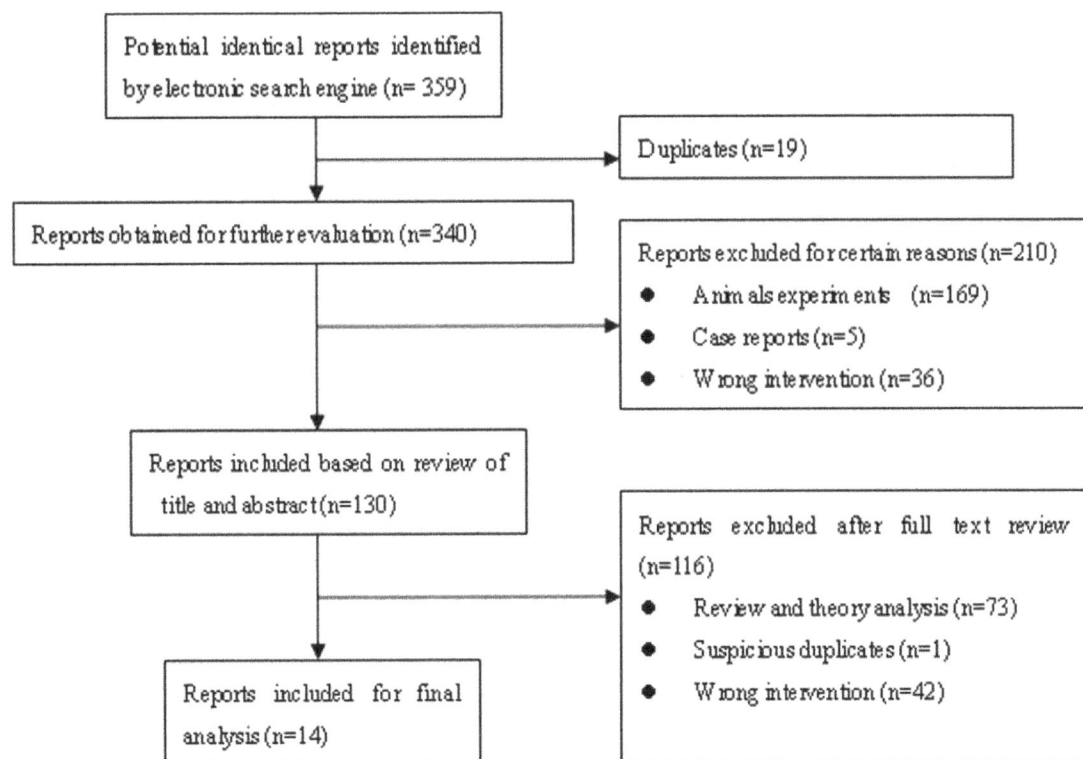

Figure 1. Flow chart of reports selection. This figure shows the process of the selection. The researchers applied the search method to find 359 reports related to the topic. One researcher (XL) picked out 19 duplications of these reports by the software NoteExpress and 169 reports of animals experiments, 5 cases and 36 reports of the wrong intervention by scanning the title and abstract of the citation retrieved by the selection search engine (first scanning). Another researcher (WJY) then viewed the full text of all potentially eligible reports obtained and picked out 73 reviews and theory analyses, one suspicious duplicate and 42 reports of the wrong intervention. At last, 14 reports are included for final analysis.

Assessment methods

We assessed the quality of these reports by CONSORT and STRICTA standards. CONSORT (consolidated standards of reporting trails) was introduced in 1996 [6] in an attempt to alleviate the problems arising from inadequate reporting, and it was revised five years later [7]. STRICTA (standards for reporting interventions in controlled trials of acupuncture) was compiled between late 2001 and early 2002 [8].

The CONSORT statement comprises a 22-item checklist including abstract, background, participants, interventions, objectives, outcome measures, sample size, sequence generation, allocation concealment, implementation, blinding, statistical methods, participant flow, recruitment, demographic data, numbers analyzed, outcomes and estimation, ancillary analyses, adverse events, interpretation and overall evidence.

STRICTA consists of 15 items including acupuncture rationale, points used, number of needle inserted depths of insertion, response elicited, needle stimulation, needle retention time, needle type, treatment regimen, co-interventions, practitioner background, duration of training, length of clinical experience, expertise, control interventions. The above information can also be found in Table 2 and Table 3.

Two researchers were required to study the CONSORT and STRICTA standards before making assessment to ensure correct understanding of every item listed in the two checklists. If they had any difficulties or disagreements in the process, they solved the problem in discussions. The 14 reports were then assessed according to the two standards respectively and each item was marked "M" (mentioned) or "NM" (not mentioned).

Results

Report selection

A total of 359 potentially relevant reports were identified from the databases for review. 229 publications were considered to be unfit for our study after a preliminary review of title and abstract. Another 74 were excluded after full-text review. At last a total of 14 full-text reports [9–22] were regarded eligible for a more systematic analysis.

Characteristics of the Reports

The characteristics of all the included reports are presented in Table 1. All the 14 reports were found in 11 different medical journals published by six different publishing houses. Sample sizes ranged from a small pilot study of 17 subjects to a large scale, and the largest sample included 104 subjects. Only one report was published in America. All the 14 studies included in our assessment were published during the year 2006–2010, while in 2009 the number of reports published reached the peak (43%) (Figure 2).

Use of CONSORT and STRICTA

At first we found that none of the reports included in the assessment explicitly mentioned the CONSORT or STRICTA statement. After referring to the official websites of the 11 journals, we found that only two journals require manuscripts to be submitted to meet the CONSORT or STRICTA standards. However, we found out later that there were 3 reports that included 19 items of CONSORT and 12 items of STRICTA

Table 1. Characteristics of the reports included (N = 14).

Report title	Journal name	Year of publication	Type of control	Number of participants	Country of publication
He 2008	JOURNAL OF PRACTICAL TRADITIONAL CHINESE MEDICINE	2008	aceglutamide	60	China
Yu 2007	SHAANXI JOURNAL OF TRADITIONAL CHINESE MEDICINE	2007	Nimodipine	67	China
Sun 2009	JOURNAL OF CLINICAL ACUPUNTURE AND MOXIBUSTION	2009	duxil tablet	60	China
Hou 2010	WORLD JOURNAL OF INTEGRATED TRADITIONAL AND WESTERN MEDICINE	2010	Sham acupuncture	36	China
Hou 2009	JOURNAL OF BEI JING UNIVERSITY OF TRADITONAL CHINESE MEDICINE	2009	Sham acupuncture	40	China
Sun 2007	Chinese Journal of Traditional Medical Science and Technology	2007	Aricept	62	China
Su 2006	LIAO NING JOURNAL OF TRADITIONAL CHINESE MEDICINE	2006	Nimodipine	100	China
Zhou 2008	SHANGHAI JOURNAL OF ACUPUNTURE AND MOXIBUSTION	2008	Sham acupuncture	60	China
Zhou 2008	GUANGXI JOURNAL OF TRADITIONAL CHINESE MEDICINE	2008	Regular treatment	60	China
Liu 2009	SHANGHAI JOURNAL OF ACUPUNTURE AND MOXIBUSTION	2009	Aricept	17	China
Chen 2008	JOURNAL OF EMERGENCY IN TRADITIONAL CHINESE MEDICINE	2008	Regular treatment	60	China
Chen 2009	Chinese Journal of Traditional Medical Science and Technology	2009	Regular treatment	60	China
Feng 2009	Jilin Journal of Traditional Chinese Medicine	2009	Sham acupuncture	104	China
Pei 2009	THE JOURNAL OF ALTERNATIVE AND COMPLEMENTARY MEDICINE	2009	Conventional rehabilitation	38	America

Table 2. Reporting quality of 14 RCTs based on CONSORT.

Total number of items	Number of reported RCTs (%)	
Abstract	7	50.00
Introduction		
Background	11	78.57
Methods		
Participants	12	85.71
Interventions	13	92.86
Objectives	12	85.71
Outcomes	13	92.86
Sample size	14	100.00
Randomization		
Sequence generation	7	50.00
Allocation concealment	2	14.29
Implementation	1	7.14
Blinding	0	0.00
Statistical methods	12	85.71
Results		
Participant flow	0	0.00
Recruitment	0	0.00
Baseline data	13	92.86
Numbers analyzed	12	85.71
Outcomes and estimation	10	71.43
Ancillary analyses	4	28.57
Adverse events	3	21.43
Discussion		
Interpretation	13	92.86
Overall evidence	7	50.00

Table 3. Reporting quality of interventions in 14 RCTs based on STRICTA.

Intervention	Number of reported RCTs (%)	
Acupuncture rationale	13	92.86
Needling details		
Points used	14	100
Number of needles inserted	3	21.43
Depths of insertion	10	71.43
Response elicited	6	42.86
Needle stimulation	11	78.57
Needle retention time	12	85.71
Needle type	7	50.00
Treatment regimen	11	78.57
Co-interventions	3	21.43
Practitioner background	0	0.00
Duration of training	0	0.00
Length of clinical experience	0	0.00
Expertise	0	0.00
Control intervention(s)	11	78.57

checklist, which means that the two statements have actually been employed by more authors.

Reporting Assessment Using CONSORT and STRICTA

The results are presented in Table 2 and Table 3. Not a single report fulfilled either all the 21 items of the CONSORT checklist or the 15 STRICTA items. Above all, the main problem we found was a lack of information concerning method of blinding, practitioner background, and participant flow and recruitment.

CONSORT. Seven CONSORT items were mentioned in less than 30% of the total reports. They are methods of blinding, participant flow and recruitment (0%), implementation of randomization (7.14%), description of allocation concealment (14.29%), adverse events of acupuncture (21.43%) and outcomes of ancillary analyses (28.57%).

Another four CONSORT items were included in more than half of all the reports, i.e., abstract, sequence generation and overall evidence in the section of discussion.

STRICTA. None of these studies gave any information about practitioner background which was made up of expertise, duration of training and length of clinical experience. Two STRICTA items, namely, number of needles inserted and co-interventions were explained in 21.43% of the reports. Another two items were made clear in less than half of the reports, i.e., needle type (50%) and response elicited.

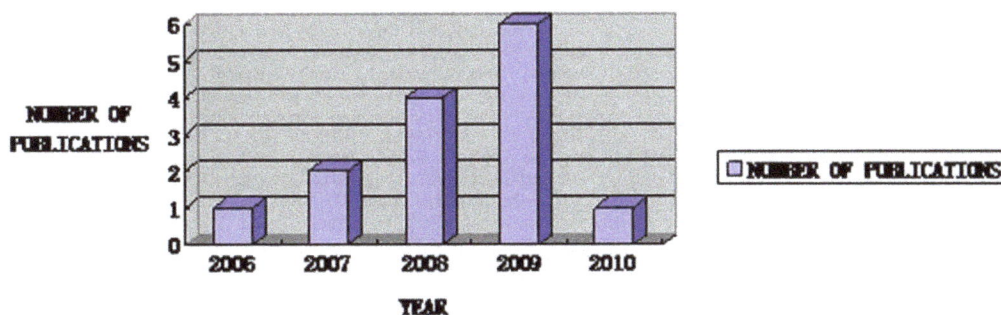

Figure 2. Number of reports published in the recent five years. According to the Table 1, the years of publication of included reports is mainly during these five years, namely from the 2006 to 2010. Figure 2 shows one report is published in 2006, two in 2007, four in 2008, six in 2009, and one in 2010.

Discussion

Summary of the study

The main strength of our study is that we have searched a total of nine databases in order to encompass all the related reports. Moreover, reports selection, data collection, reports assessment and all the other work were carefully conducted by well-trained researchers.

Another important strength of our study is that we use the CONSORT and STRICTA statement to evaluate RCTs of acupuncture. Both of them are the most widely accepted criteria for reporting quality assessment in acupuncture studies. Plain in words and ready for use, the two statements were developed in the aim of alleviating the problems arising from inadequate reporting of randomized controlled trials. They are powerful tools, as has been proved by the fact that the majority of their items were well reported, with a few exceptions (7 CONSORT items and 9 STRICTA ones were poorly reported).

We believe it is high time to call for clinical researchers to follow the two statements in conducting RCTs and in thesis writing. At present, Chinese journals set down no requirements for the author to follow the CONSORT or STRICTA statement in reporting Therefore, we recommend that mainstream Chinese journals make the application of CONSORT or STRCITA a prerequisite, so that transparency and integrity of RCTs can be ensured. More importantly, for policy makers, it is urgent to let more clinical researchers know about the CONSORT and STRICTA statement.

Limitations

Although we have assessed the 14 reports comprehensively and systematically, there are still some limitations. First, the reports included in our study were published exclusively in years between 2006 and 2010 although we didn't make any limitations on the date of publication during sample selection. The fact that the selected reports cover a narrow time span may harm the value of our study. However, it is worth mentioning that the whole concept of mild cognitive impairment was not put forward until 1999 by American scholar Petersen. Apparently it took some time for the diagnostic criteria to be introduced to China and to be widely accepted by Chinese scholars. In addition, it probably cost more time for acupuncture, a complementary and alternative intervention, to be involved in the treatment. Recently, some research groups propose the need to test the efficacy of acupuncture treatment after three or four years' clinical practice in cognitive impairment patients, thus RCTs were conducted. Nevertheless, at the beginning we didn't realize it was impossible for us to find any target report before 1999

if sample selection was conducted with "mild cognitive impairment" as a search word, which means we have done something useless and our search strategy remains to be improved.

According to resources and databases accessible to us, the earliest RCTs were carried out in 2006. However, there might be earlier articles in the database that we didn't find for certain reasons, such as language competence. We limited our search to reports written in Chinese and English, but the English report turned out to be one in number. It seems that our quality review was confined to domestic reports. Results may vary if we were able to include more reports in other languages, but this requires our team members to attain a higher level of language skills, a target we are confident to reach in the future.

Another limitation lies in that we didn't follow the rule of blinding when assessing and allocating the reports. Researches who did the scanning were directly involved in the evaluation process. This is because we believe two researchers are enough to evaluate the whole 14 selected reports and allocation was unnecessary. However, although the two researchers had studied the same version of the checklist items beforehand, they came out with different opinions on certain issues. This shows that assessment bias still exists.

Conclusion

Our study suggests that the reporting quality of recently published reports of RCTs of acupuncture treatment for mild cognitive impairment remains to be improved. However, we have found only one published report had formally appealed for the adoption of CONSORT in future research. With more articles published on this subject, it is necessary to call for the wide application of the CONSORT and STRICTA standards to improve the quality of reporting, and this study should be pursued further with a greater number of reports on this subject assessed and analyzed.

Acknowledgments

Give our thanks to the authors of the cited articles timely reply our questions and SHANG Hongcai professor's for his careful guidance.

Author Contributions

Conceived and designed the experiments: WJY XL SHC. Performed the experiments: XL WJY. Analyzed the data: HJ XL WJY. Contributed reagents/materials/analysis tools: HJ XJ. Wrote the paper: WJY XL. Resolved the disagreement and bias: SHC HJ XJ.

References

1. Gmdman M, Petemen RC, Morris JC, ADSC Cooperative Study, et al. (1996) Rate of dementia of the Alzheimer type in subjects with mild cognitive impairment[J]. Neurology 46: A403.
2. WANG Ying, HAO Guangyue, GAO Bing (2006) introduction of revised edition of CONSORT statement-the reliable standard to improve qualities reporting evaluation [J]. Journal of Baotou medicine college. pp 355–357.
3. ZHANG Xiaoli, LI Jing, ZHANG Mingming, etc (2006) Assessing the Reporting Quality of Randomized Controlled Trials on Acupuncture for Acute Ischemic Stroke Using the CONSORT Statement and STRICTA [J]. Chinese Journal of Evidence Based Medicine 6(8): 586690.
4. Altman DG, Schulz K, Moher D, et al. (2001) The Revised Statement CONSORT for Reporting Randomized Trials Explanation and Elaboration. Ann Intern Med 134(8): 663–694.
5. Mac Pherson H, White A, Cummings M, et al. (2002) STRICTA(Standards for Reporting Interventions in Controlled Trials of Acupuncture). Acupuncture in Medicine 20(1): 22–25.
6. Begg C, Cho M, Eastwood S, Horton R, Moher D, et al. (1996) Improving the quality of reporting of randomized controlled trials, the CONSORT statement JAMA 276(8): 637–639.
7. Moher D, Schula KF, Altman D, CONSORT Group (Consolidated Standards of Reporting Trials) (2001) The CONSORT statement: Revised recommendations for improving the quality of repors of parallel-group randomized trials JAMA 285(15): 1987–1991.
8. MacPherson H, White A, Cummings M, Jobst K, Rose K, et al. (2001) Standards for reporting invention in controlled trials of acupuncture: The STRICTA recommendations. Complement Ther Med(1): 216–249, 20(1):22-25, 8(1):85-89.
9. He Xia (2008) Clinical Research on Mild Cognitive Impairment Treated by Combination of Acupuncture and Medicine. JOURNAL OF PRACTICAL TRADITIONAL CHINESE MEDICINE ZYAO, 2008(11).
10. Yu Tao (2007) Acupuncture Treatment of Vascular Cognitive Impairment without Dementia in 31 Cases. SHAANXI JOURNAL OF TRADITIONAL CHINESE MEDICINE SXZY, 2007(06).
11. Sun Yuanzheng, Zhang Ying (2009) Clinical Research on Mild Cognitive Impairment Treated by Combination of Acupuncture and Duxil Tablet. JOURNAL OF CLINICAL ACUPUNCTURE AND MOXIBUSTION ZJLC, 2009(09).
12. Hou Xiaobing, et al. (2010) The Impact of Acupuncture on Mild Cognitive Impairment in Functional Magnetic Resonance Imaging. WORLD JOURNAL OF INTEGRATED TRADITIONAL AND WESTERN MEDICINE SJZX, 2010(02).
13. Hou Xiaobing (2009) Brain Functional Magnetic Resonance Imaging (fMRI) Changes in Leukoaraiosis with Mild Cognitive Impairment before and after Treatment of Acupuncture. Beijing University of Traditional Chinese Medicine.

14. Sun Yuanzheng, Zhu Pengyu, Zhang Yan (2007) 30 Cases of of Mild Cognitive Impairment Treated with Acupunture and Oral Donepezil. Chinese Journal of Traditional Medical Science and Technology. TJYY, (03).

15. Su Zhiwei, Liu Huanrong (2006) 100 Cases of Mild Cognitive Impairment Treated with Yishen Tongdu Method Liaoning Journal of Traditional Chinese Medicine LNZY, 2006(08).

16. Zhou Xiaoping, et al. (2008) Effect of the Acupunture Method of Regulating Mild and Smooth Meridian on Patients with Mild Cognitive Impairment after Cerebral infarction. Shanghai Journal of Acupunture and Moxibustion SHZJ, 2008(05).

17. Zhou Xiaoping, et al. (2008) Effect of the Acupunture Method of Regulating Mild and Smooth Meridian on Patients with Mild Cognitive Impairment. GUANGXI JOURNAL OF TRADITIONAL CHINESE MEDICINE GXZY, 2008(02).

18. Liu Jie, Liu Zhiyan (2009) Clinical Observation on Electro-acupunture Treatment for Mild Cognitive Impairment of Deficiency of Kidney Essence. Shanghai Journal of Acupunture and Moxibustion. SHZJ, 2009(06).

19. Chen Shangjie, et al. (2008) Effects of Different Acupunture Methods on Neurological Deficit Score and Quality of Life of Patients with Mild Cognitive Impairment. Journal of Emergency in Traditional Chinese Medicine ZYJZ, 2008(03).

20. Chen Shangjie, et al. (2009) Effects of Different Acupunture Methods on SMS and MBI of Patients with Mild Cognitive Impairment. Chinese Journal of Traditional Medical Science and Technology. TJYY 2009(01).

21. Feng Chunqing, et al. (2009) Effects observation of "Qi-reinforcing, Blood-regulating and Body resistance-strengthening" Acupunture Method for Treating Mild Cognitive Impairment. Lin Journal of Traditional Chinese Medicine. 2009 29(10).

22. P C, C H, L JG (2009) Effects of electroacupunture treatment on impaired cognition and quality of life in Taiwanese stroke patients. Journal of alternative and complementary medicine (New York, N.Y.), 2009(10).

4

An Updated Review of the Efficacy of Cupping Therapy

Huijuan Cao[1,2], Xun Li[2], Jianping Liu[2]*

1 Centre for Complementary Medicine Research, University of Western Sydney, Penrith, Australia, **2** Centre for Evidence-Based Chinese Medicine, Beijing University of Chinese Medicine, Beijing, China

Abstract

Background: Since 1950, traditional Chinese medicine (TCM) cupping therapy has been applied as a formal modality in hospitals throughout China and elsewhere in the world. Based on a previous systematic literature review of clinical studies on cupping therapy, this study presents a thorough review of randomized controlled trials (RCTs) to evaluate the therapeutic effect of cupping therapy.

Method: Six databases were searched for articles published through 2010. RCTs on cupping therapy for various diseases were included. Studies on cupping therapy combined with other TCM treatments versus non-TCM therapies were excluded.

Results: 135 RCTs published from 1992 through 2010 were identified. The studies were generally of low methodological quality. Diseases for which cupping therapy was commonly applied were herpes zoster, facial paralysis (Bell palsy), cough and dyspnea, acne, lumbar disc herniation, and cervical spondylosis. Wet cupping was used in most trials, followed by retained cupping, moving cupping, and flash cupping. Meta-analysis showed cupping therapy combined with other TCM treatments was significantly superior to other treatments alone in increasing the number of cured patients with herpes zoster, facial paralysis, acne, and cervical spondylosis. No serious adverse effects were reported in the trials.

Conclusions: Numerous RCTs on cupping therapy have been conducted and published during the past decades. This review showed that cupping has potential effect in the treatment of herpes zoster and other specific conditions. However, further rigorously designed trials on its use for other conditions are warranted.

Editor: German Malaga, Universidad Peruana Cayetano Heredia, Peru

Funding: Huijuan Cao and Jianping Liu were supported by the grant of international cooperation project (No. 2009DFA31460) and the 111 Project (B08006) from China. Jianping Liu was in part supported by the Grant Number R24 AT001293 from the National Center for Complementary and Alternative Medicine (NCCAM) of the US National Institutes of Health. The funders had no role in study design, data collection and analysis, decision to publish, or preparation of the manuscript.

Competing Interests: The authors have declared that no competing interests exist.

* E-mail: Jianping_l@hotmail.com

Introduction

Cupping is a traditional Chinese medicine (TCM) therapy dating back at least 2,000 years. Types of cupping include retained cupping, flash cupping, moving cupping, wet cupping, medicinal cupping, and needling cupping [1]. The actual cup can be made of materials such as bamboo, glass, or earthenware. The mechanism of cupping therapy is not clear, but some researchers suggest that placement of cups on selected acupoints on the skin produces hyperemia or hemostasis, which results in a therapeutic effect [2].

In our previous study, we conducted a systematic literature review based on available clinical studies published from 1958 through 2008 [3]. We concluded that the majority of the 550 included studies showed that cupping is of potential benefit for pain conditions, herpes zoster, and cough and dyspnea. Five other systematic reviews [4–8] on cupping therapy have also been published, focusing on pain conditions, stroke rehabilitation, hypertension, and herpes zoster, respectively. The numbers of included trials in these reviews were quite small (between 1and 8 trials). Lee et al. [9] conducted an overview of these five reviews and concluded that cupping is only effective as a treatment for pain, and even for this indication doubts remain. Extensive search did not find further related reviews.

Though the quality of included randomized controlled trials (RCTs) in the aforementioned reviews was generally poor according to the Cochrane risk of bias tool, we felt that it was still worth conducting an overview systematic review to further evaluate the therapeutic effect of cupping therapy for specific disease/conditions due to the paucity of evidence in this subject.

Methods

The flow diagram for this review and supporting CONSORT checklist are available as supporting information; see Checklist S1 and Protocol S1.

Inclusion Criteria

Eligible studies were randomized controlled trials (RCTs) that examined the therapeutic effect of cupping therapy, including one or more types of cupping methods, compared with no treatment, placebo, or conventional medication. Cupping combined with other interventions and compared with other interventions alone were also included. Studies that looked at cupping therapy combined with other TCM therapies, such as acupuncture, compared with non-TCM therapies were excluded. Multiple

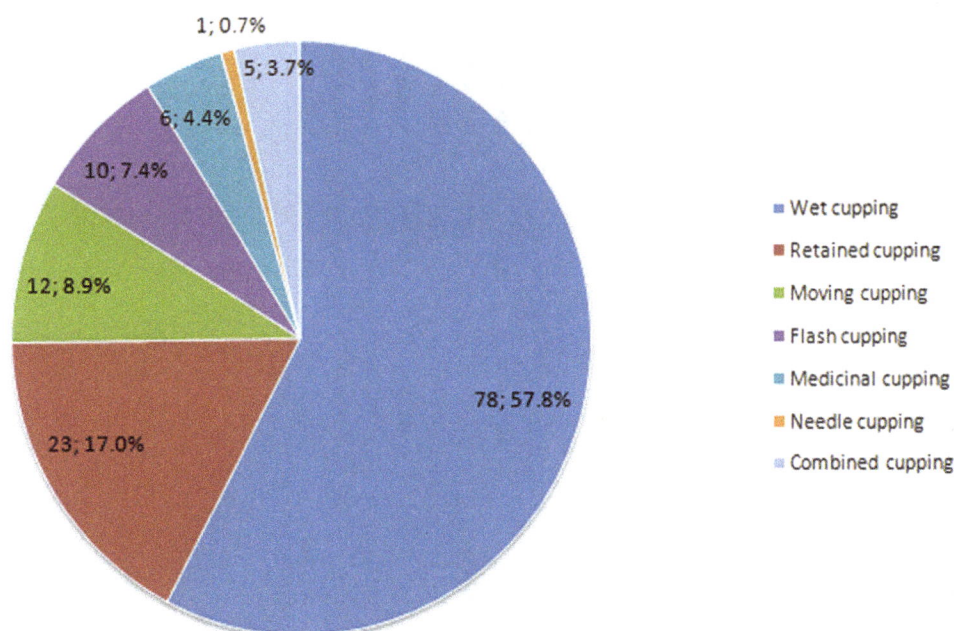

Figure 1. Constituent ratios of types of cupping therapy.

publications reporting the same patient data set were also excluded. There was no restriction on language and publication type.

Identification and Selection of Studies

Based on our previous review [3], an updated search of publications was performed using China Network Knowledge Infrastructure (CNKI) (2009 through 2010), Chinese Scientific Journal Database (VIP) (2009 through 2010), Chinese Biomedical Database (CBM) (2009 through 2010), Wanfang Database (2009 through 2010), PubMed (1966 through 2010), and the Cochrane Central Register of Controlled Trials (CENTRAL, 1800 through 2010). All searches ended at December 2010. The search terms included *cupping therapy, bleeding cupping, wet cupping, dry cupping, flash cupping, herbal cupping, moving cupping, needling cupping* and *retained cupping*. Two authors (HC and XL) independently identified and checked each study against the inclusion criteria.

Data Extraction and Quality Assessment

Two authors (HC and XL) independently extracted the data from the included trials. The extracted data included authors and title of study, year of publication, type of disease, study size, age and gender of participants, and methodological information. Other extracted data included type of cupping therapy, treatment process, control interventions, outcomes (for example, overall efficacy rate), and adverse effects.

Quality of included trials was evaluated. Methodological quality of RCTs was assessed using criteria from the *Cochrane Handbook for Systematic Reviews of Interventions* [10]. Trials were appraised according to the risk of bias for each important outcome, including adequacy of generation of the random allocation sequence, allocation concealment, blinding, and outcome reporting. Quality of each trial was categorized into low/unclear/high risk of bias. Trials that met all criteria were categorized into low risk of bias, trials that met none of the criteria were categorized into high risk of bias, and the remaining trials were categorized

into unclear risk of bias if there was insufficient information to make a judgment.

Data Analysis and Statistical Methods

Data were extracted using Microsoft Access and transferred into Microsoft Excel spreadsheets to be calculated for frequency. Outcome data were summarized using risk ratio (RR) with 95% confidence intervals (CI) for binary outcomes or mean difference (MD) with 95% CI for continuous outcomes. RevMan 5.0.20 software was used for data analyses. Meta-analysis was used if the trials had good homogeneity, which was assessed by examining I^2 (an index that describes the percentage of variation across studies that is due to heterogeneity rather than chance), on study design, participants, interventions, control, and outcome measures. Funnel plot analysis was done to determine publication bias.

Results

Basic Information of Studies

Searches of six databases identified 1,294 citations, the majority of which were deemed ineligible from reading title and abstract (Protocol S1). Full-text papers of 108 trials were retrieved. In addition to the 73 trials from our previous review, 62 new trials were included in this study. Of the 135 included trials [11–145], 132 were published in Chinese, including 3 unpublished dissertations [16,27,72].The remaining 3 trials [69,73,86] were published in English. All included studies were published from 1992 through 2010, with more than half from 2008 through 2010 (Table S1).

Description of Interventions

Among the included trials, 78 (57.78%) used wet cupping as the main intervention, 23 (17.04%) used retained cupping, 12 (8.89%) used moving cupping, 10 trials (7.40%) used flash cupping, 6 (4.44%) used medicinal cupping, and 1 (0.74%) used

Table 1. Reporting of quality components in 135 included randomized clinical trials on cupping therapy.

Year published	No. of Randomized controlled trials	Adequate sequence generation (%)	Adequate allocation concealment (%)	Blinding method reported (%)	Incomplete outcome data (yes, %)	Selective outcome reporting (yes, %)	Comparability of baseline (yes, %)	Sample size estimation (yes, %)	Inclusive criteria (yes, %)	Exclusive criteria (yes, %)	Diagnostic standard (yes, %)
1992	2	0	0	0	0	0	0	0	0	0	0
1993	1	1(100%)	0	0	0	0	0	0	0	0	0
1994	1	0	0	0	0	0	0	0	0	0	0
1995	-	-	-	-	-	-	-	-	-	-	-
1996	-	-	-	-	-	-	-	-	-	-	-
1997	2	0	0	0	0	0	0	0	0	0	0
1998	1	0	0	0	0	0	0	0	0	0	0
1999	2	0	0	0	0	0	1(50%)	0	0	0	1(50%)
2000	2	0	0	0	0	0	1(50%)	0	1(50%)	2(100%)	2(100%)
2001	-	-	-	-	-	-	-	-	-	-	-
2002	-	-	-	-	-	-	-	-	-	-	-
2003	7	0	0	0	0	0	2(28.57%)	0	0	1(14.29%)	4(57.14%)
2004	8	0	0	0	0	0	6(75%)	0	3(37.5%)	1(12.5%)	3(37.5%)
2005	10	2(20%)	0	1(10%)	0	0	7(70%)	0	6(60%)	5(50%)	8(80%)
2006	19	5(26.32%)	0	1(5.26%)	1(5.26%)	0	14(73.68%)	1(5.26%)	4(21.05%)	4(21.05%)	15(78.95%)
2007	11	4(36.37%)	0	0	2(18.19%)	0	11(100%)	0	3(27.27%)	3(27.27%)	7(63.64%)
2008	12	5(41.67%)	0	1(8.33%)	0	0	10(83.33%)	0	4(33.33%)	4(33.33%)	10(83.33%)
2009	28	5(17.86%)	3(10.71%)	1(3.57%)	1(3.57%)	1(3.57%)	24(85.71%)	2(7.14%)	11(39.29%)	12(42.86%)	25(89.29%)
2010	29	3(10.34%)	0	0	1(3.45%)	0	25(86.21%)	0	9(31.03%)	7(24.14%)	25(86.21%)
Total	135	25(18.52%)	3(2.22%)	4(2.96%)	5(3.70%)	1(0.74%)	101(74.81%)	3(2.22%)	42(31.11%)	40(29.63%)	101(74.81%)

Table 2. Effect of estimates of wet cupping treatment for herpes zoster in 15 RCTs.

Trials	Comparisons	Effect estimates ([95%CI])	P
Numbers of cured patients			
Wet cupping plus other interventions versus other interventions alone			
Wet cupping plus medication versus medications alone			
Guo L 2006 [32]	Wet cupping plus aciclovir, VitB$_1$, VitB$_{12}$ versus aciclovir, VitB$_1$, VitB$_{12}$	RR 1.48 [1.05, 2.09]	
Liu L 2003 [61]	Wet cupping plus aciclovir, VitB$_1$, VitB$_{12}$ and aciclovir cream versus aciclovir, VitB$_1$, VitB$_{12}$, and aciclovir cream	RR 3.83 [2.07, 7.06]	
Long W 2003 [64]	Wet cupping plus ultraviolet radiation versus ultraviolet radiation alone	RR 1.30 [1.06, 1.59]	
Xu L 2004 [104]	Wet cupping plus aciclovir cream, aciclovir 0.5 g and glucose 250 ml intravenous drip versus aciclovir cream, aciclovir 0.5 g and glucose 250 ml intravenous drip	RR 1.35 [0.93, 1.97]	
Zhang Q 2008 [126]	Wet cupping and bloodletting on ear apex plus aciclovir and acupuncture versus aciclovir and acupuncture	RR 4.17 [1.92, 9.05]	
Subgroup		**RR 1.93 [1.23, 3.04]***	**0.005**
Wet cupping plus acupuncture versus acupuncture alone			
Huang J 2008 [37]	Wet cupping plus acupuncture versus acupuncture alone	RR 2.38 [1.10, 5.13]	
Zhang H 2009 [122]	Wet cupping plus electroacupuncture versus electroacupuncture alone	RR 1.29 [0.95, 1.76]	
Zuo R 2010 [145]	Wet cupping plus electroacupuncture versus electroacupuncture alone	RR 1.91 [1.07, 3.42]	
Subgroup		**RR 1,65 [1.08, 2.53]**	**0.02**
Overall (Random, I^2 = 76%)		**RR 1.81 [1.33, 2.45]**	**0.0001**
Wet cupping versus medications			
Ci H 2010 [20]	Wet cupping versus aciclovir	RR 1.60 [1.24, 2.06]	
Jin M 2008 [45]	Wet cupping versus aciclovir, cimetidine, indomethacin, mecobalamin, calamine, and aciclovir cream	RR 2.15 [1.54, 3.00]	
Liu L 2003 [61]	Wet cupping versus aciclovir, VitB$_1$, VitB$_{12}$, and aciclovir cream	RR 2.83 [1.47, 5.46]	
Liu Q 2004 [63]	Wet cupping versus aciclovir and poly I-C injection	RR 2.90 [1.71, 4.91]	
Wang Y 2009 [94]	Wet cupping versus valaciclovir	RR 2.34 [1.66, 3.30]	
Overall (Fixed, I^2 = 43%)		**RR 2.07 [1.77, 2.43]**	**<0.00001**
Numbers of patients with postherpetic neuralgia after treatment			
wet cupping versus medications alone			
Jin M 2008 [45]	Wet cupping versus acyclovir, cimetidine, indomethacin, mecobalamin, 23acyclovir, andacyclovir cream	RR 0.09 [0.01, 1.60]	
Liu L 2003 [61]	Wet cupping versus acyclovir, VitB$_1$, VitB$_{12}$, and acyclovir cream	RR 0.06 [0.00, 1.09]	
Wang Y 2009 [94]	Wet cupping versus valaciclovir	RR 0.23 [0.08, 0.64]	
Xiong Z 2007 [103]	Wet cupping versus acyclovir plus normal saline 250 ml intravenous drip	RR 0.05 [0.01, 0.38]	
Overall (Fixed, I^2 = 0%)		**RR 0.12 [0.06, 0.28]**	**<0.00001**
Numbers of patients with effective symptoms after treatment			
Wet cupping plus other interventions versus other interventions alone			
Wet cupping plus medication versus medication alone			
Guo L 2006 [32]	Wet cupping plus aciclovir, VitB$_1$, VitB$_{12}$ versus aciclovir, VitB$_1$, VitB$_{12}$	RR 1.00 [0.92, 1.08]	
Liu L 2003 [61]	Wet cupping plus aciclovir, VitB$_1$, VitB$_{12}$ and aciclovir cream versus aciclovir, VitB$_1$, VitB$_{12}$, and aciclovir cream	RR 1.00 [0.95, 1.05]	
Xu L 2004 [104]	Wet cupping plus aciclovir cream, aciclovir 0.5 g and glucose 250 ml intravenous drip versus aciclovir cream, aciclovir 0.5 g, and glucose 250 ml intravenous drip	RR 1.00 [0.95, 1.05]	
Zhang Q 2008 [126]	Wet cupping and blood-letting on auditive apex plus aciclovir and acupuncture versus aciclovir and acupuncture	RR 1.00 [0.95, 1.05]	
Subgroup		**RR 1.00 [0.97, 1.03]**	**0.99**
Wet cupping plus acupuncture versus acupuncture alone			
Huang J 2008 [37]	Wet cupping plus acupuncture versus acupuncture alone	RR 1.09 [0.83, 1.43]	
Zhang H 2009 [122]	Wet cupping plus electroacupuncture versus electroacupuncture alone	RR 1.20 [0.97, 1.48]	
Zuo R 2010 [145]	Wet cupping plus electroacupuncture versus electroacupuncture alone	RR 1.11 [0.98, 1.27]	
Subgroup		**RR 1.13 [1.02, 1.25]**	**0.02**
Overall (Random, I^2 = 52%)		**RR 1.02 [0.98, 1.06]**	**0.41**
Wet cupping versus medications			

Table 2. Cont.

Trials	Comparisons	Effect estimates ([95%CI])	P
Ci H 2010 [20]	Wet cupping versus aciclovir	RR 1.22 [1.07, 1.40]	
Jin M 2008 [45]	Wet cupping versus aciclovir, cimetidine, indomethacin, mecobalamin, calamine, and aciclovir cream	RR 1.07 [0.98, 1.17]	
Liu L 2003 [61]	Wet cupping versus aciclovir, $VitB_1$, $VitB_{12}$ and aciclovir cream	RR 1.00 [0.94, 1.06]	
Liu Q 2004 [63]	Wet cupping versus aciclovir and poly I-C injection	RR 1.27 [1.05, 1.54]	
Wang Y 2009 [94]	Wet cupping versus valaciclovir	RR 1.08 [0.99, 1.17]	
Overall (Random, $I^2=82\%$)		**RR 1.11 [1.00, 1.23]**	**0.06**
Average cure time			
Wet cupping plus other interventions versus other interventions alone			
Guo L 2006 [32]	Wet cupping plus aciclovir, $VitB_1$, $VitB_{12}$ versus aciclovir, $VitB_1$, $VitB_{12}$	MD −2.10 [−3.55, −0.65]	
Liu L 2003 [61]	Wet cupping plus aciclovir, $VitB_1$, $VitB_{12}$, and aciclovir cream versus aciclovir, $VitB_1$, $VitB_{12}$, and aciclovir cream	MD −5.08 [−8.04, −2.12]	
Overall (Fixed, $I^2=68\%$)		**MD −2.67 [−3.97, −1.37]**	**<0.0001**
Wet cupping versus medications			
Liu L 2003 [61]	Wet cupping versus aciclovir, $VitB_1$, $VitB_{12}$, and aciclovir cream	MD −3.14 [−6.45, 0.17]	
Overall (Fixed, $I^2=0\%$)		**MD −3.14 [−6.45, 0.17]**	**0.06**

needle cupping. Combined cupping in which at least two types of cupping methods were applied, was used in 5 trials (3.70%) (Figure 1).

Distribution of Diseases/Conditions

In the included trials, 56 diseases or symptoms were treated by cupping therapy. Diagnostic criteria varied, some authors used international criteria, such as ICD-10, others used Chinese criteria, such as those issued by government health agencies, or criteria from Chinese language medical textbooks. Some authors did not report any sources for their diagnostic criteria. The 6 most common diseases/conditions for which cupping was applied were herpes zoster (17 trials), facial paralysis (Bell palsy) (17 trials), cough and dyspnea (8 trials), acne (6 trials), lumbar disc herniation (6 trials) and cervical spondylosis (6 trials) (Table 1). Meta-analyses were conducted on 4 diseases/conditions – herpes zoster, facial paralysis (Bell palsy), acne and cervical spondylosis (characteristics of the RCTs involving these 4 diseases are presented in Tables S2, S3, S4 and S5). Due to the heterogeneity of the RCTs of the remaining 2 diseases/conditions – lumbar disc herniation and cough and dyspnea – meta-analyses could not be completed.

Of the 6 diseases/conditions, 3 were related to pain, including herpes zoster, an inflammatory pain of the nerve; and lumbar disc herniation and cervical spondylosis, pain caused by nerve compression. Relieving pain was the main purpose of cupping therapy in these studies. Retained cupping or wet cupping was typically applied.

Facial paralysis (Bell palsy) falls under nerve, nerve root, and plexus disorders. In the studies we reviewed, flash cupping and moving cupping were commonly applied.

Respiratory diseases, such as pneumonia, bronchitis, and asthma, for which the main purpose of treatment is to alleviate the symptoms of cough and dyspnea are also treated by cupping therapy. Retained cupping or wet cupping therapy on EX-B1, a so-called extra acupoint (acupuncture point not located on one of the traditional channels), was mostly used in the studies for treating cough and dyspnea symptoms.

Acne is a skin condition that affects the face, neck, shoulders, chest, and back. In the studies we evaluated, wet cupping was primarily used to relieve the skin breakouts.

The remaining 50 diseases/conditions are presented in Table S1.

Methodological Quality of RCTs

According to our pre-defined methodological quality criteria, none of the 135 trials were low risk of bias and the majority was high risk of bias (Table 1). Three trials [23,69,73] reported sample size calculations, 25 trials [11,14,17,23,26,32,35,41,48,57,60,69,70,72,73,79,81,85,88,94,97,99,107,111,116] described randomization procedures (such as random number table or computer-generated random numbers), with only 2 [23,73] of the 25 trials using sealed envelope allocation concealment. Four trials [17,48,94,99] mentioned blinding, of which only 2 [48,94] reported that they blinded outcome assessors, the other 2 trials did not report who were blinded. Five trials [11,39,72,80,116] reported the number of dropouts, but none of these used intention-to-treat analysis.

There were 101 (74.81%) trials that reported comparability of baseline data, 42 (31.11%) trials specified the inclusion criteria, 40 (29.63%) trials specified the exclusion criteria, and 101 (74.81%) trials described diagnostic criteria. Efficacy standard was reported in 126 (93.33%) trials, but 110 of them used composite outcome measures, which categorized treatment efficacy into four grades (cured, markedly effective, effective, and ineffective) according to change in symptoms, the other 16 trials used single outcome measure for therapeutic effect. Symptoms were commonly used as outcome measures.

Estimate Effects of RCTs with Cupping

Due to insufficient number of RCTs and the variations in study quality, participants, intervention, variable control, and outcome measures, results of most of the studies could not be synthesized by quantitative methods. Though 133 of the 135 included studies showed that cupping therapy as well as cupping combined with other treatment were significantly

Table 3. Effect of estimates of cupping for facial paralysis in 15 RCTs.

Trials	Comparisons	Effect Estimates ([95%CI])	P
Numbers of cured patients			
Cupping plus other interventions versus other interventions alone			
Flash cupping plus acupuncture versus acupuncture alone			
Cao R 2009 [12]	Flash cupping plus acupuncture versus acupuncture alone	RR 2.00 [1.09, 3.66]	
Fu C 2004 [25]	Flash cupping plus acupuncture versus acupuncture alone	RR 1.73 [1.30, 2.30]	
Huang L 2009 [39]	Flash cupping plus acupuncture versus acupuncture alone	RR 1.33 [0.95, 1.86]	
Li K 2009 [49]	Flash cupping plus acupuncture versus acupuncture alone	RR 1.50 [1.02, 2.21]	
Zhao N 2010 [133]	Flash cupping plus acupuncture versus acupuncture alone	RR 1.33 [1.04, 1.68]	
Subgroup		**RR 1.51 [1.29, 1.76]**	**<0.00001**
Wet cupping plus acupuncture versus acupuncture alone			
Gao B 2010 [28]	Wet cupping plus acupuncture and mecobalamine versus acupuncture and mecobalamine alone	RR 1.68 [0.62, 4.53]	
Huang L 2010 [40]	Wet cupping plus acupuncture versus acupuncture alone	RR 1.60 [0.79, 3.23]	
Lü J 2010 [71]	Wet cupping plus acupuncture versus acupuncture alone	RR 1.29 [0.95, 1.76]	
Ren Y 2006 [77]	Wet cupping plus acupuncture versus acupuncture alone	RR 1.91 [1.32, 2.76]	
Sun H 2010 [80]	Wet cupping plus acupuncture versus acupuncture alone	RR 1.71 [1.23, 2.36]	
Wang L 2010 [89]	Wet cupping plus acupuncture versus acupuncture alone	RR 1.41 [0.85, 2.35]	
Subgroup		**RR 1.60 [1.33, 1.93]**	**<0.0001**
Medicinal cupping plus medication versus medications			
Qiu J 2003 [76]	Medicinal cupping plus neurotrophic drugs versus neurotrophic drugs alone	RR 1.44 [1.11, 1.87]	
Subgroup		**RR 1.44 [1.11, 1.87]**	**0.006**
Wet cupping plus TDP and medications versus TDP and medications			
Li W 2005 [51]	Wet cupping plus TDP, antivirus and neurotrophic drugs versus TDP and drugs alone	RR 1.18 [0.89, 1.57]	
Subgroup		**RR 1.18 [0.89, 1.57]**	**0.25**
Flash cupping plus herbal medicine and acupuncture versus herbal medicine and acupuncture			
Ou X 2009 [75]	Flash cupping plus herbal decoction and acupuncture versus herbal decoction and acupuncture	RR 1.37 [1.05, 1.80]	
subgroup		**RR 1.37 [1.05, 1.80]**	**0.02**
Overall (Fixed, $I^2 = 0\%$)		**RR 1.49 [1.35, 1.65]**	**<0.00001**
Wet cupping versus medications			
Zhu F 2009 [141]	Wet cupping versus antivirus and neurotrophic drugs	RR 1.33 [0.83, 2.14]	
Overall		**RR 1.33 [0.83, 2.14]**	**0.23**

effective for certain diseases (Table S6), interpretation of the positive findings from the individual studies needs to be incorporated with the clinical characteristics of the included studies and evidence power. Therefore, the beneficial effect of cupping therapy needs to be confirmed through large and rigorously-designed RCTs.

We conducted meta-analyses to evaluate therapeutic effect of cupping therapies for herpes zoster, facial paralysis, acne, and cervical spondylosis (Tables 2–5).

Meta-analysis of 15 RCTs [20,29,32,37,45,61,63,64,94,102–104,122,126,145] to evaluate the efficacy of wet cupping therapy for herpes zoster (2 trials [13,123] were excluded due to insufficient data), wet cupping was found to be superior to pharmaceutical medications, such as antiviral, in effecting a cure (RR 2.07, 95%CI 1.77 to 2.43, $p<0.00001$, 5 trials, random model) (Figure 2), and in lowering the incidence rate of post-herpetic neuralgia (RR 0.12, 95%CI 0.06 to 0.28, $p<0.00001$, 4 trials, fixed model). But no difference was identified in the number

Table 4. Effect of estimates of cupping for acne in 6 RCTs.

Trials	Comparisons	Effect Estimates ([95%CI])	P
Numbers of cured patients			
Wet cupping plus other interventions versus other interventions alone			
Wet cupping plus herbal medicine versus herbal medicine alone			
Huang J 2010 [38]	Wet cupping plus herbal preparation, topical cream versus herbal preparation and external cream	RR 2.06 [1.33, 3.18]	
Subgroup		**RR 2.06 [1.33, 3.18]**	**0.001**
Wet cupping plus acupuncture versus acupuncture alone			
Liu H 2009 [59]	Flash cupping plus acupuncture versus acupuncture alone	RR 1.91 [0.99, 3.72]	
Wang Q 2007 [91]	Moving and wet cupping plus acupuncture versus acupuncture alone	RR 1.67 [0.87, 3.20]	
Subgroup		**RR 1.79 [1.12, 2.86]**	**0.01**
Overall (Fixed, $I^2 = 0\%$)		**RR 1.93 [1.40, 2.65]**	**<0.0001**
Wet cupping versus medications			
Wu F 2010 [95]	Wet cupping versus tanshinone	RR 1.07 [0.45, 2.56]	
Wu Y 2008 [97]	Wet cupping versus tetracycline and ketoconazole cream	RR 2.50 [1.31, 4.77]	
Zhang K 2008 [125]	Wet cupping versus tetracycline	RR 2.75 [1.38, 5.48]	
Overall (Fixed, $I^2 = 37\%$)		**RR 2.14 [1.42, 3.22]**	**0.0003**
Average cure time			
Cupping plus other intervention versus other interventions alone			
Li W 2005 [51]	Wet cupping plus TDP, antivirus and neurotrophic drugs versus TDP and drugs alone	MD −4.14 [−5.74, −2.54]	
Qiu J 2003 [76]	Medicinal cupping plus neurotrophic drugs versus neurotrophic drugs alone	MD −8.00 [−9.78, −6.22]	
Overall (Random, $I^2 = 90\%$)		**MD −6.05 [−9.83, −2.27]**	**0.002**
Wet cupping versus medications			
Zhu F 2009 [141]	Wet cupping versus antivirus and neurotrophic drugs	MD −7.20 [−14.27, −0.13]	
Overall		**MD −7.20 [−14.27, −0.13]**	**0.05**

of patients with improved symptoms (RR 1.11, 95%CI 1.00 to 1.23, $p = 0.06$, 5 trials, random model). Wet cupping in combination with pharmaceutical medications was significantly better than medications alone in effecting a cure (RR 1.93, 95%CI 1.23 to 3.04, $p = 0.005$, 5 trials, random model), but no difference in symptom improvement was observed (RR 1.00, 95%CI 0.97 to 1.03, $p = 0.99$, 4 trials, random model) (Figure 3). Wet cupping combined with acupuncture was superior to acupuncture alone both in effecting a cure (RR 1.65, 95%CI 1.08 to 2.53, $p = 0.02$, 3 trials, random model) (Figure 3) and in improving symptoms (RR 1.13, 95%CI 1.02 to 1.25, $p = 0.02$, 3 trials, random model).

There were 17 RCTs [12,15,39,40,47,49–51,71,75–77,80, 89,133,141] that assessed the therapeutic effect of cupping therapy for facial paralysis. Two of the trials [47,50] were excluded from the meta-analysis due to the incomparability between treatment and control groups. Six trials used flash cupping therapy, 8 trials used wet cupping, and 1 trial used medicinal cupping as the main intervention. Meta-analysis showed flash cupping combined with acupuncture (RR 1.51, 95%CI 1.29 to 1.76, $p < 0.00001$, 5 trials, fixed model) and wet cupping combined with acupuncture (RR 1.60, 95%CI 1.33 to 1.93, $p < 0.0001$, 6 trials, fixed model) were markedly better than acupuncture alone in effecting a cure (Figure 4). In addition, cupping in combination with medications, such as neurotrophic drugs, was superior to medications alone in reducing average cure time (MD −6.05, 95%CI −9.83 to −2.27, $p = 0.002$, 2 trials, random model).

Six trials [38,59,91,95,97,125] evaluated the efficacy of cupping therapy for acne. Meta-analysis showed that, for improving the cure rate, wet cupping therapy was significantly better than medications, such as tanshinone, tetracycline, and ketoconazole (RR 2.14, 95%CI 1.42 to 3.22, $p = 0.0003$, 3 trials, fixed model). Furthermore, cupping therapy combined with other interventions was superior to other interventions alone (RR 1.93, 95%CI 1.40 to 2.65, $p < 0.0001$, 3 trials, fixed model). As each comparison had less than five trials, it was not meaningful to conduct a funnel plot analysis.

For cervical spondylosis, 6 trials [79,86,90,93,116,117] evaluated the efficacy of cupping therapy on this condition. Cupping therapy, especially wet cupping on GV-14 and *Ashi* points, combined with other treatment, including acupuncture and traction, was better than other treatments alone in effecting a cure (RR 1.52, 95%CI 1.20 to 1.92, $p = 0.0005$, 5 trials, fixed model) and in ameliorating symptoms (RR 3.84, 95%CI 2.19 to 6.75, $p < 0.00001$, 6 trials, fixed model). One trial [117] compared wet cupping with flunarizine for symptom improvement, and found no difference between the two groups (RR 1.18, 95%CI 0.60 to 2.32, $p = 0.63$, 1 trial).

A funnel plot analysis of 39 trials was performed to examine outcome for the number of cured patients irrespective of disease. The result showed potential asymmetry (Figure 5).

Serious adverse effects were not reported in any of the 135 included trials.

Table 5. Effect of estimates of cupping for cervical spondylosis in 6 RCTs.

Trials	Comparisons	Effect Estimates ([95%CI])	P
Numbers of cured patients			
Cupping plus other interventions versus other interventions alone			
Cupping plus acupuncture versus acupuncture alone			
Wan XW 2007 [86]	Needling cupping plus acupuncture versus acupuncture alone	RR 1.59 [1.14, 2.22]	
Subgroup		**RR 1.59 [1.14, 2.22]**	**0.007**
Wet cupping plus acupuncture versus acupuncture alone			
Shao M 2003 [79]	Wet cupping plus acupuncture versus acupuncture alone	RR 1.64 [1.04, 2.58]	
Wang PL 2010 [90]	Wet cupping plus acupuncture versus acupuncture alone	RR 1.15 [0.63, 2.12]	
Subgroup		**RR 1.46 [1.01, 2.09]**	**0.04**
Wet cupping plus electroacupuncture versus electroacupuncture alone			
Wang XM 2004 [93]	Wet cupping plus electroacupuncture versus electroacupuncture alone	RR 1.59 [0.72, 3.53]	
Subgroup		**RR 1.59 [0.72, 3.53]**	**0.25**
Wet cupping plus traction versus traction alone			
You Y 2006 [116]	Wet cupping plus traction versus traction alone	RR 1.55 [0.83, 2.91]	
Subgroup		**RR 1.55 [0.83, 2.91]**	**0.17**
Overall (Fixed, $I^2 = 0\%$)		**RR 1.52 [1.20, 1.92]**	**0.0005**
Numbers of effective patients			
Cupping plus other interventions versus other interventions alone			
Cupping plus acupuncture versus acupuncture alone			
Wan XW 2007 [86]	Needling cupping plus acupuncture versus acupuncture alone	RR 10.36 [0.53, 201.45]	
Subgroup		**RR 10.36 [0.53, 201.45]**	**0.12**
Wetcupping plus acupuncture versus acupuncture alone			
Shao M 2003 [79]	Wet cupping plus acupuncture versus acupuncture alone	RR 2.90 [1.14, 7.38]	
Wang PL 2010 [90]	Wet cupping plus acupuncture versus acupuncture alone	RR 6.83 [0.79, 59.48]	
Subgroup		**RR 3.43 [1.47, 8.01]**	**0.004**
Wet cupping plus electroacupuncture versus electroacupuncture alone			
Wang XM 2004 [93]	Wet cupping plus electroacupuncture versus electroacupuncture alone	RR 7.22 [0.72, 72.56]	
Subgroup		**RR 7.22 [0.72, 72.56]**	**0.09**
Wet cupping plus warm acupuncture versus warm acupuncture alone			
Zeng HW 2007 [117]	Wet cupping plus acupuncture and moxibustion versus acupuncture and moxibustion alone	RR 3.86 [1.12, 13.26]	
Subgroup		**RR 3.86 [1.12, 13.26]**	**0.03**
Wet cupping plus traction versus traction alone			
You Y 2006 [116]	Wet cupping plus traction versus traction alone	RR 3.24 [1.04, 10.05]	
Subgroup		**RR 3.24 [1.04, 10.05]**	**0.17**
Overall (Fixed, $I^2 = 0\%$)		**RR 3.84 [2.19, 6.75]**	**<0.00001**
Wet cupping versus medications			
Zeng HW 2007 [117]	Wet cupping versus flunarizine	RR 1.18 [0.60, 2.32]	
Overall		**RR 1.18 [0.60, 2.32]**	**0.63**

Discussion

In our previous review [3], we focused on the characteristics of the RCTs on cupping therapy. This review aimed to ascertain whether or not cupping therapy is efficacious for several conditions, especially when combined with other treatments. With this review, we expanded our search to include articles published from 2008 through 2010. The 62 new studies indicate that the ancient TCM practice of cupping remains an important therapeutic modality in China and is gaining recognition elsewhere. For diseases/conditions that are commonly treated by cupping, we conducted meta-analyses by synthesizing data from homogeneous studies to assess the therapeutic effect of cupping in treating these diseases/conditions. For studies whose data were inappropriate for synthesis, we used qualitative methods to evaluate their findings. This is the first instance that quantitative

Study	Intervention Events	Total	Control Events	Total	Weight	Risk Ratio M-H, Fixed, 95% CI
Liu L 2003	20	30	8	34	7.3%	2.83 [1.47, 5.46]
Liu Q 2004	29	32	10	32	9.7%	2.90 [1.71, 4.91]
Jin M 2008	43	45	20	45	19.4%	2.15 [1.54, 3.00]
Wang Y 2009	50	55	21	54	20.5%	2.34 [1.66, 3.30]
Ci H 2010	76	104	42	92	43.2%	1.60 [1.24, 2.06]
Total (95% CI)		**266**		**257**	**100.0%**	**2.07 [1.77, 2.43]**
Total events	218		101			

Heterogeneity: Chi² = 7.01, df = 4 (P = 0.14); I² = 43%
Test for overall effect: Z = 8.90 (P < 0.00001)

Favors control   Favors intervention

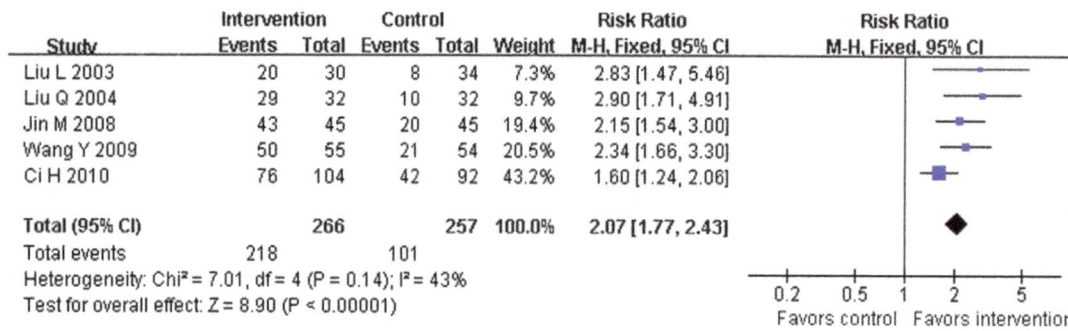

Figure 2. Effect of estimates of wet cupping versus medication on numbers of cured patients with herpes zoster.

and qualitative methods were used in a systematic review to evaluate the efficacy of cupping therapy.

Despite the large number of studies on cupping therapy, including the 62 new ones, there remains a lack of well-designed investigations. Of the 135 RCTs included in this review, 84.44% were high risk of bias. One issue is adherence to the Consolidated Standards of Reporting Trials (CONSORT) [146] in which randomization methods should be clearly described and fully reported. Another issue is blinding, which continues to be a challenge for studies involving manual healing therapies, such as acupuncture, massage, and cupping therapy. Lee et al [147] report developing a sham cupping device with a tiny opening that in effect reduces the negative pressure in the cup once it is attached to the skin. The RCT they conducted showed that the device appears to be tenable as a control for actual cupping, though confirmatory studies are needed. While blinding during studies on cupping therapy may be difficult to achieve, at the very least, blinding of outcome assessors and statistics should be attempted to minimize performance and assessment biases. Another area that researchers

should be attentive to is adapting STRICTA [148] standards when designing and reporting studies. Similar to acupuncture, cupping therapy is based on energy channels (meridians) and acupoints. Therefore, methodology details should be reported, including types of cups, acupoints used and their TCM rationale, practitioner background, number of treatment sessions and frequency, among other STRICTA-recommended information. Standardization can also be achieved by registering with and following the protocol of international organizations [149], such as WHO International Clinical Trials Registry Platform (ICTRP) [150].

As in our previous review, we continue to emphasize the importance of using standard outcome measures for specific diseases/conditions. As mentioned, 80.74% of the included trials used composite outcome measures, which categorized treatment efficacy into four grades. The classifications of "cure," "markedly effective," "effective," and "ineffective" are not internationally recognized with their exact meaning open to interpretation. This can increase clinical heterogeneity. We suggest that researchers comply with international standards,

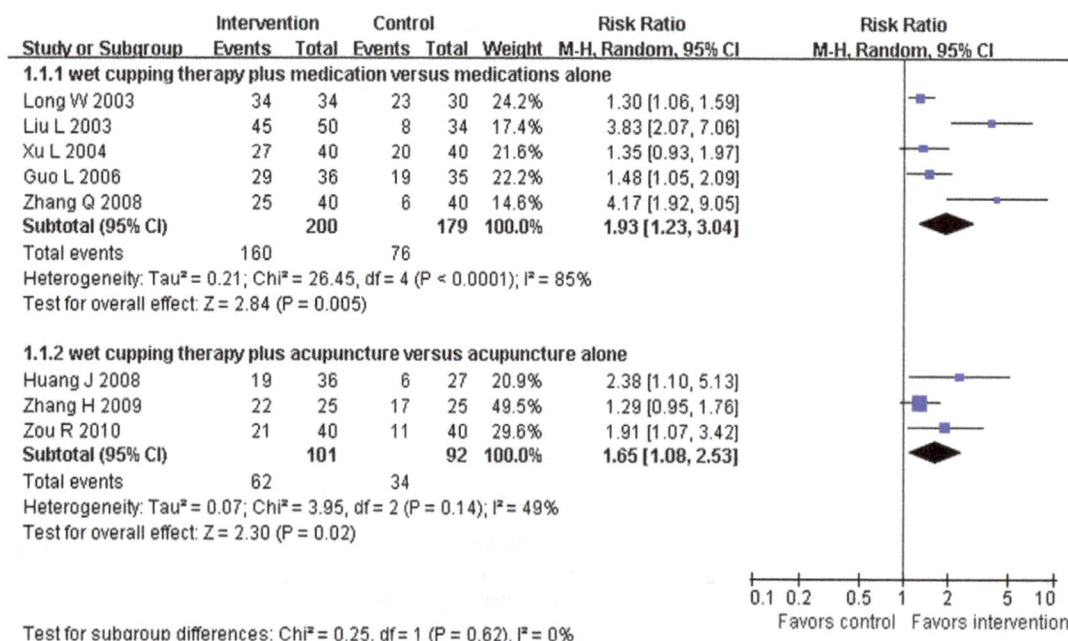

Study or Subgroup	Intervention Events	Total	Control Events	Total	Weight	Risk Ratio M-H, Random, 95% CI
1.1.1 wet cupping therapy plus medication versus medications alone						
Long W 2003	34	34	23	30	24.2%	1.30 [1.06, 1.59]
Liu L 2003	45	50	8	34	17.4%	3.83 [2.07, 7.06]
Xu L 2004	27	40	20	40	21.6%	1.35 [0.93, 1.97]
Guo L 2006	29	36	19	35	22.2%	1.48 [1.05, 2.09]
Zhang Q 2008	25	40	6	40	14.6%	4.17 [1.92, 9.05]
Subtotal (95% CI)		200		179	100.0%	1.93 [1.23, 3.04]
Total events	160		76			

Heterogeneity: Tau² = 0.21; Chi² = 26.45, df = 4 (P < 0.0001); I² = 85%
Test for overall effect: Z = 2.84 (P = 0.005)

1.1.2 wet cupping therapy plus acupuncture versus acupuncture alone						
Huang J 2008	19	36	6	27	20.9%	2.38 [1.10, 5.13]
Zhang H 2009	22	25	17	25	49.5%	1.29 [0.95, 1.76]
Zou R 2010	21	40	11	40	29.6%	1.91 [1.07, 3.42]
Subtotal (95% CI)		101		92	100.0%	1.65 [1.08, 2.53]
Total events	62		34			

Heterogeneity: Tau² = 0.07; Chi² = 3.95, df = 2 (P = 0.14); I² = 49%
Test for overall effect: Z = 2.30 (P = 0.02)

Favors control   Favors intervention

Test for subgroup differences: Chi² = 0.25, df = 1 (P = 0.62), I² = 0%

Figure 3. Effect of estimates of combination of wet cupping and other interventions versus other interventions alone on numbers of cured patients of herpes zoster.

Study or Subgroup	Intervention Events	Total	Control Events	Total	Weight	Risk Ratio M-H, Fixed, 95% CI
1.1.1 flash cupping therapy plus acupuncture versus acupuncture alone						
Fu C 2004	76	80	22	40	22.2%	1.73 [1.30, 2.30]
Li K 2009	39	80	26	80	19.7%	1.50 [1.02, 2.21]
Huang L 2009	50	115	37	113	28.3%	1.33 [0.95, 1.86]
Cao R 2009	22	48	11	48	8.3%	2.00 [1.09, 3.66]
Zhao N 2010	38	43	28	42	21.5%	1.33 [1.04, 1.68]
Subtotal (95% CI)		**366**		**323**	**100.0%**	**1.51 [1.29, 1.76]**
Total events	225		124			
Heterogeneity: Chi² = 3.37, df = 4 (P = 0.50); I² = 0%						
Test for overall effect: Z = 5.17 (P < 0.00001)						
1.1.2 wet cupping plus acupuncture versus acupuncture alone						
Ren Y 2006	39	50	20	49	22.5%	1.91 [1.32, 2.76]
Lv J 2010	22	25	17	25	19.0%	1.29 [0.95, 1.76]
Sun H 2010	36	40	19	36	22.3%	1.71 [1.23, 2.36]
Huang L 2010	16	58	10	58	11.2%	1.60 [0.79, 3.23]
Wang L 2010	24	60	17	60	19.0%	1.41 [0.85, 2.35]
Gao B 2010	10	50	5	42	6.1%	1.68 [0.62, 4.53]
Subtotal (95% CI)		**283**		**270**	**100.0%**	**1.60 [1.33, 1.93]**
Total events	147		88			
Heterogeneity: Chi² = 3.16, df = 5 (P = 0.68); I² = 0%						
Test for overall effect: Z = 4.99 (P < 0.00001)						
1.1.3 medicinal cupping plus medication versus medication alone						
Qiu J 2003	36	40	25	40	100.0%	1.44 [1.11, 1.87]
Subtotal (95% CI)		**40**		**40**	**100.0%**	**1.44 [1.11, 1.87]**
Total events	36		25			
Heterogeneity: Not applicable						
Test for overall effect: Z = 2.73 (P = 0.006)						
1.1.4 wet cupping plus TDP and medication versus TDP and medication alone						
Li W 2005	26	32	22	32	100.0%	1.18 [0.89, 1.57]
Subtotal (95% CI)		**32**		**32**	**100.0%**	**1.18 [0.89, 1.57]**
Total events	26		22			
Heterogeneity: Not applicable						
Test for overall effect: Z = 1.14 (P = 0.25)						
1.1.5 flash cupping therapy plus herbal medicine and acupuncture versus herbal medicine and acupuncture alone						
Ou X 2009	48	60	28	48	100.0%	1.37 [1.05, 1.80]
Subtotal (95% CI)		**60**		**48**	**100.0%**	**1.37 [1.05, 1.80]**
Total events	48		28			
Heterogeneity: Not applicable						
Test for overall effect: Z = 2.29 (P = 0.02)						

0.5 0.7 1 1.5 2
Favors control   Favors intervention

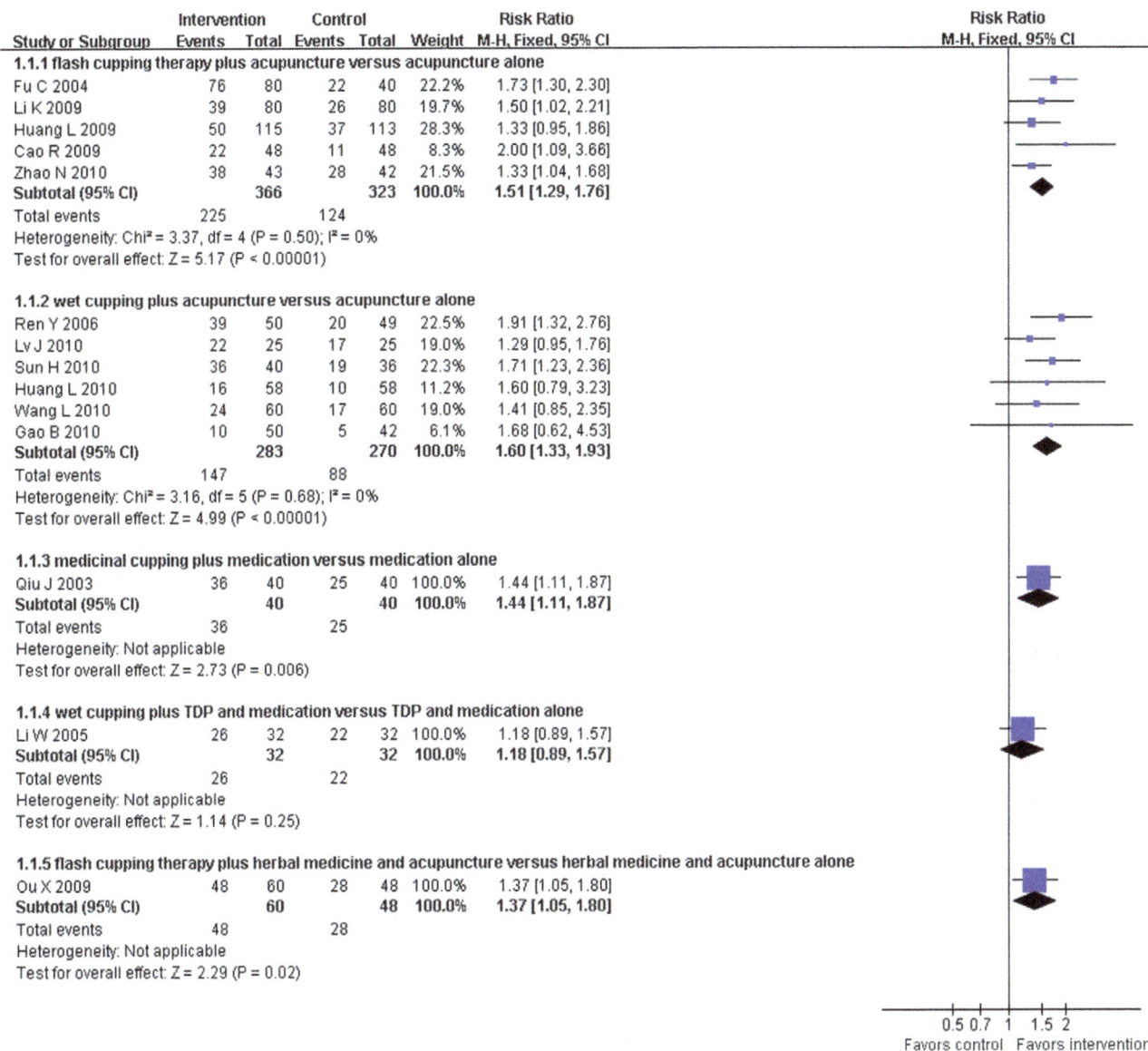

Figure 4. Effect of estimates of cupping combined with other interventions versus other interventions alone on numbers of cured patients with facial paralysis.

such as the House Brackmann score for facial nerve paralysis (Bell palsy), in the evaluation of treatment efficacy to give credibility to their work.

The potential asymmetry of the overall funnel plot test (Figure 5) of 39 RCTs that examined the outcome of the number of cured patients for 4 diseases (herpes zoster, facial paralysis, acne, and cervical spondylosis) may be caused by, small study effects, or even heterogeneity in intervention effects. Furthermore, as we did not include unpublished studies, there is high potential that our review may have publication bias. We strongly recommend that researchers plan their sample size for randomized controlled trials to ensure adequate statistical power. Furthermore, sample size calculation and analysis of outcomes should be based on the principle of intention-to-treat.

Finally, our meta-analysis revealed that cupping therapy combined with other treatments, such as acupuncture or medications, showed significant benefit over other treatments alone in effecting a cure for herpes zoster, acne, facial paralysis, and cervical spondylosis. This appears to support the common practice in China of combining TCM therapeutic modalities, either TCM with TCM, or TCM with routine western medicine, to enhance efficacy. The effect of cupping therapy over time is not known, but use of cupping is generally safe based on long-term clinical application and outcomes reported in the reviewed trials.

In conclusion, the results of this systematic review suggest that cupping therapy appears to be effective for various diseases/conditions, in particular herpes zoster, acne, facial paralysis, and cervical spondylosis. However, the main limitation of our analysis was that nearly all included trials were evaluated as high risk of bias. As such, it is necessary to conduct further RCTs that are of high quality and larger sample sizes in order to draw a definitive conclusion.

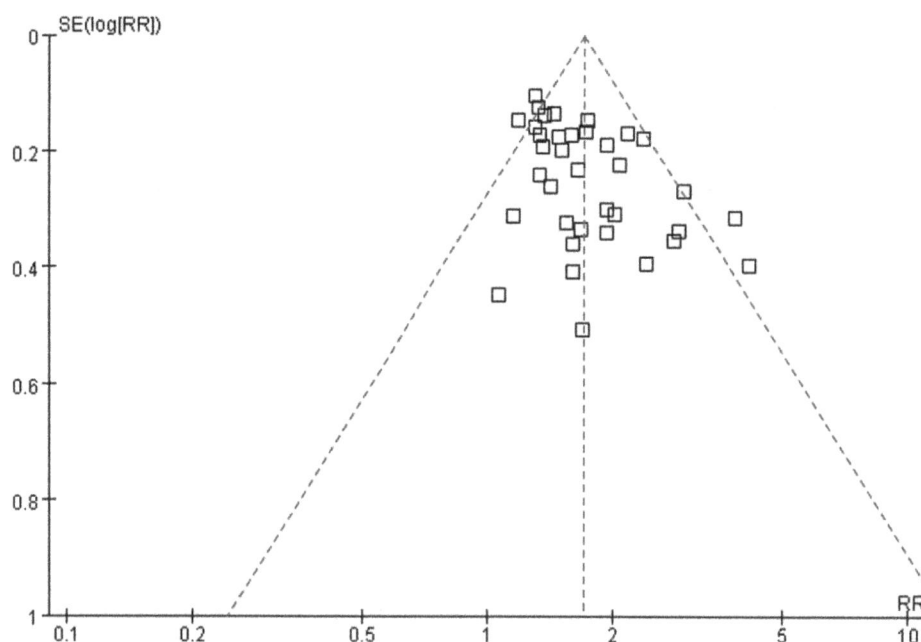

Figure 5. Funnel plot assessing outcomes of cured patients reported in 39 randomized controlled trials on 4 diseases.

Supporting Information

Table S1   Mapping of diseases/conditions reported in cupping trials (1992–2010).
(DOC)

Table S2   Characteristics of 15 included trials on cupping for herpes zoster.
(DOC)

Table S3   Characteristics of 15 included trials on cupping for facial paralysis (Bell palsy).
(DOC)

Table S4   Characteristics of 6 included trials on cupping for acne.
(DOC)

Table S5   Characteristics of 6 included trials on cupping for cervical spondylosis.
(DOC)

Table S6   Characteristics of randomized controlled trials outside meta-analysis.
(DOC)

Checklist S1   CONSORT checklist.
(DOC)

Protocol S1   Flow chart of search strategy for inclusion and exclusion of studies.
(DOC)

Acknowledgments

The authors thank Nissi S. Wang, MSc, for assisting with the English editing of this manuscript.

Author Contributions

Conceived and designed the experiments: HC JL. Analyzed the data: HC XL. Wrote the paper: HC XL JL.

References

1. Chirali IZ (1999) The cupping procedure. In:, , Chirali IZ (1999) Traditional Chinese Medicine Cupping Therapy. London: Churchill Livingstone. pp 73–86.

2. Gao LW (2004) Practical Cupping Therapy [in Chinese]. Beijing: Academy Press.

3. Cao HJ, Han M, Li X, Dong SJ, Shang YM, et al. (2010) Clinical research evidence of cupping therapy in China: A systematic literature review. BMC Complementary and Alternative Medicine 10: 70–79.

4. Cao HJ, Zhu CJ, Liu JP (2010) Wet cupping therapy for treatment of herpes zoster: A systematic review of randomized controlled trials. Altern Ther Health Med 16: 48–54.

5. Kim JI, Lee MS, Lee DH, Boddy K, Ernst E (2011) Cupping for treating pain: a systematic review. Evid Based Complement Altern Med doi: 10.1093/ecam/nep035.

6. Kwon YD, Cho HJ (2007) Systematic review of cupping including bloodletting therapy for musculoskeletal diseases in Korea. Korean J Oriental Physiol Pathol 21: 789–793.

7. Lee MS, Choi TY, Shin BC, Han CH, Ernst E (2010) Cupping for stroke rehabilitation: A systematic review. J Neurol Sci 294: 70–73.

8. Lee MS, Choi TY, Shin BC, Nam SS (2010) Cupping for hypertension: A systematic review. Clin Exp Hypertens 32: 423–425.

9. Lee MS, Kim JI, Ernst E (2011) Is cupping an effective treatment? An overview of systematic reviews. J of Acupunct Meridian Stud 4(1): 1–4.

10. Higgins JPT, Green S, eds (2009) Cochrane handbook for systematic reviews of interventions (version 5.0.2). The Cochrane Collaboration.

11. Bu TW, Tian XL, Wang SJ, Liu W, Li XL, et al. (2007) Comparison and analysis of therapeutic effects of different therapies on simple obesity [in Chinese]. Chinese Acupuncture & Moxibustion 27: 337–340.

12. Cao RL, Huang LP, Bi YF (2009) Combination of flash cupping therapy and acupuncture in treating 48 patients with peripheral facial paralysis [in Chinese]. Shanxi Journal of Traditional Chinese Medicine 30(1): 74–75.

13. Chen J, Xu HY (1993) Wet cupping therapy on 50 patients with herpes zoster [in Chinese]. The Chinese Journal of Dermatovenereology 5: 252.

14. Chen JJ (2009) Clinical observation of therapeutic effect of combination of electroacupuncture and wet cupping therapy for scapulohumeral periarthritis [in Chinese]. JCAM 25(1): 27–28.

15. Chen LA (2010) Zhi Zhi Heng Tui massage in treating 150 cases with strain of lumbar muscles by syndrome differentiation [in Chinese]. Jiangxi Journal of Traditional Chinese Medicine 41(328): 62–63.

16. Chen MX, Huang DJ (2000) Clinical study on combination of cupping therapy and moxibustion for treatment of asthenic splenonephro-yang type of colitis

gravis [in Chinese] (Master's thesis). Chengdu University of Traditional Chinese Medicine.

17. Chen YL, Liu XL, Xia JZ (2008) Clinical observation of wet cupping combined with acupuncture, tuina and traction on 30 patients with blood stasis type of prolapse of lumbar intervertebral disc [in Chinese]. Jiangsu Journal of Traditional Chinese Medicine 40(8): 47–48.

18. Cheng G (2000) Clinical report of observation of cupping therapy on lumbocrural pain caused by degenerative spondylolisthesis [in Chinese]. Journal of Clinical Acupuncture and Moxibustion1 6(7): 33–34.

19. Chi FL, Liu GL (1987) Clinical observation of therapeutic effect of cupping therapy on wound healing [in Chinese]. Chinese Primary Health Care 1(9): 24–25.

20. Ci HF (2010) Clinical observation of therapeutic effect of combination of acupuncture and cupping therapy on 104 cases with acute herpes zoster [in Chinese]. Modern Medicine & Health 26: 1550–1551.

21. Dai JY, Shao J, Wang YH, Wang L, Yin XZ (2006) Clinical comparative observations on acupuncture treatment of 200 simple obesity patients by syndrome differentiation [in Chinese]. Shanghai Journal of Acupuncture and Moxibustion 25(10): 13–15.

22. Fang X, Jin Y (2006) Clinical observation of medicinal cupping therapy on indirectly contusion injuries of temporomandibular joint [in Chinese]. Modern Journal of Integrated Traditional Chinese and Western Medicine 15: 734.

23. Farhadi K, Schiwebel DC, Saeb M, Choubsaz M, Mohammadi R, et al. (2009) The effectiveness of wet-cupping for nonspecific low back pain in Iran: A randomized controlled trial. Complement Ther Med 17: 9–15.

24. Feng WM (2004) Clinical observation of instant and forward analgesic effect of wet cupping therapy on 156 patients with soft tissue injury [in Chinese]. Chinese Journal of Traditional Medical Science and Technology 11(3): 180.

25. Fu CA, Bai ZQ (2004) Clinical observation of comparison of acupuncture and acupuncture combined with cupping therapy on facial paralysis [in Chinese]. Journal of Yanan University (Medical Science) 2(3): 59.

26. Fu L, Liu WA, Wu QM, Li XR, Li DD, et al. (2009) Observation on the efficacy of acupuncture plus pricking-cupping bloodletting in treating postapoplectic shoulder-hand syndrome [in Chinese]. Shanghai Journal of Acupuncture and Moxibustion 28: 132–134.

27. Fu Y, Jin JL (2005) Clinical observation of therapeutic effect of moving cupping therapy combined with herbal medicine on perimenopausal syndrome [in Chinese] (Master's thesis). Tianjin University of Traditional Chinese Medicine.

28. Gao BB (2010) Combination of acupuncture and wet cupping therapy on treating 92 cases with idiopathic facial palsy [in Chinese]. China Journal of Guang Ming Chinese Medicine 25: 1244–1245.

29. Gao YJ, Liu HS (2009) Combination of acupuncture and wet cupping therapy on treating 30 cases with post-herpetic neuralgia [in Chinese]. Journal of External Therapy of TCM 18(6): 34–35.

30. Ge JJ, Sun LH, Li WL (2003) Clinical observation of 48 cases on sciatica by retaining the needle and cupping [in Chinese]. Chinese Journal of the Practical Chinese with Modern Medicine 3: 823–824.

31. Guo JM, Xu CJ (1997) Wet cupping therapy on Tanzhong (RM17) for schizophrenia [in Chinese]. Shandong Journal of Traditional Chinese Medicine 16(2): 74.

32. Guo LX (2006) Clinical observation of therapeutic effect of pricking cupping bloodletting therapy on herpes zoster [in Chinese]. Shanxi Journal of Traditional Chinese Medicine 22(3): 41.

33. Guo XL, Wang XJ, Zuo WY (1992) Clinical observation of pricking-cupping bloodletting therapy on mastitis [in Chinese]. Zhen Jiu Xue Bao [vol unknown] 2: 34–35.

34. Han LX, Wang YY (1998) Observation of therapeutic effect of cupping therapy on muscle pain caused by wind-pathogen [in Chinese]. Tianjin Journal of Traditional Chinese Medicine 15(3): 122.

35. Hong YF, Wu JX, Wang B, Li H, He YC (2006) The effect of moving cupping therapy on nonspecific low back pain [in Chinese]. Chinese Journal of Rehabilitation Medicine 21: 340–343.

36. Huang GQ, Li FY, Huang Y (2004) Clinical observation on therapeutic effect of moving cupping therapy on wind-cold type of common cold [in Chinese]. Chinese Journal of Current Clinical Medicine 2: 1680–1681.

37. Huang J, Li WJ (2008) Clinical observation on acute posterior ganglionitis by method of surrounding puncture method and percussopunctator combined with cupping cup [in Chinese]. Journal of Liaoning University of Traditional Chinese Medicine 10: 168–169.

38. Huang J, Wei D, Wu JD (2010) Venesection and cupping treating acne in 76 cases [in Chinese]. China Bio-Beauty 1: 19–21.

39. Huang LP, Cao RL, Bi YF, Han ZC, Yue BA, et al. (2009) Combination of flash cupping and acupuncture on treating of 115 cases with peripheral facial paralysis [in Chinese]. Shanxi Journal of Traditional Chinese Medicine 30: 597–599.

40. Huang LP, Cao RL, Zhang XX (2010) Wet cupping therapy on Yifeng (SJ17) for 58 cases with acute peripheral facial paralysis [in Chinese]. Shanxi Journal of Traditional Chinese Medicine 31: 473–474.

41. Huang ZF, Li HZ, Zhang ZJ, Tan ZQ, Chen C, et al. (2006) Observations on the efficacy of cupping for treating 30 patients with cancer pain [in Chinese]. Shanghai Journal of Acupuncture and Moxibustion 25(8): 14–15.

42. Ji J (1992) Observation on clinical effect of vitiligo treated with medicinal cupping [in Chinese]. Chinese Acupuncture & Moxibustion 12(3): 11–12.

43. Jiang H, Hu D, Chen HY (2006) Observation and nursing for cupping along the channels of TCM to treatment chronic bronchitis with acute pulmonary infection [in Chinese]. Journal of Nursing Science 21(1): 48–49.

44. Jiang XY, Zhuo R (2008) Therapeutic effect of blood-letting puncture and cupping on upper-limb edema after mastectomy for breast cancer [in Chinese]. Journal of Nursing Science 23(8 Surgery Edition): 37–38.

45. Jin MZ, Xie ZQ, Chen XW, Chen DX, Chen DP (2008) Observations on the efficacy of blood-letting puncture and cupping in treating middle-aged and senile herpes zoster [in Chinese]. Shanghai Journal of Acupuncture and Moxibustion 27(3): 20–21.

46. Kang HQ, Li M (2005) Clinical observation of wet cupping on 48 patients with erysipelas [in Chinese]. Journal of Emergency Traditional Chinese Medicine 14(1): 51.

47. Li HT, Liu JH (2005) Clinical observation on treatment of peripheral facial paralysis with acupuncture and pricking-cupping therapy [in Chinese]. Journal of Chinese Integrated Medicine 3(1): 18, 69.

48. Li JC, Fan YS (2008) Clinical observations on treatment of subhealth with acupuncture and moxibustion plus moving cupping on the back [in Chinese]. Shanghai Journal of Acupuncture and Moxibustion 27(2): 8–9.

49. Li KZ (2009) Clinical observation on treatment of 80 cases of peripheral facial paralysis with acupuncture and flash cupping therapy [in Chinese]. Journal of Qiqihar Medical College 30(24): 3091.

50. Li P (2010) Clinical observation on treatment of 60 cases of acute peripheral facial paralysis with acupuncture and flash cupping therapy [in Chinese]. Journal of Shanxi College of Traditional Chinese Medicine 33(4): 83–84.

51. Li WH (2005) Clinical observation on plum-blossom needle therapy combined with cupping for treatment of acute facial paralysis [in Chinese]. Chinese Acupuncture and Moxibustion 25: 765–767.

52. Li X (2006) Therapeutic effect of plum-blossom needle tapping and moving cupping on lateral thigh skin neuritis: A clinical study [in Chinese]. Practical New Medicine 7: 702–703.

53. Liang SY (2009) Wet cupping therapy plus massage on treatment of 50 cases with pivot joint disturbance vertigo [in Chinese]. Fujian Journal of Traditional Chinese Medicine 40(1): 28–29.

54. Liang YL, Lu LQ, Yang XQ, Liang JL (2009) Clinical observation of wet cupping therapy plus acupuncture on treatment of insomnia [in Chinese]. Nursing Practice and Research 6(6): 79–80.

55. Liao FR (2009) Observations on the efficacy of pricking bloodletting plus cupping in treating cervical vertigo [in Chinese]. Shanghai Journal of Acupuncture and Moxibustion 28: 399–400.

56. Lin SZ (2005) Observation of wet cupping combined with electroacupuncture on 52 patients with prolapse of lumbar intervertebral disc [in Chinese]. Traditional Chinese Medicine Research 18(11): 47–49.

57. Liu BX, Xu M, Huang CJ, Ma LS, Lou YM, et al. (2008) Therapeutic effect of balance cupping therapy on non-specific low back pain [in Chinese]. Chinese Journal of Rehabilitative Theory and Practice 14: 572–573.

58. Liu BX, Xu M, Huang CJ, Tang FY, Lou YM, et al. (2010) Clinical observation on the treatment of lateral humeral epicondylitis using self-made herbal decoction cupping therapy [in Chinese]. Journal of Zhejiang University of Traditional Chinese Medicine 34: 409–10.

59. Liu HP, Liang B, He JB, Zhang CQ (2009) Therapeutic effect of acupuncture combined with flash cupping for acne vulgaris [in Chinese]. Liaoning Journal of Traditional Chinese Medicine 36: 1395–1397.

60. Liu J, Zhao Y, Zeng R, Kenedy J (2005) Randomized controlled trial on observation of wet cupping therapy on sore pain of keen joint of African people [in Chinese]. Chinese Journal of Clinical Rehabilitation 9(47): 135–136.

61. Liu L, Li ZL (2003) Curative effect observation on treating herpes zoster by Zhong Xi Medicine [in Chinese]. Chinese Journal of the Practical Chinese with Modern Medicine 3: 1088–1089.

62. Liu L, Li WL, Man W (2006) Clinical observation of wet cupping combined with auricular therapy on chloasma [in Chinese]. Journal of Hebei Traditional Chinese Medicine and Pharmacology 21(2): 30–31.

63. Liu QW, Chang HS (2004) Integrative Chinese and western medicine for herpes zoster [in Chinese]. Journal of External Therapy of Traditional Chinese Medicine 13(5): 53.

64. Long WH, Liu H (2003) 34 cases observation of combined therapy for herpes zoster [in Chinese]. Journal of Medical Theory and Practice 16: 1170.

65. Liu YZ, Liu JR, Liu LS, Sun L, Wu XX, et al. (2009) Clinical study of Wang Yan Xun Jing medicinal cupping therapy for cerebral infarction. China Foreign Medical Treatment 2: 113–114.

66. Lu HM, Ding S (2009) Clinical observation of therapeutic effect of combination of electroacupuncture and wet cupping therapy for shoulder-hand syndrome [in Chinese]. Journal of Practical Traditional Chinese Medicine 25: 320–321.

67. Lu J, Wang Y (2007) Acupuncture combined with wet cupping therapy on 63 cases of prolapse of lumbar intervertebral disc [in Chinese]. Journal of Clinical Acupuncture and Moxibustion 23(3): 16–17.

68. Lu ZX, Jin HL, Zhang P (2009) Cupping for preventing nausea and vomiting after laparoscopic gallbladder resection [in Chinese]. Journal of Zhejiang College of Traditional Chinese Medicine 33: 862–863.

69. Ludtke R, Albrecht U, Stange R, Uehleke B (2006) Brachialgia paraesthetica nocturna can be relieved by "wet cupping" – results of a randomized pilot study. Complementary Therapies in Medicine 14: 247–53.

70. Luo XX, Ma LS (2010) Clinical observation of effect of balance cupping for acute strain of lumbar muscle [in Chinese]. Chinese Journal of Information on TCM 17(9): 75–76.

71. Lü JC (2010) Combination of electroacupuncture and wet cupping therapy for intractable facial paralysis accompany with sensory disturbance of facial nerve [in Chinese]. China Higher Medical Education 10: 136–137.

72. Ma CT, Zhang J (2006) Clinical observation of moving cupping therapy on excess pattern depression [in Chinese] (Master's thesis). Beijing University of Chinese Medicine.

73. Michalsen A, Bock S, Ludtke R, Rampp T, Baecker M, et al. (2009) Effects of traditional cupping therapy in patients with carpal tunnel syndrome: A randomized controlled trial. The Journal of Pain 10: 601–618.

74. Ni ML (2010) 48 cases clinical observation of acupuncture plus flash cupping therapy on treating facial muscle spasm [in Chinese]. Heilongjiang Medicine Journal 23: 453.

75. Ou XH, Xu SC (2009) Sixty cases of refractory facial paralysis treated with traditional Chinese medicine using acupuncture and flash tank [in Chinese]. Journal of Chengdu University of Traditional Chinese Medicine 32(3): 37–38.

76. Qiu JZ, Fan CM, Wei FY, Gao CL (2003) Clinical observation of therapeutic effect of medicinal cupping on acute facial neuritis [in Chinese]. China Journal of Modern Medicine 13(21): 146.

77. Ren YJ (2006) Observation of wet cupping combined with acupuncture on 50 patients with facial paralysis [in Chinese]. Shanxi Journal of Traditional Chinese Medicine 27: 480–481.

78. Rui XG (2010) Observations on the efficacy of acupuncture plus cutaneous needle tapping in treating inflammation of superior cluneal nerves [in Chinese]. Shanghai Journal of Acupuncture and Moxibustion 29: 515–516.

79. Shao M, Liu TY (2003) Clinical observations on the treatment of 93 cervical spondylopathy by Dazhui blood-letting puncturing and cupping [in Chinese]. Shanghai Journal of Acupuncture and Moxibustion 22(8): 20–21.

80. Sun HW, Li L (2010) Observation of wet cupping therapy on treating 40 cases with post- auricular pain after peripheral facial palsy [in Chinese]. China Journal of Guang Ming Chinese Medicine 25: 1674.

81. Sun LJ, Xu XD (2007) Clinical observation of therapeutic effect of moving cupping on back shu points combined with acupuncture on 30 patients with simple obesity [in Chinese]. China Practical Medicine 2(32): 138–139.

82. Sun SQ, Xu SX (2006) 67 cases suffered from erysipelas on lower legs cured by means of integration of traditional Chinese medicine and western medicine [in Chinese]. Journal of Chinese Practical Medicine 1(5): 109–110.

83. Tang CR (2003) Acupuncture combined with moving cupping therapy for diabetic peripheral neuropathy [in Chinese]. Sichuan Journal of Traditional Chinese Medicine 21(7): 89–90.

84. Tao Q, Lu HX (2007) Clinical observation of electroacupuncture combined with wet cupping therapy on abdominal aorta calcification related to lumbar intervertebral disc prolapse [in Chinese]. Journal of Clinical Acupuncture and Moxibustion 23(8): 46–47.

85. Wan XW (2005) Clinical observation on acupuncture combined with cupping therapy for treatment of ankylosing spondylitis [in Chinese]. Chinese Acupuncture and Moxibustion 25: 551–552.

86. Wan XW (2007) Clinical observation on treatment of cervical spondylosis with combined acupuncture and cupping therapies [in Chinese]. Journal of Acupuncture and Tuina Science 5: 345–347.

87. Wang J (2010) Combination of acupuncture and moving cupping therapy for 42 cases with functional dyspepsia [in Chinese]. China Science and Technology Information 15: 176.

88. Wang L (2010) Clinical observation of flash cupping for treating chronic obstructive pulmonary disease in remission [in Chinese]. Chinese General Nursing 8: 2574–1575.

89. Wang LR, Liu HF, Li QY (2010) Observation on the clinical efficacy of meridian cupping plus acupuncture in treating 60 cases of acute peripheral facial paralysis. Sichuan Journal of Traditional Chinese Medicine 28(1): 110–112.

90. Wang PL (2010) Clinical observation on therapeutic effects of abdominal acupuncture combined with blood-letting acupuncture and cupping for treating nerve-root cervical spondylosis. Clinical Journal of Chinese Medicine 9(2): 15–17.

91. Wang QF, Wang GY (2007) Observation on the efficacy of acupuncture and moxibustion plus blood-letting puncture and moving cupping in treating acne [in Chinese]. Shanghai Journal of Acupuncture and Moxibustion 26(12): 20–21.

92. Wang SP (2009) Observation of cupping therapy in treating 62 cases of bronchial asthma [in Chinese]. Guiding Journal of Traditional Chinese Medicine and Pharmacology 15(10): 56.

93. Wang XM, Zhou ZX (2004) Electroacupuncture combined with wet cupping therapy on 66 patients with cervical spondylotic radiculopathy [in Chinese]. Shanxi Journal of Traditional Chinese Medicine 25(1): 60–61.

94. Wang YH, Huang SX, Liu BY, Guo YF, Ding X, et al. (2009) Clinical observation of therapeutic effect of acupuncture for herpes zoster [in Chinese]. Chinese Journal of Basic Medicine in Traditional Chinese Medicine 15: 774–777.

95. Wu FF, Yang SQ, Zhang SJ (2010) Wet cupping therapy on back shu points on treatment of acne [in Chinese]. Journal of Qiqihar Medical College 31: 1596.

96. Wu PX, Ma WL, Zhao XX (2010) Clinical observation of acupuncture plus cupping therapy for chronic urticaria [in Chinese]. Guiding Journal of Tradtional Chinese Medicine and Pharmacology 16(11): 79.

97. Wu YT (2008) Therapeutic effects on acne by bloodletting with cupping therapy on the back [in Chinese]. Journal of Practical Traditional Chinese Internal Medicine 22(10): 61–62.

98. Xiao W, Wang Y, Kong HB, Wang X, Wang J, et al. (2009) Observation of cupping therapy on back-shu points for chronic obstructive pulmonary disease [in Chinese]. Chinese Journal of Traditional Chinese Medicine 21: 420–421.

99. Xiao W, Wang Y, Kong HB, Wang J, Wang Z, et al. (2010) Effect of cupping at back-shu acupoints on immunologic function in patients with chronic obstructive pulmonary disease during stable stage [in Chinese]. Journal of Anhui College of Traditional Chinese Medicine 29(5): 37–39.

100. Xin KP (2006) Cupping on Dazhui on 30 children with fever caused by heat stroke [in Chinese]. Jiangxi Journal of Traditional Chinese Medicine 37(285): 53–54.

101. Xiong JF (2010) Observation of wet cupping therapy for 60 cases with acute prolapse of lumbar intervertebral disc [in Chinese]. Journal of External Therapy of Traditional Chinese Medicine 19(5): 28–29.

102. Xiong SY, Hu Y, Gong LP (2007) Observation of therapeutic effect of cupping therapy on herpes zoster pain [in Chinese]. Journal of Nurses Training 22: 948–949.

103. Xiong ZL, Zhang GH (2007) Cupping therapy combined with acupuncture on 48 patients with acute herpes zoster [in Chinese]. Journal of Clinical Acupuncture and Moxibustion 23(7): 38–39.

104. Xu L, Yang XJ (2004) Therapeutic effect of acyclovir in combination with meridian acupuncture and cupping in the treatment of 40 cases of herpes zoster [in Chinese]. Tianjin Pharmacy 16(3): 23–24.

105. Xu M, Liu BX, Huang CJ, Tang FY, Lou YM, Liang Z, et al. (2009) The therapeutic effects of balance cupping therapy on chronic lumbar muscle strain [in Chinese]. Liaoning Journal of Traditional Chinese Medicine 36: 1007–1008.

106. Xu MY (2006) Clinical observation of therapeutic effect of cupping on Zhong Ji (RM3) in the treatment of post-operative uroschesis [in Chinese]. Liaoning Journal of Traditional Chinese Medicine 33: 719.

107. Xu SW (2008) Observation on the therapeutic effect of acupuncture on generalized osteoarthritis [in Chinese]. Shanghai Journal of Acupuncture and Moxibustion 27(4): 11–12.

108. Xu SX (1999) Application of cupping therapy in treatment of furuncles [in Chinese]. The Chinese Journal of Dermatoneurology 21(2): 21–22.

109. Xu WD, Zhang YJ, Yang J, Chen XX, Liu YX (2006) Cupping on back shu points for acute bronchitis [in Chinese]. Journal of Clinical Acupuncture and Moxibustion 22(8): 39–40.

110. Xu Y, Ge HZ (2010) Clinical observation on treating acute lumbar sprain by cupping plus acupuncture. Clinical Journal of Chinese Medicine 10(2): 70–71.

111. Xue WH, Wang JL, Wang GR (2005) Clinical observation of wet cupping therapy on rotaviral enteritis [in Chinese]. Liaoning Journal of Traditional Chinese Medicine 32: 826.

112. Yang JH, Guo LZ, Xiong J (2007) Clinical observation on the treatment of 46 cases of acute ankle sprain with acupuncture combined with venesection and ventouse [in Chinese]. Guiding Journal of Traditional Chinese Medicine 13(4): 57–58.

113. Yao X (2006) Clinical observation of cupping therapy combined with acupuncture on chronic diarrhea [in Chinese]. Jilin Medical Journal 27: 1403–1404.

114. Yin GZ, Zheng LJ (2009) Observation of 72 cases of psoriasis treated by wet cupping therapy [in Chinese]. Xinjiang Journal of Traditional Chinese Medicine 27(5): 13–15.

115. You Y, Lan CY, Liang W, Yang ZH, Xu S, et al. (2006) Wet cupping combined with traction for prolapse of lumbar vertebral disc [in Chinese]. Chinese Journal of Convalescent Medicine 15(1): 14–15.

116. You Y, Yang ZH, Sun DZ, Lan CY (2006) Effect of plum-blossom needle therapy and cupping therapy combined with traction on cervical spondylosis of vertebral artery type [in Chinese]. Chinese Journal of Rehabilitative Theory and Practice 12: 1037–1038.

117. Zeng HW, Nie B, Huang NB (2007) Analysis of the efficacy of blood-letting puncture and cupping plus warming acupuncture for treating cervical spondylopathy of vertebral artery type [in Chinese]. Shanghai Journal of Acupuncture and Moxibustion 26(6): 8–10.

118. Zha BG, Wang ZY (2005) Cupping therapy on accelerating thenar wound healing: Clinical trial of 28 cases [in Chinese]. Hunan Journal of Traditional Chinese Medicine 21(3): 81.

119. Zhang DD, Li JB (2009) Combination of wet cupping therapy and acupuncture on treatment of post-stroke shoulder-hand syndrome [in Chinese]. Jilin Journal of Traditional Chinese Medicine 29: 796–797.

120. Zhang FY, Liu XH (2006) Acupuncture combined with moving cupping therapy on 30 cases of simple obesity and hyperlipidemia [in Chinese]. Journal of External Therapy of Traditional Chinese Medicine 15(5): 42–43.

121. Zhang HB (2010) Clinical observation of acupuncture combined with venesection and ventouse on periarthritis of the shoulder: Report of 60 cases [in Chinese]. Shanxi Journal of Traditional Chinese Medicine 26(10): 28–29.

122. Zhang HX, Liu YN, Huang GF, Zou R, Wei W (2009) Observation of different types of acupuncture on pain reduction of herpes zoster of the head and face [in Chinese]. Journal of Emergency Traditional Chinese Medicine 18: 1979–1981.

123. Zhang JW, Wang XL, Zhou SH (2004) Clinical observation of combination of acyclovir and acupuncture in the treatment of 41 cases of herpes zoster [in Chinese]. Chinese General Practice 7: 1179–1180.
124. Zhang JX, Diao J, Yu SP (2007) Traditional cupping therapy with syndrome differentiation on insomnia [in Chinese]. Chinese Journal of Clinical Medicinal Professional Research 13: 3444.
125. Zhang KX, Song SJ (2008) Clinical observation of wet cupping therapy on back shu points for acne [in Chinese]. World Health Digest 5: 193–194.
126. Zhang Q, Liang XS, Guo TZ, Li TN (2008) Observation on treatment of head-face herpes zoster [in Chinese]. Liaoning Journal of Traditional Chinese Medicine 35: 602.
127. Zhang QL, Fu XH (2009) Clinical observation of cupping therapy plus electroacupuncture on treatment of lumbar vertebral disc prolapse with blood stasis syndrome [in Chinese]. Acta Chinese Medicine and Pharmacology 37(5): 79–80.
128. Zhang XY (2009) Sixteen cases with refractory hiccup treated by moving cupping on back shu points [in Chinese]. Journal of the Chinese Acupuncture and Moxibustion 25(7): 45–46.
129. Zhang YB, Yan CY (2010) Clinical observation of medicinal cupping therapy on treating chronic gastritis. Guangxi Journal of Traditional Chinese Medicine 33(2): 17–18.
130. Zhang YC, Yan XY (2004) Clinical observation of and nursing care for the treatment of bronchiolitis by auxliary glass cupping [in Chinese]. Journal of Qilu Nursing 10(1): 28.
131. Zhang YD (2005) Observation of moving and retained cupping therapy on 30 pediatric cases with recurrent respiratory tract infection [in Chinese]. Journal of External Therapy of Traditional Chinese Medicine 14(6): 40–41.
132. Zhao J (2010) Combination of cupping therapy and antibiotictreatment of 220 pediatric cases with cough after acute upper respiratory infection [in Chinese]. Shanxi Journal of Traditional Chinese Medicine 26(8): 34.
133. Zhao NX, Shi HJ, Ren TY, Guo RL (2010) Observation of flash cupping therapy for acute peripheral facial neuritis [in Chinese]. Journal of Guiyang College of Traditional Chinese Medicine 32(2): 72–73.
134. Zhao XQ, Zheng JH, Wang GC, Lu YK, Su JY (2003) Treatment of 40 cases of intracranial hypertension syndrome by pricking GV14 acupoint plus cupping [in Chinese]. Chinese Acupuncture and Moxibustion 23(2): 75–76.
135. Zheng L (2008) Clinical observation of wet cupping therapy on osteoarthritis [in Chinese]. Chinese Journal of Traditional Medical Traumatology and Orthopedics 16(10): 27–28.
136. Zheng ZH, Liu QQ, Xiao YL, Jia SL, Chen L, et al. (1999) Clinical observation of therapeutic effect of medicinal cupping therapy on prevention and treatment of bronchial asthma [in Chinese]. Hebei Journal of Traditional Chinese Medicine 14(2): 29–30.
137. Zhong JR, Zhao YS, Liang QS, Gao E, Yu PN (2010) Observation of ventouse therapy immediately following venomous snake bite [in Chinese]. China Modern Medicine 17(4): 19–21.
138. Zhou LW (2007) Moving cupping therapy on 45 cases of myofasciitis causing rigidity of the neck and back [in Chinese]. Clinical Journal of Traditional Chinese Medicine 19: 170–171.
139. Zhou Y, Wu RM, Cao Y (2010) Observation of cupping therapy for pneumonia [in Chinese]. Journal of Guiyang College of Traditional Chinese Medicine 32(4): 54–55.
140. Zhou YM (1994) Moving cupping therapy on 100 cases of common cold [in Chinese]. Chinese Acupuncture and Moxibustion 14(S1): 292.
141. Zhu F, Chen SJ, Feng DR, Xu QY (2009) Observation of wet cupping therapy on treatment of acute peripheral facial neuritis [in Chinese]. Journal of Emergency Traditional Chinese Medicine 18: 702–703.
142. Zhu Y, Zhang FX (2009) Observation of wet cupping therapy plus auricular acupressure for chloasma [in Chinese]. Chinese Medicine Modern Distance Education of China 7(3): 97.
143. Zhu Y (2010) Combination of acupuncture and wet cupping therapy for 50 cases of chloasma [in Chinese]. Shanxi Journal of Traditional Chinese Medicine 31: 476–478.
144. Zou LY, Hu JY (2009) Cupping therapy on treatment of 40 cases with acute lumbar muscle strain [in Chinese]. Henan Traditional Chinese Medicine 29: 802–803.
145. Zou R, Zhang HX, Huang GF, Zhou L, Li X, et al. (2010) Analgesic effect of electroacupuncture at EX-B2 combined with press needles and ventouse for patients with herpes zoster [in Chinese]. Chinese Journal of Rehabilitation 25: 205–206.
146. The CONSORT Group. CONSORT Statement 2001-Checklist: Items to include when reporting a randomized trial. Available: http://www.consort-statement.org.
147. Lee MS, Kim JI, Kong JC, Lee DH, Shin BC (2010) Developing and validating a sham cupping device. Acupunct Med 28: 200–204.
148. MacPherson H, Altman DG, Hammerschlag R, Youping L, Taixiang W, et al. (2010) Revised STandards for Reporting Interventions in Clinical Trials of Acupuncture (STRICTA): Extending the CONSORT Statement. PLoS Med 7(6): e1000261. doi:10.1371/journal.pmed.1000261.
149. Laine C, Horton R, DeAngelis CD, Drazen J, Frizelle F, et al. (2007) Clinical trial registration looking back and moving ahead. N Engl J Med 356: 2734–2736.
150. Viergever RF, Ghersi D (2011) The Quality of Registration of Clinical Trials. PLoS ONE 6(2): e14701.

5

Characterizing Acupuncture Stimuli Using Brain Imaging with fMRI - A Systematic Review and Meta-Analysis of the Literature

Wenjing Huang[1,2], Daniel Pach[1], Vitaly Napadow[4,5], Kyungmo Park[6], Xiangyu Long[8], Jane Neumann[8,9], Yumi Maeda[4,5], Till Nierhaus[7,8], Fanrong Liang[2], Claudia M. Witt[1,3]*

1 Institute for Social Medicine, Epidemiology and Health Economics, Charité University Medical Center, Berlin, Germany, 2 Chengdu University of Traditional Chinese Medicine, Chengdu, China, 3 Center for Integrative Medicine, University of Maryland School of Medicine, Baltimore, Maryland, United States of America, 4 Athinoula A. Martinos Center for Biomedical Imaging, Department of Radiology, Massachusetts General Hospital, Charlestown, Massachusetts, United States of America, 5 Department of Radiology, Logan College of Chiropractic, Chesterfield, Missouri, United States of America, 6 Department of Biomedical Engineering, Kyung Hee University, Yongin, Republic of Korea, 7 Berlin NeuroImaging Center and Department Neurology, Charité, Berlin, Germany, 8 Max Planck Institute for Human Cognitive and Brain Sciences, Leipzig, Germany, 9 Leipzig University Medical Center, IFB Adiposity Diseases, Leipzig, Germany

Abstract

Background: The mechanisms of action underlying acupuncture, including acupuncture point specificity, are not well understood. In the previous decade, an increasing number of studies have applied fMRI to investigate brain response to acupuncture stimulation. Our aim was to provide a systematic overview of acupuncture fMRI research considering the following aspects: 1) differences between verum and sham acupuncture, 2) differences due to various methods of acupuncture manipulation, 3) differences between patients and healthy volunteers, 4) differences between different acupuncture points.

Methodology/Principal Findings: We systematically searched English, Chinese, Korean and Japanese databases for literature published from the earliest available up until September 2009, without any language restrictions. We included all studies using fMRI to investigate the effect of acupuncture on the human brain (at least one group that received needle-based acupuncture). 779 papers were identified, 149 met the inclusion criteria for the descriptive analysis, and 34 were eligible for the meta-analyses. From a descriptive perspective, multiple studies reported that acupuncture modulates activity within specific brain areas, including somatosensory cortices, limbic system, basal ganglia, brain stem, and cerebellum. Meta-analyses for verum acupuncture stimuli confirmed brain activity within many of the regions mentioned above. Differences between verum and sham acupuncture were noted in brain response in middle cingulate, while some heterogeneity was noted for other regions depending on how such meta-analyses were performed, such as sensorimotor cortices, limbic regions, and cerebellum.

Conclusions: Brain response to acupuncture stimuli encompasses a broad network of regions consistent with not just somatosensory, but also affective and cognitive processing. While the results were heterogeneous, from a descriptive perspective most studies suggest that acupuncture can modulate the activity within specific brain areas, and the evidence based on meta-analyses confirmed some of these results. More high quality studies with more transparent methodology are needed to improve the consistency amongst different studies.

Editor: Ben J. Harrison, The University of Melbourne, Australia

Funding: Funding provided by Carstens Foundation and Chinese Scholarship Council. The funders had no role in study design, data collection and analysis, decision to publish, or preparation of the manuscript.

Competing Interests: The authors have declared that no competing interests exist.

* E-mail: claudia.witt@charite.de

Introduction

Acupuncture is a therapy of inserting and manipulating fine filiform needles into specific body locations (acupuncture points) to treat diseases. Acupuncture is an ancient Chinese treatment that has been systematically used for over 2000 years [1]. Currently, acupuncture is used widely all over the world, but its biological mechanism is not well understood. From a neurophysiological aspect acupuncture can be regarded as a complex somatosensory stimulation [2]. Although the clinical effect of acupuncture is generally accepted for certain diagnoses [3], such as knee pain, low back pain etc., there exists controversy regarding the specific effect of acupuncture, especially for the specificity of acupuncture points and meridians. In clinical studies large effects produced by sham acupuncture were observed [4–6].

Interest in investigating acupuncture mechanisms with imaging techniques has been growing since the mid 1990 s [7,8]. Positron emission tomography (PET), single photon emission computed tomography (SPECT), and magnetic resonance imaging (MRI) have been used and, there is also interest in electro-encephalography (EEG). Functional MRI (fMRI), investigating the hemodynamic blood oxygenation level dependent (BOLD) effect, has come to dominate the brain mapping field due to its minimal invasiveness, lack of radiation exposure, excellent spatial resolution and relatively wide availability.

In the previous decade, an increasing number of studies applied fMRI to investigate acupuncture stimulation. The aim of this review was to give a systematic overview about the fMRI research on acupuncture regarding the following four aspects: 1) differences between verum and sham acupuncture, 2) differences due to various methods of acupuncture manipulation, 3) differences between patients and healthy volunteers, 4) differences between different acupuncture points.

Methods

The search strategy, research questions, inclusion and exclusion criteria and data extraction and analysis were predefined in our protocol. During the study, the database search was extended for the Japanese and Korean databases.

Searching

We searched the following sources:

1.PubMed (1948–2009.09) 2.EMBASE (1980–2009.09) 3. CNKI (China National Knowledge Infrastructure) (1915–2009.09) 4.Japanese Ichushi-Web (1983–2009.09) 5.Korean NDSL (National Digital Science Links) (1946–2009.09); KTKP (Korean Traditional Knowledge Portal) (1997–2008)

We searched these databases in the appropriate language using the following MeSH terms and search strategies:

English: 1.fMRI; 2.Functional MRI; 3.MRI, Functional; 4. Magnetic Resonance Imaging, Functional; 5.acupuncture; 6.#1 or #2 or #3 or #4; 7.#5 and #6;

Chinese: 1.针刺(acupuncture); 2.磁共振成像(Magnetic Resonance Imaging); 3.#1 and #2

Japanese: 1.1.鍼(acupuncture); 2.機能的磁気共鳴画像法 (Functional Magnetic Resonance Imaging); 3.#1 and #2

Korean: 1.기능적 자기공명영상 (fMRI, functional Magnetic Resonance Imaging); 2.침 (acupuncture); 3.#1 and #2

We screened the bibliographies of identified trials and reviewed articles for further potentially relevant publications.

Selection

In this review we included all studies using fMRI to investigate the effect of acupuncture on the human brain. Each study had to have at least one group, which received an intervention with any type of needle-based acupuncture. We included trials on healthy volunteers as well as patients and all types of needle acupuncture were accepted. There were no language restrictions and no limitations on outcome measures. Reviews, editorials and trials on animals were excluded.

The available abstracts of all identified references were screened and we excluded all citations that clearly did not fit the inclusion criteria. Full copies of all remaining articles and those references without available abstracts were obtained. Subsequently the three researchers (WJH: Pubmed, Embase and CNKI, KP: Korean databases, YM: Japanese databases) screened the full texts and assessed whether these trials met the inclusion criteria.

In the meta-analysis, we included studies investigating only verum acupuncture or both verum and sham acupuncture by fMRI using whole brain acquisition. Studies were excluded if 1) the number of study participants was less than five; 2) results were not reported as 3-dimensional coordinates in standard stereotactic space; 3) only the results from regions of interest (ROI) were reported or 4) only single subject data instead of group data were reported.

Data extraction and analysis

The three researchers (WJH: Pubmed, Embase and CNKI, KP: Korean databases, YM: Japanese databases) extracted the data for all descriptive information from the publications, namely published journals, language, study place, study type, subjects, handedness, objective, interventions, control groups, block-design, fMRI device type, software for fMRI data analysis, sample size, and results. The extracted data were discussed with three supervisors (CW, DP and VN). Any inconsistencies were discussed and reconsidered until consensus was reached.

Results were structured according to the four research questions. Studies that matched multiple research questions were displayed more than once, but only with the part of the study relevant to the respective research question.

Furthermore, one figure for different acupuncture points from publications in Talairach coordinates was generated by one author (XYL) using Analysis of Functional NeuroImages (AFNI, http://afni.nimh.nih.gov) and MRIcron software (http://www.cabiatl.com/mricro). The anatomical image was generated using MRIcron software.

The meta-analyses were conducted (JN, XYL, WJH) in Talairach space, using the activation likelihood estimation technique (ALE) implemented in GingerALE 2.1.1 software [9–11]. This technique assesses the convergence between activation foci from different experiments. Prior to the analysis, coordinates reported in MNI (Montreal Neurological Institute) space were converted to Talairach anatomical space using the Lancaster transform [12]. For each experiment, every reported activation maximum was modeled by a 3-dimensional Gaussian probability distribution centered at the given coordinate. The width of the Gaussian probability distribution was determined individually for each experiment based on empirical estimates of between-subject variability, taking into account the number of subjects in each experiment [9]. Voxel-wise ALE scores were calculated from the union of the Gaussian probability distributions within and across experiments. In a random effects analysis, ALE scores were tested against a null hypothesis of random distribution across the brain, thereby identifying those regions where empirical ALE values were higher than could be expected by chance. Resulting ALE maps were thresholded at $p < 0.05$ (corrected for multiple comparisons by False Discovery Rate). The minimum cluster volume was chosen to exceed the number of voxels corresponding to 5% possible false positives. The contrast studies analysis (subtraction analysis which compares two ALE maps) was performed with randomization testing with 10,000 permutations. As there exists no correction for multiple comparison with this approach, the threshold was set at $p < 0.05$ (uncorrected) with a min. cluster size = 200 mm^3 [13].

ALE maps were computed for the following statistical comparisons. From all studies included in the meta-analysis: 1a) greater activation of verum acupuncture points compared to baseline (verum>rest), 1b) greater deactivation of verum acupuncture points compared to baseline (rest>verum). From the studies which provided direct contrasts between verum and sham acupuncture: 2a) greater activation from verum than sham acupuncture (or greater deactivation for sham, i.e. verum>sham), 2b) greater deactivation from verum than sham acupuncture (or greater activation for sham, i.e. sham>verum). From the studies which had both verum and sham acupuncture groups: 3a) greater activation of verum acupuncture points than baseline (verum>

rest), 3b) greater deactivation of verum acupuncture points than baseline (rest>verum), 3c) greater activation of sham acupuncture points than baseline (sham>rest), 3d) greater deactivation of sham acupuncture points than baseline (rest>sham), 3e) comparison ALE map of greater activation of verum than sham acupuncture relative to rest ("verum>rest" - "sham>rest"), 3f) comparison ALE map of greater deactivation of verum than sham acupuncture relative to rest ("rest>verum" - "rest>sham").

Results

Study characteristics

The 149 studies were published between 1999 and 2009 (trial flow see Figure 1), Figure 2 shows the number of publications per year in corresponding countries in the last 11 years. Most of the studies were performed in China, US and Korea and predominantly published in Chinese and English (50.3% Chinese, 38.9% English, 9.4% Korean, 0.7% German and 0.7% Japanese). The median number of subjects per study was 17 (min. 1 to max. 67), and the total number of all studies included 2469 subjects. 24 studies reported parallel group randomized trials. 128 studies were on healthy volunteers, 13 studies on patients, 8 studies on the comparison of patients and healthy volunteers. Most of the trials applied a block design for fMRI data acquisition, with a time range for each block of 8 sec to 6 min, and the number of blocks

ranged from one to 12 blocks. 105 studies included right-handed subjects while only 3 studies included also left-handed subjects. 34 studies were included in the meta-analyses.

Descriptive findings of differences between verum and sham acupuncture

51 publications explored four kinds of sham acupuncture including a) a placebo needle (Streitberger needle [14]: with a blunt tip, which when it touches the skin causes a pricking sensation for the patient, simulating the puncturing of the skin. The needle moves inside the handle, and appears to be shortened.); b) needling at non-acupuncture points in close proximity to acupuncture points; c) needling at non-acupuncture points distant to acupuncture points; d) cutaneous stimulation at the same acupuncture points or sham point/area (Table S1). Two of the studies [15,16] are referenced more than once in the table because of the different sham acupuncture methods evaluated in these studies. The studies included mainly healthy volunteers, but four publications [17–20] included patients with Parkinson's disease or stroke.

A placebo needle: Streitberger Needle. The four studies which compared verum acupuncture with the Streitberger Needle were all from the US and showed heterogeneous results [16,19,21,22]. Yoo et al. [16] found more activation associated

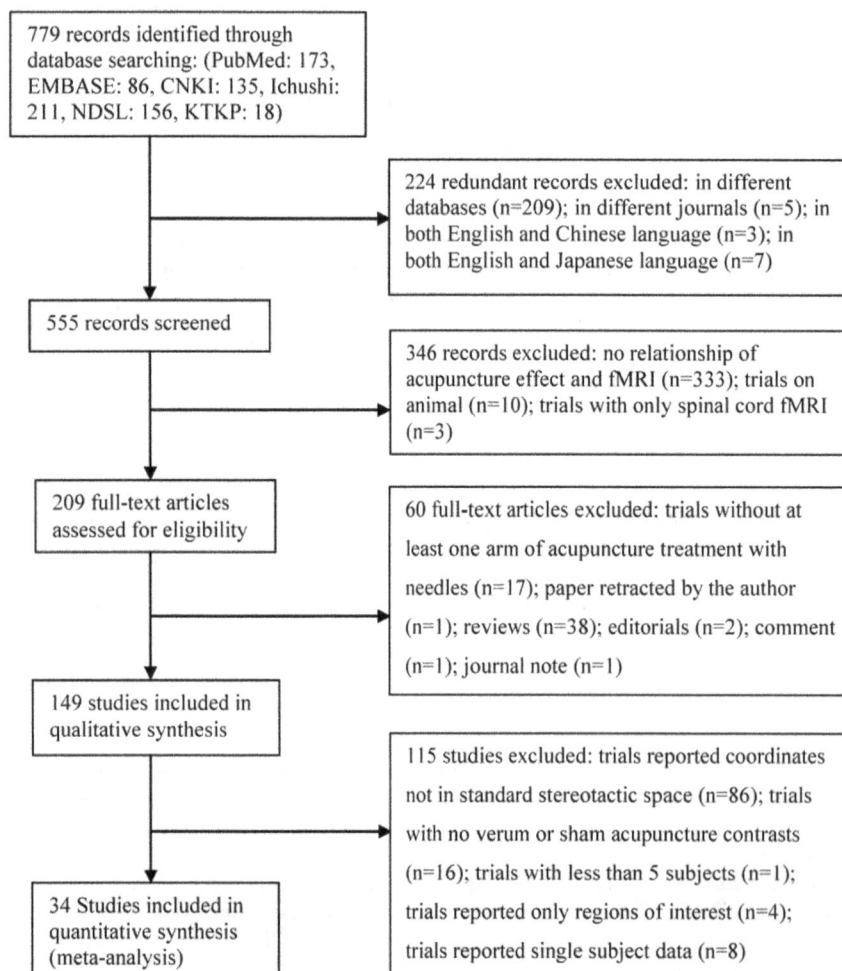

Figure 1. Flow of information through the different phases of the systematic review.

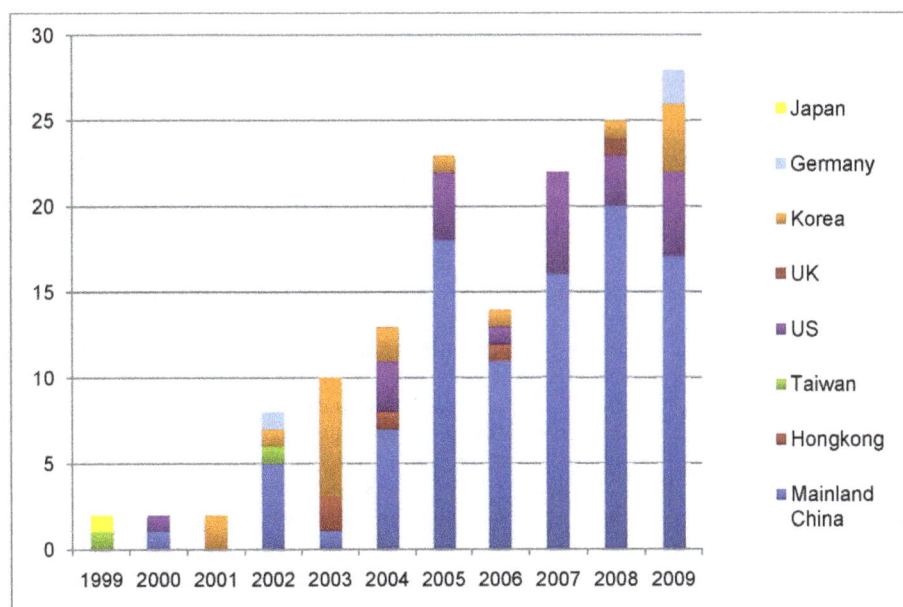

Figure 2. Number of publications on acupuncture and fMRI identified in the last 11 years.

with verum acupuncture in the somatosensory areas and motor areas. Dougherty et al. [21] reported that acupuncture produced more activation in the medial orbitofrontal cortex and more deactivation in brainstem and insula, while the Streitberger needle showed higher activation in the language area (Wernicke), pons, operculum and insula. According to Deng et al. [22] verum acupuncture resulted in more activation in insula and operculum compared to the Streitberger needle placed at a non-acupuncture point. A study with stroke patients [19] (scan during passive finger movement pre and -post 10 weeks treatment of verum acupuncture or the Streitberger placebo needle) showed a trend toward a greater maximum activation change in the motor cortical area for the verum acupuncture group.

Acupuncture at non-acupuncture points in close proximity to acupuncture points. Two third (64%) [15,23–37] of 25 studies showed that acupuncture treatments were associated with more activation, mainly in the somatosensory areas, motor areas, basal ganglia, cerebellum, limbic system and higher cognitive areas (e.g. prefrontal cortex). Three studies [28,37,38] showed also more deactivations in the limbic system in response to acupuncture. In contrast, one study [39] found greater activation in the supplementary motor area in response to sham acupuncture. Five other studies [40–44] found no significant difference between verum and sham acupuncture. One experiment was analyzed twice [45,46] and came to different results.

Acupuncture at non-acupuncture points distant to acupuncture points. Of six studies, two studies [47,48] showed no differences between verum and sham acupuncture. Four studies [49–52] showed more activation associated with acupuncture in the somatosensory areas, brainstem, basal ganglia, higher cognitive areas and part of the limbic system (hypothalamus, nucleus accumbens), and one study [52] showed more activation associated with sham acupuncture in the motor area and operculum. Verum acupuncture showed also more deactivation in part of the limbic system (amygdala, hippocampus, cingulate gyrus/cortex) [47,52]. In addition, Napadow et al. [51] found that both verum and sham acupuncture showed linearly

decreasing activation over repeated stimulus blocks in the sensorimotor areas, while verum acupuncture produced bimodal activity in a limbic midbrain region - activation in early blocks, but deactivation in later stimulus blocks.

Cutaneous stimulation at the same acupuncture point or sham point/area. There are 18 studies (15 on healthy volunteers). Only one study [16] on healthy volunteers found greater activation in the somatosensory area during verum acupuncture, whereas in four studies [53–56] somatosensory activation was greater with cutaneous stimulation. For motor areas and higher cognitive areas, five studies [15,16,55,57,58] showed that acupuncture was associated with more activation. For brainstem, basal ganglia, cerebellum and limbic system the results were complex or contradictory: in the basal ganglia, brainstem and cerebellum, two studies [53,59] found that acupuncture was associated with more deactivation while three other studies [15,57,60] found acupuncture associated with more activation; thalamus and insula [15,16,54,58] were activated more while hypothalamus, hippocampus, amygdala and temporal pole [53,54,58,59] were deactivated more by acupuncture. In addition, when eliciting deqi, Hui et al. [53] found extensive deactivation in the cerebrum, brainstem and cerebellum, while eliciting deqi mixed with pain, activation was the predominant pattern. Five Chinese studies [61–65] found almost no significant differences between verum and sham, though two of them found greater activation intensity in the cerebellum or parietal lobe for verum acupuncture [61,62]. Among the three publications on patients, Schockert et al. [20] found more activation in the motor area on stroke patients during acupuncture while Li et al. [17] found more activation in the somatosensory and motor areas with a control, brushing stimulation on stroke patients. In patients with Parkinson's disease Chae et al. [18] showed that acupuncture was associated with more activation than covert cutaneous stimulation in the motor area, basal ganglia, visual and higher cognitive area; and more activation in the motor, visual, higher cognitive areas and limbic system, compared to overt cutaneous stimulation.

Descriptive findings of differences due to various methods of acupuncture manipulation

Manipulation methods can differ in the depth of needling, forms of needle stimulation (e.g. manual versus electrical), intensity of stimulation, and stimulus timing parameters (e.g. duration, frequency, etc.). Here, we summarized the results from those studies comparing different methods of manipulation at acupuncture points in healthy volunteers (see Table 1). Two of the studies [58,66] are displayed more than once in the table as they explored multiple comparisons.

Comparison of different needling depths. Of four studies, two studies [67,68] found no significant difference between deep and superficial needling. Whereas Zhang et al. [25] found more activation in almost all brain areas from deep needling and Wu et al. [52] found more activation from superficial needling in the somatosensory area, motor area and language areas (Broca and Wernicke areas), and from deep needling more deactivation in the limbic system.

Comparison of electro-acupuncture vs. manual acupuncture. Overall, the results of three studies showed that electro-acupuncture tends to produce more activation and less deactivation compared to manual acupuncture. Regarding brain activations, two studies [58,69] found more activation associated with electro-acupuncture in somatosensory areas, motor area, brainstem, cingulate or insula and one study [66] found no significant difference. Regarding brain deactivations, two studies [66,69] showed manual acupuncture was associated with more deactivation in the limbic system [69], cuneus [66], transverse temporal gyrus [66] or middle frontal gyrus [66], yet two studies [58,69] also showed more deactivation from electro-acupuncture in the septal area or precuneus.

Comparison of different frequencies of electro-acupuncture stimulation. Two studies compared different electro-acupuncture frequencies. Napadow et al. [58] found that the brainstem was more activated at 2 Hz than at 100 Hz. But Li et al. [66] found no significant difference between 2 Hz and 20 Hz.

Comparison of different intensities of manual acupuncture stimulation. Of six studies one study [70] observed that a longer duration of manipulation induced more activation in the inferior frontal, temporal, parietal gyrus, occipital lobe, cerebellum or temporal pole and more deactivation in the prefrontal cortex, orbital gyrus or pons than shorter manipulation. Four studies [42,71–73] found more activation in the somatosensory areas, limbic system, visual, language areas or higher cognitive areas in response to stimulation compared to no stimulation. The last study [74] showed that stimulation which induced deqi by maximum manipulation was associated with more activation in the postcentral gyrus and the limbic system than stimulation that didn't induce deqi with minimum manipulation.

Descriptive findings of differences between patients and healthy volunteers

All seven studies comparing healthy volunteers with patients showed that patients responded differently (See Table 2). According to Wang et al. [75] the frontal lobe was activated in stroke patients while motor areas were activated in healthy volunteers. Fu et al. [76] found patients with Alzheimer's disease had more activation in the cingulate gyrus and cerebellum. Liu et al. [77] found more robust activation in the hypothalamus in heroin addicts. Wu et al. [78] found deactivation in primary motor cortex (M1), parahippocampal gyrus, and higher cognitive areas and more activation in the cuneus and the insula in children with spastic cerebral palsy but not in healthy children. Conversely,

more activation in caudate nucleus, thalamus and cerebellum was found in healthy children. Napadow et al. [79] compared patients with carpal tunnel syndrome (CTS) before and after five weeks' acupuncture to healthy volunteers receiving no treatment. Following acupuncture, a significant decrease in the activation area was found in contralateral primary somatosensory cortex (SI) and M1 in the CTS patients, as well as, increased separation between digit 3 and digit 2 cortical representations in SI, suggesting acupuncture-induced neuroplasticity. In addition, Napadow et al. compared manual acupuncture to cutaneous stimulation on both CTS patients and healthy volunteers. They found that CTS patients responded to verum acupuncture with less deactivation in the amygdala and greater activation in the lateral hypothalamic area [80], compared to healthy subjects. Moreover, CTS patients responded to sham acupuncture with greater activation in the somatosensory areas, cognitive and affective areas. Li et al. [17] found that stroke patients had more activation in the SI than healthy volunteers when both groups underwent both verum and sham acupuncture.

Descriptive findings of differences between different acupuncture points

The data on acupuncture point specific changes in brain activation and deactivation are shown in Table S2, originating from 76 publications [15,16,22,24,27,31,33,42,45–47,51–53,55,57–59,61,63,64,67,69,81–107] [29,34,37,39,40,43,73,108–126] addressing 37 acupuncture points. Acupuncture points along the 12 regular meridians and one extra meridian (Du meridian) were assessed. The data showed changes in brain activity for each individual acupuncture point from respective publications. The most studied points were LI4, ST36, PC6, LR3 and GB34. These points have a wide clinical applicability and are frequently used in clinical practice. Overall the data showed that acupuncture stimulation mainly influenced the brain activity of the somatosensory areas, motor areas, auditory areas, visual areas, cerebellum, the limbic system and higher cognitive areas.

Furthermore, we generated on a descriptive level map (Figure 3) of 18 acupuncture points from 46 publications, which reported pre-post data on Talairach coordinates. These 18 points were located along 9 meridians. The brain maps of each acupuncture point differ considerably from each other. However, the acupuncture points on the same meridian showed some similarities among the activation/deactivation pattern. For example, the points on the stomach meridian showed activation in the supramarginal gyrus and deactivation in the posterior cingulate, hippocampus, and parahippocampus. In addition, the vision related points GB37 and UB60 showed deactivation in the visual areas such as the cuneus.

Descriptive findings of other comparisons and results

Besides our four main research questions, there are more research findings worth mentioning: comparisons between acupuncture and other stimulations; comparisons of acupuncture under different consciousness states; acupuncture at different time points; acupuncture at group of points; acupuncture effect correlated to expectation. Moreover, resting state functional connectivity was also investigated in several recently published papers.

Acupuncture vs. visual stimulation. Of four studies, Bai et al. [127] compared the stimulation phase and the resting phase of acupuncture stimulation and visual stimulation and found the BOLD signal returned to near-baseline values shortly after the visual stimulus, but for acupuncture stimulation the resting phase activities might be even higher than that of the stimulation phases.

Table 1. Descriptive analysis of differences due to various methods of acupuncture manipulation.

Author (year)	Language	Studyplace	Study design	Case NO.	Group NO.	Intervention	Control	Points	Statistic	Group differences which result in more activation	Group differences which result in more deactivation
a) Comparison of Different Needling Depths											
Li et al. 2000	C	CN	NCT	26	2	MA (muscle layer)	MA (round tip, non-penetrating, stimulating between the epidermis and dermis)	ST36, ST32	NA	NSD	NSD
MacPherson et al. 2008	E	UK	RIO, PB	17	2	MA (8–12 mm)	MA (1–2 mm)	LI4 (R)	Y	NSD	NSD
Zhang et al. 2007	E	CN	NCT,PB	12	2	EA (2–3 cm)	EA (subcutaneous)	GB34, GB39 (L)	Y	EA (2–3 cm)>EA (subcutaneous): Con. SI, SII, MC, ant. CingC, IN, Th, H, OC, Ce; Bil. PFG, Cau and P	NSD
Wu et al. 1999	E	CN	Semi-RIO, PB	18	2	MA (2 cm)	MA (1 mm)	ST36 (L)	NA	1) MA (2 cm)>MA (1 mm): Con. Hyp. Nac; 2) MA (1 mm)>MA (2 cm): SI, Th, ant. CingC (BA 32, 34); Con. SMA; Bil. Fop (BA44 and SMA), PO (BA40)	1)MA (2 cm)>MA (1 mm): Bil. Ant. CingC (rostral part, BA 24B), Ipsi. OG, BG, Con. Amyg. H
b) Comparison of Electro-acupuncture vs. Manual Acupuncture											
Kong et al. 2002	E	CN	RIO	11	2	MA (3 Hz, 180 rpm)	EA (3 Hz)	LI4 (L)	Y	EA>MA: Con. preCG; SII (CO, PO); Ipsi. Put/In	1) MA>EA: Con. STG and Put/IN, post. Cing, STG and Ipsi. LN/In; 2) EA>MA: Con. preCun
Li et al. 2003	E	CN	NCT	20	3	MA	1) EA (2 Hz); 2) EA (20 Hz)	BL60, 65, 66, 67 (R)	Y	NSD	MA>2 EA groups: Bil. Cun(BA18), TTG (BA41), MFG (BA46)
Napadow et al. 2005	E	US	NCT, PB	13	3	MA (ERRM, 1 Hz)	1) EA (2 Hz); 2) EA (100 Hz)	ST36 (L)	Y	1) EA 2 Hz >MA: SI, Con. Cing-am, NRP; 2) EA 100 Hz>MA: SI, Con. Cing-am	EA>MA: septal area
c) Comparison of Different Frequencies of Electro-acupuncture Stimulation											
Li et al. 2003	E	CN	NCT	20	2	EA (2 Hz)	EA (20 Hz)	BL60, 65, 66, 67 (R)	Y	NSD	NSD
Napadow et al. 2005	E	US	NCT, PB	13	2	EA (2 Hz)	EA (100 Hz)	ST36 (L)	Y	EA 2 Hz>EA 100 Hz: NRP	NA
d) Comparison of Different Intensities of Manual Acupuncture Stimulation											
Li et al 2006	E	CN	RCT/P	18	3	MA (30 s)	1) MA (60 s); 2) MA (180 s)	LI4 (R)	Y	1) 60 s>30 s: Ipsi. IFG,ITG; 2) 180 s>60 s: Bil. Tpole, Ce, OL; 3) 180 s>30 s: Bil. Tpole, Ce, IPL	1) 60 s>30 s: Bil. OG, Ipsi. TL, P; 2) 180 s>60 s: Bil. diPFC, MEFG; 3) 180 s>30 s: Bil. diPFC, MEFG
Gareus et al. 2002	E	DE	NCT	21	2	MA (twisting)+visual stimu (Bil.)	MA (no stimu)+visual stimu (L)	GB37	NA	1) MA(twisting+visual)>MA(no stimu+visual): IN, PO, PTC, IPL, supCol, Cun, MOG, CingG	NA

Table 1. Cont.

Author (year)	Language	Studyplace	Study design	Case NO.	Group NO.	Intervention	Control	Points	Statistic	Group differences which result in more activation	Group differences which result in more deactivation
Hu et al. 2005	C	CN	RCT	19	3	MA(twirling, 120–200 rpm) (Bil.)	1) MA (no stimu) +visual stimu (L); 2) MA (no stimu)+visual stimu (Bil.)	GB37, LR3	Y	MA>MA (no stimuli)+ visual stimuli (L/Bil.): V1	NA
Fang et al. 2004	E	CN	RIO, PB	15	2	MA (ERRM, rotating, 2 Hz)	MA (no stimu)	LR3, GB40 (L)	Y	*MA(rotating)>MA (no stimu): Bil. SII; Ipsi. FOP(BA10), Ce; Con. Th*	NA
Cheng et al. 2009	C	CN	NCT	12	2	MA (rotating, 1.5 Hz)	MA (no stimu)	KI3 (R)	Y	*MA(rotating)>MA(no stimu): Ipsi. STGNA (BA22); Con. MFG(BA46),IFG(BA45), IPL(BA40); Bil. postCG(BA2,3)*	NA
Gong et al. 2003	C	CN	NCT, PB, OB	64	2	MA (with deqi, 1 cun deep, thrusting and lifting at 0.3– 0.5 cun)	MA (no deqi, 0.4 cun deep, thrusting and lifting at 0.1–0.2 cun)	ST36, ST39 (R)	Y	*deqi>no deqi: Bil. CingC, IN, upper wall of latS, Con. postCG*	NA

Words in italics means statistically significant;

Amyg = Amygdala, ant. = anterior, BA = Brodmann area, BG = basal gyrus, Bil. = bilateral, C = Chinese, Cau = caudate nucleus, Ce = cerebellum, Cing = cingulate gyrus, Cing-am = anterior middle cingulate, CingC = cingulate cortex, CingG = cingulate gyrus, CN = China, CO = central operculum, Con. = contralateral, Cun = cuneus, DE = Germany, dlPFC = dorsolateral prefrontal cortex, E = English, EA = electro-acupuncture, ERRM = even reinforcing and reducing method, Fop = frontal operculum, H = hippocampus, Hyp = hypothalamus, IFG = inferior frontal gyrus, IN = insula, Ipsi = ipsilateral, IPL = inferior parietal lobule, ITG = inferior temporal gyrus, L = left, latS = lateral sulcus, LN = lenticular nucleus, MA = manual acupuncture, MC = motor cortex, MEFG = medial frontal gyrus, MFG = middle frontal gyrus, MOG = middle occipital gyrus, NA = information unavailable, Nac = nucleus accumbens, NCT = non-randomized controlled trial, NRP = nucleus raphe pontis, NSD = non statistically different, OB = observer blinded, OC = occipital cortex, OG = orbital gyrus, OL = occipital lobe, P = pons, PB = patient blinded, PFG = prefrontal gyrus, PO = parietal operculum, postCG = postcentral gyrus, preCG = precentral gyrus, preCun = precuneus, PTC = parieto-temporal cortex, Put = putamen, R = right, RCT/P = parallel group randomized trial, RIO = randomized intervention order, rpm = rotations per minute, SI = primary somatosensory area, SII = second somatosensory area, SMA = supplementary motor area, stimu = stimulation, STG = superior temporal gyrus, supCol = superior colliculi, Th = thalamus, TL = temporal lobe, Tpole = temporal pole, TTG = transverse temporal gyri, V1 = primary visual cortices, Y = yes.

Table 2. Descriptive analysis of differences between patients and healthy volunteers.

Author (year)	Language	Studyplace	Studydesign	Pat.NO.	HVNO.	Disease	Intervention	Control	Statistic	Response for both groups	Differences for both groups
Wang et al. 2004	C	CN	NCT	17	20	lesions in left central sulcus	EA (1 Hz, 0.1–03mA) ST36, GB34 (R)	N	Y	NA	Activation:1) Pat.Con. FL (the areas which are near the lesions and 3 cm anterior to central sulcus); 2) HV: SMA, MC
Fu et al. 2005	C	CN	NCT	6	6	Alzheimer's disease	EA (1 Hz) PC6 (R)	N	Y	Activation:Bil. TL, FL	Activation: Pat.>HV: CingG, Ce
Liu et al. 2007	E	CN	NCT	6	6	heroin addicts	MA ST36 (L)	N	Y	Activation:Con. Hyp, Th, paraHG	Activation:1)Pat.>HV: Con. Hyp; 2)HV>Pat. Con. Th, paraHG
Napadow et al. 2007*	E	US	NCT	13	12	Carpal tunnel syndrome	Electro-stimuli 100 Hz (Digit2, Digit3, Digit5) (Pat.: affected side; HV: dominant hand side)	N	Y	NA	1) Pat.: stimulating Digit3, decreased extent of activation: BA1, BA4; 2) no significant change in HV
Wu et al. 2008	E	CN	NCT	11	10	spastic cerebral palsy	MA (ERRM, rotating 2 Hz) LR3 (L)	N	Y	Activation:Con. STG(BA22); Ipsi. H	1) Deactivation:Pat.>HV:Bil. MFG (BA10),preCG(BA4); Con. MTG(BA21), paraHG; Ipsi. SFG(BA8), IFG(BA46); 2) Activation:Pat.>HV: Bil. OL(Cunl): Ipsi. IN ; HV> Pat.:Bil. Cau, Th, Ce
Napadow et al. 2007	E	US	NCT	13	12	Carpal tunnel syndrome	MA (1.5 cm 1 Hz) LI4 (Pat.:affected side, HV: dominant hand side)	CS (1 Hz, monofilament) LI4 (Pat.:affected side, HV: dominant hand side)	Y	1)Activation:Con.LHA; 2) Deactivation:Con Amyg; pgACC, amACC, rspPCC, dlPFC, vmPFC, ant. IN, septal area, SI, SMA, Th	1) Activation:Pat.>HV: LHA; 2) Deactivation:HV> Pat. :Amyg
Li et al. 2006	E	CN	NCT	12	12	Stroke	EA (2 Hz) LI4,LI11 (L)	CS (1 Hz rough sponge brushing finger and palm) (L)	Y	Activation:CS> EA:Con. M1, SI	Activation: Pat.>HV: SI (for both CS and EA)

*published in Human Brain Mapping.
Words in italics means statistically significant;

amACC = anterior-middle anterior cingulate cortex, Amyg = Amygdala, BA = Brodmann area, Bil. = bilateral, C = Chinese, Cau = caudate nucleus, Ce = cerebellum, CingG = cingulate gyrus, CN = China, Con. = contralateral, CS = cutaneous stimulation, dlPFC = dorsolateral prefrontal cortex, EA = electro-acupuncture, ERRM = even reinforcing and reducing method, FL = frontal lobe, H = hippocampus, HV = healthy volunteers, Hyp = hypothalamus, IFG = inferior frontal gyrus, IN = insula, Ipsi. = ipsilateral, L = left, LHA = lateral hypothalamic area, M1 = primary motor cortex, MA = manual acupuncture, MC = motor cortex, MFG = middle frontal gyrus, MTG = middle temporal gyrus, N = no, NA = information unavailable, NCT = non-randomized controlled trial, OL = occipital lobe, paraHG = parahippocampal gyrus, Pat. = patient, pgACC = pregenual cingulate cortex, preCG = precentral gyrus, R = right, rspPCC = retrosplenial posterior cingulate cortex, SI = primary somatosensory area, SFG = superior frontal gyrus, SMA = supplementary motor area, STG = superior temporal gyrus, Th = thalamus, TL = temporal lobe, vmPFC = ventromedial prefrontal cortex, Y = yes.

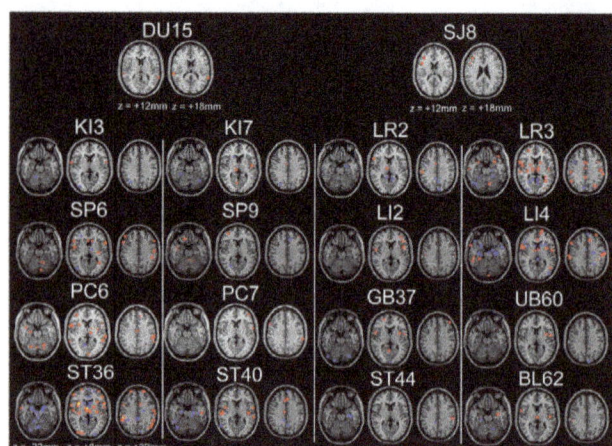

Figure 3. Map of brain response to 18 different acupuncture points. Red: activation; Blue: deactivation; Yellow: overlap.

Hu et al. [71] and Gareus et al. [72] had contradictory results. Surprisingly, Hu et al. [71] reported no significant activation in the visual cortex during visual stimulation but from acupuncture stimulation, whereas Gareus et al. [72] found no activation in the visual cortex during acupuncture stimulation, and activation from visual stimulation. Li et al. [66] found both visual stimulation and acupuncture could activate the visual cortex.

Acupuncture vs. word generation paradigm. One study from Li et al. [29] found acupuncture at language specific acupuncture points SJ8 and Du15 did not activate the typical language areas in the left inferior frontal cortex which were activated during a word-generation task.

Acupuncture vs. finger tapping. Of three studies, both Kong et al. [39] and Hu et al. [81] found finger-tapping task can produce more reliable fMRI signal changes than that evoked by electro-acupuncture stimulation. However, Wang et al. [128] found no significant difference between electro-acupuncture at ST36, GB34 and a finger-tapping task.

Acupuncture in different states of consciousness (awake or anesthetized). One study from Wang et al. [129] compared healthy subjects who underwent acupuncture at ST36 in two different consciousness states. The result showed activation in the awake state was greater than under anesthetic in the somatosensory area, the limbic system and basal ganglia.

Acupuncture at different time points. One study from Zeng et al. [130] compared acupuncture at KI3 and KI7 at two different time points – "open point time" and "closed point time" (the open or closed time point is determined by the Chinese medicine theory "Zi-Wu-Liu-Zhu"—the body's Qi and blood circulation schedule; acupuncture at the open point time results in maximum clinical effect and vice versa) [1]. The result showed acupuncture at "open point time" was associated with more deactivation in the frontal lobe, temporal lobe, cingulate cortex and cerebellum than acupuncture at the "closed point time".

Acupuncture of group of points. In 29 papers [25,35,38,44,49,62,65,68,71,74,75,93,100,109,130–144] more than one acupuncture point was stimulated simultaneously. Of these groups of points, some were functional related, some were on the same meridian, some had close locations for electric stimulation, few were real acupuncture clinical formula. 15 of these 29 papers were included among our first four main questions. Overall the results of these studies were very

heterogeneous and only three studies [93,109,136] reported an interaction effect between acupuncture points.

Acupuncture effect correlated to expectations. Three studies by Kong et al. [145–147] applied an expectancy model, and found positive expectation can increase acupuncture analgesia based on the objective fMRI signal changes in response to noxious stimuli. The study indicated that different mechanisms exist between acupuncture analgesia and expectancy evoked placebo analgesia. For the verum acupuncture group, there were only a few small differences (in primary motor cortex and middle frontal gyrus) between the high expectancy side and low expectancy side. However, for the sham acupuncture group, more differences were observed in contralateral operculum, ipsilateral insula, inferior frontal gyrus, medial frontal gyrus and superior frontal gyrus. So this result suggested expectancy might involve distinct mechanisms between verum acupuncture and sham acupuncture.

Functional connectivity modulated by acupuncture. Eight studies investigated functional connectivity of resting state. One of the first such studies (Dhond et al. study [57]) found that verum acupuncture, but not monofilament tapping increased resting state connectivity of the default mode network (DMN) to pain, affective and memory related regions of the brain. Verum acupuncture also increased sensorimotor network (SMN) connectivity to pain-related brain regions. Zhang et al. [148] and Bai et al. [149] found that acupuncture stimulation may induce the modulation of the "acupuncture-related" network, represented by significant changes of functional connectivity in several regions of the brain, such as the bilateral frontal gyrus, bilateral temporal gyrus, inferior parietal lobe, middle occipital gyrus, pre- and postcentral gyrus, anterior cingulate cortex (ACC), parahippocampus, insula, tonsil, pyramis, culmen, precuneus and cuneus. Qin et al. [150,151] identified an amygdala-related network during the resting state both after verum and penetrating sham acupuncture at a nearby point. Compared to sham, verum acupuncture increased the connectivity between the amygdala, the PAG (periaqueductal gray) and the insula, and decreased the connectivity between the amygdala with the middle frontal cortex, the postcentral gyrus and the posterior cingulate cortex (PCC). Zhang et al. [119] compared the visual related functional networks between pre- and post- electro-acupuncture on the visual-related point GB37 and the non-visual related point KI8 and described a positive correlation between the pre-post resting states in visual networks for the GB37 group while an anti-correlation for the KI8 group. Liu et al. [152] found a similar result when comparing electro-acupuncture at GB37 and KI8. In addition, in a later study Liu et al. [153] reported that the DMN could be modulated after electro-acupuncture at the three acupuncture points (GB37, BL60 and KI8) and at a nearby sham point. As for intrinsic connectivity, the PCC and precuneus strongly interacted with other nodes during the pre- and post-stimulation states. The correlation was interrupted between the PCC/precuneus and the ACC. The orbital prefrontal cortex negatively interacted with the left medial temporal cortex only at the acupuncture points.

Results from the ALE meta-analysis

A total of 34 studies were eligible for the inclusion criteria for the ALE meta-analyses (Table 3). A total of 10 meta-analyses were performed.

The meta-analysis for verum acupuncture stimuli on greater activation of verum acupuncture points compared to baseline (1a, verum>rest) included 36 experiments, 377 subjects and 470 foci. The result showed significant convergence in the supramarginal gyrus, secondary somatosensory cortex (SII), pre-supplementary

Table 3. Studies included in the ALE meta-analyses.

Author (year)	Intervention (verum)	Control (sham)	Subjects Intervention	Subjects Control	Contrast Pre-post	Contrast Between group	Included in following meta-analyses
Wang et al. 2007	EA(5 Hz random wave, 1–3mA) LI4 (R)	sham EA (5 Hz random wave, 1–3mA), NAP (1 cm apart from the right corner of the mouth) (R)	5	5	verum>rest; rest>verum; sham>rest; rest>sham		1a/b; 3a/b/c/d/e/f
Wang et al. 2006	MA (2.54 cm, ERRM, 1 Hz) LR3 (R)	sham MA, NAP (near LR3) (R)	10	10	verum>rest; sham>rest		1 a; 3a/c/e
Zhang et al. 2005	EA (3 cm, 2 Hz, 10 V), GB34, GB39 (L)	sham EA (3 cm, 2 Hz, 10 V), NAPs (3–4 cm lateral to GB34, GB39 respectively) (L)	16	18	verum>rest; rest>verum; sham>rest; rest>sham		1a/b; 3a/b/c/d/e/f
Hui et al. 2005	MA (2–3 cm, rotating 60 rpm) ST36 (R)	CS (tapping, monofilament), ST36 (R)	11	11	verum>rest; rest>verum; sham>rest; rest>sham		1a/b; 3a/b/c/d/e/f
Yoo et al. 2004	MA (1 cm, rotating, 2 Hz) PC6 (R)	1) sham MA (1 cm, rotating, 2 Hz), NAP (1.5–2 cm interior to PC6) (R); 2) CS (brushing, 2 Hz, monofilament) area unclear	12	12	verum>rest; sham>rest	verum>sham	1a; 2a; 3a/c/e
Wu et al. 1999	MA (1 cm, ERRM, 1–2 Hz) LI4 (L)	sham MA (5 mm, manipulation lightly), NAP (2–3 cm lateral fromST35) (L)	9	9	verum>rest; rest>verum; sham>rest		1a/b; 3a/b/c/e/f
Wu et al. 2002	EA (2–3 cm, 4 Hz) GB34 (L)	1) sham EA (2–3 cm, 4 Hz) NAP (4–5 cm lateral from GB34) (L); 2) mini EA (0.3–0.5 cm, 4 Hz, mini CUR), NAP (4–5 cm from sham point)	15	15	verum>rest; sham>rest	verum>sham	1a; 2a; 3a/c/e
Wang et al. 2009	EA (2 Hz, 0.8–1.8mA, continuous wave) ST42, ST36 (R)	sham EA (2 Hz, 0.8–1.8mA, continuous wave), NAP (at the depression inferior and posterior to the Capitula fibula), NAP (1 cun below GB 40)	30	10	verum>rest; rest>verum; sham>rest;		1a/b; 3a/b/c/e/f
Fang et al. 2008	MA (2–4 mm, rotating 160 rpm) LR3, LR2, ST44 (L)	sham MA(2–4 mm, rotating 160 rpm), NAP (metatarsal III and IV on the dorsum of the left foot) (L)	10	10	verum>rest; rest>verum; sham>rest; rest>sham		1a/b; 3a/b/c/d/e/f
Guan et al. 2008	EA (2 Hz, 10–20mA) GB37 (Bil)	sham EA (2 Hz, 10–20mA), NAP (Bil)	8	8	verum>rest; sham>rest		1a; 3a/c/e
Kong et al. 2007	EA (2 Hz) UB60, GB37 (R)	sham EA (2 Hz), NAP(1.5 cm post. and inf. to the small head of the fibula) (R)	6	6	verum>rest; rest>verum; sham>rest; rest>sham		1a/b; 3a/b/c/d/e/f
Fukunaga et al. 1999	EA (10–15 mm, 4 Hz) LI4 (R)	CS (brushing, cosmetic brush 4 Hz) LI4 (R)	17	17	verum>rest; sham>rest		1a; 3a/c/e
Napadow et al. 2005	MA (ERRM, 1 Hz/ 2 Hz/100 Hz) ST36 (L)	CS (tapping, 1 Hz, monofilament) ST36 (L)	13	13	verum>rest; rest>verum; sham>rest;		1a/b; 3a/b/c/e/f
Chae et al. 2009	MA (0.8 cm, rotating 1 Hz) LR2 (L)	CS (unclear) LR2 (L)	10	10		verum>sham	2a
Chae et al. 2009	MA (0.8 cm, rotating 1 Hz) LR2 (L)	1) CS: covert (rotating 1 Hz) LR2 (L); 2) CS: overt (rotating 1 Hz) LR2 (L)	10	10		verum>sham	2a

Table 3. Cont.

Author (year)	Intervention (verum)	Control (sham)	Subjects Intervention	Control	Contrast Pre-post	Between group	Included in following meta-analyses
Li et al. 2008	1) MA ST36 (R); 2) MA ST43 (R); 3) MA LR3 (R) 4) MA LR6 (R)	1) sham MA, NAP (dorsum between the first and second metatarsals, approximately 10 mm from the 2 real acupoints: ST43, LR3) (R); 2) sham MA, NAP (near ST36 and LR6) (R), same manipulation	1)9; 2) 9; 3)10; 4)8	1)7; 2)8		verum>sham	2a
Li et al. 2008	1) MA (15 mm, rotating,1 Hz) ST43 (R); 2) MA (15 mm, rotating,1 Hz) ST44 (R)	sham MA (15 mm, rotating,1 Hz) NAP (10 mm beside the two points)	1)9; 2)9	7		verum>sham	2a
Yan et al. 2005	1) MA (15 mm, ERRM, 1 Hz; 2)) MA (15 mm, ERRM, 1 Hz) LR3 (R)	1)sham MA (15 mm, ERRM, 1 Hz), NAP1 (10 mm anterior to LR3) (R); 2) sham MA (15 mm, ERRM, 1 Hz), NAP2(10 mm anterior to LI4) (R)	1)8; 2)10	1)7; 2)9		verum>sham; sham>verum	2a/b
Lu et al. 2008	MA (15 mm, ERRM, 1 Hz) LR6 (R)	sham MA (15 mm, ERRM, 1 Hz), NAP (lateral to LR6) (R)	8	8		verum>sham	2a
Dougherty et al. 2008	MA (ERRM, 180 rpm) LI4 (R)	Streitberger needle LI4 (R), manipulation gentely	6	6		verum>sham; sham>verum	2a/b
Napadow et al. 2009	MA (1.5 cm, rotating, 0.5 Hz) PC6 (L)	CS (tapping, 0.5 Hz, monofilament) PC6 (L)	15	15		verum>sham	2a
Wang et al. 2005	MA (rotating, 2 Hz) BL62 (R)		6		verum>rest; rest>verum;		1a/b
Hou et al. 2002	MA (rotating, 2 Hz) LI4 (R)		6		verum>rest; rest>verum		1a
Kong et al. 2002	1)MA (rotating, 3 Hz) LI4 (L); 2) EA (3 Hz) LI4 (L)		11		verum>rest; rest>verum;		1a/b
Zhang et al. 2007	MA (25 mm) LI4, PC6, SP6, ST36 (R)		11		verum>rest; rest>verum;		1a/b
Li et al. 2005	MA (15 mm, ERRM, 1 Hz) LI4 (R)		6		verum>rest; rest>verum;		1a/b
MacPherson et al. 2008	MA (8–12 mm) LI4 (R)		17		verum>rest; rest>verum;		1a/b
Wu et al. 2007	MA (1.2cun) ST36 (R)		11		verum>rest; rest>verum;		1a/b
Chen et al. 2008	MA (0.3–0.5 cm, ERRM, 1–2 Hz) PC7 (R)		8		verum>rest		1a
Wang et al. 2007	EA (5 Hz, 1–3mA) LI4 (R)		6		verum>rest; rest>verum;		1a/b
Wu et al. 2008	MA (1.2cun) ST36, ST40 (R)		12		verum>rest		1a
Li et al. 2003	1) EA (2 Hz) SJ8 2) EA (2 Hz) DU15		18		verum>rest		1a

Table 3. Cont.

Author (year)	Intervention (verum)	Control (sham)	Subjects		Contrast		Included in following meta-analyses
			Intervention	Control	Pre-post	Between group	
Deng et al. 2008	MA LI2 (non-dominant hand side)		13		verum>rest		1a
Li et al. 2006	MA (15 mm, ERRM, 1 Hz, 30 s/60 s/180 s) LI4 (R)		18		verum>rest; rest>verum;		1a/b

CS = cutaneous stimulation, CUR = current, EA = electro-acupuncture, ERRM = even reinforcing and reducing method, L = left, MA = manual acupuncture, NAP = non-acupuncture point, R = right.

motor area (pre-SMA), middle cigulate gyrus, insula, thalamus and precentral gyrus. The meta-analysis for greater deactivation of verum acupuncture points compared to baseline (1b, rest>verum) included 22 experiments, 219 subjects and 265 foci and the result revealed significant convergence in the subgenual anterior cingulate, subgenual cortex, amygdala/hippocampal formation, ventromedial prefrontal cortex (vmPFC), nucleus accumbens, and PCC (Table 4, Figure 4A).

For the direct contrast of verum and sham acupuncture on greater activation from verum than sham acupuncture or greater deactivation for sham acupuncture (2a, verum>sham) we included in the meta-analysis 17 experiments, 156 subjects and 171 foci, resulting in significant convergence in fusiform gyrus, cerebellum, SI and middle cingulate gyrus. Whereas, on greater deactivation from verum than sham acupuncture or greater activation for sham (2b, sham>verum, 21 subjects, 3 experiments and 27 foci) the result showed significant convergence in supramarginal gyrus, superior temporal gyrus and cuneus (Table 5, Figure 4B).

The Subtraction analysis for verum versus sham acupuncture included in the first step analyses 3a–d for the pre-post contrast on verum or sham acupuncture compared to baseline (Table 5, Figure 4C). The analysis of greater activation of verum acupuncture than baseline (3a, verum>rest) included 234 subjects, 20 experiments and 305 foci and revealed significant convergence in middle cingulate gyrus, pre-SMA, superior temporal gyrus, supramarginal gyrus, SII, thalamus and insula. The analysis of greater deactivation of verum acupuncture compared to baseline (3b, rest>verum, 172 subjects, 15 experiments and 222 foci) came to the following significant convergence: subgenual anterior cingulate, amygdala/hippocampal formation, vmPFC and PCC. Comparing results on greater activation of sham acupuncture points than baseline (3c, sham>rest) from 164 subjects, 15 experiments and 200 foci, showed significant convergence in cerebellum, supramarginal gyrus, superior temporal gyrus and thalamus. Including data on greater deactivation of sham acupuncture points compared to baseline (3d, rest>sham) from 50 subjects, 5 experiments and 52 foci, resulted in significant convergence in pregenual anterior cingulate, subgenual cortex and parahippocampal gyrus.

Finally, in the contrast (subtraction) comparing the between-group differences for verum and sham acupuncture, significant differences between "verum>rest" and "sham>rest" (3e) as well as between "rest>verum" and "rest>sham" (3f) were identified. The subtraction analysis for "verum>rest" - "sham>rest" showed convergent activations in pre-SMA, middle cingulate gyrus, claustrum, insula, supramarginal gyrus, SII and dorsolateral prefrontal cortex (dlPFC). The subtraction analysis for "rest>verum" - "rest>sham" revealed convergence in amygdala/hippocampal formation (Table 5, Figure 4D).

Discussion

Overall the results indicate that studies on acupuncture neuroimaging are very heterogeneous in terms of the study question, methodology and quality, this is the case in the descriptive analysis as well as in the meta-analysis.

From the descriptive view on the data it seems that compared to sham, verum acupuncture tended to be associated with more activation in the basal ganglia, brain stem, cerebellum, and insula and more deactivation was seen in the so-called "default mode network" and limbic brain areas, such as the amygdala and the hippocampus. In addition, a trend for more robust brain activation with greater intensity of acupuncture stimulation seems to be there. However, electro-acupuncture at low frequency also

Table 4. Clusters showing significant convergence for verum acupuncture points (FDR pN corrected at the cluster level, p<0.05) from ALE meta-analyses.

Brain region	BA	Talairach coordinates			ALE value	Volume (mm³)
		X	y	z		
Verum>rest (1a)						
Supramaginal gyrus/insula/SII	40	54	−26	24	0.0460	15440
	40	−54	−24	20	0.0565	8072
Pre-supplementary motor area/middle cingulate	6	−2	6	48	0.0318	9576
Thalamus		08	−16	8	0.0323	3776
Precentral gyrus	44	−46	−2	8	0.0259	3696
Rest>verum (1b)						
Anterior cingulate	32	0	34	−8	0.0406	6032
Subgenual cortex	25	2	8	−4	0.0202	1304
Amygdala/hippocampal formation		−28	−8	−24	0.0253	3240
Ventromedial prefrontal cortex	10	−2	60	10	0.0261	1728
Posterior cingulate	31	−6	−56	22	0.0188	1120

tended to activate a broader range of brain areas than electro-acupuncture at high frequencies. Furthermore, it looks like that patients responded to acupuncture stimulation with a more robust fMRI response compared to healthy volunteers. Acupuncture at different acupuncture points showed in the studies both similarities and differences between points. Finally, studies also suggested that acupuncture modulated the resting state connectivity within several noted networks including the default mode network, sensorimotor network, and amygdala-related network etc.

From the meta-analyses focusing only on brain response to verum acupuncture stimuli, activation was noted in supramarginal gyrus, SII, pre-SMA, middle cigulate gyrus, insula, thalamus and precentral gyrus, while deactivation was noted in pregenual anterior cingulate, subgenual cortex, amygdala/hippocampal formation, vmPFC, nucleus accumbens and PCC. Acupuncture specific effects were noted by meta-analyses of differences between verum and sham, which showed greater response in middle cingulate for verum compared to sham acupuncture. However, the results were variant within the different meta-analyses. The meta-analyses of direct contrast between verum and sham showed significant convergence for "verum>sham" in fusiform gyrus, cerebellum and SI, while for "sham>verum" in superior temporal gyrus, supramarginal gyrus and cuneus. Whereas, the subtraction meta-analyses of group-derived contrast showed greater activation from verum in pre-SMA, claustrum, insula, supramarginal gyrus, SII, dlPFC, greater deactivation from verum in amygdala/hippocampal formation. This heterogeneity suggests that group-derived contrast for verum and sham acupuncture tended to be above threshold in consistently specific brain areas, but were not significantly different in those areas, when assessed at the single study level.

Strengths and limitations

To our knowledge this is the first systematic and extensive review on fMRI and acupuncture without any language restrictions. Besides the internationally well known databases such as Pubmed and EMBASE, less well known international databases such as the Chinese CNKI, the Japanese Ichushi WEB, and the Korean NDSL and KTKP were searched and the publications found were included in this review. Therefore, this very extensive review provides a transparent and detailed overview of the current literature available. In addition we structured the publications according to the research questions, such as the differences in brain activity associated with acupuncture stimuli between patients and healthy volunteers, to provide a good overview and a strong basis for future study designs, interventions, measurement methods, and possible diagnoses. Moreover, we complemented the systematic and comprehensive literature review with several ALE meta-analyses, providing analytic results for stronger evidence that are supported statistically. However, some studies reported direct contrast between verum and sham acupuncture groups, while some others reported pre-post contrast for each group, resulting in the fact that several meta-analyses had to be performed. The studies included in the descriptive review and the meta-analyses were highly heterogeneous regarding their study design, their aims and their quality of reporting. The reasons for these heterogeneous results are numerous, such as the varying acupuncture manipulation methods, different types of control arms, different methods of acquisition and analyzing the imaging data, the mainly investigated brain regions (region of interest) and the statistical analysis. The large variability between subjects and sessions with respect to the imaging data also needs to be taken into consideration [39,154]. The imprecise nomenclature [155] is sometimes misleading, such as activation, deactivation, changes, baseline. We did not formally assess the quality of the publications, because no valid checklist for this type of research is available, though reporting guidelines are available and should be consulted by future research publications [156]. A narrative review including only studies that are considered to be of high quality would have overcome this problem. However the aim of this paper was to provide a systematic and broad overview for the first time using the publications currently available. We believe that many trials included in this review have limitations regarding their study design, analysis and reporting of their results. Hence, our results have to be interpreted with care. This is underlined by the multitude of contradictory results. Lastly, the field of research on brain imaging for acupuncture is evolving rapidly which may indeed lessen the relevance of older results using sub-optimal methodologies and analysis techniques.

Figure 4. Results from the ALE meta-analyses. Meta-analyses were performed to evaluate brain response to acupuncture across studies, and contrast verum and sham acupuncture. (A) Brain response to verum acupuncture demonstrated activation in sensorimotor and affective/salience processing brain regions and deactivation in the amygdala and DMN brain regions. (B) Differences in brain response for verum and sham acupuncture from direct contrast showed significance in somatosensory areas, limbic regions, visual processing regions and cerebellum. (C) Brain response to verum and sham acupuncture individually demonstrated activation in sensorimotor and affective/salience processing brain regions and deactivation in the amygdala and DMN brain regions associated with verum acupuncture; while sham acupuncture produced activation in somatosensory regions, affective/salience processing regions, cerebellum and deactivation in limbic regions. (D) Differences in brain response between verum and sham acupuncture from subtraction analysis showed more activation in the sensorimotor affective/cognitive processing brain regions and more deactivation in the amygdala/hippocampal formation for verum acupuncture. For subfigures A–C, p<0.05, cluster level FDR corrected, color bar showed ALE value; for subfigure D, p<0.05, cluster level uncorrected, color bar showed Z value. Amyg: amygdala; Ce: cerebellum; dlPFC: dorsolateral prefrontal cortex; FG: fusiform gyrus; H: hippocampal formation; IN: insula; MCC: middle cingulate cortex; Nac: nucleus accumbens; paraHG: parahippocampal gyrus; PCC: posterior cingulate cortex; preCG: precentral gyrus; pre-SMA: pre-supplementary motor area; SI: primary somatosensory cortex; SII: secondary somatosensory cortex; sgACC: subgenual anterior cingulate cortex; SMG: supramarginal gyrus; Th: thalamus; vmPFC: ventromedial prefrontal cortex.

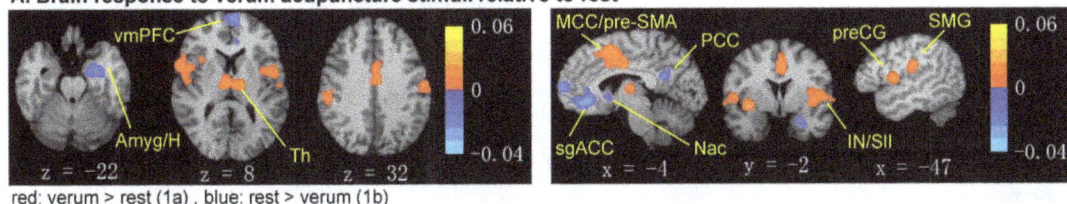

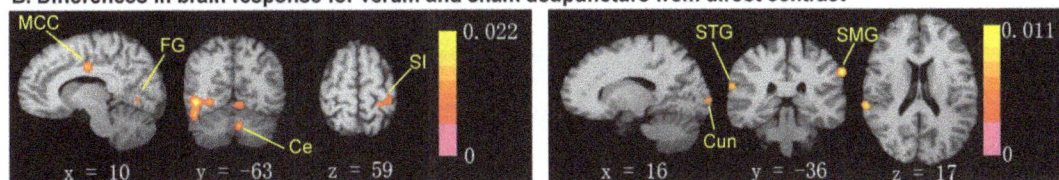

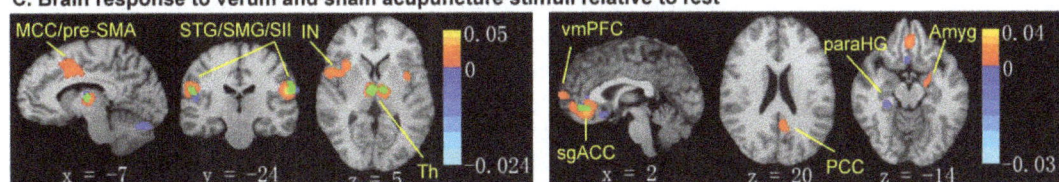

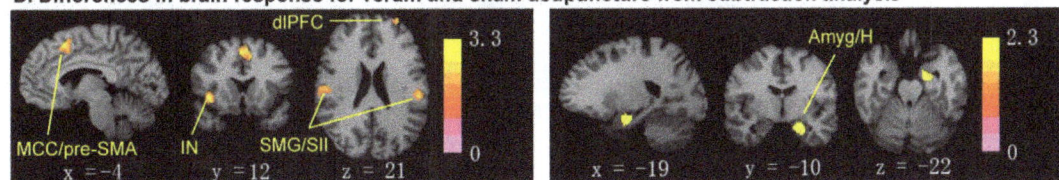

Discussion of results

The studies on BOLD activation and deactivation from a single point or a group of points came mainly from China and Korea. The controlled studies, including sham acupuncture as a control, were mainly from China and the US: the Chinese studies mainly used penetrating sham at a nearby non-acupuncture point as a control while the US studies mainly applied the non-penetrating Streitberger needle or monofilament tapping at the same acupuncture points. Studies on patients were mainly from China. Although we did not evaluate the quality of the publications, the papers published in English used a clearer reporting style than those published in other languages. The most innovative studies came from the US. These studies had clear study questions and

explored acupuncture neurocorrelates with a pain matrix, expectation, autonomic regulation, somatosensory perception and deqi related brain response.

While in the descriptive analysis similarities were observed in the brain response to stimulation at different acupuncture points, some differences across points were also noted. For example, brain deactivation observed in the visual areas (precuneus, cuneus) appeared not only when the vision related points (GB37, UB60) were needled, but also when several non-vision related points (LR2, LR3, ST36) were needled, but not with the other points. One could argue, based on TCM theory, that for the two points on liver meridian (LR2, LR3), the liver opens into the eyes, reflecting its physiological and pathological conditions [157]. The

Table 5. Clusters showing significant convergence for verum versus sham acupuncture (FDR pN corrected at the cluster level, p<0.05) from ALE meta-analyses.

Brain region	BA	Talairach coordinates			ALE value	Z value	Volume (mm³)
		x	y	z			
Direct comparision verum>sham (2a)							
Fusiform gyrus	37	44	−64	−6	0.0197		3720
Culmen of Vermis		−2	−66	−10	0.0160		1520
Cerebellar tonsil		−4	−58	−32	0.0224		1240
Postcentral gyrus	3	−20	−36	64	0.0116		992
Middle cingulate	24	10	−12	34	0.0165		904
Direct comparision sham>verum (2b)							
Supramarginal gyrus	40	−62	−34	34	0.0108		1120
Superior temporal gyrus	42	64	−34	20	0.0088		552
Cuneus	18	18	−98	0	0.0069		400
Verum>rest (3a)							
Middle cingulate/Pre-supplementary motor area	24	−2	2	38	0.0353		7392
Superior temporal gyrus	22	50	6	2	0.0262		6232
Supramarginal gyrus/SII	40	−54	−22	18	0.0484		6040
	40	56	−26	22	0.0402		4080
Thalamus		−8	−16	6	0.0326		4504
Insula	13	−38	−4	0	0.0177		2056
Sham>rest (3c)							
Tuber of vermis		0	−70	−24	0.0239		2664
Supramarginal gyrus/SII	40	−60	−22	22	0.0159		2424
Superior temporal gyrus	41	50	−32	16	0.0168		2320
	22	−52	10	−2	0.0180		808
Thalamus		6	−14	8	0.0206		1848
Rest>verum (3b)							
Anterior cingulate	32	0	32	−8	0.0413		5400
Amygdala/hippocampal formation	34	−18	−8	−20	0.0262		2632
Ventromedial prefrontal cortex	10	−2	60	10	0.0260		1784
Posterior cingulate	31	−6	−56	22	0.0193		1288
Rest>sham (3d)							
Anterior cingulate	32	−4	40	−2	0.0128		1720
Parahippocampal gyrus	36	28	−32	−14	0.0110		392
Subcallosal gyrus	25	4	14	−12	0.0108		360
"Verum>rest" – "sham>rest" (3e)*							
Pre-supplementary motor area/middle cingulate	6	4	12	46		2.7822	2120
Claustrum/insula		32	5	−1		3.2905	1848
Supramarginal gyrus/SII	40	−52	−26	22		2.4181	1728
	40	54	−18	24		2.2904	1168
Dorsolateral prefrontal cortex	10	−28	57	23		2.2383	568
"Rest>verum" – "rest>sham" (3f)*							
Amygdala/hippocampal formation	34	−14	−9	−20		2.2768	1104

*uncorrected p<0.05.

stimulation of different acupoints in the same spinal segment could induce different fMRI activation patterns in the brain [142] while acupoints on the same meridian show some similarities in the activation/deactivation pattern [23].

The meta-analyses could only be done for publications that provided Talairach data, which was not the case for all of our study questions. The meta-analyses on the specific effect of acupuncture that compared verum and sham acupuncture came up with heterogeneous results. The subtraction analyses reflected descriptive results more than the direct contrast analyses. For example, subtraction meta-analyses confirmed more activation from verum in basal ganglia and insula, more deactivation in the limbic region of amygdala/hippocampal formation associated with verum, while meta-analyses of direct contrast for verum and sham confirmed more activation in cerebellum associated with verum. The convergence of brain regions shown for these meta-analyses comparing verum and sham acupuncture overlapped for middle cingulate gyrus. The first reason for the heterogeneous results might be the literature heterogeneity. Only two publications had both pre-post and between-group comparison results [15,37]. Also, the different methods of acupuncture stimuli may have a strong impact of the result. Moreover, the direct contrast "verum>sham" included either more activation from verum or more deactivation from the sham. Thus, the results of direct contrast "verum>sham" and subtraction analysis "verum>rest" – "sham>rest" are not directly comparable. The ALE subtraction analysis for the comparison of verum versus sham acupuncture should be interpreted with caution because the groups are disparate in total number of foci. However, we refrained from randomly extracting experiments from the larger foci set [10], as this might have biased our results substantially. In particular, for the "rest>verum" – "rest>sham", extracting 5 experiments out of 15 from "rest>verum" could most probably influence the result by chance. The meta-analysis of direct contrast for "sham> verum" included only three experiments and 27 foci. Hence this analysis might be with not enough power and doesn't represent the general. Nevertheless, we could see that brain regions such as SII, insula, cingulate gyrus, amygdala/hippocampal formation and prefrontal cortices might be important when differentiating the acupuncture specific effect from sham acupuncture. Acupuncture analgesia is considered as one of the most important indications for clinical acupuncture treatment [158], and those brain regions mentioned above are associated with the pain neuromatrix and might contribute in explaining the mechanism of acupuncture specific analgesia.

Comparisons with other reviews

Some of the previous reviews [7,8,159–161] focused on a broader topic of neuroimaging techniques including EEG, PET, SPECT or MEG. Those reviews summarized research questions underlying certain acupuncture mechanisms, such as acupuncture analgesia, acupuncture placebo effect, specificity of meridian and acupuncture points, and acupuncture modulation on brain networks. They displayed the evidence for each research question and cited the relevant literature accordingly. However, in most cases the literature search was not transparently displayed. The other reviews [162–168] focusing on acupuncture and fMRI, had other emphases: Beissner et al. [162] focused on methodological problems, Cho et al. [163] explored neural substrates for hypothalamus-pituitary-adrenal axis and Chae et al. [164] reviewed traditional Korean acupuncture. The four Chinese narrative reviews on fMRI and acupuncture [165–168] discussed several research questions on the specific effects of acupuncture, such as different acupuncture points, manipulation methods, deqi or not deqi, and sham acupuncture. Our systematic literature review aimed to display the available studies as broad as possible and should offer a better and deeper overview on this topic, thus supporting future studies.

Methodological consideration regarding future studies

One of the advantages for fMRI is that there are multiple possibilities by which experiments can be designed and data analyzed, providing information on different aspects of brain physiology. However, the inherent heterogeneity can complicate subsequent reviews and meta-analyses. Certain basic guidelines on proper statistical analyses of fMRI data should be followed, such as calculating difference maps if two conditions, such as brain response to stimulation at different acupoints, are to be contrasted. Furthermore, as suggested by Poldrack et al., publications relating to fMRI investigations of acupuncture should report all pertinent information relating to both imaging and acupuncture procedures [156]. Important topics include design and task specification, planned group comparisons, behavioral performance metrics, imaging details, data pre-processing, intersubject registration, statistical modeling details for both the individual and group level, and statistical inference including approach to multiple comparisons correction. Adoption of these guidelines will improve manuscript reviews and shorten the time to acceptance (or rejection), as well as facilitate the inclusion of publications in future reviews and meta-analyses.

Conclusion

Brain response to acupuncture stimuli encompasses a broad network of regions consistent with not just somatosensory, but also affective and cognitive processing. While published results on acupuncture and fMRI were heterogeneous, from a descriptive perspective most studies suggest that acupuncture can modulate the brain activity within specific brain areas, and the evidence based on meta-analyses confirmed part of these results. Future studies should further improve methodological aspects and reporting related to both fMRI and acupuncture, and strictly control experimental conditions for more robust inference. Specifically, direct contrast analyses should be used to contrast different stimulus conditions (e.g. verum versus sham acupuncture) when evaluating research questions concerning acupuncture specificity.

Supporting Information

Table S1   Descriptive analysis of differences between verum and sham acupuncture.
(DOCX)

Table S2   Descriptive analysis of changes related to cortical and sub-cortical activation and deactivation at verum acupuncture points.
(DOCX)

Acknowledgments

We would like to thank the authors who provided us further details about their trial for our meta-analyses.

Author Contributions

Conceived and designed the experiments: WJH CW DP. Analyzed the data: WJH DP VN KP XYL JN YM CW. Wrote the paper: WJH DP VN KP XYL JN YM TN FRL CW. Data extraction: WJH DP KP YM.

References

1.   Liang F (2006) Acupuncture and Moxibustion. Shanghai: Shanghai Scientific and Technical Publishers.

2.   Backer M, Hammes M, Sander D, Funke D, Deppe M, et al. (2004) Changes of cerebrovascular response to visual stimulation in migraineurs after repetitive sessions of somatosensory stimulation (acupuncture): a pilot study. Headache 44: 95–101.

3.   WHO (2002) Acupuncture: Review and Analysis of Reports on Controlled Clinical Trials: World Health Organization. . 87 p.

4.   Linde KSA, Jürgens S, Hoppe A, Brinkhaus B, Witt C, et al. (2005) Acupuncture for Patients with Migraine - A Randomized Trial (ART Migraine). JAMA 293: 2118–2125.

5. Brinkhaus BWC, Jena S, Linde K, Streng A, Wagenpfeil S, et al. (2006) Acupuncture in Patients with Chronic Low Back Pain - A Randomised Controlled Trial. Arch Intern Med 166: 450–457.

6. Melchart D, Streng A, Hoppe A, Brinkhaus B, Witt C, et al. (2005) Acupuncture in patients with tension-type headache: randomised controlled trial. BMJ 331: 376–382.

7. Dhond RP, Kettner N, Napadow V (2007) Neuroimaging acupuncture effects in the human brain. J Altern Complement Med 13: 603–616.

8. Lewith GT, White PJ, Pariente J (2005) Investigating acupuncture using brain imaging techniques: the current state of play. Evid Based Complement Alternat Med 2: 315–319.

9. Eickhoff SB, Laird AR, Grefkes C, Wang LE, Zilles K, et al. (2009) Coordinate-based activation likelihood estimation meta-analysis of neuroimaging data: a random-effects approach based on empirical estimates of spatial uncertainty. Hum Brain Mapp 30: 2907–2926.

10. Laird AR, Fox PM, Price CJ, Glahn DC, Uecker AM, et al. (2005) ALE meta-analysis: controlling the false discovery rate and performing statistical contrasts. Hum Brain Mapp 25: 155–164.

11. Turkeltaub PE, Eden GF, Jones KM, Zeffiro TA (2002) Meta-analysis of the functional neuroanatomy of single-word reading: method and validation. Neuroimage 16: 765–780.

12. Lancaster JL, Tordesillas-Gutierrez D, Martinez M, Salinas F, Evans A, et al. (2007) Bias between MNI and Talairach coordinates analyzed using the ICBM-152 brain template. Hum Brain Mapp 28: 1194–1205.

13. Eickhoff SB, Bzdok D, Laird AR, Roski C, Caspers S, et al. (2011) Co-activation patterns distinguish cortical modules, their connectivity and functional differentiation. Neuroimage 57: 938–949.

14. Streitberger K, Kleinhenz J (1998) Introducing a placebo needle into acupuncture research. Lancet 352: 364–365.

15. Yoo SS, Teh EK, Blinder RA, Jolesz FA (2004) Modulation of cerebellar activities by acupuncture stimulation: evidence from fMRI study. Neuroimage 22: 932–940.

16. Yoo SS, Kerr CE, Park M, Im DM, Blinder RA, et al. (2007) Neural activities in human somatosensory cortical areas evoked by acupuncture stimulation. Complement Ther Med 15: 247–254.

17. Li G, Jack CR, Jr., Yang ES (2006) An fMRI study of somatosensory-implicated acupuncture points in stable somatosensory stroke patients. J Magn Reson Imaging 24: 1018–1024.

18. Chae Y, Lee H, Kim H, Kim CH, Chang DI, et al. (2009) Parsing brain activity associated with acupuncture treatment in Parkinson's diseases. Mov Disord 24: 1794–1802.

19. Schaechter JD, Connell BD, Stason WB, Kaptchuk TJ, Krebs DE, et al. (2007) Correlated change in upper limb function and motor cortex activation after verum and sham acupuncture in patients with chronic stroke. J Altern Complement Med 13: 527–532.

20. Schockert T, Schnitker R, Boroojerdi B, Vietzke K, Qua Smith I, et al. (2009) Kortikale Aktivierungen durch Yamamoto Neue Schädelakupunktur (YNSA) in der Behandlung von Schlaganfallpatienten: Eine Sham-kontrollierte Studie mit Hilfe der funktionellen Kernspintomographie (fMRI). Deutsche Zeitschrift für Akupunktur 52: 21–29.

21. Dougherty DD, Kong J, Webb M, Bonab AA, Fischman AJ, et al. (2008) A combined [11C]diprenorphine PET study and fMRI study of acupuncture analgesia. Behav Brain Res 193: 63–68.

22. Deng G, Hou BL, Holodny AI, Cassileth BR (2008) Functional magnetic resonance imaging (fMRI) changes and saliva production associated with acupuncture at LI-2 acupuncture point: a randomized controlled study. BMC Complement Altern Med 8: 37.

23. Li L, Liu H, Li YZ, Xu JY, Shan BC, et al. (2008) The human brain response to acupuncture on same-meridian acupoints: evidence from an fMRI study. J Altern Complement Med 14: 673–678.

24. Xiao YY, Du L, Hong BK, et al. (2008) Study on fMRI brain map in patients undergoing needling at Zusanli (ST36) by reinforcing method. Zhongguo Zhong Xi Yi Jie He Za Zhi 28: 122–125.

25. Zhang JH, Cao XD, Lie J, Tang WJ, Liu HQ, et al. (2007) Neuronal specificity of needling acupoints at same meridian: a control functional magnetic resonance imaging study with electroacupuncture. Acupunct Electrother Res 32: 179–193.

26. Hu KM, Wang CP, Xie HJ, Henning J (2006) Observation on activating effectiveness of acupuncture at acupoints and non-acupoints on different brain regions. Zhongguo Zhen Jiu 26: 205–207.

27. Wang W, Li KC, Shan BC, Xu JY, Yan B, et al. (2006) Study of acupuncture point Liv 3 with funcitonal MRI. Chin J Radiol 40: 29–35.

28. Yan B, Li K, Xu J, Wang W, Liu H, et al. (2005) Acupoint-specific fMRI patterns in human brain. Neurosci Lett 383: 236–240.

29. Li G, Liu HL, Cheung RT, Hung YC, Wong KK, et al. (2003) An fMRI study comparing brain activation between word generation and electrical stimulation of language-implicated acupoints. Hum Brain Mapp 18: 233–238.

30. Lu N, Zhao JG, Shan BC, Li KC (2008) Study of acupuncture point Liv6 with functional MRI. Chin J Med Imaging Technol 24: 46–48.

31. Huang Y, Li GL, Lai XS, Tang CZ, Yang JJ (2009) An fMRI cerebral functional imaging comparison on needling in Zhigou (SJ6) vs a sham point. Journal of Chengdu University of TCM 32: 3–6.

32. Li L, Xu JY, Li YZ, Liu H, Yuan XL, et al. (2008) fMRI study of acupuncture at adjacent acupoints located on the stomach meridian of Foot-Yanming. Chin J Med Imaging Technol 24: 1001–1003.

33. Lai XS, Su PZ, Huang Y, Zou YQ, Wu JX, et al. (2009) Comparison of fMRI cerebral functional imaging between needling Waiguan (SJ5) and combined SJ5 and sham point. Tianjin Journal of Traditional Chinese Medicine 26: 113–115.

34. Jeun SS, Kim JS, Kim BS, Park SD, Lim EC, et al. (2005) Acupuncture stimulation for motor cortex activities: a 3T fMRI study. Am J Chin Med 33: 573–578.

35. Choi N-g, Han J-b, Jang S-j (2009) Comparaison of brain activation iamges associated with sexual arousal induced by visual stimulation and SP6 acupucnture : fMRI at 3 tesla. JOURNAL OF RADIOLOGICAL SCIENCE AND TECHNOLOGY 32: 183–194.

36. Choe B-y (2002) Clinical Application of Functional MRI : Motor Cortex Activities by Acupuncture. Journal of the Korean Magnetic Resonance Society 6: 89–93.

37. Wu MT, Sheen JM, Chuang KH, Yang P, Chin SL, et al. (2002) Neuronal specificity of acupuncture response: a fMRI study with electroacupuncture. Neuroimage 16: 1028–1037.

38. Zhang JH, Feng XY, Li J, Tang WJ, Li Y (2005) Functional MRI studies of acupoints and non-acupoints electroacupuncture analgesia modulating within human brain. Chinese computed medical imaging 11: 10–16.

39. Kong J, Gollub RL, Webb JM, Kong JT, Vangel MG, et al. (2007) Test-retest study of fMRI signal change evoked by electroacupuncture stimulation. Neuroimage 34: 1171–1181.

40. Kong J, Kaptchuk TJ, Webb JM, Kong JT, Sasaki Y, et al. (2007) Functional neuroanatomical investigation of vision-related acupuncture point specificity-A multisession fMRI study. Hum Brain Mapp.

41. Cho Z-H, Hwang S-c, Son Y-d, Kang C-k, Wong EK, et al. (2004) Acupuncture Analgesia : A Sensory Stimulus Induced Analgesia Observed by functional Magnetic resonance Imaging. The Journal of Korean Acupuncture & Moxibustion Society 21: 57–71.

42. Fang JL, Krings T, Weidemann J, Meister IG, Thron A (2004) Functional MRI in healthy subjects during acupuncture: different effects of needle rotation in real and false acupoints. Neuroradiology 46: 359–362.

43. Wesolowski T, Lotze M, Domin M, Langner S, Lehmann C, et al. (2009) Acupuncture reveals no specific effect on primary auditory cortex: a functional magnetic resonance imaging study. Neuroreport 20: 116–120.

44. Wang GB, Liu C, Wu LB, Yan B, Gao SZ, et al. (2009) Functional magnetic resonance imaging on acupuncturing Yuan-Source and He-Sea acupoints of stomach meridian of foot Yangming. ACTA ACADEMIAE MEDICINAE SINICAE 31: 171–176.

45. Fang JL, Jin Z, Wang Y, Li K, Zeng YW, et al. (2005) Comparison of central effects of acupuncturing Taichong and nearby two acupoints by functional MRI. Chin J Med Imaging Technol 21: 1332–1336.

46. Fang J, Jin Z, Wang Y, Li K, Kong J, et al. (2008) The salient characteristics of the central effects of acupuncture needling: Limbic-paralimbic-neocortical network modulation. Hum Brain Mapp.

47. Wang W, Liu L, Zhi X, Huang JB, Liu DX, et al. (2007) Study on the regulatory effect of electro-acupuncture on hegu point (LI4) in cerebral response with functional magnetic resonance imaging. Chin J Integr Med 13: 10–16.

48. Ai L, Dai JP, Zhao BX, Tian J, Fan YP, et al. (2004) Investigation of analgesic mechanism of acupuncture : a fMRI study. Chin J Med Imaging Technol 20: 1197–1200.

49. Li G, Huang L, Cheung RT, Liu SR, Ma QY, et al. (2004) Cortical activations upon stimulation of the sensorimotor-implicated acupoints. Magn Reson Imaging 22: 639–644.

50. Liu WC, Feldman SC, Cook DB, Hung DL, Xu T, et al. (2004) fMRI study of acupuncture-induced periaqueductal gray activity in humans. Neuroreport 15: 1937–1940.

51. Napadow V, Dhond R, Park K, Kim J, Makris N, et al. (2009) Time-variant fMRI activity in the brainstem and higher structures in response to acupuncture. Neuroimage 47: 289–301.

52. Wu MT, Hsieh JC, Xiong J, Yang CF, Pan HB, et al. (1999) Central nervous pathway for acupuncture stimulation: localization of processing with functional MR imaging of the brain–preliminary experience. Radiology 212: 133–141.

53. Hui KK, Liu J, Marina O, Napadow V, Haselgrove C, et al. (2005) The integrated response of the human cerebro-cerebellar and limbic systems to acupuncture stimulation at ST 36 as evidenced by fMRI. Neuroimage 27: 479–496.

54. Hui KK, Marina O, Claunch JD, Nixon EE, Fang J, et al. (2009) Acupuncture mobilizes the brain's default mode and its anti-correlated network in healthy subjects. Brain Res 1287: 84–103.

55. Napadow V, Dhond RP, Kim J, LaCount L, Vangel M, et al. (2009) Brain encoding of acupuncture sensation–coupling on-line rating with fMRI. Neuroimage 47: 1055–1065.

56. Fukunaga M (1999) Brain activation under electro-acupuncture stimulation using functional magnetic resonance imaging. The bulletin of Meiji University of oriental medicine 25: 7–19.

57. Dhond RP, Yeh C, Park K, Kettner N, Napadow V (2008) Acupuncture modulates resting state connectivity in default and sensorimotor brain networks. Pain 136: 407–418.

58. Napadow V, Makris N, Liu J, Kettner NW, Kwong KK, et al. (2005) Effects of electroacupuncture versus manual acupuncture on the human brain as measured by fMRI. Hum Brain Mapp 24: 193–205.

59. Hui KK, Liu J, Makris N, Gollub RL, Chen AJ, et al. (2000) Acupuncture modulates the limbic system and subcortical gray structures of the human brain: evidence from fMRI studies in normal subjects. Hum Brain Mapp 9: 13–25.

60. Chae Y, Lee H, Kim H, Sohn H, Park JH, et al. (2009) The neural substrates of verum acupuncture compared to non-penetrating placebo needle: an fMRI study. Neurosci Lett 450: 80–84.

61. Huang Y, Zeng TJ, Wang YJ, Lai XS, Zhang YZ, et al. (2009) A comparison of functional magnetic resonance imaging of cerebral regions activated by cutaneous needling and regular needling at Waiguan (SJ5) acupoint. Journal of Anhui TCM college 28: 25–28.

62. Wu JX, Huang Y, Lai XS, Zou YQ, Tang CZ, et al. (2009) The fMRI comparative study on cutaneous or routine needling in acupoints Waiguan (SJ5) and Neiguan (PC6). Chinese archives of traditional Chinese medicine 27: 1625–1627.

63. Huang Y, Song YB, Lai XS, Tang CZ, Yang JJ (2009) Comparison study between shallowly skin needling and routine needling in Neiguan (PC6) by fMRI. Journal of Shandong University of TCM 33: 243–245.

64. Huang Y, LI XX, Lai XS, Zou YQ, Wu JX (2009) Study of fMRI of cerebral functional regions induced by cutaneous and routine needling in Zhigou (SJ6). Hebei J TCM 31: 254–256.

65. Zou YQ, Huang Y, Lai XS, Tang CZ, Yang JJ (2008) The fMRI comparative study on cutaneous or routine needling in acupoints Waiguan (SJ5) and Zhigou (SJ6). Journal of Yunnan University of traditional Chinese medicine 31: 44–47.

66. Li G, Cheung RT, Ma QY, Yang ES (2003) Visual cortical activations on fMRI upon stimulation of the vision-implicated acupoints. Neuroreport 14: 669–673.

67. MacPherson H, Green G, Nevado A, Lythgoe MF, Lewith G, et al. (2008) Brain imaging of acupuncture: comparing superficial with deep needling. Neurosci Lett 434: 144–149.

68. Li DZ, Li XZ (2000) Comparative study of pricking the cutaneous region of acupoint and needling its depth by means of fMRI. Zhongguo Zhen Jiu. pp 491–492.

69. Kong J, Ma L, Gollub RL, Wei J, Yang X, et al. (2002) A pilot study of functional magnetic resonance imaging of the brain during manual and electroacupuncture stimulation of acupuncture point (LI-4 Hegu) in normal subjects reveals differential brain activation between methods. J Altern Complement Med 8: 411–419.

70. Li K, Shan B, Xu J, Liu H, Wang W, et al. (2006) Changes in FMRI in the human brain related to different durations of manual acupuncture needling. J Altern Complement Med 12: 615–623.

71. Hu KM, Wang CP, Henning J (2005) Observation on relation of acupuncture at Guangming (GB 37) and Taichong (LR 3) with central nervous reaction. Zhongguo Zhen Jiu 25: 860–862.

72. Gareus IK, Lacour M, Schulte AC, Hennig J (2002) Is there a BOLD response of the visual cortex on stimulation of the vision-related acupoint GB 37? J Magn Reson Imaging 15: 227–232.

73. Cheng HJ, Chen SJ, Zhu F (2009) Magnetic resonance imaging study of twisting or untwisting Taixi acupoint (KI3) on brain function. Journal of clinical rehabilitative tissue engineering research 13: 5020–5022.

74. Gong HH, Wang YZ, Xiao XZ, Qiu CM, Wang LY, et al. (2003) Investigation of cerebral cortical functional areas of the acupoints in zu-san li and xia ju xu by fMRI. Journal of diagnostic imaging & interventional radiology 12: 133–136.

75. Wang W, Qi JP, Xia YL, Huang XL, Li WX, et al. (2004) The response of human motor cortex to acupuncture of S36 and G34 as revealed by functional MRI. Chin J Phys Med Rehabil 26: 472–475.

76. Fu P, Jia JP, Zhu J, Huang JJ (2005) [Effects of acupuncture at Neiguan (PC 6) on human brain functional imaging in different functional states]. Zhongguo Zhen Jiu 25: 784–786.

77. Liu S, Zhou W, Ruan X, Li R, Lee T, et al. (2007) Activation of the hypothalamus characterizes the response to acupuncture stimulation in heroin addicts. Neurosci Lett 421: 203–208.

78. Wu Y, Jin Z, Li K, Lu ZL, Wong V, et al. (2008) Effect of acupuncture on the brain in children with spastic cerebral palsy using functional neuroimaging (FMRI). J Child Neurol 23: 1267–1274.

79. Napadow V, Liu J, Li M, Kettner N, Ryan A, et al. (2007) Somatosensory cortical plasticity in carpal tunnel syndrome treated by acupuncture. Hum Brain Mapp 28: 159–171.

80. Napadow V, Kettner N, Liu J, Li M, Kwong KK, et al. (2007) Hypothalamus and amygdala response to acupuncture stimuli in Carpal Tunnel Syndrome. Pain 130: 254–266.

81. Hu JP, Li YG, Cao DR, Gong SB (2008) Reproducibility of functional MR imaging during electroacupuncture stimulation at PC6 (Neiguan). ACTA ACADEMIAE MEDICINAE MILITARIS TERTIAE 30: 1878–1882.

82. Fu P, Jia JP, Min BQ (2005) Acupuncture at Neiguan acupoint for brain functional MRI of patients with Alzheimer disease. Chin J Neurol. pp 118–119.

83. Ha C-h, Lee H, Lim Y-k, Hong K-e, Lee B-r, et al. (2003) A fMRI study on the cerebral activity induced by Electro-acupuncture on Taichong(Liv3). The Journal of Korean Acupuncture & Moxibustion Society 20: 187–207.

84. Xu FM, Xie P, Lv FJ, Mou J, Li YM, et al. (2007) The fMRI study of acupuncture at the five transport points of liver meridian. Journal of Nanjing TCM University 23: 224–227.

85. Yan LP, Sun ZR, Xie B, Ma X (2005) Brain functional response after electroacupuncture at Quchi point with fMRI method. JCAM 21: 61–63.

86. Hong K-e, Lee B-r, Lee H, Yim Y-k, Kim Y-j (2003) A fMRI study on the cerebral activity induced by Electro-acupuncture on Sanyinjiao(Sp6). The Journal of Korean Acupuncture & Moxibustion Society 20: 86–103.

87. Parrish TB, Schaeffer A, Catanese M, Rogel MJ (2005) Functional magnetic resonance imaging of real and sham acupuncture. Noninvasively measuring cortical activation from acupuncture. IEEE Eng Med Biol Mag 24: 35–40.

88. Kim J-h, Lee H, Lim Y-k, Hong K-e, Lee B-r, et al. (2003) A fMRI study on the cerebral activity induced by Electro-acupuncture on Sp9(Yinlingquan). The Journal of Korean Acupuncture & Moxibustion Society 20: 114–133.

89. Zhu MJ, Hu KM (2004) A fMRI study of the TCM theory "the liver connects eye links". Journal of Hainan medical college 10: 169–170.

90. Bae E-j, Hong K-e, Lee H, Lee B-r, Yim Y-k, et al. (2003) A fMRI study on the cerebral activity induced by Electro-acupuncture on Fenglong(St40). The Journal of Korean Acupuncture & Moxibustion Society 20: 208–226.

91. Chi X (2009) A fMRI study of acupuncture on Zhongzhu (SJ3) point. Acta Chinese medicine and pharmacology 37: 37–38.

92. Chi X, Ju YL, Sun ST (2007) Study of acupuncture Zhongzhu (SJ3) Houxi (SI3) by functional MRI (fMRI). Chinese archives of traditional Chinese medicine 25: 843–844.

93. Huang Y, Li TL, Lai XS, Zou YQ, Wu JX, et al. (2009) Functional brain magnetic resonance imaging in healthy people receiving acupuncture at Waiguan versus Waiguan plus Yanglingquan points: a randomized controlled trail. Journal of Chinese integrative medicine 7: 527–531.

94. Zhang R, Zou YQ, Huang SQ, Chen ZG, Liang BL, et al. (2007) MRI cerebral function imaging following acupuncture at Hegu, Zusanli, Neiguan and Sanyinjiao points. Journal of clinical rehabilitative tissue engineering research 11: 4271–4274.

95. Hou JW, Huang WH, Wang Q, Feng JW, Pu YL, et al. (2002) Functional MRI studies of acupuncture analgesia modulating within the human brain. Chin J Radiol 36: 206–210.

96. Wang W, Xu HB, Kong XQ, Huang JB, Zhi X, et al. (2009) Experimental study on fMRI in human brain with electroacupuncture. J Pract Radiol 25: 305–308.

97. Li K, Shan BC, Liu H, Wang W, Xu JY, et al. (2005) fMRI study of acupuncture at large intestine 4. Chin J Med Imaging Technol 21: 1329–1331.

98. Liu H, Shan BC, Gao DS, Xu JY, Wang W, et al. (2006) Different cerebellar responding to acupuncture at Liv3 and LI4: an fMRI study. Chin J Med Imaging Technol 22: 1165–1167.

99. Yin L, Jin XL, Shi X, TIan JH, Ma L, et al. (2002) Imaging with PET and fMRI on brain function in acupuncturing the ST36 (Zusanli). Chin J Rehabil Theory Practice 8: 523–524.

100. Xu JY, Wang FQ, Wang H, Shan BC, Lv J, et al. (2004) Control study on effects of acupuncture at Hegu (LI4) and Taichong (LR3) points on fMRI cerebral function. Zhongguo Zhen Jiu 24: 263–265.

101. Long Y, Liu B, Liu X, Yan CG, Chen ZG, et al. (2009) Resting-state functional MRI evaluation of after-effect of acupuncture at Zusanli point. Chin J Med Imaging Technol 25: 373–376.

102. Xiao YY, Wu RH, Pei RQ, Lin R, Rao HB (2004) Functional MR imaging (fMRI) of acupuncture: observation of stimulating the acu-point ST36 (zusanli). J Pract Radiol 20: 106–108.

103. Fu P, Jia JP, Xu M, Wang M (2005) Changes of brain function in different areas of cerebral cotices due to electroacupuncture at the point ST36 through MRI. Chinese journal of clinical rehabilitation 9: 92–93.

104. Wu ZY, Miao F, Xiang QY, Hao J, Cao Y, et al. (2007) The MRI research of brain function on acupuncture at Zusanli (ST36) point. Chinese journal of traditional medical science and technology 14: 305–307.

105. Fang SH, Zhang SZ, Liu H (2006) Study on brain response to acupuncture by functional magnetic resonance imaging–observation on 14 healthy subjects. Zhongguo Zhong Xi Yi Jie He Za Zhi 26: 965–968.

106. Tian LF, Zhou C, Chen M, Zhou TG, Cai K, et al. (2006) Using functional magnetic resonance imaging to study the correlation between the acupoint and cerebral region. Zhen Ci Yan Jiu 31: 113–115.

107. Kim Y-i, Kim Y-h, Lim Y-k, Lee H, Lee B-r, et al. (2003) A fMRI study on the cerebral activity induced by Electro-acupuncture on Zusanli(St36). The Journal of Korean Acupuncture & Moxibustion Society 20: 133–150.

108. Chi X, Sun ST (2007) Cerebral functional magnetic resonance imaging study of point Waiguan acupuncture. Shanghai J Acu-mox 26: 30–31.

109. Park T-g, Kim Y-I, Hong K-e, Yim Y-k, Lee H, et al. (2004) A study on Brain activity induced by electro-acupuncture on Taechung(LR3) and Hapkok(LI4) using functional Magnetic Resonance Imaging. The Korean Journal of Meridian & Acupoint 21: 29–46.

110. Chen WJ, Shou YQ, Li JH, Xu ZS, Liu H (2007) The effect of acupuncture at the acupoint Sanyinjiao on brain function as revealed by the functional magnetic resonance imaging. Chin J Phys Med Rehabil 29: 774–779.

111. Wu ZY, Miao F, Xiang QY, Hao J, Ge LB, et al. (2008) Comparative study on acupuncting the different acupoints of the same meridian with functional magnetic resonance imaging. Chinese J Med Imaging 16: 101–105.

112. Cai K, Chen M, Wang WC, Zhou C, Zhou TG, et al. (2007) fMRI of cortical activation by acupuncture. Information of medical equipment 22: 84–86.

113. Guan YQ, Yang XZ (2008) Brain BOLD-fMRI study of electroacupuncture stimulating the acupoint related visual. Hebei J TCM 30: 1065–1068.

114. Chen P, Zhao BX, Qin W, Chen HY, Tian J, et al. (2008) Study on the mechanism of acupuncture at Daling (PC 7) for mental diseases by fMRI. Zhongguo Zhen Jiu 28: 429–432.

115. Park K-y, Lee B-r, Lee H, Yim Y-k, Hong K-e, et al. (2003) A fMRI study on the cerebral activity induced by Electro-acupuncture on Taixi(K3). The Journal of Korean Acupuncture & Moxibustion Society 20: 194–208.

116. Yoon J-h, Hwang M-s, Bae G-t, Lee S-h, Lee S-d, et al. (2001) The new finding on BOLD response of motor acupoint KI6 by fMRI. The Journal of Korean Acupuncture & Moxibustion Society 18: 60–69.

117. Kwon C-h, Lee J-b, Hwang M-s, Yoon J-h (2004) The New Finding on BOLD Response of Moter Acupoint KI6 by fMRI. The Journal of Korean Acupuncture & Moxibustion Society 21: 177–186.

118. Kang J-h, Lee H, Lee B-r, Hong K-e, Yim Y-k, et al. (2003) A fMRI study on the cerebral activity induced by Electro-acupuncture on K7(Fuliu). The Journal of Korean Acupuncture & Moxibustion Society 20: 66–84.

119. Zhang Y, Liang J, Qin W, Liu P, von Deneen KM, et al. (2009) Comparison of visual cortical activations induced by electro-acupuncture at vision and nonvision-related acupoints. Neurosci Lett 458: 6–10.

120. Chi X, Sun ST, Bao DP (2006) fMRI study of acupuncture at Houxi (SI3) point. JCAM 22: 37–38.

121. Chen SJ, Liu B, Fu WB, Wu SS, Chen J, et al. (2008) A fMRI observation on different cererbral regions activated by acupuncture of Shenmen (HT 7) and Yanglao (SI 6). Zhen Ci Yan Jiu 33: 267–271.

122. Chen HD, Ying GL, Jiang B, He WL (2006) Studding effect of acupuncturing Baihui point for brain function with fMRI method. Journal of Zhejiang University of traditional Chinese medicine 30: 656–659.

123. Wang AC, Wang YL, Jiang T, Ma B, Chen JF, et al. (2005) Observation on changes of cerebral images after acupuncture of Shenmai (BL62) by using fMRI. Zhen Ci Yan Jiu 30: 43–47.

124. Deng ZS, Qiu ML, C. F-S SL (2005) A study on response of the specific functional areas of the human brain to acupuncture stimulating visual-ralated acupoints using BOLD fMRI. J Pract Radiol 21: 1240–1242.

125. Rheu K-h, Choi I-h, Park H-j, Lim S (2006) fMRI Study on the Brain Activity Induced by Manual Acupuncture at BL62. The Korean Journal of Meridian & Acupoint 23: 89–103.

126. Fu P, Jia JP, Wang M (2005) Acupuncture at Shenmen acupoint for brain functional MRI of patients with Alzheimer disease. Chinese journal of clinical rehabilitation. pp 120–121.

127. Bai L, Qin W, Tian J, Liu P, Li L, et al. (2009) Time-varied characteristics of acupuncture effects in fMRI studies. Hum Brain Mapp 30: 3445–3460.

128. Wang W, Zhu F, Qi JP, Xia YL, Xia LM, et al. (2002) Comparison study of human brain response to acupuncture stimulation vs finger tapping task by using real time fMRI. Chin J Radiol 36: 211–214.

129. Wang SM, Constable RT, Tokoglu FS, Weiss DA, Freyle D, et al. (2007) Acupuncture-induced blood oxygenation level-dependent signals in awake and anesthetized volunteers: a pilot study. Anesth Analg 105: 499–506.

130. Zhen JP, Liu C, He JZ, Wang BG, Yang DH, et al. (2008) The research of brain fMRI in acupuncture of KI in different time. Chinese imaging journal of integrated traditional and western medicine 6: 325–331.

131. Park J-m, Gwak J-y, Cho S-y, Park S-u, Jung W-a, et al. (2008) Effects of Head Acupuncture Versus Upper and Lower Lims Acupuncture on Signal Activation of Blood Oxygen Level Dependent (BOLD) fMRI on the Brain and Somatosensory Cortex. The Journal of Korean Acupuncture & Moxibustion Society 25: 151–165.

132. Teng J, Wang YL, Wang AC, Zhao JN, Liu M (2008) Study on cerebral images with frontal-three-needle penetration by functional magnetic resonance imaging. Journal of Shandong University of TCM 32: 104–106.

133. Zhou Y, Jin J (2008) Effect of acupuncture given at the HT 7, ST 36, ST 40 and KI 3 acupoints on various parts of the brains of Alzheimer' s disease patients. Acupunct Electrother Res 33: 9–17.

134. Li J, Zhang JH, Dong JC (2007) Influence of acupuncture analgesia on cerebral function imaging in sciatica patients. Shanghai J Acu-mox 26: 3–6.

135. Chang JL, Gao Y, Zhang H, Tan ZJ, Jiang GD (2007) A preliminary discussion of the effect of electroacupuncture at acupoints HT5 and GB39 on lingual function and fMRI changes in a case of subcortical aphasia. Chinese journal of rehabilitation medicine 22: 13–17.

136. Wang W, Li KC, Shan BC, Yan B, Hao J, et al. (2006) fMRI study of acupuncture at "four gate points" on normal aging people. Chin J Med Imaging Technol 22: 829–832.

137. Zhou C, Wang JZ, Chen M, Zhou TG, Cai K, et al. (2005) The correlative study between acupoint stimulations and corresponding brain cortices on functional MRI. Chin J Radiol 39: 252–255.

138. He YZ, Wang LN, Huang L, Wang XH, Liu SR, et al. (2006) Effects of acupuncture on the cortical functional areas activated by index finger motion in the patient with ischemic stroke. Zhongguo Zhen Jiu 26: 357–361.

139. Xu FM, Xie P, Lu FJ, Mou J, Li YM, et al. (2007) Study on corresponding areas the liver and lung channels in brain with fMRI. Zhongguo Zhen Jiu 27: 749–752.

140. Qiu MG, Wang J, Xie B, Wu BH, Zhang SX, et al. (2005) Establishment of analyzing methods for functional MR images when electroacupuncture stimulation on Guangming and Waiguan acupoints. ACTA ACADEMIAE MEDICINAE MILITARIS TERTIAE 27: 1970–1972.

141. Xu JY, Wang FQ, Shan BC, Chen Y, Wang H, et al. (2004) PET and fMRI to evaluate the results of acupuncture treatment of the cognition of alzheimer's disease. Chinese imaging journal of integrated traditional and western medicine 2: 85–87.

142. Zhang WT, Jin Z, Luo F, Zhang L, Zeng YW, et al. (2004) Evidence from brain imaging with fMRI supporting functional specificity of acupoints in humans. Neurosci Lett 354: 50–53.

143. Cho Z-h, Kim K-y, Kim H-k, Lee B-r, Wong EK, et al. (2001) Correlation between acupuncture stimulation and cortical activation - further evidence. The Journal of Korean Acupuncture & Moxibustion Society 18: 105–113.

144. Chang SX, Feng GS, Kong XQ, Li G, Liu DX, et al. (2002) Functional MRI study of cortical function area activation with electronic acupuncture stimulation of multiple acupoints. Lin Chuang Fang She Xue Za Zhi 21: 99–102.

145. Kong J, Kaptchuk TJ, Polich G, Kirsch I, Vangel M, et al. (2009) An fMRI study on the interaction and dissociation between expectation of pain relief and acupuncture treatment. Neuroimage 47: 1066–1076.

146. Kong J, Kaptchuk TJ, Polich G, Kirsch I, Vangel M, et al. (2009) Expectancy and treatment interactions: a dissociation between acupuncture analgesia and expectancy evoked placebo analgesia. Neuroimage 45: 940–949.

147. Kong J, Gollub RL, Rosman IS, Webb JM, Vangel MG, et al. (2006) Brain activity associated with expectancy-enhanced placebo analgesia as measured by functional magnetic resonance imaging. J Neurosci 26: 381–388.

148. Zhang Y, Qin W, Liu P, Tian J, Liang J, et al. (2008) An fMRI study of acupuncture using independent component analysis. Neurosci Lett.

149. Bai L, Tian J, Qin W, Pan X, Yang L, et al. (2007) Exploratory analysis of functional connectivity network in acupuncture study by a graph theory mode. Conf Proc IEEE Eng Med Biol Soc 2007: 2023–2026.

150. Qin W, Tian J, Bai L, Pan X, Yang L, et al. (2008) FMRI Connectivity Analysis of Acupuncture Effects on an Amygdala-Associated Brain Network. Mol Pain 4: 55.

151. Qin W, Tian J, Pan X, Yang L, Zhen Z (2006) The correlated network of acupuncture effect: a functional connectivity study. Conf Proc IEEE Eng Med Biol Soc 1: 480–483.

152. Liu P, Qin W, Zhang Y, Tian J, Bai L, et al. (2009) Combining spatial and temporal information to explore function-guide action of acupuncture using fMRI. J Magn Reson Imaging 30: 41–46.

153. Liu P, Zhang Y, Zhou G, Yuan K, Qin W, et al. (2009) Partial correlation investigation on the default mode network involved in acupuncture: an fMRI study. Neurosci Lett 462: 183–187.

154. Yeo S, Kim Y, Choe I-h, Rheu C-h, Choi Y-g, et al. (2009) Reproducibility Between two physicians of fMRI study on the Brain Activity Induced by Acupuncture. Journal of Meridian & Acupoint 26: 39–51.

155. Raichle ME, Mintun MA (2006) Brain work and brain imaging. Annu Rev Neurosci 29: 449–476.

156. Poldrack RA, Fletcher PC, Henson RN, Worsley KJ, Brett M, et al. (2008) Guidelines for reporting an fMRI study. Neuroimage 40: 409–414.

157. Sun G (2008) Basic Theroy of Traditional Chinese Medicine. Beijing: China Press of Traditional Chinese Medicine. 315 p.

158. Han JS (2011) Acupuncture analgesia: areas of consensus and controversy. Pain 152: S41–48.

159. Dhond RP, Kettner N, Napadow V (2007) Do the neural correlates of acupuncture and placebo effects differ? Pain 128: 8–12.

160. Li X, Liu X, Liang F (2008) Functional brain imaging studies on specificity of meridian and acupoints. Neural Regen Res 3: 777–781.

161. Campbell A (2006) Point specificity of acupuncture in the light of recent clinical and imaging studies. Acupunct Med 24: 118–122.

162. Beissner F, Henke C (2009) Methodological Problems in fMRI Studies on Acupuncture: A Critical Review With Special Emphasis on Visual and Auditory Cortex Activations. Evid Based Complement Alternat Med.

163. Cho ZH, Hwang SC, Wong EK, Son YD, Kang CK, et al. (2006) Neural substrates, experimental evidences and functional hypothesis of acupuncture mechanisms. Acta Neurol Scand 113: 370–377.

164. Chae Y, Park HJ, Hahm DH, Hong M, Ha E, et al. (2007) fMRI review on brain responses to acupuncture: the limitations and possibilities in traditional Korean acupuncture. Neurol Res 29 Suppl 1: S42–48.

165. Zhao L, You ZL, Tang Y, Liang FR (2009) Observation of brain response to acupuncture stimuli using fMRI. Lishizhen medicine and materia medica research 20: 1343–1345.

166. Li XT, Song XG (2009) An overview of the application of functional MRI technique on clinical acupuncture. Journal of Anhui TCM College 4: 78–80.

167. Jiang C, Zhou SY, Zhao L, Li Y (2010) To evaluate the application of fMRI technique in acupuncture research. Journal of practical traditional Chinese medicine 26: 275–277.

168. Hu T, Hu KM (2009) The application progress on brain response to acupuncture using functional MRI. Med J West China 21: 1987–1988.

6

Effects of Long-Term Acupuncture Treatment on Resting-State Brain Activity in Migraine Patients: A Randomized Controlled Trial on Active Acupoints and Inactive Acupoints

Ling Zhao[1], Jixin Liu[2]*, Fuwen Zhang[3], Xilin Dong[1], Yulin Peng[1], Wei Qin[2], Fumei Wu[1], Ying Li[1], Kai Yuan[2], Karen M. von Deneen[2], Qiyong Gong[4], Zili Tang[5], Fanrong Liang[1]*

1 Acupuncture and Tuina School, Chengdu University of Traditional Chinese Medicine, Chengdu, Sichuan, China, 2 School of Life Science and Technology, Xidian University, Xi'an, Shaanxi, China, 3 School of Clinical Medicine, Chengdu University of Traditional Chinese Medicine, Chengdu, Sichuan, China, 4 Department of Radiology, The Center for Medical Imaging, Huaxi MR Research Center, West China Hospital of Sichuan University, Chengdu, Sichuan, China, 5 German Cancer Consortium (DKTK), Heidelberg, Germany

Abstract

Background: Acupuncture has been commonly used for preventing migraine attacks and relieving pain during a migraine, although there is limited knowledge on the physiological mechanism behind this method. The objectives of this study were to compare the differences in brain activities evoked by active acupoints and inactive acupoints and to investigate the possible correlation between clinical variables and brain responses.

Methods and Results: A randomized controlled trial and resting-state functional magnetic resonance imaging (fMRI) were conducted. A total of eighty migraineurs without aura were enrolled to receive either active acupoint acupuncture or inactive acupoint acupuncture treatment for 8 weeks, and twenty patients in each group were randomly selected for the fMRI scan at the end of baseline and at the end of treatment. The neuroimaging data indicated that long-term active acupoint therapy elicited a more extensive and remarkable cerebral response compared with acupuncture at inactive acupoints. Most of the regions were involved in the pain matrix, lateral pain system, medial pain system, default mode network, and cognitive components of pain processing. Correlation analysis showed that the decrease in the visual analogue scale (VAS) was significantly related to the increased average Regional homogeneity (ReHo) values in the anterior cingulate cortex in the two groups. Moreover, the decrease in the VAS was associated with increased average ReHo values in the insula which could be detected in the active acupoint group.

Conclusions: Long-term active acupoint therapy and inactive acupoint therapy have different brain activities. We postulate that acupuncture at the active acupoint might have the potential effect of regulating some disease-affected key regions and the pain circuitry for migraine, and promote establishing psychophysical pain homeostasis.

Trial Registration: Chinese Clinical Trial Registry ChiCTR-TRC-13003635

Editor: Mario D. Cordero, University of Sevilla, Spain

Funding: This study was supported by the National Basic Research Program of China (973 Program, No. 2012CB518501), National Natural Science Foundation of China (Nos. 30901900, 30930112, 81101108), the Project of Administration of Traditional Chinese Medicine of Sichuan Province (No. 2012-E-038), and the Project of Innovative Research Team Research Fund of Sichuan Provincial Education Department (No. 12TD002). The funders had no role in study design, data collection and analysis, decision to publish, or preparation of the manuscript.

Competing Interests: The authors have declared that no competing interests exist.

* E-mail: acuresearch@126.com (FL); liujixin@life.xidian.edu.cn (JL)

Introduction

Migraine is a common neurological disorder that typically manifests as repeated episodes of moderate or severe unilateral, pulsating headache aggravated by routine physical activity and is associated with nausea and/or phonophobia and photophobia [1]. Migraine has attracted more and more attention worldwide as a public health issue because of its high prevalence, frequent attack history, significant medical burden, and a serious reduction in quality of life (QOL) and productivity [2,3]. Although the exact

mechanism of migraine is still unclear, there is plenty of neuroimaging evidence showing that migraine is a central nervous system disorder [4–6]. Our research group involving migraine without aura patients showed that abnormal structure and function was possibly associated with an impaired pain processing and modulatory process, such as in the anterior cingulate cortex (ACC), insula, basal ganglia, thalamus, supplementary motor area (SMA), prefrontal cortex, etc. [7–9].

Acupuncture has a long history in China as one of the treatment modalities of Traditional Chinese Medicine (TCM) and is increasingly being adopted in the West as a complementary and alternative treatment to prevent migraine attacks and to relieve pain during a migraine. The latest Cochrane meta-analysis suggests that acupuncture as a migraine prophylaxis is safe and at least as effective, if not more effective, than prophylactic drug treatment [10]. During the past decade, a considerable number of high quality clinical studies have indicated that acupuncture is able to alleviate headache degree and/or improve the QOL [11–13]. However, despite the popularity of acupuncture in migraine therapy, there persists limited knowledge on the physiological mechanisms behind this method, and some controversy on the superiority of verum acupuncture over sham control. Some studies suggested that the obvious influence of acupuncture on pain symptoms was either insignificant or a placebo effect [12,14].

With the development of neuroimaging techniques, this has provided a brand new view to explore the central mechanisms of acupuncture, and has been a global trend in acupuncture research. We detected cerebral glucose metabolism after short periods of acupuncture stimulation in migraineurs through positron emission tomography (PET) with computed tomography examination, and found that transientapp:addword:transient acupuncture stimulation induced different levels of cerebral glucose metabolism in some pain-related brain regions [15]. In fact, one session of acupuncture stimulation did not fully model the clinical situation, and was hardly enough to achieve the expected effect in clinical practice. Therefore, the cumulative therapeutic effect of long-term acupuncture would help to reveal the underlying mechanisms of acupuncture treatment in more depth.

In the current study, we performed a ReHo approach [16] to compare the blood oxygen level-dependent (BOLD) signals in the brains of migraine patients during the resting-state. ReHo is based on a data-driven approach and thus requires no prior knowledge and has good test-retest reliability [17]. It was originally proposed for measuring the degree of regional synchronization of functional magnetic resonance imaging (fMRI) time courses and focused on the similarities or coherence of the intraregional spontaneous low-frequency (<0.08 Hz) BOLD signal, which enables a novel perspective to understand the functional regulation in particular brain regions. An important advantage of using the ReHo method over other methods is that it detects changes or modulations that are induced by different conditions across the whole brain in a voxel-by-voxel manner. ReHo analysis has been used to study migraine in our group [7,18], and other diseases like Alzheimer's disease [19], Parkinson's disease [20], attention-deficit/hyperactivity disorder [21], and so on.

We hypothesized that if acupuncture therapy is effective, it would modulate disease-affected brain regions and dysfunctional pain modulatory circuitry in migraine patients. In the current study, a randomized controlled trial and resting-state fMRI were adopted to compare the difference in brain activation patterns evoked by active acupoints and inactive acupoints for migraine patients. Furthermore, a correlation analysis was performed to investigate the possible correlation between clinical variables and brain activity.

Methods

The protocol for this trial and supporting CONSORT checklist are available as supporting information; see Checklist S1 and Protocol S1. This trial was performed at the Teaching hospital of Chengdu University of TCM. The study protocol was registered with the Chinese Clinical Trial Registry (ChiCTR) (Identifier: ChiCTR-TRC-13003635). The study was performed according to the principles of the Declaration of Helsinki (Edinburgh version,

2000), and was approved by the ethics committee at the Teaching Hospital of Chengdu University of TCM. Based on the previous report about minimum sample size in neuroimaging studies [22], a sample size of 16 per group was needed (total N = 32). Considering a conservative dropout rate of 25%, a total sample size of 40 migraineurs was determined. However, during the period of recruitment, a large number of eligible migraine patients (far more than the originally planned sample size) were willing to receive acupuncture treatment. According to a previous study [11], the difference in mean score of VAS between the acupuncture group and sham acupuncture group at 8 weeks was 1 ($\delta = 1$). For this study, it was determined prospectively that $\alpha = 0.05$(two-sided), $1-\beta = 0.9$, and that the standard deviation would be 1.2 according to the two group subsets. Thirty-one participants were required for each group (1:1 allocation). Thus, we decided to enroll a total of 80 participants (after attrition) and randomly selected 40 migraineurs to implement the fMRI experiment.

2.1 Participants

All subjects gave written, informed consent after the experimental procedures had been fully explained. Subjects were enrolled from the neurology department of the Teaching Hospital of Chengdu University of TCM. Recruitment took place June 2012 through March 2013. The diagnosis of migraine without aura was established according to the classification criteria of the International Headache Society (IHS) [1]. The inclusion criteria were as follows: (1) all subjects were right-handed and had 2 to 6 migraine attacks per month during the last 3 months and during the baseline period (4 weeks before enrollment); (2) all subjects were 18 to 55 years of age; in addition, the start of headache needed to be before the age of 50; (3) received education for more than 6 years and completed the baseline headache diary; (4) had not taken any prophylactic headache medicine or any acupuncture treatment during the last 3 months; (5) no record of long-term analgesics consumption; and (6) had no contraindications to exposure to a high magnetic field. General exclusion criteria were: (1) existence of neurological diseases; (2) hypertension, diabetes mellitus, hypercholesteremia, vascular/heart disease, and major systemic conditions; (3) pregnant or lactating women; (4) alcohol or drug abuse; (5) any neuroimaging research study participation during the last 6 months; and (6) inability to understand the doctor's instructions.

2.2 Study Design

We performed a single-blind, randomized controlled trial with two groups: active acupuncture group and inactive acupuncture group. The primary objective of this study was to compare the difference in resting-state brain activation patterns evoked by active acupoints and inactive acupoints in migraine patients via fMRI assessment. The secondary objective was to investigate the possible correlation between brain responses and clinical efficacy. The total observation period within this study was 12 weeks for each patient, including a baseline period of 4 weeks, and a treatment period of 8 weeks. Headache diaries were given to recruited patients to record the details of migraine attacks for 4 weeks (−4 to 0 weeks) during the baseline period. After the initial assessment and screening, patients who met the inclusion criteria were randomly assigned into the active acupoint group or the inactive acupoint group in a 1:1 ratio. All patients were asked to document their headache diaries, and the outcome measurement was completed both for the baseline, 4 and 8 weeks after randomization. Additionally, 20 migraineurs in each group were randomly selected to receive fMRI examinations at the end of baseline and at the end of the treatment period respectively.

2.3 Randomization

Randomization numbers of 80 patients were generated through computerized block-randomization with the SAS procedure PROC PLAN in the SAS package (SAS Version 9.0, SAS Institute, Inc., Cary, NC) by an independent statistician. In this study, the block size was set to 4, and the number of blocks was 20. Opaque, sealed envelopes with consecutive numbers were used for allocation concealment. Investigators who selected the eligible participants after baseline screening opened the envelopes according to the patients' screening sequence numbers, and placed the patients into either the active group or the inactive group. Additionally, we used Microsoft Excel's sampling tool to generate a random sample of 20 from 40 eligible migraineurs for each group. In the new random list, each number represented the enrolled sequence number in the subgroup. Next, the corresponding patients were selected to perform the fMRI scans.

2.4 Intervention

In this study, traditional Chinese style acupuncture was used and treatments were manipulated by two specialized acupuncturists with at least five years of training and three years of experience. They received special training prior to the study to ensure they had consistent manual acupuncture therapy. The training program included some standard operation procedures on the locations of the acupoints, acupuncture manipulation techniques, and so on. They implemented acupuncture therapy in both groups by turns. The active acupuncture points were selected according to traditional classic and systematic reviews of ancient and modern literature of acupuncture for migraine upon several consensus meetings with experts based on the experience from our previous study [11,23]. Moreover, the control group was given inactive acupoints which were chosen according to their anatomical locations, corresponding to Chinese meridians, proximity to verum acupoints and role in treating diseases [24]. The active treatment (group A) was performed on bilateral SJ5 (Waiguan), GB20 (Fengchi), GB34 (Yanglingquan), and GB40 (Qiuxu); and the inactive control (group B) was implemented on bilateral SJ22 (Erheliao), PC7 (Daling), GB37 (Guangming), and SP3 (Taibai) (figure 1).

All acupoints were punctured bilaterally using single-use stainless steel filiform needles (Hwato Needles, Sino-foreign Joint Venture Suzhou Hua Tuo Medical Instruments Co., China), 25 mm–40 mm in length and 0.25 mm–0.30 mm in diameter. The depths of the inserted needles differed but were approximately 2.5 cm–3.5 cm. Needles were twisted with rotation ($90° < $ amplitude $< 180°$) at a frequency of 1–2 Hz. Stimulation was repeated 1–3 times to acquire the de-qi sensation ("de-qi sensation" is a complex feeling including soreness, numbness, heaviness, distention and dull pain at the site of needle placement). Each group's treatment consisted of 32 sessions of acupuncture over a period of 8 weeks (once every other day, preferably 4 times a week), and each session lasted 30 minutes.

2.5 Blinding

Due to the procedure of the acupuncture technique, two acupuncturists in this study were not blinded. Investigators in charge of patient screening and randomized distribution were not involved in treatment and data analyses. They knew the group assignment, but they did not know the corresponding treatment schedule. The outcome assessor, who was not involved in acupuncture treatment and data analyses, was blinded throughout the study.

To guarantee that the patients were blinded during the treatment period, several approaches were performed for migraine patients in both groups: they were informed that they would receive one of two types of acupuncture treatment, which depended on different traditional Chinese acupuncture theories; acupuncture treatment was achieved in a large independent single-room with screen dividers for patient blinding and privacy; and two groups of patients received bilateral and equivalent number of acupoint stimulations each time.

2.6 Outcome Measures in Clinical Efficacy

All patients were required to fill out headache diary records for 12 weeks, including a 4-week baseline, and 4 and 8 weeks after randomization. The headache diary recorded the severity, frequency and duration of headache according to the guidelines of the IHS for Clinical Trials in Migraine [25]. VAS score 0–10 as a primary clinical outcome measured the intensity of headache. As secondary clinical outcome measures, the number of days with a migraine per 4 weeks and frequency of migraines per 4 weeks (defined as the number of migraine separated by pain free intervals of at least 48 hours) measured the duration and severity of headache respectively. In addition, the HIT-6 questionnaire [26] was adopted to assess the severity and impact of headache on a patient's life.

It is worth mentioning that the feelings of de-qi were collected after removing needles during the 8th, 16th, 24th, and 32nd sessions. Migraineurs were interviewed by an acupuncturist who did not know the treatment allocation. Patients were asked to evaluate each component of the de-qi sensations they had experienced during the acupuncture stimulation period, and the intensity used a VAS ranging from 0 (none) to 10 (max), which has been commonly used to measure the feelings of de-qi [27,28]. The score for the VAS was the sum of all component scores. The overall de-qi score was the mean score from all sessions.

2.7 fMRI data acquisition

Resting-state fMRI scans were performed on each group at the baseline and after 8 weeks' treatment to detect the local features of spontaneous brain activity. The imaging data were carried out in a 3 Tesla Siemens MRI system (Allegra, Siemens Medical System, Erlangen, Germany) at the Huaxi MR Research Center, West China Hospital of Sichuan University, Chengdu, China. A standard eight-channel phase-array head coil was used, along with restraining foam pads to minimize head motion and to diminish scanner noise. The resting-state functional images were obtained with echo-planar imaging (EPI) (30 continuous slices with a slice thickness $= 5$ mm, repetition time $= 2000$ ms, echo time $= 30$ ms, flip angle $= 90°$, field of view $= 240$ mm $\times 240$ mm, matrix $= 64 \times 64$). During the 6-min fMRI scanning, participants were instructed to keep their eyes closed, relax, move as little as possible, and stay awake. It needs to be emphasized that if there was an attack for migraine patients during the scan or examination, they could not be scanned and the scan would be postponed. In this study, records in the headache diary were checked to ensure every patient did not suffer from a migraine attack at least 72 hours prior to the brain scan.

2.8 Data Analysis

2.8.1 Clinical data analysis. The statistical analysis was performed by an independent statistician blinded to treatment allocation in the Teaching Hospital of Chengdu University of TCM. SPSS statistical package program (Version 14.0, SPSS Inc., Chicago, IL, USA) was used. Baseline characteristics and clinical outcomes were analyzed by the intention-to-treat (ITT) population which included all participants who had randomized allocation. Missing data of dropped-out participants were replaced by the last

Active acupoints

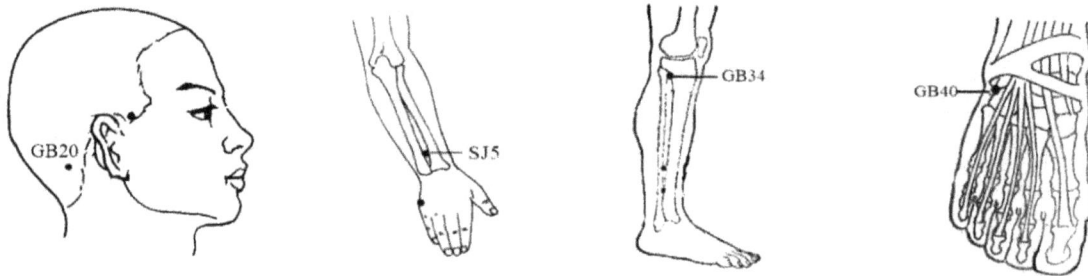

Inactive acupoints

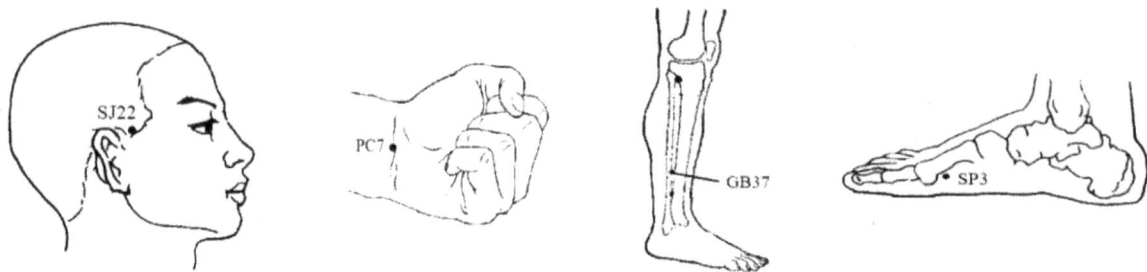

Locations of active acupoints and inactive acupoints

Figure 1. Locations of active acupoints and inactive acupoints. The active acupoints were located as follows: SJ5, on the dorsal aspect of the forearm on the line connecting SJ4 and the tip of the elbow, 2 cun above the transverse crease of the wrist between the ulna and radius; GB20, in a depression between the upper portion of the sternocleidomastoid muscle and the trapezius; GB34, on the lateral aspect of the lower leg in the depression anterior and inferior to the head of the fibula; GB40, anterior and inferior to the external malleolus in a depression on the lateral side of the tendon of the extensor digitorum longus. The inactive acupoints were located as follows: SJ22, on the side of the head on the posterior border of the hairline at the temple at the level with the root of the auricle, posterior to the superficial temporal artery; PC7, in the middle of the transverse crease of the wrist between the tendons of the palmaris longus and flexor carpi radialis; GB37, on the lateral aspect of the lower leg 5 cun above the tip of the external malleolus on the anterior border of the fibula; SP3, proximal and inferior to the head of the 1st metatarsal-phalangeal joint in a depression at the junction of the red and white skin.

observation carried forward (LOCF) method. The significant level used for the statistical analysis with 2-tailed testing was 5%. Continuous variables were presented as the mean (standard deviation) with 95% confidence intervals (CI). Categorical variables were described as n (percentage). Treatment effects such as VAS, frequency of migraine attack per 4 weeks, number of days with migraine per 4 weeks, and HIT-6 were evaluated using a repeated-measures analysis of variance (ANOVA) model with a between-subjects factor Therapy (levels: active and inactive) and a within-subjects repeated measures factor TIME (levels: baseline, 1–4 weeks, and 5–8 weeks). For the change in VAS, analysis of covariance with baseline VAS as a covariate was used to compare the difference between two groups at the end of treatment. The general linear model repeated measures procedure was used to test the differences in the repeated continuous variables (*de-qi* sensations) between the two groups.

2.8.2 Imaging data preprocessing. In the functional image data preprocessing, the first five scans were discarded to eliminate nonequilibrium effects of magnetization and to allow participants to become familiar with the scanning circumstances. Data preprocessing was done using Statistical Parametric Mapping (SPM5, http://www.fil.ion.ucl.ac.uk/spm). The images were corrected for the acquisition delay between slices, aligned to the first image of each session for motion correction and spatially normalized to the standard Montreal Neurological Institute (MNI) template in SPM5. We calculated the maximum excursion movement values for each of the translation planes (x, y, and z) and each of the rotation planes (roll, pitch, and yaw) for every participant. None of them had head movements exceeding 1 mm on any axis and head rotation greater than 1° during the entire fMRI scan. Finally, a band-pass filter ($0.01\ \text{Hz} < f < 0.08\ \text{Hz}$) was applied to remove physiological and high-frequency noise.

2.8.3 MRI data analysis. ReHo, a method proposed by Zang et al. [29], was performed in the Resting-state fMRI Data Analysis Toolkit (http://www.restfmri.net) [16]. First, the Kendall's coefficient of concordance (KCC) of each voxel was calculated by the time series of the voxel and its nearest 26 neighboring voxels (cluster size = 27). Second, the KCC maps were standardized by their own mean KCC within the whole brain mask. Third, the resulting maps were smoothed with a Gaussian kernel with a full-width at half-maximum (FWHM) of 4 mm. In the statistical analysis, an independent-sample *t*-test was used to explore ReHo differences between the two groups with age as a covariate. Results were assumed to be statistically significant at $P < 0.05$ after false discovery rate (FDR) correction within the whole brain. The correlation analysis was performed based on different clusters in the brain after acupuncture treatments relative to the baseline for each group. Within each cluster, we extracted the ReHo values after acupuncture and baseline respectively. The mean of their subtraction (end of treatment-baseline) was correlated with the changes in the clinical variables, and Bonferroni correction was used.

Results

3.1 Participants

Eighty eligible patients were equally allocated into the active treatment group and inactive treatment group (40 in each group). Two patients from the active acupuncture group and five from the inactive acupuncture group dropped out during the study because of private reasons: noncompliance with treatment schedule or inability to be contacted (figure 2). In total, 80 patients who received acupuncture therapies were included in the ITT analysis of the clinical outcome measures. The baseline and demographics with the ITT population are shown in table 1, which showed that the two groups were comparable at baseline. Furthermore, 40 patients (20 in each group) finished the fMRI scans, and the baseline characteristics did not differ between the two groups (table 2).

3.2 Neuroimaging results

In the active acupoint group, migraine patients showed significantly higher ReHo values in the bilateral ACC (Brodmman area (BA) 24, BA32), insula (BA13), thalamus, SMA (BA6), superior temporal gyrus (STG) (BA22), cuneus (BA17, BA18), lingual gyrus (BA18), cerebellum, and brainstem after acupuncture treatment. A decrease in ReHo values was observed after treatment in the bilateral posterior cingulate cortex (PCC) (BA31), middle frontal gyrus (MFG) (BA10), angular gyrus (BA39), precuneus (BA7), middle temporal gyrus (MTG) (BA39), left hippocampus, inferior parietal lobule (BA39), inferior temporal gyrus (ITG) (BA20), and right postcentral gyrus (BA40) ($P<0.05$, FDR corrected with a minimal cluster size of 20 voxels) (table 3 and figure 3).

In the control group, an increase in ReHo values was observed after inactive treatment in the left ACC (BA32) and medial frontal gyrus (MeFG) (BA10). A signal decrease in ReHo values was detected in the right MFG (BA6) ($P<0.05$, FDR corrected with a minimal cluster size of 20 voxels) (table 3 and figure 3).

Additionally, we have performed a direct comparison of the ReHo changes between the active and inactive group. The active acupoint group showed higher ReHo in the thalamus, ACC, STG, SMA and lower ReHo in the hippocampus, MFG, and MTG than the inactive group ($P<0.001$, uncorrected) (as shown in figure 4).

3.3 Clinical outcomes and comparison of de-qi sensations

Comparison within each group, both the active acupoint group and inactive group showed significant decreases in the VAS score, frequency of migraine attack per 4 weeks, number of days with migraine per 4 weeks and HIT-6 score after 8 weeks' treatment ($P<0.05$). Based on this study, a significant difference was found in the VAS scores between the two groups by analysis of variance for repeated measures ($P=0.015$) (table 4). The difference in VAS between the active group and inactive group was more than 0.9 in week 8 ($P=0.006$). However, no significant differences were observed between the two groups for the frequency of migraine attack per 4 weeks, number of days with migraine per 4 weeks, and HIT-6 score at the end of treatment ($P>0.05$) (table 4). Furthermore, analysis of variance of repeated measures indicated

that there was no significant difference between the two groups in de-qi sensations ($P>0.05$) (table 5).

3.4 Correlation coefficients of the brain response and clinical variable results

In the active acupoint group, the decrease in the VAS score was significantly related to the increased average ReHo values in the ACC ($r = -0.6619$, $P<0.05$) and insula ($r = -0.7407$, $P<0.05$, Bonferroni corrected). In the inactive control group, the decrease in the VAS score was only significantly related to the increased average ReHo values in the ACC ($r = -0.6611$, $P<0.05$, Bonferroni corrected) (figure 5).

3.5 Adverse events

No serious adverse events happened during the study. One case in the active acupuncture group suffered acupuncture fainting during acupuncture treatment. The patient was told to lie down and rest. The symptoms of dizziness and sweating disappeared in 15 minutes. Two cases in each group reported having minor hemorrhage at the needling site. They were told to put pressure on the needling areas for about 5 minutes, and recovered in a short time. All of the patients with adverse events completed the study process.

Discussion

In this RCT study, we focused on the difference in brain activation patterns evoked by active acupoints and inactive acupoints in migraine patients via fMRI assessment, and determined the potential physiological mechanism behind this therapy. An inactive acupoint is a validated sham control method in acupuncture research [30–32] with the advantage of minimizing bias from patients. By the way, non-acupoints are thought to have no therapeutic influence and are usually adopted as a placebo control in previous clinical trials and neuroimaging studies. In addition, minimal acupuncture or superficial insertion was often employed to stimulate non-acupoints producing inconspicuous de-qi sensations [11,23], but this might significantly cause bias among Chinese subjects. To ensure comparability between the two groups during acupuncture manipulation, de-qi sensations were assessed several times during the treatment session. Needling at inactive acupoints could effectively reduce the aforementioned bias, and evenly control non-specific factors such as expectancy effects during the period of study. In this experiment, the overall de-qi sensations in the active acupoint group and inactive acupoint group were comparable and had no statistical difference.

4.1 Similarities and differences in clinical efficacy between active acupuncture and inactive acupuncture

Based on the clinical outcomes of this RCT, both active and inactive acupuncture methods were helpful in treating migraine after 8 weeks of therapy ($P<0.05$). Both treatments remarkably alleviated the clinical symptoms of migraine (intensity of pain, attack frequency, and days with migraine) and improved the QOL. Furthermore, acupuncture at active acupoints was significantly superior to acupuncture at inactive acupoints in alleviating pain intensity ($P=0.015$) in the current study. This result was similar with our previous RCT report on the efficacy of acupuncture at true acupoints compared with non-acupoints for migraine prevention [11]. We inferred that similar clinical effects of both treatments might partly result from placebo and psychological effects. The placebo response is an essential part of pain treatment, especially in the improvement of headache sufferers. A systematic review has shown that when clinicians

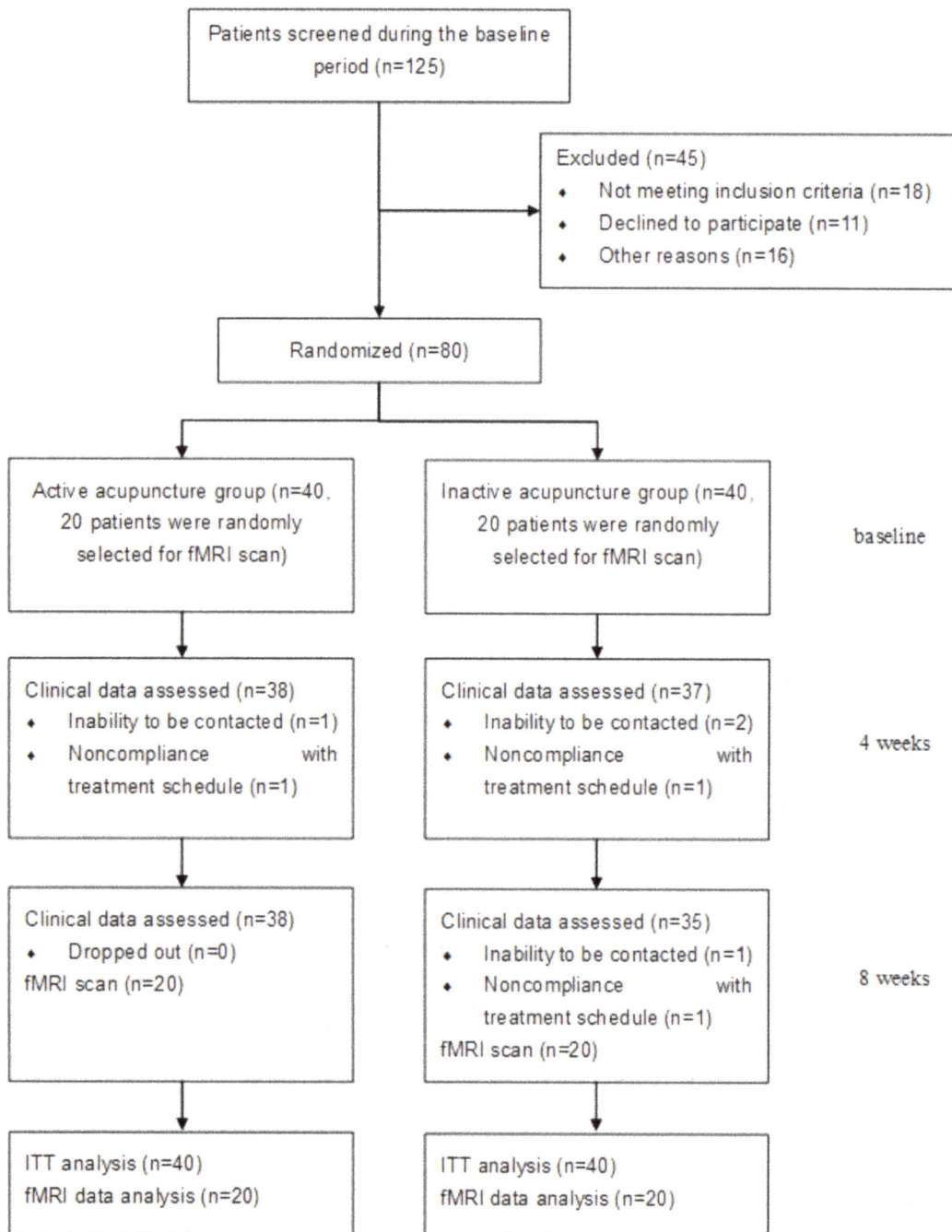

Figure 2. The flow chart of study. The flow chart of this study according to the CONSORT Statement.

Table 1. Baseline and demographics for migraine patients without aura (ITT).

Items	Active acupoint Group (n = 40)	Inactive acupoint Group (n = 40)
Mean age (SD), (years)	33.35 (11.69)	33.23 (9.73)
Female, n (%)	28 (70.0)	29 (72.5)
Mean education(SD), (years)	12.70 (3.29)	13.68 (3.74)
Mean duration of illness (SD), (years)	10.58 (7.40)	9.93 (5.73)
Family history (Y (%)/N (%))	8 (20.0)/32 (80.0)	9 (22.5)/31 (77.5)

Notes: ITT, intention-to-treat; SD, Standard deviation; Y, yes; N, no.

Table 2. Baseline characteristics of 40 migraineurs who participated in the fMRI scan.

Items	Active acupoint Group (n = 20)	Inactive acupoint Group (n = 20)
Mean age (SD), (years)	32.90 (10.99)	37.25 (9.68)
Female, n (%)	14 (70.0)	12 (60.0)
Mean education(SD), (years)	12.95 (3.52)	13.35 (4.12)
Mean duration of illness (SD), (years)	8.55 (6.49)	10.40 (7.40)
Family history (Y (%)/N (%))	2(10.0)/18 (90.0)	0 (0)/20 (100.0)
VAS score (SD)	5.28 (2.03)	5.44 (1.48)
Frequency of migraine attacks per 4 weeks*	7.90 (4.88)	5.45 (4.33)
Number of days with migraine (days) per 4 weeks	11.45 (9.30)	8.75 (9.21)
HIT-6 score	60.45 (8.13)	61.55 (7.98)

Notes: SD, Standard deviation; Y, yes; N, no.;
*Frequency of migraine attack, the number of episodes of migraine attacks separated by pain-free intervals of at least 48 hours.

stated positive outcome expectancies as opposed to uncertain expectancies, most studies found improvements in patient self-reports on pain, anxiety, and distress [33]. During the process of the study, two acupuncturists were responsible for the treatments alternately, and another experienced doctor who did not know the treatment allocation took charge of the efficacy evaluation. As we know, acupuncture treatment could create enhanced placebo effects, such as patient expectations, longer patient-doctor appointments, and the power of touch and suggestion, so both the active treatment and inactive treatment evenly ameliorated the headache degree and frequency originating from patients' self-reports which may be explained by the aforementioned nonspecific effects.

4.2 The similarities in resting-state brain activity evoked by active and inactive treatment

Based on the resting-state fMRI results, common brain regions responding to the acupuncture active treatment and inactive treatment included the ACC, MFG, and MTG. Among these areas, there was a significant negative correlation between the increased average ReHo values of the ACC and a decrease in the VAS score in both groups ($P < 0.05$, corrected). The results suggested that the increase in ReHo values in the ACC might be the common mechanism of acupuncture treatment for migraine patients, despite the needled active acupoints or inactive acupoints.

The ACC is a key region composed of the "pain matrix" and is involved in the medial pain system. It is one of the common "brain signature" structures in chronic pain diseases, and is thought to be

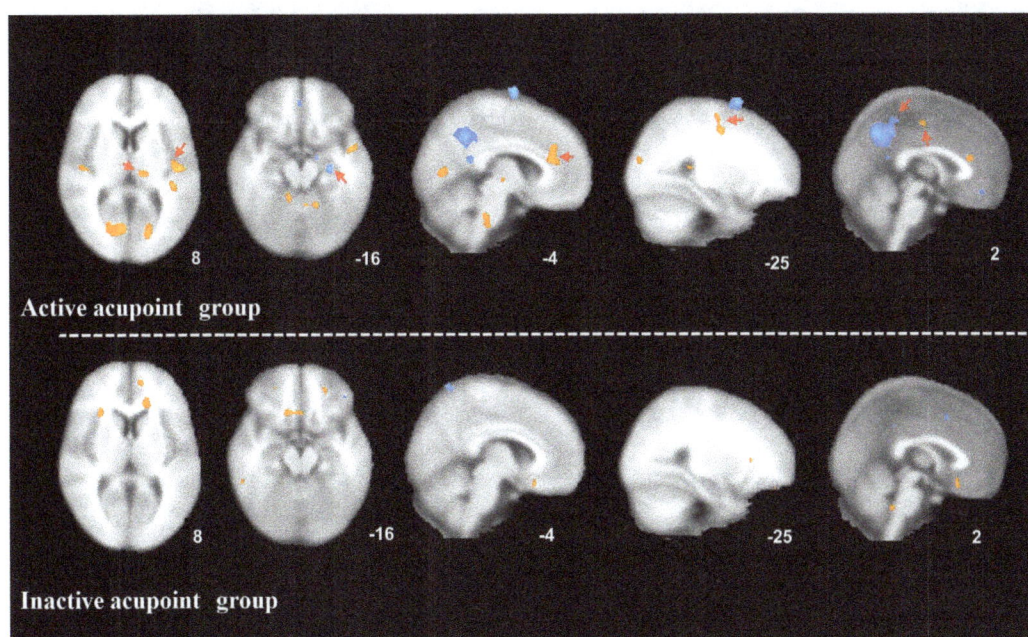

Figure 3. Brain activity in migraineurs without aura after different acupuncture treatment. Long-term active acupoint therapy elicited a more extensive and remarkable cerebral response compared with acupuncture at inactive acupoints.

Table 3. The cerebral ReHo changes in migraine patients without aura after active or inactive acupuncture treatment.

Region	Hemi	Active acupoint Group (n=20) Talairach x	y	z	t value	BA	Sign	Cluster size	Inactive acupoint Group (n=20) Talairach x	y	z	t value	BA	Sign	Cluster size
Limbic System															
ACC	L	-3	30	12	3.52	BA24/32	↑	33	-6	46	-5	3.47	BA32	↑	23
ACC	R	6	33	23	3.86		↑	52							
PCC	L	-3	-45	41	-3.78	BA31	→	39							
PCC	R	3	-48	38	-3.78		→	61							
Hippocampus	L	-30	-18	-14	-3.84	-	→	21							
Hippocampus	R														
Insula	L	-42	-11	6	3.26	BA13	↑	21							
Insula	R	36	-14	20	4.04		↑	23							
Thalamus	L	-15	-20	4	3.95	VPM	↑	26							
	R	15	-20	7	2.89		↑	21							
	L	-18	-20	4	3.05	VPL	↑	22							
	R	15	-17	4	3.34		↑	27							
Frontal Cortex															
MFG	L	-21	62	22	-3.37	BA 10	→	40							
MFG	R	42	59	14	-4.47		→	79	45	2	44	-4.43	BA6	→	32
MeFG	L								-6	49	-5	3.69	BA10	↑	26
	R														
SMA	L	-27	-9	50	2.9	BA6	↑	26							
	R	33	-9	53	3.78		↑	47							
Temporal Cortex															
STG	L	-45	-18	-2	4.76	BA 22	↑	67							
	R	50	-9	0	5.38		↑	87							
MTG	L	-50	-63	28	3.56	BA 39	→	30							
	R	50	-63	28	4.2		→	53							
ITG	L	-56	-10	-27	-3.29	BA 20	→								
	R														
Occipital Cortex															
Cuneus	L	-18	-78	9	3.71	BA 17/18	↑	51							
	R	21	-86	21	3.94		↑	85							
Lingual gyrus	L	-15	-73	4	2.84	BA 18	↑	16							
	R	12	-73	4	3.55		↑	71							

Table 3. Cont.

Region	Hemi	Active acupoint Group (n = 20)						Inactive acupoint Group (n = 20)						
		Talairach			t value	BA	Sign	Cluster size	Talairach			t value	BA	Sign	Cluster size
		x	y	z					x	y	z				
Parietal Lobe															
Inferior parietal lobule	L	−45	−65	42	−3.94	BA39	↓	37							
	R														
Angular gyrus	L	−48	−71	31	−4.21	BA39	↓	39							
	R	50	−65	31	−3.67		↓	31							
Postcentral gyrus	L														
	R	56	−33	49	−3.11	BA 40	↓	28							
Precuneus	L	−3	−44	46	−3.72	BA7	↓	153							
	R	3	−54	36	−4.58		↓	47							
Cerebellum	L	−15	−53	−12	3.89	-	↑	73							
	R	12	−47	−13	3.61		↑	37							
Brainstem	L					-									
	R	6	−34	−31	3.96		↑	51							

Notes: P<0.05, FDR corrected with a minimal cluster size of 20 voxels; Hemi, Hemisphere; BA, Brodmann Area; Up or down arrow (↑ / ↓) indicates whether the structure showed a signal increase or decrease respectively; L, left; R, right.

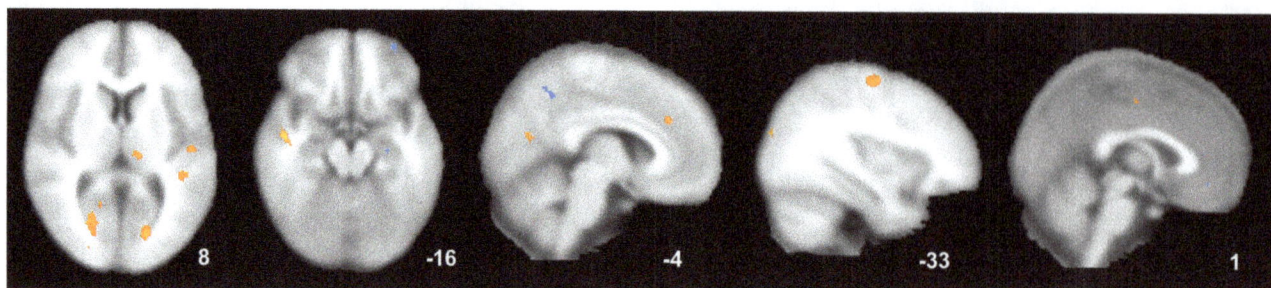

Figure 4. Direct comparison of the ReHo changes between the active and inactive group. The active acupoint group showed higher ReHo in the thalamus, ACC, superior temporal gyrus, SMA and lower ReHo in the hippocampus, middle frontal gyrus, and middle temporal cortex than the inactive group ($P<0.001$, uncorrected).

engaged with both cognitive-attentional and affective dimensions of pain. The ACC has been recognized in playing a deterministic role in endogenous pain control, which is mediated by endogenous opioid systems [34]. In previous neuroimaging studies, the ACC was the most consistently deactivated region in PET and fMRI migraine studies [35,36], and also had a decrease in gray matter [37,38]. Our research group verified that compared with healthy controls, migraineurs showed a significant decrease in ReHo values and amplitude of low-frequency fluctuation (ALFF) in the ACC [7,9], and showed aberrant functional connectivity which had the ACC involved [8,39]. In the present study, acupuncture-induced reduction in pain intensity ratings was negatively associated with increased average ReHo values in the ACC which illustrated that acupuncture treatment could promote pain reduction successfully by modulating the migraine-affected dysfunction region, the ACC, to some extent.

On the other hand, we inferred that the similarities in both clinical improvements and cerebral responses between active treatment and inactive treatment were possibly due to the placebo effect. During the process of treatment, migraineurs had positive expectations towards acupuncture therapy independent of whether or not the treatments were active or inactive, and moreover,

Table 4. Clinical outcome measures in each group (ITT).

Outcome measure	Active acupoint Group (n = 40)		Inactive acupoint Group (n = 40)		$P^\P$	$P^\dagger$
	Mean (SD)	95% CI	Mean (SD)	95% CI		
VAS score						
−4–0 weeks	5.11 (1.75)	(4.55–5.67)	5.23 (1.78)	(4.66–5.80)	0.7484	$P_T = 0.0000$
1–4 weeks	3.80 (1.62)	(3.28–4.32)	4.64 (1.17)	(4.27–5.01)	0.0094	$P_{T*G} = 0.0888$
5–8 weeks	3.07 (1.57)	(2.57–3.57)	4.07 (1.54)	(3.58–4.56)	0.0052	$P_G = 0.0150$
Difference from baseline in VAS$^\parallel$	2.096 (0.25)	(1.61–2.58)	1.110 (0.25)	(0.62–1.60)	0.006$^\parallel$	-
Frequency of migraine attacks per 4 weeks*						
−4–0 weeks	6.83 (4.21)	(5.48–8.17)	5.98 (3.72)	(4.79–7.16)	0.3412	$P_T = 0.0000$
1–4 weeks	4.35 (2.63)	(3.51–5.19)	3.92 (1.69)	(3.38–4.46)	0.3802	$P_{T*G} = 0.3168$
5–8 weeks	2.85 (2.19)	(2.15–3.55)	3.10±2.00	(2.46–3.74)	0.5983	$P_G = 0.4742$
Number of days with migraine (days) per 4 weeks						
−4–0 weeks	9.85 (7.94)	(7.31–12.39)	9.73 (7.62)	(7.29–12.16)	0.9429	$P_T = 0.0000$
1–4 weeks	5.56 (4.25)	(4.20–6.92)	4.91 (2.36)	(4.16–5.66)	0.4043	$P_{T*G} = 0.6459$
5–8 weeks	3.51 (2.66)	(2.66–4.36)	3.91 (2.82)	(3.01–4.82)	0.5122	$P_G = 0.8835$
HIT-6 score						
−4–0 weeks	58.10 (6.81)	(55.92–60.28)	58.13 (7.12)	(55.85–60.40)	0.4224	$P_T = 0.0000$
1–4 weeks	47.25 (9.55)	(44.20–50.30)	49.69 (9.35)	(46.70–52.68)	0.2515	$P_{T*G} = 0.3834$
5–8 weeks	47.86 (8.42)	(45.17–50.55)	50.39 (6.67)	(48.26–52.52)	0.1395	$P_G = 0.2232$

Notes: ITT, intention-to-treat;
CI, confidence interval;
*Frequency of migraine attack, the number of episodes of migraine attacks separated by pain-free intervals of at least 48 hours;
¶P values based on t-test between the two groups;
†P values based on repeated measures;
$^\parallel$based on analysis of covariance analysis;
P_T, values for comparison between different time points;
P_{T*G}, values for Time*Group interaction;
P_G, values for comparison between different groups.

Table 5. Comparison of *de-qi* sensations during treatment period (ITT).

Time points	Active acupoint Group (n = 40)	Inactive acupoint Group (n = 40)	*P* value
1st	8.70±4.16	10.31±4.26	0.1070
2nd	8.61±4.63	8.09±4.64	0.6372
3rd	9.13±3.89	8.18±3.70	0.2890
4th	10.62±4.45	10.42±4.42	0.8461

Notes: Comparison between different time points: F = 4.128, *P* = 0.007; Time*Group: F = 1.384, *P* = 0.249; Comparison between different groups: F = 0.001, *P* = 0.9790.

migraineurs were blinded to their groups and acquired comparable *de-qi* sensations throughout the duration of therapy. The ACC was commonly activated by acupuncture stimulation [40,41], and it plays an important role during placebo modulation of pain perception. Recent papers have described the effect of the placebo and expectancy on acupuncture analgesia, and certain findings were similar to our results. For example, some researchers found that reductions in pain intensity ratings were associated with placebo and opioid analgesia coinciding with increased activity in the ACC [42]. Additionally, active acupoint treatment induced a more prominent cerebral response in the ACC, thus we considered that the differences in both clinical variables and neuroimaging data between the two groups indicated that the placebo effect could not fully explain the neurobiological underpinning of active acupuncture therapy.

4.3 The difference in resting-state brain activity evoked by active and inactive treatment

Compared with acupuncture at inactive acupoints, long-term active acupoint therapy elicited a more extensive and remarkable cerebral response in the present study. The following cerebral regions exhibited increases in ReHo values only in the active acupoint group: the bilateral insula, thalamus, SMA, STG, cuneus, lingual gyrus, cerebellum, and brainstem. Meanwhile, decreases in ReHo values in the bilateral PCC, MTG, angular gyrus, precuneus, left hippocampus, ITG, inferior parietal lobule, and right postcentral gyrus were observed only in the active acupoint group (table 3 and figure 3). A further direct between-group comparison indicated that the active acupoint group showed higher ReHo in the thalamus, ACC, SMA, STG and lower ReHo in the hippocampus, MFG, and MTG than the inactive group (figure 4). In general, we found that active acupoint

treatment for a longitudinal course had major effects on the pain matrix, lateral pain system, medial pain system, default mode network (DMN), and some regions closely related to the cognitive components of pain processing.

In our results, active acupoint treatment elicited dramatic and extensive ReHo changes in the bilateral thalamus, including the ventral posterolateral nucleus (VPL) and ventral posteromedial nucleus (VPM). These nuclei are key intermediates in the lateral pain system, and play an important role in processing spatial and intensity aspects of noxious stimuli. The thalamus commonly had a dysfunction in migraine patients in previous documents [5,43], and its abnormalities were deemed to contribute to migraine pathophysiology. Pharmacological studies demonstrated that successful migraine preventive treatments modulated thalamic activity [5]. We speculated that the correlation between the VAS score and ReHo values was not detected in the thalamus, but was attributed to its relay function between a variety of subcortical areas and the cerebral cortex. Our results indicated that active acupoint treatment may play a major role in the sensory-discriminative component of pain and also in the appropriate modulation of the emotional aspect of pain.

In addition, as the core regions of the DMN, the PCC and precuneus were found to have decreased ReHo values after active acupuncture treatment. These findings were consistent with previous evidence which supports the position that genuine acupuncture leads to stronger DMN deactivation than sham acupuncture on healthy subjects [44]. Previous resting-state fMRI studies have shown that various pain diseases were associated with abnormal connectivity patterns among DMN regions [45,46], and our research group confirmed that migraine patients without aura had a DMN abnormality compared with healthy controls [39]. The DMN has previously been suggested as a potential neural

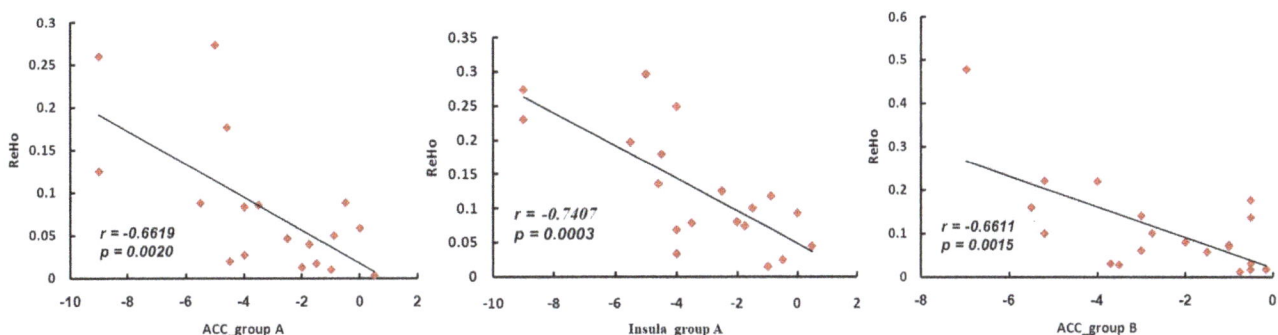

Figure 5. Correlation coefficients of brain response and VAS score. A. Active acupoint group; B. Inactive acupoint group. The decrease in the VAS score was significantly related to the increased average ReHo values in the ACC in the two groups (*P*<0.05, Bonferroni corrected). Moreover, the decrease in the VAS score was associated with increased average ReHo values in the insula (*P*<0.05, Bonferroni corrected) which could be detected in the active acupoint group.

marker of treatment efficacy in chronic pain, and our findings demonstrated that active acupuncture analgesia could be achieved by regulating the migraineurs' resting state and changing the dysfunctional architecture of the DMN.

Based on our results, we detected that a long course of acupuncture treatment on active acupoints affected the hippocampus, which is associated with cognitive components of pain processing, as well as a major component of the human brain that links affective states with memory processing. The hippocampus was described as having increased gray matter volume in patients suffering chronic pain in a meta-analysis [47], and this was confirmed in a recent migraine study [6]. It seems to frequently participate in the central effects of acupuncture. The cerebellum has anatomical connections with multiple areas of the frontal cortex and limbic regions, which are critical for its involvement in emotional and cognitive processing. A previous animal study indicated that the cerebellum contributes more to pain processing than just motor control [48]. Decreased gray matter volume in the cerebellum has been recently described in migraine patients without aura in a voxel-brain morphometry study in our research group [49], and another study also verified the migraineurs' cerebellar microstructural abnormalities [50]. Several independent functional imaging studies have reinforced the fact that the dysfunction of the brain stem is related to the pathogenesis of migraine [51–53]. The brain stem serves as a lower center in functions such as pain sensitivity control and consciousness. In our study, the modulation of active acupuncture treatment on the hippocampus, cerebellum and brain stem might be related to regulating the process of nociceptive information and homeostatic emotion originating from pain processing.

4.4 The potential mechanism of active acupuncture therapy for migraineurs

In order to better explore the possible physiological mechanism underlying different acupuncture treatments for migraine patients, a correlation analysis was employed. Except for the ACC, which is a co-related brain area for the two groups, we further noted that VAS reduction following active acupoint treatment was associated with the insula. The insula is a functionally heterogeneous brain region that participates in pain perception, emotional processing and interoception. It was commonly revealed that there was a difference in gray matter volume in chronic pain patients compared with healthy controls [47]. The insular networks were found to be altered by migraine headache [54,55], and our research team demonstrated that migraine patients have dysfunctional connectivity involved with the insula [8,39]. We were interested in the active acupuncture-induced reduction in pain intensity ratings which were negatively associated with increased

average ReHo values in the insula, as well as the ACC in the present study. These two regions belong to the "homeostatic afferent pathway", which carries information about the physiological status of tissues in the body. Pain is both an aspect of interoception and a behavioral drive caused by a physiological imbalance that homeostatic systems alone cannot rectify [56,57]. Our results illustrated that active acupuncture treatment could alleviate migraine intensity by modulating the disordered homeostatic afferent network back to physiological balance.

Limitations

The main limitations of the present study included the following: we expanded the number of eligible participants involved in the RCT, but the fMRI examinations were performed for 40 migraineurs who were randomly selected from 80 eligible migraineurs, so the correlation analysis of clinical measures and brain responses involved only 40 participants who completed the fMRI detections. Lack of an index to access and quantify the expectancy during the acupuncture treatment session is another limitation. Further studies need to quantify the patients' expectation and explore the effect on clinical efficacy and physiological mechanism of some non-specific factors during long-term acupuncture treatment.

Conclusions

In conclusion, the current study showed that long-term active acupoint therapy and inactive acupoint therapy have different brain activities. Acupuncture at active acupoints might have the potential effect of regulating some disease-affected key regions and the pain circuitry for migraine. More importantly, our results provided some evidence that active acupuncture treatment as a holistic therapy promotes psychophysical pain homeostasis.

Supporting Information

Checklist S1   CONSORT Checklist.
(DOCX)

Protocol S1   Trial Protocol.
(DOCX)

Author Contributions

Conceived and designed the experiments: LZ FL YL JL WQ QG. Performed the experiments: LZ XD YP FW. Analyzed the data: LZ JL FZ KY WQ ZT. Contributed reagents/materials/analysis tools: QG KY. Wrote the paper: LZ JL WQ KMvD.

References

1. (2004) The International Classification of Headache Disorders: 2nd edition. Cephalalgia 24 Suppl 1: 9–160.
2. Manack AN, Buse DC, Lipton RB (2011) Chronic migraine: epidemiology and disease burden. Curr Pain Headache Rep 15: 70–78.
3. Buse DC, Lipton RB (2013) Global perspectives on the burden of episodic and chronic migraine. Cephalalgia 33:885–890.
4. Schwedt TJ, Dodick DW (2009) Advanced neuroimaging of migraine. Lancet Neurol 8: 560–568.
5. Granziera C, Daducci A, Romascano D, Roche A, Helms G, et al. (2014) Structural abnormalities in the thalamus of migraineurs with aura: A multiparametric study at 3 T. Hum Brain Mapp 35:1461–1468.
6. Maleki N, Becerra L, Brawn J, McEwen B, Burstein R, et al. (2013) Common hippocampal structural and functional changes in migraine. Brain Struct Funct 218: 903–912.
7. Yu D, Yuan K, Zhao L, Dong M, Liu P, et al. (2012) Regional homogeneity abnormalities in patients with interictal migraine without aura: a resting-state study. NMR Biomed 25: 806–812.

8. Yuan K, Zhao L, Cheng P, Yu D, Dong T, et al. (2013) Altered Structure and Resting-State Functional Connectivity of the Basal Ganglia in Migraine Patients Without Aura. J Pain 14:836–844.
9. Xue T, Yuan K, Cheng P, Zhao L, Yu D, et al. (2013) Alterations of regional spontaneous neuronal activity and corresponding brain circuit changes during resting state in migraine without aura. NMR Biomed 26:1051–1058.
10. Linde K, Allais G, Brinkhaus B, Manheimer E, Vickers A, et al. (2009) Acupuncture for migraine prophylaxis. Cochrane Database Syst Rev 1: CD001218.
11. Li Y, Zheng H, Witt CM, Roll S, Yu SG, et al. (2012) Acupuncture for migraine prophylaxis: a randomized controlled trial. CMAJ 184: 401–410.
12. Diener HC, Kronfeld K, Boewing G, Lungenhausen M, Maier C, et al. (2006) Efficacy of acupuncture for the prophylaxis of migraine: a multicentre randomised controlled clinical trial. Lancet Neurol 5: 310–316.
13. Wang LP, Zhang XZ, Guo J, Liu HL, Zhang Y, et al. (2011) Efficacy of acupuncture for migraine prophylaxis: a single-blinded, double-dummy, randomized controlled trial. Pain 152: 1864–1871.

14. Linde M, Fjell A, Carlsson J, Dahlof C (2005) Role of the needling per se in acupuncture as prophylaxis for menstrually related migraine: a randomized placebo-controlled study. Cephalalgia 25: 41–47.

15. Yang J, Zeng F, Feng Y, Fang L, Qin W, et al. (2012) A PET-CT study on the specificity of acupoints through acupuncture treatment in migraine patients. BMC Complement Altern Med 12: 123.

16. Zang Y, Jiang T, Lu Y, He Y, Tian L (2004) Regional homogeneity approach to fMRI data analysis. Neuroimage 22: 394–400.

17. Zuo XN, Xu T, Jiang L, Yang Z, Cao XY, et al. (2013) Toward reliable characterization of functional homogeneity in the human brain: preprocessing, scan duration, imaging resolution and computational space. Neuroimage 65: 374–386.

18. Zhao L, Liu J, Dong X, Peng Y, Yuan K, et al. (2013) Alterations in regional homogeneity assessed by fMRI in patients with migraine without aura stratified by disease duration. J Headache Pain 14: 85.

19. Zhang Z, Liu Y, Jiang T, Zhou B, An N, et al. (2012) Altered spontaneous activity in Alzheimer's disease and mild cognitive impairment revealed by Regional Homogeneity. Neuroimage 59: 1429–1440.

20. Sheng K, Fang W, Su M, Li R, Zou D, et al. (2014) Altered spontaneous brain activity in patients with Parkinson's disease accompanied by depressive symptoms, as revealed by regional homogeneity and functional connectivity in the prefrontal-limbic system. PLoS One 9: e84705.

21. Zhu CZ, Zang YF, Cao QJ, Yan CG, He Y, et al. (2008) Fisher discriminative analysis of resting-state brain function for attention-deficit/hyperactivity disorder. Neuroimage 40: 110–120.

22. Friston K (2012) Ten ironic rules for non-statistical reviewers. Neuroimage 61: 1300–1310.

23. Li Y, Liang F, Yang X, Tian X, Yan J, et al. (2009) Acupuncture for treating acute attacks of migraine: a randomized controlled trial. Headache 49: 805–816.

24. Choi EM, Jiang F, Longhurst JC (2012) Point specificity in acupuncture. Chin Med 7: 4.

25. Tfelt-Hansen P, Block G, Dahlof C, Diener HC, Ferrari MD, et al. (2000) Guidelines for controlled trials of drugs in migraine: second edition. Cephalalgia 20: 765–786.

26. Kosinski M, Bayliss MS, Bjorner JB, Ware JE Jr., Garber WH, et al. (2003) A six-item short-form survey for measuring headache impact: the HIT-6. Qual Life Res 12: 963–974.

27. Kou W, Gareus I, Bell JD, Goebel MU, Spahn G, et al. (2007) Quantification of DeQi sensation by visual analog scales in healthy humans after immunostimulating acupuncture treatment. Am J Chin Med 35: 753–765.

28. Xu SB, Huang B, Zhang CY, Du P, Yuan Q, et al. (2013) Effectiveness of strengthened stimulation during acupuncture for the treatment of Bell palsy: a randomized controlled trial. CMAJ 185: 473–479.

29. Song XW, Dong ZY, Long XY, Li SF, Zuo XN, et al. (2011) REST: a toolkit for resting-state functional magnetic resonance imaging data processing. PLoS One 6: e25031.

30. Tjen ALSC, Li P, Longhurst JC (2004) Medullary substrate and differential cardiovascular responses during stimulation of specific acupoints. Am J Physiol Regul Integr Comp Physiol 287: R852–862.

31. Zhou W, Fu LW, Tjen ALSC, Li P, Longhurst JC (2005) Afferent mechanisms underlying stimulation modality-related modulation of acupuncture-related cardiovascular responses. J Appl Physiol 98: 872–880.

32. Li P, Ayannusi O, Reid C, Longhurst JC (2004) Inhibitory effect of electroacupuncture (EA) on the pressor response induced by exercise stress. Clin Auton Res 14: 182–188.

33. Crow R, Gage H, Hampson S, Hart J, Kimber A, et al. (1999) The role of expectancies in the placebo effect and their use in the delivery of health care: a systematic review. Health Technol Assess 3: 1–96.

34. Wager TD, Rilling JK, Smith EE, Sokolik A, Casey KL, et al. (2004) Placebo-induced changes in FMRI in the anticipation and experience of pain. Science 303: 1162–1167.

35. Kim JH, Kim S, Suh SI, Koh SB, Park KW, et al. (2010) Interictal metabolic changes in episodic migraine: a voxel-based FDG-PET study. Cephalalgia 30: 53–61.

36. Aderjan D, Stankewitz A, May A (2010) Neuronal mechanisms during repetitive trigemino-nociceptive stimulation in migraine patients. Pain 151: 97–103.

37. Rocca MA, Ceccarelli A, Falini A, Colombo B, Tortorella P, et al. (2006) Brain gray matter changes in migraine patients with T2-visible lesions: a 3-T MRI study. Stroke 37: 1765–1770.

38. Jin C, Yuan K, Zhao L, Yu D, von Deneen KM, et al. (2012) Structural and functional abnormalities in migraine patients without aura. NMR Biomed 26: 58–64.

39. Xue T, Yuan K, Zhao L, Yu D, Dong T, et al. (2012) Intrinsic brain network abnormalities in migraines without aura revealed in resting-state fMRI. PLoS One 7: e52927.

40. Napadow V, Makris N, Liu J, Kettner NW, Kwong KK, et al. (2005) Effects of electroacupuncture versus manual acupuncture on the human brain as measured by fMRI. Hum Brain Mapp 24: 193–205.

41. Dhond RP, Yeh C, Park K, Kettner N, Napadow V (2008) Acupuncture modulates resting state connectivity in default and sensorimotor brain networks. Pain 136: 407–418.

42. Etkin A, Egner T, Kalisch R (2011) Emotional processing in anterior cingulate and medial prefrontal cortex. Trends Cogn Sci 15: 85–93.

43. Afridi SK, Giffin NJ, Kaube H, Friston KJ, Ward NS, et al. (2005) A positron emission tomographic study in spontaneous migraine. Arch Neurol 62: 1270–1275.

44. Bai L, Qin W, Tian J, Dong M, Pan X, et al. (2009) Acupuncture modulates spontaneous activities in the anticorrelated resting brain networks. Brain Res 1279: 37–49.

45. Napadow V, LaCount L, Park K, As-Sanie S, Clauw DJ, et al. (2010) Intrinsic brain connectivity in fibromyalgia is associated with chronic pain intensity. Arthritis Rheum 62: 2545–2555.

46. Otti A, Guendel H, Wohlschlager A, Zimmer C, Noll-Hussong M (2013) Frequency shifts in the anterior default mode network and the salience network in chronic pain disorder. BMC Psychiatry 13: 84.

47. Smallwood RF, Laird AR, Ramage AE, Parkinson AL, Lewis J, et al. (2013) Structural brain anomalies and chronic pain: a quantitative meta-analysis of gray matter volume. J Pain 14: 663–675.

48. Dey PK, Ray AK (1982) Anterior cerebellum as a site for morphine analgesia and post-stimulation analgesia. Indian J Physiol Pharmacol 26: 3–12.

49. Jin C, Yuan K, Zhao L, Yu D, von Deneen KM, et al. (2013) Structural and functional abnormalities in migraine patients without aura. NMR Biomed 26: 58–64.

50. Granziera C, Romascano D, Daducci A, Roche A, Vincent M, et al. (2013) Migraineurs Without Aura Show Microstructural Abnormalities in the Cerebellum and Frontal Lobe. Cerebellum 12:812–818.

51. Bahra A, Matharu MS, Buchel C, Frackowiak RS, Goadsby PJ (2001) Brainstem activation specific to migraine headache. Lancet 357: 1016–1017.

52. Moulton EA, Burstein R, Tully S, Hargreaves R, Becerra L, et al. (2008) Interictal dysfunction of a brainstem descending modulatory center in migraine patients. PLoS One 3: e3799.

53. Stankewitz A, May A (2011) Increased limbic and brainstem activity during migraine attacks following olfactory stimulation. Neurology 77: 476–482.

54. Maleki N, Becerra L, Brawn J, Bigal M, Burstein R, et al. (2012) Concurrent functional and structural cortical alterations in migraine. Cephalalgia 32: 607–620.

55. Maleki N, Linnman C, Brawn J, Burstein R, Becerra L, et al. (2012) Her versus his migraine: multiple sex differences in brain function and structure. Brain 135: 2546–2559.

56. Craig AD (2003) Interoception: the sense of the physiological condition of the body. Curr Opin Neurobiol 13: 500–505.

57. Craig AD (2002) How do you feel? Interoception: the sense of the physiological condition of the body. Nat Rev Neurosci 3: 655–666.

7

Decreased Risk of Stroke in Patients with Traumatic Brain Injury Receiving Acupuncture Treatment: A Population-Based Retrospective Cohort Study

Chun-Chuan Shih[1], Yi-Ting Hsu[2], Hwang-Huei Wang[3], Ta-Liang Chen[4,5,6], Chin-Chuan Tsai[1], Hsin-Long Lane[1], Chun-Chieh Yeh[7], Fung-Chang Sung[8], Wen-Ta Chiu[9], Yih-Giun Cherng[10,⦾], Chien-Chang Liao[4,5,6,11]*,⦾

1 School of Chinese Medicine for Post-Baccalaureate, I-Shou University, Kaohsiung, Taiwan, 2 Neuroscience Laboratory, Department of Neurology, China Medical University Hospital, Taichung, Taiwan, 3 Graduate Institute of Integrated Medicine, College of Chinese Medicine, China Medical University, Taichung, Taiwan, 4 Department of Anesthesiology, Taipei Medical University Hospital, Taipei, Taiwan, 5 Health Policy Research Centre, Taipei Medical University Hospital, Taipei, Taiwan, 6 School of Medicine, College of Medicine, Taipei Medical University, Taipei, Taiwan, 7 Graduate Institute of Clinical Medical Science, China Medical University, Taichung, Taiwan, 8 Department of Public Health, China Medical University, Taichung, Taiwan, 9 Graduate Institute of Injury Prevention and Control, Taipei Medical University, Taipei, Taiwan, 10 Department of Anesthesiology, Shuang Ho Hospital, Taipei Medical University, New Taipei City, Taiwan, 11 Management Office for Health Data, China Medical University Hospital, Taichung, Taiwan

Abstract

Background: Patients with traumatic brain injury (TBI) face increased risk of stroke. Whether acupuncture can help to protect TBI patients from stroke has not previously been studied.

Methods: Taiwan's National Health Insurance Research Database was used to conduct a retrospective cohort study of 7409 TBI patients receiving acupuncture treatment and 29,636 propensity-score-matched TBI patients without acupuncture treatment in 2000–2008 as controls. Both TBI cohorts were followed until the end of 2010 and adjusted for immortal time to measure the incidence and adjusted hazard ratios (HRs) with 95% confidence intervals (CIs) of new-onset stroke in the multivariable Cox proportional hazard models.

Results: TBI patients with acupuncture treatment (4.9 per 1000 person-years) had a lower incidence of stroke compared with those without acupuncture treatment (7.5 per 1000 person-years), with a HR of 0.59 (95% CI = 0.50–0.69) after adjustment for sociodemographics, coexisting medical conditions and medications. The association between acupuncture treatment and stroke risk was investigated by sex and age group (20–44, 45–64, and ≥65 years). The probability curve with log-rank test showed that TBI patients receiving acupuncture treatment had a lower probability of stroke than those without acupuncture treatment during the follow-up period (p<0.0001).

Conclusion: Patients with TBI receiving acupuncture treatment show decreased risk of stroke compared with those without acupuncture treatment. However, this study was limited by lack of information regarding lifestyles, biochemical profiles, TBI severity, and acupuncture points used in treatments.

Editor: Cesar V. Borlongan, University of South Florida, United States of America

Funding: This study is supported in part by a Grant from the Committee on Chinese Medicine and Pharmacy, Department of Health, Taiwan (CCMP98-RD-038 and CCMP99-RD-035), the National Science Council, Taiwan (102-2314-B-038-021-MY3), and Taiwan Department of Health Clinical Trial and Research Center of Excellence (DOH102-TD-B-111-004). The funder had no role in study design, data collection and analysis, decision to publish, or preparation of the paper.

Competing Interests: The authors have declared that no competing interests exist.

* E-mail: jacky48863027@yahoo.com.tw

⦾ These authors contributed equally to this work.

Introduction

Traumatic brain injury (TBI) is a common cause of disability and death in every age group and both sexes worldwide [1–3]. Health problems after TBI include neurologic deficit, cognitive impairment, psychiatric illness, poor social functioning, and other significant adverse outcomes such as brain tumors and mortality [2,4–7]. This burden of disease calls for further investigation to prevent and treat complications after TBI [8].

Stroke is the second leading cause of death worldwide and the leading cause of acquired disability in adults in most regions [9]. An international multicenter study has identified cardiac diseases, hypertension, diabetes, smoking, alcohol intake, unhealthy diet, abdominal obesity, lack of exercise, psychosocial stress and depression as risk factors associated with 90% of stroke risk [10]. Prevention is an important way to reduce stroke incidence and mortality.

An increased risk of stroke among individuals who survive TBI has been documented [11,12]. Acupuncture is a traditional Chinese medicine (TCM) treatment that is commonly used in Taiwan [13–17]. Acupuncture has been found to improve cognition and sleep quality for patients with TBI [18], and our previous report found that patients with TBI who receive acupuncture treatment had reduced use of emergency care and hospitalization in the first year after injury [19]. Acupuncture has been documented as part of rehabilitation for patients with TBI [20]. However, whether acupuncture is effective in preventing stroke for patients with TBI is unknown. This study investigates the effectiveness of acupuncture in decreasing stroke risk among patients with TBI using multivariate and immortal time adjustment in a nationwide population-based cohort study.

Methods

Ethics Statement

Insurance reimbursement claims used in this study were from Taiwan's National Health Insurance Research Database, which is available for public access. This study was conducted in accordance with the Helsinki Declaration. To protect personal privacy, the electronic database was decoded with patient identifications scrambled for further public access for research. Although National Health Research Institutes regulations do not require informed consent due to decoded and scrambled patient identification, this study was approved by Taiwan's National Health Research Institutes.

Study Design and Population

Taiwan's National Health Research Institutes set up the National Health Insurance Research Database to allow access to all medical claims for insured beneficiaries since 1996. With patient identification numbers scrambled, data files can be secured to protect patient privacy. Information available for this study included gender, birth date, disease codes, health care rendered, medicines prescribed, diagnoses for admissions and discharges, and medical institutions and physicians providing services. This database was described in detail in our previous studies [1–3,19,21–25].

From a longitudinal cohort population-based database of a randomly selected one million insured subjects in 2000, we identified persons aged ≥20 years old with newly diagnosed TBI who made visits for medical care in 2000–2008 as our eligible study patients. In order to confirm that all patients with TBI in our study were incident cases, only new-onset TBI cases were included in this study; people with previous medical records of TBI within five years before the index date were excluded. The diagnosis of TBI was validated in previous studies [1–3]. Overall, we identified 37,045 new-onset TBI survivors aged ≥20 years; 7409 of them had used at least two courses (one course including six consecutive treatments) of acupuncture after TBI. We compared TBI patients receiving at least two courses of acupuncture treatment with patients without acupuncture treatment. TBI patients with only one course of treatment were excluded from this study. Each TBI patient was either followed up from the index date until 31 December 2010 or was censored. The follow-up time, in person-years, was calculated for each TBI patient until the diagnosis of stroke or until being censored due to death, withdrawal from the insurance system or loss to follow-up. The non-acupuncture group included patients with TBI who did not have acupuncture treatment before the end-point of follow-up. The person-years of TBI patients with acupuncture were calculated from the beginning of receiving acupuncture treatment corrected by immortal time [26].

Criteria and Definition

We defined TBI according to the *International Classification of Diseases, 9th Revision, Clinical Modification* (ICD-9-CM 800–805, 850–854) [1–3,19]. The primary outcome as the incident event of stroke was defined as ICD-9-CM 430–438. Coexisting medical conditions – hypertension (ICD-9-CM 401–405), mental disorders (ICD-9-CM 290–319), diabetes (ICD-9-CM 250), ischemic heart disease (ICD-9-CM 410–414), hyperlipidemia (ICD-9-CM 272.0–272.4), migraine (ICD-9-CM 346), and epilepsy (ICD-9-CM 345) – were considered as confounding factors due to documented increased risk of stroke in patients with these coexisting medical conditions [10,11,27]. TCM physicians were defined as physicians licensed by Taiwan's Department of Health who practiced TCM in regulated clinics or hospitals. We calculated the density of TCM physicians (TCM physicians/10,000 persons) using the number of TCM physicians per 10,000 residents for each administrative unit. The first, second, and third tertiles were considered as areas with low, moderate, and high physician density.

We identified stroke-related medications such as anticoagulants, antiplatelet agents, and lipid-lowering agents as potential confounding factors in the association between acupuncture treatment and stroke. National Health Insurance-covered anticoagulant included warfarin, dabigatran, heparin, and enoxaparin. Antiplatelet agents included aspirin, dipyridamole, ticlopidine, cilostazol, clopidogrel, tirofiban, aggrenox, abciximab, and eptifibatide. Lipid-lowering agents included atorvastatin simvastatin, rosuvastatin, fluvastatin, lovastatin, pitavastatin, pravastatin, vytorin (ezetimibe with simvastatin), gemfibrozil, and fenofibrate.

The selection of acupuncture point was determined by TCM doctors who made clinical assessment in accordance with TCM principles, such as the GV26 (Shuigou) point at the junction of the upper and middle third of the philtrum. [28] Acupuncturists used commercially available, single-use, sterile, and disposable stainless steel needles [18]. After the needles placed manually, they were left in place for around 15 minutes. All of this group of doctors obey these standard TCM guidelines to perform acupuncture treatments in the licensed clinical settings.

Statistical Analysis

To reduce confounding effects, we developed a non-parsimonious multivariable logistic regression model to estimate a propensity score for acupuncture treatment. Clinical significance guided the initial choice of covariates, which included age, sex, low-income status, density of TCM physicians, types of TBI, mental disorders, hypertension, diabetes mellitus, ischemic heart disease, hyperlipidemia, migraine, and epilepsy. We used a structured iterative approach to refine this logistic regression model to achieve balance of covariates within the matched pairs. We then matched (without replacement) patients who had acupuncture treatment to those who did not by using a greedy matching algorithm with a calliper width of 0·2 SD of the log odds of the propensity score. Nearest-neighbor algorithm was applied to construct matched pairs, assuming that the proportion of 0·95 to 1·0 is perfect.

The chi-square tests were used to analyze categorized data (age group, sex, low income, density of TCM physicians, types of TBI, mental disorders, hypertension, diabetes mellitus, ischemic heart disease, hyperlipidemia, migraine, epilepsy, anticoagulants, antiplatelet agents, lipid-lowering agents, and new-onset stroke events) between patients with TBI who had received acupuncture treatment and those who had not. The mean and standard deviation of age for TBI patients with and without acupuncture treatment was compared by t-tests. We performed the multivariable Cox proportional hazard model to analyze the adjusted hazard ratios (HRs) and 95% confidence intervals (CIs) of stroke associated with acupuncture treatment in patients with TBI. All analyses were performed using Statistical Analysis Software version 9.1 (SAS Institute Inc., Cary, North Carolina, USA). A two-sided probability value of <0.05 was considered significant.

Results

After propensity-score matching procedure (**Table 1**) there was no significant difference in age, sex, low income, area with TCM physician density, types of TBI, mental disorders, hypertension, diabetes, ischemic heart disease, hyperlipidemia, migraine and epilepsy between TBI patients with and without acupuncture treatment. Patients with acupuncture treatment had higher proportions of using anticoagulants (2.3% vs. 1.7%, p = 0.0003), antiplatelet agents (28.7% vs. 22.3%, p<0.0001), and lipid-lowering agents (24.7% vs. 18.4%, p<0.0001) compared with those had no acupuncture treatment. TBI patients who underwent acupuncture treatment had a lower proportion of new-onset stroke events than those without acupuncture treatment (2.2% vs. 4.2%, p<0.0001).

During the follow-up period (**Table 2**), TBI patients with acupuncture treatment (4.9 per 1000 person-years) had a lower incidence of new-onset stroke than those without acupuncture treatment (7.5 per 1000 person-years), with a HR of 0.59 (95% CI = 0.50–0.69) after adjustment for age, gender, low income, TCM physician density, type of TBI, diabetes mellitus, hypertension, hyperlipidemia, mental disorder, ischemic heart disease, migraine, epilepsy, anticoagulants, antiplatelet agents, and lipid-lowering agents. Among patients with TBI, the decreased risk of new-onset stroke associated with acupuncture treatment showed no significant gender difference in (men, HR = 0.57, 95% CI = 0.46–0.71; women, HR = 0.62, 95% CI = 0.48–0.79). The age stratified results showed that the adjusted HR of stroke associated with acupuncture treatment for TBI patients was the lowest in the younger group aged 20–44 years. The further log-rank test (**Figure 1**) showed that TBI patients with acupuncture treatment had a lower probability of new-onset stroke events than those without acupuncture treatment (p<0.0001).

Discussion

Using Taiwan's National Health Insurance Research Database, we conducted a retrospective cohort study with comprehensive design (matching procedure of propensity score) and showed significantly decreased risk of new-onset stroke events for patients with TBI who received acupuncture treatment. The present study is the first to report that acupuncture treatment was associated with reduced stroke risk for patients with TBI.

Confounding Effects

Male, older age, low income and coexisting medical conditions are risk factors for TBI and post-TBI outcomes [1–3]. The use of TCM or acupuncture was associated with age, sex, low-income status and chronic diseases such as hypertension, mental disorders, diabetes, stroke, ischemic heart diseases, hyperlipidemia, migraine, and epilepsy. [13–17,19]. To properly evaluate whether acupuncture treatment is associated with reduced stroke risk in TBI patients, we used propensity score to match the difference of age, sex, low income, and density of TCM physicians, mental disorders, hypertension, diabetes, ischemia heart disease, hyper-

Table 1. Baseline characteristics and stroke events for traumatic brain injury patients with and without acupuncture treatment.

	Acupuncture		p-value
	No (N = 29636)	Yes (N = 7409)	
Sex	n (%)	n (%)	1.00
Female	14056 (47.4)	3514 (45.4)	
Male	15580 (52.6)	3895 (52.6)	
Age, years			1.00
20–29	9068 (30.6)	2267 (30.6)	
30–39	5824 (19.7)	1456 (19.7)	
40–49	5544 (18.7)	1386 (18.7)	
50–59	3804 (12.8)	951 (12.8)	
60–69	2844 (9.6)	711 (9.6)	
70–79	2080 (7.0)	520 (7.0)	
≥80	472 (1.6)	118 (1.6)	
Mean±SD	42.6±17.1	42.5±16.9	0.52
Low income			1.00
No	29228 (98.6)	7307 (98.6)	
Yes	408 (1.4)	102 (1.4)	
Density of TCM physicians			1.00
Low	4352 (14.7)	1088 (14.7)	
Moderate	11744 (39.6)	2936 (39.6)	
High	13540 (45.7)	3385 (45.7)	
Type of TBI			1.00
Mild	12868 (43.4)	3217 (43.4)	
Moderate	5780 (19.5)	1445 (19.5)	
Severe	10988 (37.1)	2747 (37.1)	
Coexisting medical conditions			
Mental disorders	2708 (9.1)	677 (9.1)	1.00
Hypertension	3084 (10.4)	771 (10.4)	1.00
Diabetes mellitus	1324 (4.5)	331 (4.5)	1.00
Ischemic heart disease	608 (2.1)	152 (2.1)	1.00
Hyperlipidemia	452 (1.5)	113 (1.5)	1.00
Migraine	124 (0.4)	31 (0.4)	1.00
Epilepsy	60 (0.2)	15 (0.2)	1.00
Stroke-related medications			
Anticoagulants	493 (1.7)	169 (2.3)	0.0003
Antiplatelet agents	6617 (22.3)	2127 (28.7)	<0.0001
Lipid-lowering agents	5462 (18.4)	1826 (24.7)	<0.0001
New stroke events	1250 (4.2)	163 (2.2)	<0.0001

lipidemia, migraine and epilepsy between TBI patients with and without acupuncture treatment. To accurately estimate risk of stroke after TBI for patients with and without acupuncture treatment, residual confounding effects were adjusted in the multivariable Cox proportional hazard models.

Possible Explanations

Our previous study found that patients with TBI who received acupuncture treatment had less emergency care and hospitalization in the first year after injury compared with control [19]. In a

Table 2. Incidence, adjusted hazard ratios and confidence intervals of new-onset stroke for TBI patients with and without acupuncture treatment in the stratification of sex and age.

	Non-acupuncture				Acupuncture treatment				IRR (95% CI)	HR (95% CI)
	n	Events	Person-years	Incidence*	n	Events	Person-years	Incidence*		
Overall[†]	29636	1250	173682	7.5	7409	163	33071	4.9	0.68 (0.58–0.81)	0.59 (0.50–0.69)
Sex[‡]										
Female	14056	550	84939	6.5	3514	73	15890	4.6	0.71 (0.55–0.91)	0.62 (0.48–0.79)
Male	15580	700	88743	7.9	3895	90	17181	5.2	0.66 (0.53–0.83)	0.57 (0.46–0.71)
Age[§]										
20–44	17781	235	109647	2.1	4420	24	20054	1.2	0.56 (0.35–0.85)	0.46 (0.30–0.71)
45–64	7854	480	45206	10.6	1997	66	8953	7.4	0.69 (0.53–0.90)	0.64 (0.50–0.83)
≥65	4001	535	18829	28.4	992	73	4064	18.0	0.63 (0.49–0.81)	0.60 (0.47–0.76)

*Per 1000 person-years with calculated by correcting immortal time.
[†]Adjusted for age, gender, low income, density of TCM physicians, types of TBI, diabetes mellitus, hypertension, hyperlipidemia, mental disorders, ischemic heart disease, migraine, epilepsy, anticoagulants, antiplatelet agents, and lipid-lowering agents.
[‡]Adjusted for all covariates in the full model except gender.
[§]Adjusted for all covariates in the full model except age.
CI, confidence interval; HR, hazard ratio; IRR, incidence rate ratio; TBI, traumatic brain injury; TCM traditional Chinese medicine.

small sample of patients with TBI, Zollman et al. proved that acupuncture improves cognition and perception of sleep or sleep quality [18]. A clinical trial showed the intervention of acupuncture combined with point-injection in TBI patients improved post-TBI aphasia, hemiplegia, and injuries of cranial nerves (including injuries of the facial, oculomotor and abducent nerves) [29]. This study found that TBI patients who had acupuncture had decreased risk of stroke.

We propose two possible explanations. First, acupuncture has biological benefits for TBI patients. Several studies show acupuncture's effectiveness in improving stroke patients' physical abilities [30,31]. It has been shown that acupuncture is useful in lowering blood pressure [32,33], reducing inflammatory mediators [34], and improving lipid profile [35,36]. Acupuncture may also mediate anti-pain, anti-anxiety, and other therapeutic effects via intrinsic neural circuits that influence the affective and cognitive dimensions of pain [37]. Modulation of subcortical structures may also be an important mechanism by which acupuncture exerts complex multisystem effects [38]. This modulation and sympathy-vagal response may relate to acupuncture's analgesia and other potential therapeutic effects [39]. These findings implied that acupuncture might improve physical activity to reduce the risk of stroke. Second, patients with TBI who choose acupuncture treatment may have better knowledge, attitudes and practices regarding physical rehabilitation and disease prevention, which we believe could also contribute to reduce new-onset stroke event after TBI.

Study Strengths

Among this study's strengths is its large sample, as it uses a representative sample of one million subjects from Taiwan's National Health Insurance Research Database. Second, our study design was a retrospective cohort; this provides more evidence than case-control or cross-sectional designs. Third, to eliminate the interference of sociodemographics and coexisting medical conditions between TBI patients with or without acupuncture treatment, we used propensity score matching procedure to select acupuncture treatment and non-treatment controls. To control residual confounding effects in the association between decreased risk of stroke after TBI and acupuncture treatment, we applied the

multivariable Cox proportional hazard models to calculate adjusted HRs and 95% CIs of stroke associated with acupuncture treatment. Finally, immortal time in observational studies can bias the results in favor of the treatment group, but it is difficult to identify and avoid [27]. To reduce such bias, we calculated person-years to correct immortal time in the group with acupuncture treatment.

Study Limitations

This study has several limitations. First, we used retrospective medical claims data from health insurance that lacked detailed patient information on lifestyle as well as physical, psychiatric, and laboratory examinations. Second, we used ICD-9-CM codes claimed by physicians for TBI without clarifying the severity of disease using means such as the Glasgow coma scale. Third, the data provided by insurance claims might underestimate the prevalence of TBI due to cases in which patients with very minor

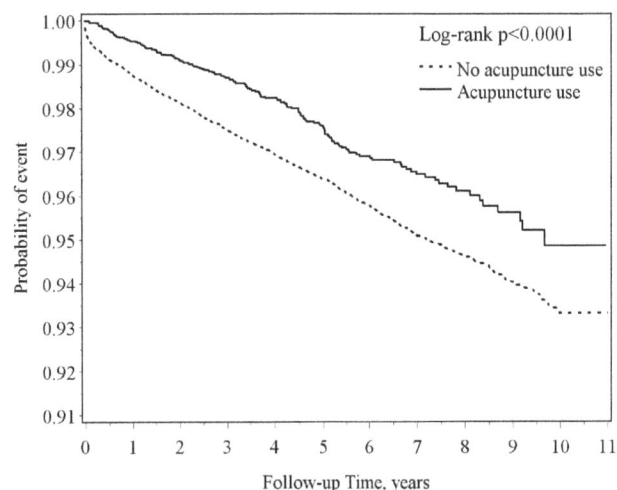

Figure 1. The stroke-free proportions estimated for TBI patients with and without acupuncture treatment using the Kaplan-Meier method.

TBI might not seek medical treatment. In addition, the beneficial effects from acupuncture were somewhat different from individual acupuncture points [40]. Our study could not validate the actual acupuncture points used in treatment due to the limited information from the National Health Insurance Research Database. Finally, the mode of acupuncture treatment for patients with TBI varied with TCM physicians. We could not confirm every TCM physician performed the same procedures and acupuncture points for patients with TBI.

Conclusions

From the results of this nationwide retrospective cohort study with matching procedure by propensity score, multivariable adjustment and immortal time correction, we suggested that TBI patients with acupuncture treatment had lower risk of new-onset stroke compared with TBI patients without acupuncture treatment. The association between acupuncture treatment and decreased risk of stroke among TBI patients existed in both sexes and among all age groups. However, further investigation is needed on specific acupuncture points to detail the mechanisms for such effects.

Acknowledgments

This study is based in part on data from the National Health Insurance Research Database provided by the National Health Research Institutes. The interpretation and conclusions contained herein do not represent those of the National Health Research Institutes.

Author Contributions

Conceived and designed the experiments: Chun-Chuan Shih, Yi-Ting Hsu, Hwang-Huei Wang, Ta-Liang Chen, Chin-Chuan Tsai, Hsin-Long Lane, Chun-Chieh Yeh, Fung-Chang Sung, Wen-Ta Chiu, Yih-Giun Cherng, Chien-Chang Liao. Performed the experiments: Chun-Chuan Shih, Hsin-Long Lane, Chien-Chang Liao. Analyzed the data: Chun-Chuan Shih, Hsin-Long Lane, Chien-Chang Liao. Contributed reagents/materials/analysis tools: Chun-Chuan Shih, Hsin-Long Lane, Chien-Chang Liao. Wrote the manuscript: Chun-Chuan Shih, Hsin-Long Lane,Yih-Giun Cherng, Chien-Chang Liao. Revising the manuscript: Chun-Chuan Shih, Yi-Ting Hsu, Hwang-Huei Wang, Ta-Liang Chen, Chin-Chuan Tsai, Hsin-Long Lane, Chun-Chieh Yeh, Fung-Chang Sung, Wen-Ta Chiu, Yih-Giun Cherng, Chien-Chang Liao.

References

1. Liao CC, Chiu WT, Yeh CC, Chang HC, Chen TL (2012) Risk and outcomes for traumatic brain injury in patients with mental disorders. J Neurol Neurosurg Psychiatry 83: 1186–1192.
2. Yeh CC, Chen TL, Hu CJ, Chiu WT, Liao CC (2013) Risk of epilepsy after traumatic brain injury: a retrospective population-based cohort study. J Neurol Neurosurg Psychiatry 84: 441–445.
3. Liao CC, Chang HC, Yeh CC, Chou YC, Chiu WT, et al. (2012) Socioeconomic deprivation and associated risk factors of traumatic brain injury in children. J Trauma Acute Care Surg 73: 1327–1231.
4. Hesdorffer DC, Rauch SL, Tamminga CA (2009) Long-term psychiatric outcomes following traumatic brain injury: a review of the literature. J Head Trauma Rehabil 24: 452–459.
5. Bazarian JJ, Cernak I, Noble-Haeusslein L, Potolicchio S, Temkin N (2009) Long-term neurologic outcomes after traumatic brain injury. J Head Trauma Rehabil 24: 439–451.
6. Dikmen SS, Corrigan JD, Levin HS, Machamer J, Stiers W, et al. (2009) Cognitive outcome following traumatic brain injury. J Head Trauma Rehabil 24: 430–438.
7. Ishibe N, Wlordarczyk RC, Fulco C (2009) Overview of the Institute of Medicine Committee's search strategy and review process for "Gulf War and Health: Long-term Consequences of Traumatic Brain Injury." J Head Trauma Rehabil 24: 424–429.
8. Engberg AW (2007) A Danish national strategy for treatment and rehabilitation after acquired brain injury. J Head Trauma Rehabil 22: 221–228.
9. Feigin VL (2007) Stroke in developing countries: can the epidemic be stopped and outcomes improved? Lancet Neurol 6: 94–97.
10. O'Donnell MJ, Xavier D, Liu L, Zhang H, Chin SL, et al. (2010) Risk factors for ischaemic and intracerebral haemorrhagic stroke in 22 countries (the INTERSTROKE study): a case-control study. Lancet 376: 112–123.
11. Chen YH, Kang JH, Lin HC (2011) Patients with traumatic brain injury: population-based study suggests increased risk of stroke. Stroke 42: 2733–2739.
12. Burke JF, Stulc JL, Skolarus LE, Sears ED, Zahuranec DB, et al. (2013) Traumatic brain injury may be an independent risk factor for stroke. Neurology 81: 33–39.
13. Liao CC, Lin JG, Tsai CC, Lane HL, Su TC, et al. (2012) An investigation of the use of traditional Chinese medicine in stroke patients in Taiwan. Evid Based Complement Alternat Med 2012: 387164.
14. Shih CC, Liao CC, Su YC, Tsai CC, Lin JG (2012) Gender differences in the use of traditional Chinese medicine among adults in Taiwan. PLoS One 7: e32540.
15. Shih CC, Su YC, Liao CC, Lin ZG (2012) The association between socioeconomic status and the utilization of traditional Chinese medicine among children in Taiwan. BMC Health Serv Res 12: 27.
16. Shih CC, Su YC, Liao CC, Lin ZG (2010) Patterns of medical pluralism among adults: results from the 2001 National Health Interview Survey in Taiwan. BMC Health Serv Res 10: 191.
17. Shih CC, Lin JG, Liao CC, Su YC (2009) The utilization of traditional Chinese medicine and associated factors in Taiwan in 2002. Chin Med J 122: 1544–1548.
18. Zollman FS, Larson EB, Wasek-Throm LK, Cyborski CM, Bode RK (2012) Acupuncture for treatment of insomnia in patients with traumatic brain injury: a pilot intervention study. J Head Trauma Rehabil 27: 135–142.
19. Shih CC, Lee HH, Chen TL, Tsai CC, Lane HL, et al. (2013) Reduced use of emergency care and hospitalization in patients with traumatic brain injury receiving acupuncture treatment. Evid Based Complement Alternat Med 2013: 262039.
20. Wong V, Cheuk DK, Lee S, Chu V (2013) Acupuncture for acute management and rehabilitation of traumatic brain injury. Cochrane Database Syst Rev 3: CD007700.
21. Yeh CC, Wang HH, Chou YC, Hu CJ, Chou WH, et al. (2013) High risk of gastrointestinal hemorrhage in patients with epilepsy: a nationwide cohort study. Mayo Clin Proc 88: 1091–1098.
22. Yeh CC, Liao CC, Chang YC, Jeng LB, Yang HR, et al. (2013) Adverse outcomes after non-cardiac surgery for patients with diabetes: a nationwide population-based retrospective cohort study. Diabetes Care 36: 3216–3221.
23. Lin JA, Liao CC, Lee YJ, Wu CH, Huang WQ, et al. (2013) Postoperative adverse outcomes in surgical patients with systemic lupus erythematosus: A nationwide population-based study. Ann Rheumatol Dis. [Epub ahead of print].
24. Liao CC, Shen WW, Chang H, Chang CC, Chen TL (2013) Surgical adverse outcomes in patients with schizophrenia: a population-based study. Ann Surg 257: 433–438.
25. Chang CC, Chang HC, Wu CH, Chang CY, Liao CC, et al. (2013) Postoperative adverse outcomes in surgical patients with idiopathic thrombocytopenic purpura: a population-based study. Br J Surg 100: 684–692.
26. Lévesque LE, Hanley JA, Kezouh A, Suissa S (2010) Problem of immortal time bias in cohort studies: example using statins for preventing progression of diabetes. BMJ 340: b5087.
27. Liao CC, Su TC, Sung FC, Chou WH, Chen TL (2012) Does hepatitis C virus infection increase risk for stroke? A population-based cohort study. PLoS One 7: e31527.
28. Tseng YJ, Hung YC, Hu WL (2013) Acupuncture helps regain postoperative consciousness in patients with traumatic brain injury: a case study. J Altern Complement Med 19: 474–477.
29. He J, Wu B, Zhang Y (2005) Acupuncture treatment for 15 cases of post-traumatic coma. J Tradit Chin Med 25: 171–173.
30. Wu P, Mills E, Moher D, Seely D (2010) Acupuncture in poststroke rehabilitation: A systematic review and meta-analysis of randomized trials. Stroke 41: e171–e179.
31. Sze FK, Wong E, Or KK, Lau J, Woo J (2002) Does acupuncture improve motor recovery after stroke? A meta-analysis of randomized controlled trials. Stroke 33: 2604–2619.
32. Flachskampf FA, Gallasch J, Gefeller O, Gan J, Mao J, et al. (2007) Randomized trial of acupuncture to lower blood pressure. Circulation 115: 3121–3129.
33. Kim DD, Pica AM, Duran RG, Duran WN (2006) Acupuncture reduces experimental renovascular hypertension through mechanisms involving nitric oxide synthases. Microcirculation 13: 577–585.
34. Choi DC, Lee JY, Moon YJ, Kim SW, Oh TH, et al (2010) Acupuncture-mediated inhibition of inflammation facilities significant functional recovery after spinal cord injury. Neurobiol Dis 39: 272–282.
35. Cabioğlu MT, Ergene N (2005) Electroacupuncture therapy for weight loss reduces serum total cholesterol, triglycerides, and LDL cholesterol levels in obese women. Am J Chin Med 33: 525–533.
36. Hsieh CH (2010) The effects of auricular acupuncture on weight loss and serum lipid levels in overweight adolescents. Am J Chin Med 38: 675–682.

37. Fang J, Jin Z, Wang Y, Li K, Kong J, et al. (2009) The salient characteristics of the central effects of acupuncture needling: limbic-paralimbic-neocortical network modulation. Hum Brain Mapp 30: 1196–1206.

38. Hui KK, Liu J, Makris N (2000) Acupuncture modulates the limbic system and subcortical gray structures of the human brain: evidence from fMRI studies in normal subjects. Hum Brain Mapp 9: 13–25.

39. Dhond RP, Yeh C, Park K, Kettner N, Napadow V (2008) Acupuncture modulates resting state connectivity in default and sensorimotor brain networks. Pain 136: 407–418.

40. Quah-Smith I, Sachdev PS, Wen W, Chen X, Williams MA (2010) The brain effects of laser acupuncture in healthy individuals: an FMRI investigation. PLoS One 5: e12619.

8

How Well Do Randomized Trials Inform Decision Making: Systematic Review Using Comparative Effectiveness Research Measures on Acupuncture for Back Pain

Claudia M. Witt[1,2]*, **Eric Manheimer[1]**, **Richard Hammerschlag[3]**, **Rainer Lüdtke[4]**, **Lixing Lao[1]**, **Sean R. Tunis[5]**, **Brian M. Berman[1]**

1 University of Maryland School of Medicine, Center for Integrative Medicine, Baltimore, Maryland, United States of America, 2 Charité University Medical Center, Institute for Social Medicine, Epidemiology and Health Economics, Berlin, Germany, 3 Research Department, Oregon College of Oriental Medicine, Portland, Oregon, United States of America, 4 Carstens Foundation, Essen, Germany, 5 Center for Medical Technology Policy, Baltimore, Maryland, United States of America

Abstract

Background: For Comparative Effectiveness Research (CER) there is a need to develop scales for appraisal of available clinical research. Aims were to 1) test the feasibility of applying the pragmatic-explanatory continuum indicator summary tool and the six CER defining characteristics of the Institute of Medicine to RCTs of acupuncture for treatment of low back pain, and 2) evaluate the extent to which the evidence from these RCTs is relevant to clinical and health policy decision making.

Methods: We searched Medline, the AcuTrials™ Database to February 2011 and reference lists and included full-report randomized trials in English that compared needle acupuncture with a conventional treatment in adults with non-specific acute and/or chronic low back pain and restricted to those with ≥30 patients in the acupuncture group. Papers were evaluated by 5 raters.

Principal Findings: From 119 abstracts, 44 full-text publications were screened and 10 trials (4,901 patients) were evaluated. Due to missing information and initial difficulties in operationalizing the scoring items, the first scoring revealed inter-rater and inter-item variance (intraclass correlations 0.02–0.60), which improved after consensus discussions to 0.20–1.00. The 10 trials were found to cover the efficacy-effectiveness continuum; those with more flexible acupuncture and no placebo control scored closer to effectiveness.

Conclusion: Both instruments proved useful, but need further development. In addition, CONSORT guidelines for reporting pragmatic trials should be expanded. Most studies in this review already reflect the movement towards CER and similar approaches can be taken to evaluate comparative effectiveness relevance of RCTs for other treatments.

Editor: Laxmaiah Manchikanti, University of Louisville, United States of America

Funding: CMW received a travel grant by the Institute for Integrative Health a non-profit organization, Baltimore, United States of America. The funders had no role in study design, data collection and analysis, decision to publish, or preparation of the manuscript. No additional external funding received for this study.

Competing Interests: The authors have declared that no competing interests exist.

* E-mail: claudia.witt@charite.de

Introduction

Comparative Effectiveness Research (CER) has considerable potential to help health care providers as well as patients and clinicians to choose among currently available therapeutic options. Different definitions for CER have been published. In this paper we use the working definition as established by the Institute of Medicine (IOM) Committee, which defines CER as "the generation and synthesis of evidence that compares the benefits and harms of alternative methods to prevent, diagnose, treat, and monitor a clinical condition or to improve the delivery of care. The purpose of CER is to assist consumers, clinicians, purchasers, and policy makers to make informed decisions that will improve health care at both the individual and population levels" [1].

However, to date, the majority of clinical trials have assessed the efficacy of medical interventions rather than their effectiveness. To support more informed decision-making, there has been a call for more evidence on real world effectiveness from CER [2]. Available systematic reviews generally do not assess available evidence from a CER perspective – in other words, to examine the extent to which published trials are relevant to clinical and health policy decision making. On the contrary, appraisal of internal validity plays one of the most prominent roles in systematic reviews. For example, Cochrane reviews provide systematic information about possible bias within each study, but do not provide systematic information about the relevance of the study results for clinical and health policy decision-making.

For a better understanding of CER, it is essential to distinguish between 'efficacy' and 'effectiveness'. 'Efficacy' refers to "the extent to which a specific intervention is beneficial under ideal conditions" [3]. Many randomized controlled trials are efficacy trials, particularly those conducted for regulatory drug approval. They aim to produce the expected result for an intervention under carefully controlled conditions chosen to maximize the likelihood of observing an effect if it exists. The trial population and setting of efficacy trials can differ in important ways from the clinical settings in which the interventions are likely to be used [4]. By contrast, 'effectiveness' is a measure of the extent to which an intervention, when deployed in the field in routine circumstances, does what it is intended to do for a specific population [3], and therefore can often be more relevant to policy evaluation and the health care decisions of providers and patients.

For randomized trials, the distinction between explanatory and pragmatic randomized trials was introduced in the 1960 s by Schwarz and Lelloch [5] and is also used in the CONSORT extension [6], another milestone publication on practical trials [7] and the pragmatic-explanatory continuum indicator summary (PRECIS) [8]. However, the term 'explanatory' can be misleading since pragmatic trials can also use an explanatory (confirmatory) statistical approach. Because of this potential confusion, we will use the terms 'efficacy' and 'effectiveness' for labeling the ends of this continuum. It is important to note that there is no sharp distinction between efficacy and effectiveness trials. Rather these terms exist in a continuum and the site along this continuum may differ for different features of the trial design.

This is reflected in the PRECIS tool [8] that was primarily developed to guide the design of RCTs along 10 dimensions of the efficacy-effectiveness continuum. In addition, the IOM has described six characteristics of CER (see Table 1) [1]. Both sets of criteria share the intent of describing the features of research that help inform clinical and health policy decisions. Use of these tools to assess existing trials may offer insights about the specific ways in which existing research has fallen short, and provide specific ideas about how to improve the quality and relevance of future trials. It is of major interest whether the available research can inform stakeholders. Do the existing criteria that define 'pragmatism' and CER that were developed for planning trials that inform clinical decision could be applied to the published trials as a means of evaluating and strengthening the evidence base for CER? Licensing drug trials usually have their main focus on efficacy, using placebo controls and objective outcome measures whenever possible. Because of these regulatory aspects, non-pharmacological studies would serve as better examples to show the whole range of an existing efficacy-effectiveness continuum.

CER is especially valuable for those disorders that are the most common and most costly to society, have the highest morbidity rates, and a great degree of variation in their practice [9]. Low back pain has a high lifetime prevalence, is one of the most common reasons for visits to a physician [10] and results in high health care expenses [11]. An estimated 8 million Americans have used acupuncture as a treatment for persistent disabling pain conditions that include chronic low back pain [12], and clinical relevance of acupuncture for chronic low back pain in usual care is highlighted by a recent clinical expertise paper on acupuncture for chronic low back pain in the New England Journal of Medicine [13]. In this paper, we explore the efficacy/effectiveness continuum in the context of RCTs that assess the impact of acupuncture on low back pain.

This systematic review aims to 1) test the feasibility of applying the PRECIS tool and the IOM CER characteristics to RCTs of acupuncture for treatment of low back pain, and 2) evaluate the extent to which the evidence from these RCTs is relevant to clinical and health policy decision making.

Methods

Data sources and searches

We identified trials using the following search strategy:

- AcuTrials™ Database [14] Feb 10, 2011 searched for low back pain and a comparator group, which was standard care/ usual care or no treatment. This database was created by the Research Department, Oregon College of Oriental Medicine, Portland, OR as a comprehensive database that includes all RCTs and systematic reviews on acupuncture published in English.

- Medline 1966 to Feb 17, 2011 searched for 'back pain and acupuncture' or 'back pain and Chinese Medicine' or 'back pain and Traditional Chinese Medicine' using the limits Clinical Trial, Meta-Analysis, Randomized Controlled Trial, English.

- Hand-searching for applicable trials, including the two most recent meta-analyses [15,16].

Study selection

Types of trials. We included controlled trials in which allocation to treatment was explicitly randomized. Trials were excluded that used an inappropriate method of randomization, e.g. open alternation or lottery.

Types of participants. Trials conducted among adult patients suffering from non-specific acute and/or chronic low back pain were included. Trials including patients with specific low back pain, e.g., sciatica or pelvic and lumbar pain during pregnancy, were excluded.

Types of interventions. The treatments considered had to at least involve needle insertion at acupuncture points, pain points or trigger points, and be described as acupuncture. The control interventions considered were conventional treatments (drugs, relaxation, physical therapies, self care etc.). Trials with additional acupuncture interventions based on usual care or other conventional interventions were included. Trials in which patients in the control group had no treatment or only rescue medication or TENS were excluded because they were not considered adequate conventional treatment interventions.

Types of publications. We included only English-language full papers that reported results of single trials. Follow-up publications, protocol publications, diagnostic trials, publications on intervention details, and publications that reported only economic results were excluded.

Sample size. Because we were mainly interested in the efficacy-effectiveness continuum and due to higher variance it is difficult to assess effectiveness with very small samples, we predefined arbitrary to include only those RCTs with ≥ 30 patients in the acupuncture group.

Data Extraction and Quality Assessment

Selection of trials and preliminary data extraction were performed by one rater (CMW). As a first step, references retrieved from Medline and the AcuTrials database were combined and duplicates were removed. All remaining abstracts were screened and trials that were clearly irrelevant were excluded (e.g., specific low back pain, only sham control or no control group, see Figure 1 for details). In addition, reference lists of recent systematic reviews [15,16] were checked, but did not reveal further unique trials. For the abstracts meeting inclusion criteria, the full papers were obtained and were formally re-checked to exclude ineligible papers. Information on methods, patients, interventions,

Table 1. Rating details using the PRECIS criteria and the IOM characteristics.

criteria	Rating# max. diff. points	Intraclass-correlation before/ after	operationa-lization* good/ moderate/ difficult	comment	suggestions
PRECIS criteria					
1) eligibility criteria	1	−.12/.59	moderate	raters need good medical knowledge about the range of patients with this diagnosis in usual care	treatment guidelines could be used to aid decision making
2) treatment flexibility intervention group	0	.82/1.00	good	usual care situation differs in countries and even US States, number of treatment always limited in interventional trials	more details in CONSORT guidelines
3) practitioner expertise intervention group	1	.10/.69	moderate	expertise range differs between countries and even US States, often no data about usual care setting and limited information about selection procedure	more details in CONSORT guidelines
4) treatment flexibility control group	1	.58/.95	moderate	publications often don't provide enough information about co-interventions, number of treatment always limited in interventional trials	more details in CONSORT guidelines
5) practitioner expertise control group	1	.60/.92	moderate	publications don't provide enough information, expertise range differs between countries and even US States, often no data about usual care setting and limited information about selection procedure	more details in CONSORT guidelines
6) follow up intensity	1	.02/.36	difficult	trial situation always differs from usual care, influence of telephone interviews, or questionnaires is difficult to operationalize	clear operationalization needed
7) outcomes	1	−.20/−.20	difficult	raters need good knowledge about valid outcomes for the diagnosis, usual care situation on one end of the scale with no interference was difficult	more diagnoses specific standards e.g. in treatment guidelines needed
8) patients' compliance	2	.28/.62	difficult	publications don't provide enough information	could be included in CONSORT guidelines
9) practitioners' protocol adherence	1	.29/.68	difficult	publications don't provide enough information	could be included in CONSORT guidelines
10) primary analysis	1	−.12/.77	good	older publications do not provide this information systematic, most trials do ITT and the relevant topic of subgroup analyses is missing in PRECIS	aspect of subgroup analysis should be included (see IOM)
IOM criteria					
1) directly informing a specific clinical decision from the patient perspective or a health policy decision from the population perspective	3	−.17/.03	moderate	depends on health system, interpreted differently from different perspectives	
2) comparing at least two alternative interventions, each with the potential to be "best practice	2	−.09/.24	moderate	raters need good medical knowledge about treatments options and standards, treatment standards differ between countries, alternatives could be whole treatment packages and also usual care	treatment guidelines could be used to aid decision making
3) describing results at the population and subgroup levels	0	−.21/1.00	moderate	publications provide often none only partial results (e.g. p value for effect modification), items can be easily clearer operationalized	Data on effect modification, but also results for subgroups needed, should be included in CONSORT guidelines
4) measuring outcomes—both benefits and harms—that are important to patients	2	−.19/1.00	moderate	raters need good knowledge about valid outcomes for the diagnosis, difficult to decide which emphasis outcome and safety has in the rating	more diagnoses specific standards e.g. in treatment guideline needed that could linked

Table 1. Cont.

criteria	Rating# max. diff. points	Intraclass-correlation before/ after	operationa-lization* good/ moderate/ difficult	comment	suggestions
5) employing methods and data sources appropriate for the decision of interest	1	−.03/.03	moderate	publications don't provide enough information about the rational and setting for trial question	
6) conducted in settings that are similar to those in which the intervention will be used in practice.	2	.37/.69	moderate	publications don't provide enough information about usual setting for the intervention, setting differs between countries	more details in CONSORT guidelines

#after consensus max difference of points (scale 1–5, 1 = max. efficacy to 5 = max. effectiveness) for each of the trials for this criteria,
*qualitative result from the discussion within the consensus procedure.

outcomes and results was extracted from the included trials and entered into an Excel spreadsheet. Special attention was given to sample size, details and rationale of the intervention and comparator groups, the terminology used (efficacy or effectiveness), the test hypothesis (non-inferiority or superiority) and the effect size. If the effect size was not given in the original publications, it was extracted from published meta-analysis.

Data syntheses and analyses

The protocol of the systematic review was predefined. For all included trials, the efficacy-effectiveness continuum was assessed using both the ten PRECIS criteria [8] and the six Institute of Medicine (IOM) defining characteristics of CER [17] To allow a clearer approach, we converted the terminology from 'explanatory/pragmatic' to 'efficacy/effectiveness.' Assessment of trials (Table 2) was performed independently by 5 raters using an enhanced quantified version of the PRECIS and IOM characteristics with a scale of 1–5 for each criterion (1 = maximal efficacy to 5 = maximal effectiveness). This allowed calculation of inter-rater correlations and to present results in figures. The five raters came from different backgrounds (MD and PhD), each had more than 10 years of experience in clinical research, had worked on aspects of research methodology, and had experience in systematic reviews and acupuncture trials. Rating was done independently, results were sent from each rater to CMW, and RL performed the statistics. For the final results, each item was discussed in a conference call between all raters until a consensus was reached.

Agreements between raters (inter-rater reliability) were calculated separately for each item and each time point (before and after the consensus conference) by intraclass-correlations as defined by Shrout and Fleiss [18].

Results

Search Results

Altogether, 119 abstracts were identified: 115 from Medline and 4 additional from the AcuTrials™ database; no further unique abstracts were identified from the recent systematic reviews. Of these abstracts, 44 full papers were screened, and 10 trials, including 4901 total patients (2482 acupuncture and 2419 control) met the eligibility criteria and were subjected to data extraction (see Figure 1).

Included trials

One trial focused on acute low back pain [19], while all the others were on chronic pain low back pain. One trial included two

acupuncture groups: a standardized group and an individualized acupuncture group [20]. For this analysis, we used the individualized acupuncture group because we assumed this group to be closer to usual care. Within the 10 trials, four included a sham acupuncture group [21–24] and four included an economic analysis [22,25–27]. Only two trials used a complex intervention. In the trial by Cherkin [28], other Chinese medicine interventions such as cupping and moxibustion, were allowed. However, in the trial by Szczurko [29], acupuncture was delivered within a naturopathic treatment, which included exercise and dietary advice. All trials tested for superiority of acupuncture treatment. None of the trials aimed to evaluate the non-inferiority of acupuncture compared to conventional care. All ten trials were published in peer reviewed medical journals with relevant impact (Arch Int Med, BMJ, Am J Epi, Pain, PLOS One, Rheumatology, Spine).

Interrater Reliability of Ratings

Raters judged the general difficulty of applying the criteria on a scale from 0–10 (0 = very easy; 10 = very difficult) as 6 (median; range 2–7) for PRECIS and 8 (median; range 6–10) for the IOM criteria. The first independent ratings of the efficacy-effectiveness continuum were highly heterogeneous between trials and between raters. This resulted in low inter-rater reliability estimates (Table 2). Missing information in the publications and difficulties in operationalizing the criteria were cited most frequently as the main reasons for the high rater variation in initial scoring of the trials (Table 1). Improved inter-rater reliability was found after the consensus discussion. The consensus process benefitted from each rater's experience in conducting and/or assessing trials on low back pain and acupuncture. Although there was still no full consensus between raters, the maximum difference was 2 points.

Mean Ratings of the Efficacy – Effectiveness Continuum

Details on the trials are presented in Table 2. The trials by Thomas et al [27] and Witt et al [26] that compared adjunctive acupuncture to usual care alone had high effectiveness scores on the efficacy-effectiveness continuum and could serve as examples for trials that aim to represent a usual care situation, whereas those trials which included an additional sham control arm [20,21,23,24] had higher efficacy scores representing a more experimental approach. This corresponded to the wording in the papers: Only those trials that included a sham control arm used the term 'efficacy;' all other trials used the term 'effectiveness'. Interestingly, most trials that scored higher on the efficacy side of the continuum were less standardized than usually observed in

PRISMA 2009 Flow Diagram

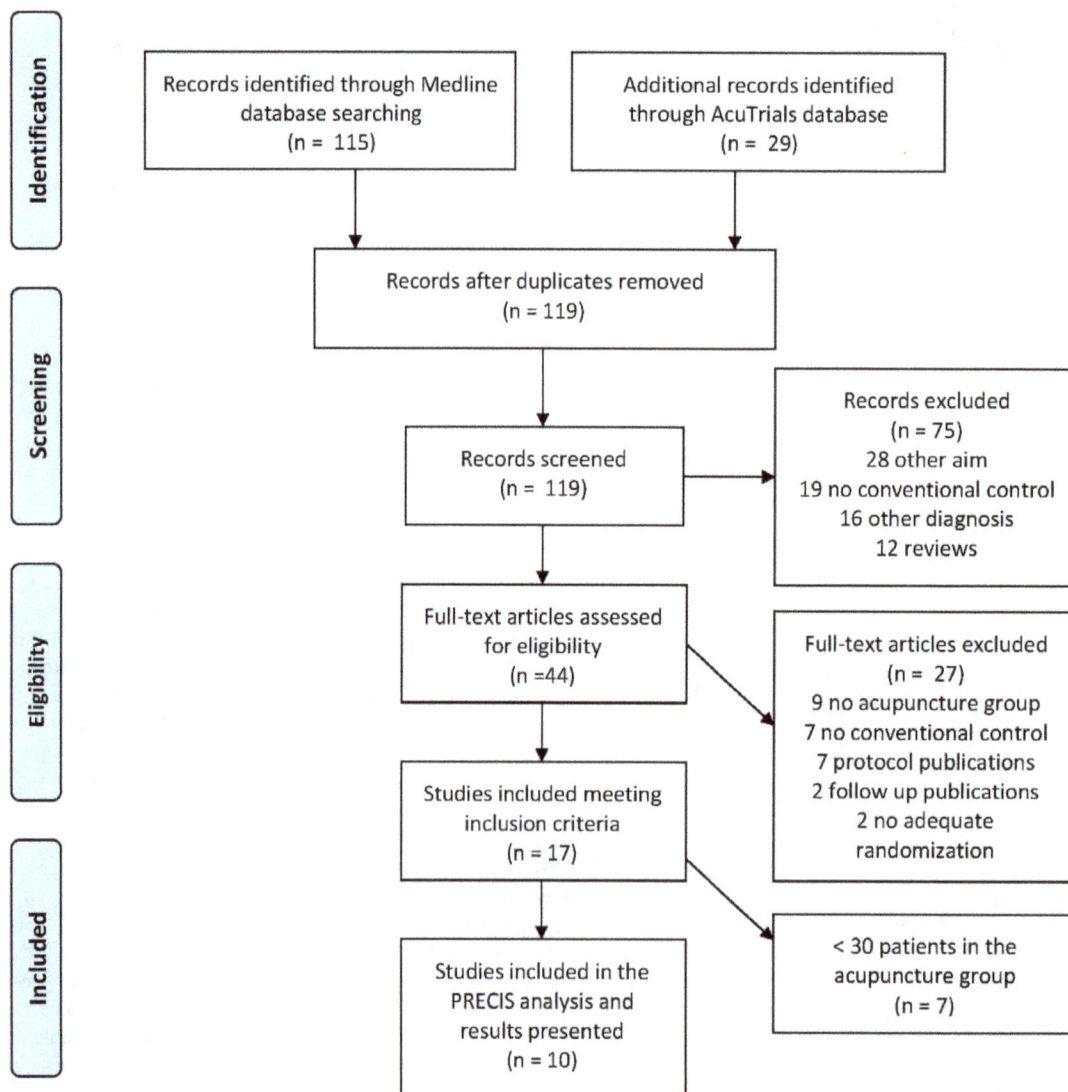

From: Moher D, Liberati A, Tetzlaff J, Altman DG, The PRISMA Group (2009). *Preferred Reporting Items for Systematic Reviews and Meta-Analyses: The PRISMA Statement.* PLoS Med 6(6): e1000097. doi:10.1371/journal.pmed1000097

For more information, visit www.prisma-statement.org.

Figure 1. Study selection.

drug research. The results showed that, for each trial, the placement along the efficacy-effectiveness continuum is multidimensional and varied for the different criteria within a given trial (Figure 2). Overall, when evaluating acupuncture as an adjunctive treatment that allowed more flexible treatment protocols, trials had higher effectiveness scores than trials that evaluated acupuncture as a treatment alternative and used a more standardized treatment protocol (Figure 2).

An interesting exploratory observation is that those trials that reported more narrow eligibility criteria and a more standardized acupuncture intervention [23,24,30] resulted in larger effect sizes (≥ 0.5, Table 2) than trials that reported a more heterogeneous

Table 2. Trials on non specific low back pain with a conventional treatment comparator and >30 patients in the acupuncture group.

Author	N Acu/Con	Result SMD	Acupuncture#	Acu rational	Setting	Comparator details	Cointervention	Ad comparator on details presented	Rating PRECIS criteria (5=effectiveness/1=efficacy)									Rating IOM criteria (5-1)						
									1	2	3	4	5	6	7	8	9	10	1	2	3	4	5	6
Acute non specific low back pain																								
Eisenberg 2007 (19)	58/150	na	free, max 10 sessions	as usual	physicians, practitioners outpatient practices	treatment follows hospital guideline care (NSAID, muscle relaxants, education, activity alteration)	treatment follows hospital guideline care (NSAID, muscle relaxants, education, activity alteration)	yes number of visits	3.4	4.0	3.6	4.0	3.6	2.4	4.2	4.8	5.0	4.0	4.6	4.6	2.0	4.8	4.8	4.2
Chronic non specific low back pain																								
Witt 2006 (26)	1451/1390	0.43* (0.38;0.49)	needle, free, max 15 sessions	as usual	physicians outpatient practices	patients were free to seek care in the health insurance system	usual care	yes pain medication in both groups reported	4.4	5.0	4.0	5.0	5.0	3.6	4.4	4.4	5.0	4.0	4.6	4.0	2.8	4.6	4.8	4.0
Haake 2007 (21)	387/387	0.56* (0.43;0.70)	needle, semi-standard, 10 or 15 session	consensus	physicians outpatient practices	German guideline based treatment (physiotherapy, exercise, NSAID)	rescue medication	no conventional group type and frequency of treatment	3.0	2.0	3.0	4.0	3.8	2.8	4.4	4.2	3.2	4.0	4.4	4.6	1.0	4.2	4.8	4.0
Thomas 2006 (27)	160/81	0.34* (0.03;0.65)	needle, free, max 10 sessions	as usual	practitioners outpatient practices	treatment as provided by their GPs	treatment as provided by their GPs	yes both groups type of treatment	4.4	5.0	3.8	5.0	5.0	3.6	4.4	4.6	5.0	3.4	4.4	4.4	2.0	4.6	4.8	4.0
Cherkin 2009 (20)	157/161	na	needle, free, 10 sessions	by one diagnostician	2 research clinics, outpatients	treatment as provided by their physicians	self care book, usual care	yes % of patients with physician and practitioner visits	3.4	3.0	3.0	5.0	5.0	2.8	4.4	4.2	4.2	3.4	4.4	4.2	1.0	4.4	4.8	3.0
Cherkin 2001 (22)	94/90	0.24* (0.00;0.48)	needle +E-stim, max 10 sessions	consensus	practitioners outpatient practices	self care materials (book, videotapes)	usual care	yes treatments both groups; % patients with as non study visits	3.0	5.0	3.4	2.0	na	2.8	4.4	4.4	4.2	4.0	4.4	3.4	2.0	4.6	4.6	4.0
Molsberger 2002 (23)	65/60	0.62** (0.26;0.97)	needle, standard, 12 sessions	literature	rehabilitation clinic, inpatients	physiotherapy, exercise, education, mud packs, IR-heat, diclofenac (3×50 mg on demand)	physiotherapy, exercise, education, mud packs, IR-heat, diclofenac (3×50 mg on demand)	yes not presented	2.6	3.0	2.6	2.0	3.0	3.4	4.4	4.9	na	3.2	4.4	4.4	1.0	4.2	4.6	3.0
Leibing 2002 (24)	40/46	0.86** (0.42;1.31)	needle, standard, 20 sessions	literature	university hospital outpatient clinic	physiotherapy	physiotherapy	yes not presented	3.4	1.0	2.0	2.4	2.2	3.2	4.4	4.8	na	3.2	4.0	4.4	1.0	4.2	4.8	2.8

Table 2. Cont.

Author	N Acu/Con	Result SMD	Acupuncture #	Acu rational	Setting	Comparator details	Cointervention	Ad comparator on details presented	Rating PRECIS criteria (5-effectiveness/1=efficacy)	Rating IOM criteria (5-1)
Szczurko 2007 (29)	39/30	na	needle, standard, 24 sessions	unclear	practitioners on site at a plant	self care booklet and physiotherapy advice and relaxation techniques		no	3.4 1.0 2.8 2.4 2.4 3.0 4.4 2.4 4.2 5.0	3.6 3.8 1.0 4.0 4.2 3.2
Meng 2003 (30)	31/24	0.50** (0.08;1.09)	needle, standard, 10 sessions	unclear	aneastesiologists at hospital, outpatients	treatment as before provided by their physicians (NSAID, aspirin, non narcotic analgesics)	treatment as before provided by their physicians (NSAID, aspirin, non narcotic analgesics)	yes patients with medication and use of other CAM treatments	2.6 2.0 2.8 3.4 5.0 3.0 4.6 3.8 na 3.0	4.0 4.6 3.0 4.2 4.6 3.2

Acu = acupuncture, Con = control, na = not available,

*primary endpoint from individual patient data meta-analysis (Vickers Trials 2010),

**short term effect on pain scales from recent meta-analysis (Yuan Spine 2008),

#standard = standardized treatment protocol, free = acupuncture as usual PRECIS: 1) Eligibility criteria, 2) Flexibility acu, 3) Practitioner expertise acu, 4) Flexibility control, 5) Practitioner Expertise control, 6) follow up, 7) Outcomes, 8)Patient compliance, 9) Practitioner adherence, 10) primary analysis IOM: 1) Informing decision making, 2) Comparing at least two alternatives, 3) Results for population and subgroups, 4) Patient relevant outcomes incl. safety, 5) Appropriate methods, 6) Setting close to reality.

patient sample and a flexible acupuncture treatment (effect size≤0.5, Table 2) [26,27].

Discussion

Using available criteria for planning CER to evaluate the efficacy-effectiveness continuum of published trials resulted in large heterogeneity between raters and items, which was partly solved by a consensus procedure. This was mainly due to information missing from the publications and to difficulties in operationalizing the criteria. Our focus on RCTs assessing acupuncture for low back pain allowed the inclusion of a number of high quality trials representing a broad spectrum of clinical research in the efficacy-effectiveness continuum. Trials that have a more flexible acupuncture treatment protocol and no further placebo control arm scored closer to effectiveness.

This is a systematic analysis that has tested the feasibility of appraising the efficacy-effectiveness continuum of randomized controlled trials. Advantages of the systematic review include its innovative scope on the process of appraisal, high quality studies covering the efficacy-effectiveness continuum, and that the scoring was done by 5 independent raters using two different sets of criteria. The review process benefitted from the experience of the selected raters in the design, performance and/or assessment of the field of research. Discussions between raters improved the inter-rater reliability significantly. This underlines the complex aspects of the efficacy-effectiveness continuum and the need for rater training. Limitations were that only one rater selected the papers, that secondary papers (e.g., on treatment details) were not included, and that randomized trials are only one part of CER and do not represent the whole spectrum of evidence. However, Cochrane reviews, which are often used to assist in decision-making, also focus on RCTs and primarily concentrate on the main paper presenting the results. Another limitation is that both criteria lists (PRECIS and IOM) were developed to guide new trials and not to assess published trials. However, the present study provides insights into the advantages and limitation of single items and indicates that, following the definition and main character-istics of CER, the ten PRECIS criteria and six IOM characteristics seem plausible candidates for the evaluation of existing research and could form a basis for a future evaluation instrument. That the items of the PRECIS tool have relevance for appraising published studies is supported by the very recent review by Koppenaal et al [31]. The authors used the PRECIS tool on two meta-analyses, scored the single items, and came to the conclusion that PRECIS can provide useful estimates on how single studies and the whole review are placed within the efficacy effectiveness continuum. Interestingly the authors used a similar scale from 1 to 5. However, they did either provide information on inter-rater variability nor details on advantages and limitations of single PRECIS items which can inform its further development.

The origin of some of the effect sizes presented in this review could be seen as a limitation. It was not the aim of this review to perform a meta-analysis and because of this effect sizes were taken from the literature and only used as an exploratory aspect for orientation.

The present findings reveal that the place of a trial in the efficacy-effectiveness continuum is multidimensional, indicating it is even more complicated to unambiguously label a trial as efficacy or effectiveness. From the scoring of the trials, it is clear that two of the RCTs [26,27] were designed mainly as effectiveness trials, whereas others were designed more as efficacy trials [23,24,29]. Interestingly, two of the trials [20,21], both including a sham control, standardized their acupuncture intervention much more

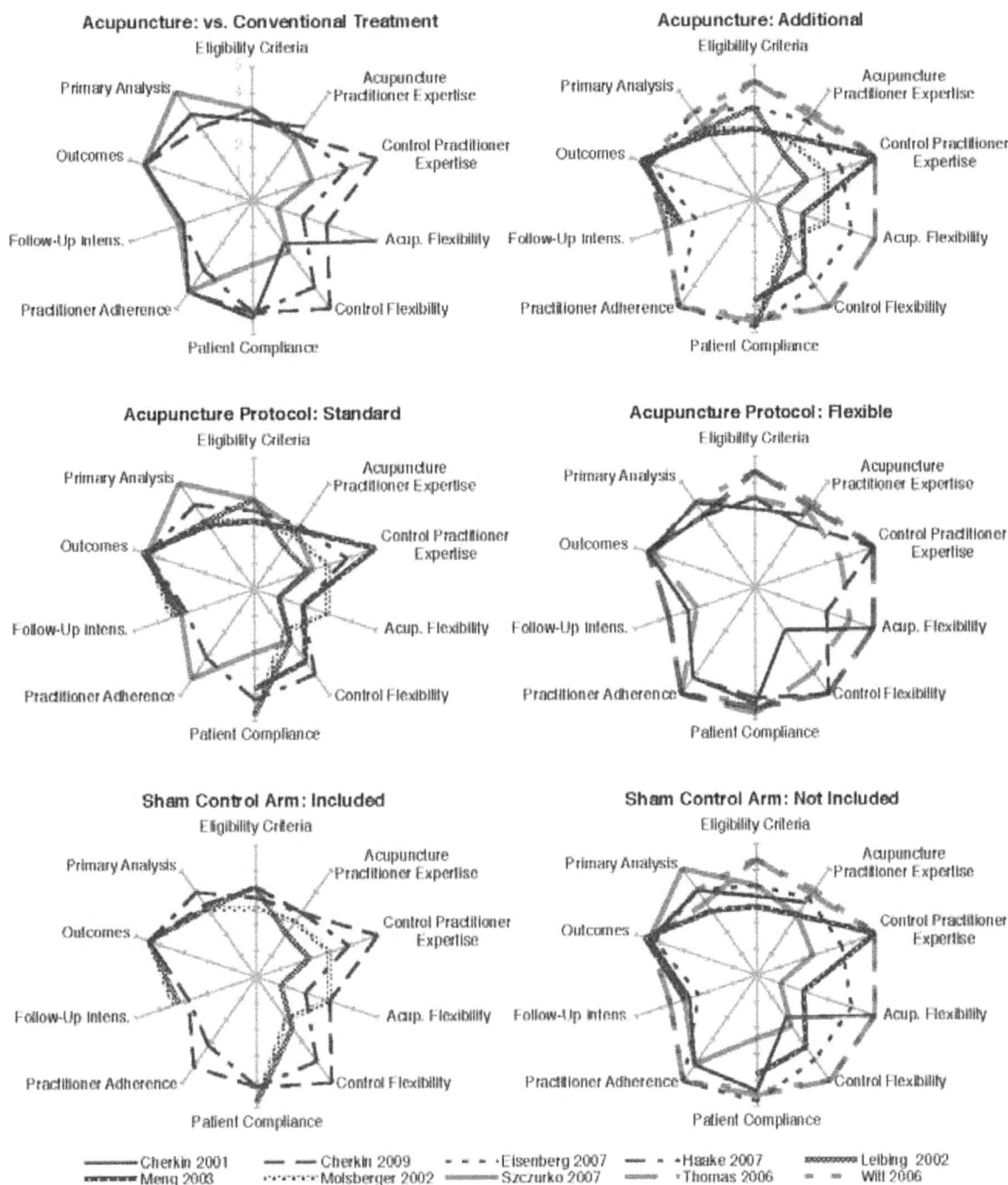

Figure 2. PRECIS scoring for the 10 included trials comparing different methodological aspects (second rating after consensus procedure), a larger rounder figure would correlate with a higher score on PRECIS representing more the effectiveness side.

than their conventional treatment control. None of the trials included all available patients, but eligibility criteria varied from relatively narrow to relatively wide.

In the early 1970's, when Asian medicine including acupuncture began its most recent migration to the West, researchers adopted the randomized controlled trial to investigate acupuncture without knowing Asian medicine had a long history [32]. Because of this evidence from those trials was often rejected as invalid and was therefore ignored. The discussion and demand for evidence that is generated in a way that satisfies decision-making

started early [33] and most studies in this review already reflect the movement toward an evidence base that can inform decisions makers. Acupuncture for low back pain can serve as a good example for different options of randomized studies within CER. On one hand, both large studies that evaluated acupuncture as adjunct to usual care represent a unique way that RCTs can more closely reflect the reality of a usual care setting [26,27]. On the other hand, those trials that had both a standard care/usual care control and a sham control arm, but still tried to keep their acupuncture intervention more flexible are good examples for a middle ground in the efficacy-effectiveness continuum [21]. Overall, the last decade of the acupuncture studies on low back pain provides useful information for the design of future randomized trials in other fields of non-pharmacological research.

In the scoring process of the trials appraising the eligibility criteria was not always easy. Therefore, it would be useful to analyze heterogeneity in addition to get better knowledge about the population in the studies [34]. It is important that trials with more heterogeneous populations result in higher outcome variances and smaller effect sizes, which must be taken into account when planning the sample sizes for future trials assessing CER.

Furthermore, CER is susceptible to systematic error [35]. The attempt to achieve methodological purity can result in clinically meaningless results, while attempting to achieve full generalizability can result in invalid and unreliable results. Achieving a creative tension between the two is crucial [36] and the relevance of the results has to be put into accordance with the rigor of the results. In CER, the evaluation of effect modifications and stratifications play a crucial role [37] to allow for conclusions on specific subgroups. This is one of the IOM criteria, but was not represented in the PRECIS score. Although the trials in our analysis were mainly published in high-ranking journals, none of the trials that scored more on the effectiveness side of the continuum gave detailed information about subgroups. For decision-making, this aspect should be strengthened in future trials and should be included in the criteria list for evaluation of the efficacy-effectiveness continuum.

One problem that came up during the rater consensus procedure was the information missing from the main publications. It is highly recommended to include in future review processes also all available secondary papers. However, in the case of the included studies information on selection procedure of practitioners, as well as for patient compliance measures and practitioner adherence to protocol would not have been complete. In addition, it would be helpful to know more about the setting in which the treatment is typically carried out in each respective country and how much the trial setting differs from the clinical treatment setting. Although standards for reporting clinical trials (CONSORT [6], STRICTA [38]) mention the most relevant aspects, the above mentioned aspects, such as describing the usual setting for this treatment in detail and providing clear information on patients' compliance and practitioner adherence, are not adequately represented in the CONSORT guidelines and should be discussed in future revisions.

Conclusion

It is of high relevance for stakeholders to appraise the extent to which published trials are relevant to clinical and health policy decision-making. A systematic instrument, which can be also used in systematic reviews, needs further development. The available instruments for planning randomized studies for CER could provide a basis for this, but would need further development that includes more defined operational criteria and a rater's training manual. In addition, CONSORT guidelines for reporting RCTs should be more extended, fostering on reporting more details on CER relevant aspects. Most studies in this review already reflect the movement toward an evidence base that can inform both decision-makers and provide useful information for the design of randomized trials for other non-pharmacological treatments.

Author Contributions

Conceived and designed the experiments: CMW BB. Performed the experiments: RH EM RL LL CMW. Analyzed the data: CMW RL. Wrote the paper: CMW EM RH RL LL SRT BB.

References

1. Committee on Comparative Effectiveness Research Prioritization (2009) What is Comparative Effectiveness Research? In:, , Institute of Medicine (2009) Initial National Priorities for Comparative Effectiveness Research. Washington D.C.: The National Academies Press. 29 p.
2. Conway PH, Clancy C (2009) Comparative-Effectiveness Research – Implications of the Federal Coordinating Council's Report. N Engl J Med 361: 330.
3. Last J, Spasoff RA, Harris S (2001) A dictionary of epidemiology. Oxford: Oxford University Press.
4. Committee on Comparative Effectiveness Research Prioritization (2009) Optimizing Evidence. In: Institute of Medicine, ed. Initial National Priorities for Comparative Effectiveness Research. Washington D.C.: The National Academies Press. 31 p.
5. Schwarz D, Lelloch J (1967) Explanatory and pragmatic attitudes in therapeutical trials. J Chronic Dis 20: 637–647.
6. Zwarenstein M, Treweek S, Gagnier JJ, Altman DG, Tunis S, et al. (2008) Improving the reporting of pragmatic trials: an extension of the CONSORT statement. BMJ 337: a2390.
7. Tunis SR, Stryer DB, Clancy CM (2003) Practical clinical trials: increasing the value of clinical research for decision making in clinical and health policy. JAMA 290: 1624–1632.
8. Thorpe KE, Zwarenstein M, Oxman AD, Treweek S, Furberg CD, et al. (2009) A pragmatic-explanatory continuum indicator summary (PRECIS): a tool to help trial designers. CMAJ 180: E47–E57.
9. Fineberg H (2009) Foreword. In:, , Institute of Medicine (2009) Initial National Priorities for Comparative Effectiveness Research. Washington D.C.: The National Academies Press.
10. Deyo RA, Mirza SK, Martin BI (1976) Back pain prevalence and visit rates: estimates from U.S. national surveys, 2002. Spine 31: 2724–2727.
11. Luo X, Pietrobon R, Sun SX, Liu GG, Hey L (1976) Estimates and patterns of direct health care expenditures among individuals with back pain in the United States. Spine 29: 79–86.
12. Barnes PM, Powell-Griner E, McFann K, Nahin RL (2004) Complementary and alternative medicine use among adults: United States, 2002. Adv Data. pp 1–19.
13. Berman BM, Langevin HM, Witt CM, Dubner R (2010) Acupuncture for chronic low back pain. N Engl J Med 363: 454–461.
14. Oregon College of Oriental Medicine (2011) AcuTrials® Database. Available: http://acutrials.ocom.edu. Accessed 2011 Feb 10.
15. Yuan J, Purepong N, Kerr DP, Park J, Bradbury I, et al. (1976) Effectiveness of acupuncture for low back pain: a systematic review. Spine 33: E887–E900.
16. Rubinstein SM, van MM, Kuijpers T, Ostelo R, Verhagen AP, et al. (2010) A systematic review on the effectiveness of complementary and alternative medicine for chronic non-specific low-back pain. Eur Spine J 19: 1213–1228.
17. Committee on Comparative Effectiveness Research Prioritization (2009) Characteristics of CER. In: Institute of Medicine, ed. Initial National Priorities for Comparative Effectiveness Research. Washington D.C.: The National Academies Press. pp 37–39.
18. Shrout PE, Fleiss JL (1979) Interclass Correlations: Uses in Assessing Rater Reliability. Psychological Bulletin 86: 420–428.
19. Eisenberg DM, Post DE, Davis RB, Connelly MT, Legedza AT, et al. (2007) Addition of choice of complementary therapies to usual care for acute low back pain: a randomized controlled trial. Spine 32: 151–158.
20. Cherkin DC, Sherman KJ, Avins AL, Erro JH, Ichikawa L, et al. (2009) A randomized trial comparing acupuncture, simulated acupuncture, and usual care for chronic low back pain. Arch Intern Med 169: 858–866.
21. Haake M, Muller HH, Schade-Brittinger C, Basler HD, Schafer H, et al. (2007) German Acupuncture Trials (GERAC) for chronic low back pain: randomized, multicenter, blinded, parallel-group trial with 3 groups. Arch Intern Med 167: 1892–1898.
22. Cherkin DC, Eisenberg D, Sherman KJ, Barlow W, Kaptchuk TJ, et al. (2001) Randomized trial comparing traditional Chinese medical acupuncture, therapeutic massage, and self-care education for chronic low back pain. Arch Intern Med 161: 1081–1088.
23. Molsberger A, Diener HC, Krämer J, Michaelis J, Schäfer H, et al. (2002) GERAC-Akupunktur-Studien. Deutsches Ärzteblatt 99: B 1539–1541.
24. Leibing E, Leonhardt U, Koster G, Goerlitz A, Rosenfeldt JA, et al. (2002) Acupuncture treatment of chronic low-back pain – a randomized, blinded, placebo-controlled trial with 9-month follow-up. Pain 96: 189–196.
25. Eisenberg DM, Kessler RC, Van Rompay MI, Kaptchuk TJ, Wilkey SA, et al. (2001) Perceptions about complementary therapies relative to conventional therapies among adults who use both: results from a national survey. Ann Intern Med 135: 344–351.

26. Witt CM, Jena S, Selim D, Brinkhaus B, Reinhold T, et al. (2006) Pragmatic randomized trial of effectiveness and cost-effectiveness of acupuncture for chronic low back pain. American Journal of Epidemiology 164: 487–496.

27. Thomas KJ, MacPherson H, Thorpe L, Brazier J, Fitter M, et al. (2006) Randomised controlled trial of a short course of traditional acupuncture compared with usual care for persistent non-specific low back pain. BMJ 333: 623–626.

28. Cherkin DC, Deyo RA, Sherman KJ, Hart LG, Street JH, et al. (2002) Characteristics of visits to licensed acupuncturists, chiropractors, massage therapists, and naturopathic physicians. J Am Board Fam Pract 15: 463–472.

29. Szczurko O, Cooley K, Busse JW, Seely D, Bernhardt B, et al. (2007) Naturopathic care for chronic low back pain: a randomized trial. PLoS ONE 2: e919.

30. Meng CF, Wang D, Ngeow J, Lao L, Peterson M, et al. (2003) Acupuncture for chronic low back pain in older patients: a randomized, controlled trial. Rheumatology (Oxford) 42: 1–10.

31. Koppenaal T, Linmans J, Knottnerus JA, Spigt M (2011) Pragmatic vs. explanatory: An adaptation of the PRECIS tool helps to judge the applicability of systematic reviews for daily practice. J Clin Epidemiol.

32. Witt CM, MacPherson H, Kaptchuk TJ, Wahlberg A (2011) Efficacy, effectiveness and efficiency. In: Scheid V, MacPherson H, eds. Integrating East Asian Medicine into Contemporary Health Care. London: Churchill Livingstone.

33. Mason S, Tovey P, Long AF (2002) Evaluating complementary medicine: methodological challenges of randomised controlled trials. BMJ 325: 832–834.

34. Kent DM, Rothwell PM, Ioannidis JP, Altman DG, Hayward RA (2010) Assessing and reporting heterogeneity in treatment effects in clinical trials: a proposal. Trials 11: 85.

35. Strom BL (2007) Methodologic challenges to studying patient safety and comparative effectiveness. Med Care 45: S13–S15.

36. Godwin M, Ruhland L, Casson I, MacDonald S, Delva D, et al. (2003) Pragmatic controlled clinical trials in primary care: the struggle between external and internal validity. BMC Med Res Methodol 3: 28.

37. Witt CM, Schützler L, Lüdtke R, Wegscheider K, Willich SN (2011) Patient Characteristics and Variation in Treatment Outcomes: Which Patients Benefit Most From Acupuncture for Chronic Pain? Clin J Pain 27: 550–555.

38. MacPherson H, Altman DG, Hammerschlag R, Youping L, Taixiang W, et al. (2010) Revised STandards for Reporting Interventions in Clinical Trials of Acupuncture (STRICTA): extending the CONSORT statement. PLoS Med 7: e1000261.

9

Acupuncture Modulates Resting State Hippocampal Functional Connectivity in Alzheimer Disease

Zhiqun Wang[1], Peipeng Liang[1,5], Zhilian Zhao[1], Ying Han[2], Haiqing Song[2], Jianyang Xu[3], Jie Lu[1]*, Kuncheng Li[1,4,5]*

1 Department of Radiology, Xuanwu Hospital of Capital Medical University, Beijing, China, 2 Department of Neurology, Xuanwu Hospital of Capital Medical University, Beijing, China, 3 General Hospital of Chinese People's Armed Police Forces, Beijing, China, 4 Key Laboratory for Neurodegenerative Diseases, Ministry of Education, Beijing, China, 5 Beijing Key Laboratory of Magnetic Resonance Imaging and Brain Informatics, Beijing, China

Abstract

Our objective is to clarify the effects of acupuncture on hippocampal connectivity in patients with Alzheimer disease (AD) using functional magnetic resonance imaging (fMRI). Twenty-eight right-handed subjects (14 AD patients and 14 healthy elders) participated in this study. Clinical and neuropsychological examinations were performed on all subjects. MRI was performed using a SIEMENS verio 3-Tesla scanner. The fMRI study used a single block experimental design. We first acquired baseline resting state data during the initial 3 minutes and then performed acupuncture stimulation on the Tai chong and He gu acupoints for 3 minutes. Last, we acquired fMRI data for another 10 minutes after the needle was withdrawn. The preprocessing and data analysis were performed using statistical parametric mapping (SPM5) software. Two-sample t-tests were performed using data from the two groups in different states. We found that during the resting state, several frontal and temporal regions showed decreased hippocampal connectivity in AD patients relative to control subjects. During the resting state following acupuncture, AD patients showed increased connectivity in most of these hippocampus related regions compared to the first resting state. In conclusion, we investigated the effect of acupuncture on AD patients by combing fMRI and traditional acupuncture. Our fMRI study confirmed that acupuncture at Tai chong and He gu can enhance the hippocampal connectivity in AD patients.

Editor: Daqing Ma, Imperial College London, Chelsea & Westminster Hospital, United Kingdom

Funding: This work was supported by the Project Sponsored by the Scientific Research Foundation for the Returned Overseas Chinese Scholars, the Natural Science Foundation of China (Grant No. 81000606, 81370037, 61105118, 81141018, 81030028, and 81225012), China Postdoctoral Science Foundation funded project (No. 201003142), and Key Work of Special Project supported by the city government (Z101107052210002 and Z111107067311036).The funders had no role in study design, data collection and analysis, decision to publish, or preparation of the manuscript.

Competing Interests: The authors have declared that no competing interests exist.

* E-mail: lujie@xwh.ccmu.edu.cn (JL); likuncheng@xwh.ccmu.edu.cn (KL)

Introduction

Alzheimer disease (AD) is the most common cause of dementia, and there is currently no effective therapy for the disease. Acupuncture has shown promise in treating AD patients by mobilizing the neurophysiological system to modulate cognitive function [1]. However, the neural mechanism underlying the effects of acupuncture is still unknown.

Recently, a promising resting-state functional magnetic resonance imaging (fMRI) method has provided insight into brain activity or connectivity and can be used to assess the effects of acupuncture. Accumulating neuroimaging evidence suggests that acupuncture can modulate resting state brain activity or connectivity [2–6]. However, the majority of these studies have focused on healthy subjects. Only two papers have investigated acupuncture's effects on AD patients. One study found that acupuncture activates several temporal lobe and parietal lobe regions in AD patients [1]. Another study found that several brain regions, temporal lobe regions in particular, are activated after acupuncture in AD patients [7]. These fMRI studies suggest that acupuncture may activate regions associated with cognition, which contribute to the treatment's specific therapeutic effect. However, these AD-related acupuncture studies did not examine connectiv-

ity changes among brain regions; instead, they explored activation of brain regions.

In order to better understand the pathophysiology of AD, it is necessary to study acupuncture's effect on the functional connectivity of the hippocampus. Previous neuroimaging studies have shown that the hippocampus is one of the earliest pathological sites of AD and plays a crucial role in memory processes [8–10]. By using MRI method, many studies have demonstrated AD-related hippocampal abnormalities including atrophy [11,12] hypometabolism [13], and decreased activity [14]. Furthermore, several fMRI studies reported markedly reduced functional connectivity in hippocampus-related memory networks in early-stage AD [15,16] as well as mild cognitive impairment [17–19]. One recent resting-state fMRI study found stronger recovery of hippocampal functional connectivity after donepezil treatment in AD patients [20], which indicates there is some plasticity in hippocampal connectivity. Therefore, we selected the hippocampus as the region of interest to conduct functional connectivity analysis and to explore the effects of acupuncture.

Considering the important role of the hippocampus and acupuncture's probable effects, we chose to observe how hippocampal activity – which is abnormal in AD patients at rest – might be affected by acupuncture. Few studies have reported changes in hippocampal connectivity in AD patients when measuring resting-state fMRI and the effects of acupuncture. Here, we hypothesized that abnormal resting-state hippocampal connectivity with vital brain regions would be enhanced in AD patients following acupuncture.

The fMRI experiment was performed after acupuncture at the acupoints Tai chong and He gu. According to traditional Chinese medicine, AD belongs to the category of dementia. When a lesion is located in the brain, acupuncture point selection should be based on inducing resuscitation and coordinating yin and yang. Huangdi Neijing says "the viscera of the disease, all take its original point". He gu is the original point of the large intestine channel of hand yangming (LI4), and it is one of the most commonly used acupoints in the clinical therapy, playing an important role in dispelling wind and analgesia and restoring consciousness. Taichong is the original point of the liver channel of foot jueyin (Liv3), which functions to relieve the depressed liver and subdue the endogenous wind and sedatives. He gu and Tai chong are collectively named the Si Guan (four gates) point. Combined use of these two acupoints can harmonize yin and yang, regulate qi and blood, finally improve the cognitive ability of AD patients. Therefore, we choose these two acupoints.

In the present study, we sought to investigate the effects of acupuncture on hippocampal functional connectivity in AD patients compared to healthy controls. We first explored hippocampal functional connectivity during the resting state and then identified regions in AD patients showing connectivity that was significantly different compared to controls. Finally, we tested whether interregional connectivity could be modulated by acupuncture in AD patients.

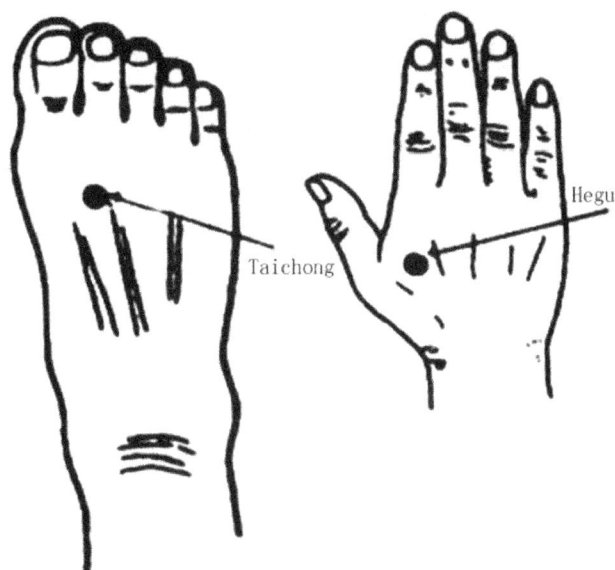

Figure 1. Location of acupoints used in the experiment. The left acupoint represent Taichong, which is located in the dorsal foot, the first and second metatarsal cavity before integration. The right acupoint represent Hegu, which is located in the dorsal hand, between the first and second metacarpal and the midpoint of the second metacarpal radial side.

Materials and Methods

Subjects

Twenty-eight right-handed subjects participated in this study, including 14 patients with AD and 14 healthy controls. The AD subjects were recruited from patients who had consulted in the memory clinic at Xuanwu Hospital for memory complaints. Healthy elderly controls were recruited from the local community. This study was approved by the Medical Research Ethics Committee of Xuanwu Hospital. All subjects gave their written informed consent. The details of the consent form included the study's aim, inclusion and exclusion criteria, procedures, potential harm and benefits, medical care, privacy rights, and withdrawal process. They were informed of their right to discontinue participation at any time. All potential participants who declined to participate or otherwise did not participate were still eligible for treatment (if applicable) and were not disadvantaged in any other way for not participating in the study.

All AD patients underwent a complete physical and neurological examination, standard laboratory tests and an extensive battery of neuropsychological assessments. The diagnosis of AD fulfilled the Diagnostic and Statistical Manual of Mental Disorders 4th Edition criteria for dementia [21] and the National Institute of Neurological and Communicative Disorders and Stroke/Alzheimer Disease and Related Disorders Association (NINCDS-ADRDA) criteria for possible or probable AD [22]. The subjects were classified according to Clinical Dementia Rating (CDR) scores [23]; patients with CDRs of 1 and 2 were designated AD patients.

Healthy controls met the following criteria: a) no neurological or psychiatric disorders such as stroke, depression or epilepsy; b) no neurological deficiencies such as visual or hearing loss; c) no abnormal findings such as infarction or focal lesion in conventional brain MR imaging; d) no cognitive complaints; e) mini-mental state examination (MMSE) score of 28 or higher; and f) CDR score of 0.

Participants with contraindications for MRI such as pacemakers, cardiac defibrillators, implanted material with electric or magnetic systems, vascular clips or mechanical heart valves, cochlear implants or claustrophobia were excluded. In addition, patients with a history of stroke, psychiatric disease, drug abuse, severe hypertension, systematic diseases and intellectual disability were excluded.

Data Acquisition

MRI data acquisition was performed using a SIEMENS verio 3-Tesla scanner (Siemens, Erlangen, Germany). The subjects were instructed to remain still, keep their eyes closed and think of nothing in particular. fMRI was acquired axially using echo-planar imaging (EPI) [repetition time (TR)/echo time (TE)/flip angle (FA)/field of view (FOV) = 2000 ms/40 ms/90°/24 cm, image matrix = 64×64, slice number = 33, thickness = 3 mm, gap = 1 mm and bandwidth = 2232 Hz/pixel]. In addition, 3D T1-weighted magnetization-prepared rapid gradient echo (MPRAGE) sagittal images were obtained (TR/TE/inversion time (TI)/FA = 1900 ms/2.2 ms/900 ms/9°, image matrix = 256×256, slice number = 176 and thickness = 1 mm).

Our study used a single block experimental design. We first acquired baseline resting state data during the initial 3 minutes; we then performed acupuncture stimulation for the following 3 minutes. A silver needle that was 0.30 mm in diameter and 25 mm long was inserted and twirled at four acupoints of the human body, which were Tai chong on the dorsum of the left and right feet and He gu on the dorsum of the left and right hands. We

Table 1. Characteristics of the AD patients and Normal controls.

Characteristics	AD	NOR	P value
N (M/F)	14(4/10)	14(6/8)	–
Age, years	66.92±8.91	66.07±5.78	0.86*
Education, years	10.07±3.38	11.00±4.52	0.61*
MMSE	15.92±4.32	28.00±1.41	<0.01*
AVLT(immediate)	11.35±3.95	26.86±5.24	<0.01*
AVLT(delayed)	2.64±1.59	11.07±2.76	<0.01*
AVLT(recognition)	3.35±1.55	12.71±2.09	<0.01*
CDR	1–2	0	–

MMSE, Mini-Mental State Examination; Plus-minus values are means ± S.D. AVLT, Auditory verbal learning test; immediate, immediate recall of learning verbal; delayed; delayed recall of learning verbal; recognition, recognition of learning verbal; CDR, clinical dementia rate. *The P values were obtained by one-way analysis of variance tests.

acquired fMRI for another 10 minutes after the needle was withdrawn. The location of Tai chong and He gu see the Figure 1.

Imaging Preprocess

Unless otherwise stated, all analyses were conducted using a statistical parametric mapping software package (SPM5, http://www.fil.ion.ucl.ac.uk/spm). The first 10 volumes of functional images were discarded to allow the signal to reach equilibrium and to let participants adapt to the scanning noise. The remaining 229 fMRI images were first corrected for within-scan acquisition time differences between slices and then realigned to the first volume to correct for inter-scan head motion. No participant had head motion of more than 1.5 mm displacement in any of the x, y, or z directions or $1.5°$ of any angular motion throughout the course of scan. The individual structural image was co-registered to the mean functional image after motion correction using a linear transformation. The transformed structural images were then segmented into gray matter (GM), white matter (WM) and cerebrospinal fluid (CSF) using a unified segmentation algorithm [24]. The motion corrected functional volumes were spatially normalized to the Montreal Neurological Institute (MNI) space and re-sampled to 3 mm isotropic voxels using the normalization parameters estimated during unified segmentation. Subsequently, the functional images were spatially smoothed with a Gaussian kernel of $4×4×4$ mm^3 full width at half maximum (FWHM) to decrease spatial noise. Following this, temporal filtering (0.01 Hz< f <0.08 Hz) was applied to the time series of each voxel to reduce the effect of low-frequency drifts and high-frequency noise [25,26] using the Resting-State fMRI Data Analysis Toolkit (http://resting-fmri.sourceforge.net). To further reduce the effects of confounding factors, we also regressed out the following confounding sources [27]: (1) six motion parameters, (2) linear drift, (3) white matter signal and (4) CSF signal.

Region of Interest Definition

Bilateral hippocampus region of interests (ROIs) were generated using the free software WFU_PickAtlas Tool Version 2.4 (http://www.ansir.wfubmc.edu) [28], which has been used in previous studies [18,29]. For each seed region, the blood oxygenation level dependent (BOLD) time series of the voxels within the seed region was averaged to generate the reference time series.

Functional Connectivity Analysis

For each subject and each seed region (bilateral hippocampus), a correlation map was produced by computing the correlation coefficients between the reference time series and the time series from all the other brain voxels. Correlation coefficients were then converted to z values using Fisher r-to-z transformation to improve normality [30].

Statistical Analysis

The individual z value was entered into a random effect one sample t-test in a voxel-wise manner to determine brain regions showing significant connectivity with the left and right hippocampus within each group under a combined threshold of P<0.01 and cluster size = 405 mm^3. This yielded a corrected threshold of P< 0.001, determined by Monte Carlo simulation using the AlphaSim program with the following parameters: FWHM = 4 mm, within the GM mask (http://afni.nimh.nih.gov/pub/dist/doc/manual/AlphaSim.pdf). This procedure produced significant hippocampal functional connectivity z-statistic maps for the two groups (AD

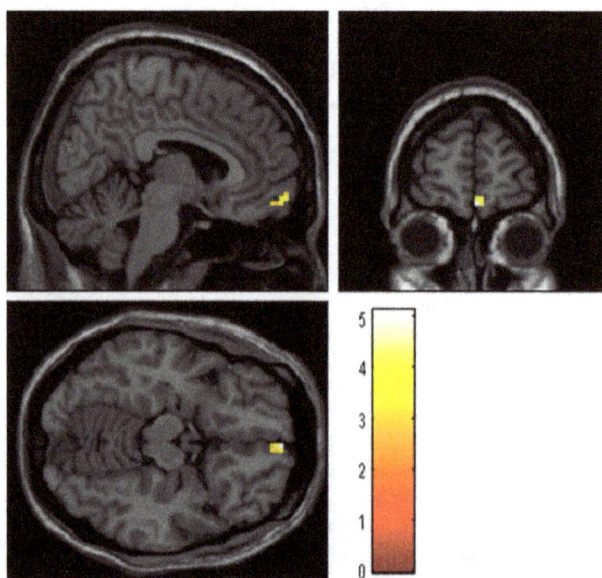

Figure 2. Brain regions showing decreased connectivity to left hippocampus in AD group comparing to control group. Left in picture is left in the brain. The color scale represents t values. Warm color represents decreased connectivity.

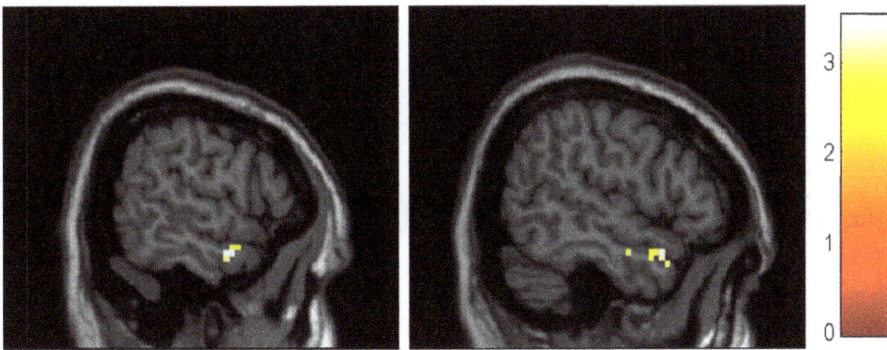

Figure 3. Brain regions showing decreased connectivity to right hippocampus in AD group comparing to control group. Left in picture is left in the brain. The color scale represents t values. Warm color represents decreased connectivity.

patients and controls). We then made masks showing the bilateral hippocampus by combining the corresponding two z-statistic maps (i.e., AD patients and controls) and then used this mask for analyzing the corresponding group differences.

The z values were also entered into a random effect two-sample t-test to identify regions showing significant differences between AD patients and controls in connectivity with the bilateral hippocampus. Voxels that passed a corrected threshold of $P<$ 0.01 (group differences between AD patients and healthy controls: single voxel threshold of $P<0.01$ and cluster size 270 mm^3, using the AlphaSim program with parameters FWHM = 4 mm with mask) indicated a significant difference between the two groups.

Based on the group differences (between AD and healthy controls) of the baseline resting state, we would define functional ROIs according to activated clusters. Our aim was to determine if the effect of acupuncture can ameliorate the functional pathways. First, we extracted the z values for the pre-acupuncture and post-acupuncture stage for both AD and controls. Then, an independent-sample t-test was run for each of the ROIs (pre-acupuncture versus post-acupuncture).

Results

Clinical Data and Neuropsychological Test

Demographic characteristics and neuropsychological scores are shown in Table 1. There were no significant differences between the two groups in gender, age, or years of education, but the neuropsychological test scores, such as the MMSE and auditory verbal learning test (AVLT) scores, were significantly different ($P<$ 0.01) between the two groups.

Comparisons of the Hippocampal Connectivity between AD Patients and Healthy Controls in the Resting State

We compared the AD vs. control group resting state data to find the regions in AD patients that showed abnormal functional connectivity (shown in Table 2, Figures 2 and 3). When comparing left hippocampus connectivity between the AD and control groups, the right medial prefrontal cortex (MPFC) showed significantly decreased connectivity with the left hippocampus in the AD group. There were no regions showing increased connectivity with the left hippocampus in the AD group.

Table 2. Regions showing decreased and increased hippocampal connectivity in AD subjects during resting state.

Brain Regions	BA	Cluster size	Coordinates (MNI) x	y	z	T-score
Left hippocampus						
NC>AD						
R MPFC	11	12	3	60	−5	5.12
AD>NC						
None						
Right hippocampus						
NC>AD						
R ITG	21	12	60	0	−21	3.51
	20		51	−6	−21	3.06
R STG	38	13	54	12	−21	3.22
AD>NC						
None						

$P<0.01$, uncorrected, extent threshold = 10. BA Broadman area. MNI, Montreal Neurological Institute; x, y, z, coordinates of primary peak locations in the MNI space. T value represents differences of hippocampal connectivity in AD and normal controls. MPFC, medial prefrontal cortex; MTG, middle temporal gyrus; ITG, inferior temporal gyrus; STG, superior temporal gyrus.

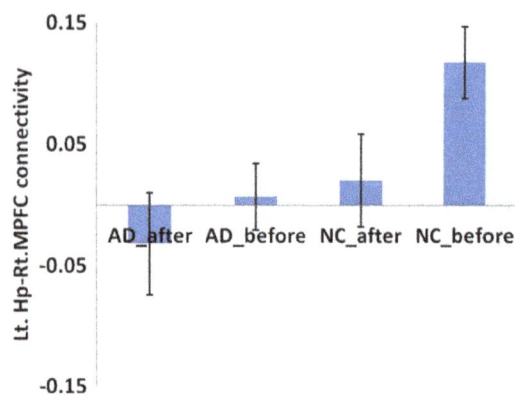

Figure 4. Comparison of connectivity of left hippocampus-right MPFC between pre and post acupuncture among AD patients and controls. There is a significant decreased connectivity following acupuncture for healthy controls (t = 1.942, p = 0.033). However, the AD patients showed negative connectivity after acupuncture, the different is not significant for the AD patients (t = 0.774, p = 0.225),

When comparing the right hippocampal connectivity between the AD and control groups, there was significantly decreased hippocampal connectivity with the right superior temporal gyrus (STG) and the inferior temporal gyrus (ITG) in the AD group. No regions showed increased connectivity with the right hippocampus in the AD group.

Comparisons of the ROI Functional Connectivity between Post-acupuncture and Pre-acupuncture in the AD Patients

There was a significant decrease in the connectivity between the left hippocampus and right MPFC in healthy controls following acupuncture (t = 1.942, p = 0.033). The AD patients showed decreased connectivity between the left hippocampus and right MPFC, but the difference was not significant in the AD patients (t = 0.774, p = 0.225). For detailed data on the regions, see Figure 4.

Connectivities between the right hippocampus and right ITG and STG were lower following acupuncture in the control group, but the differences were not significant (right ITG: t = 0.403, p = 0.345; right STG: t = 0.675, p = 0.254); the AD patients showed higher connectivity after acupuncture (right ITG: t = 1.61, p = 0.056; right STG: t = 1.458, p = 0.08) and these results did not reach but approach significance. For the details of the regions, see Figures 5 and 6.

Comparisons of the Whole Brain Hippocampal Connectivity Post-acupuncture and Pre-acupuncture in AD Patients

We also compared the whole brain connectivity post-and pre-acupuncture in AD patients. In the AD group, we found that the right middle frontal lobe (MFG) showed significantly higher connectivity with the left hippocampus following acupuncture. There were no other regions showing altered connectivity with the left or right hippocampus in the AD group. For the details of the regions, see Table 3 and Figures 7.

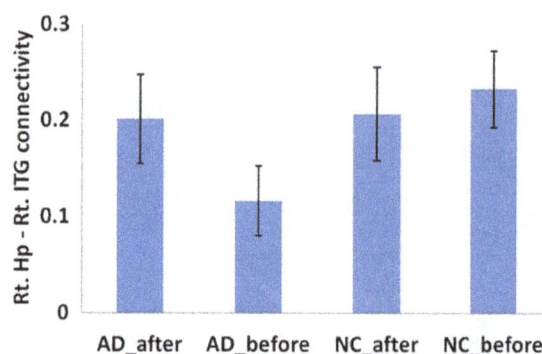

Figure 5. Comparison of connectivity of right hippocampus and right ITG between pre and post acupuncture among AD patients and controls. The acupuncture induced increased functional connectivity for the AD patients (t = 1.61, p = 0.056). There was no significant difference for healthy controls (t = 0.403,p = 0.345).

Comparisons of the Whole Brain Hippocampal Connectivity Post-acupuncture and Pre-acupuncture in Normal Control Subjects

For reference, we also made a comparison of the post- and pre-acupuncture hippocampal connectivity in the normal control subjects. We found that the bilateral thalamus showed significantly higher connectivity with the left hippocampus, while the MPFC showed significantly lower connectivity with the left hippocampus. In addition, the left thalamus, MFG and insula showed significantly higher connectivity with the right hippocampus following acupuncture in the control group. For the details of the regions, see Table 4 and Figures 8 and 9.

In order to see if there is any enhancement in the acupuncture group comparing with the non acupuncture group among patients with the same illness, we selected another non acupuncture AD group as reference to compare the differences of hippocampal connectivity. To keep the structure of the paper, we put the results into the supplementary material. As the results, we found several regions such as the bilateral medial temporal gyrus (MTG), left ITG and fusiform gyrus (FG) showed increased hippocampal connectivity when comparing acupuncture AD group to the non-acupuncture AD group. The results are consistent with our other results. The details see Table S1, S2 and Figure S1, S2 in File S1.

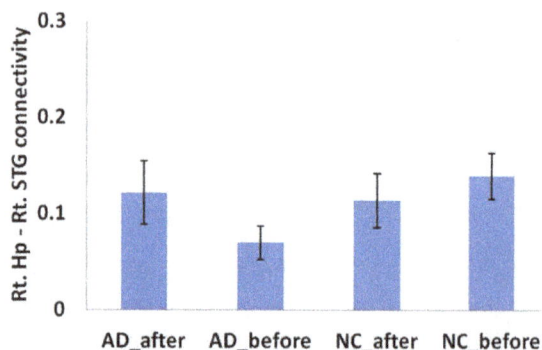

Figure 6. Comparison of connectivity of right hippocampus and right STG between pre and post acupuncture among AD patients and controls. The acupuncture induced increased functional connectivity for the AD patients (t = 1.458, p = 0.08). There was no significant difference for healthy controls (t = 0.675, p = 0.254).

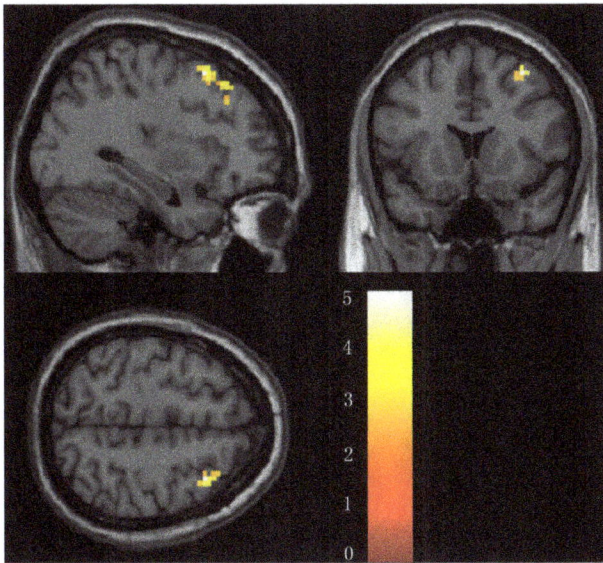

Figure 7. Brain regions showing altered connectivity to left or right hippocampus in AD group after acupuncture comparing to before acupuncture. The right MFG showed increased connectivity to left hippocampus in AD patients after acupuncture. Left in picture is left in the brain. The color scale represents t values.

Discussion

Recently, several researchers have begun to pay attention to the sustained effect of acupuncture and its influence on the resting brain. For the first time, we used fMRI hippocampal connectivity analysis to explore the sustained effect of acupuncture on AD patients. The following are the two main findings of the present study: first, multiple regions show disrupted connectivity in the hippocampus in AD patients. Most of these regions are involved in the hippocampal–cortical memory system. Second, hippocampal connectivity with the frontal and lateral temporal regions in AD patients showed enhancement after acupuncture.

During the resting state, we found abnormal hippocampal functional connectivity in the AD patients relative to controls. The right MPFC showed decreased connectivity with the left hippocampus in the AD patients. The MPFC is considered an important component of human default-mode networks (DMN) [25,31–32]. In previous resting fMRI studies, it has been suggested that a disrupted connection between the MPFC and hippocampus may represent decreased activity of the DMN and contribute to memory impairment in AD patients [15–16,33]. In addition, the right temporal regions (STG and ITG) showed decreased connectivity with the right hippocampus in AD patients. According to previous studies, the lateral temporal cortex, including the STG and ITG, is consistently involved with the DMN, though connectivity is less robust [31]. The STG and ITG regions are important components of the DMN, and AD patients present with amyloid deposits, hypometabolism and atrophy in those regions of the brain [12]. Using resting-state fMRI analysis, disrupted connections between the right hippocampus and temporal regions have also been reported in early-stage AD patients [15–16,18]. Together, our results are largely consistent with those reported by previous studies.

When comparing connectivity of the ROIs post and pre-acupuncture, we found enhanced connectivity between the right temporal regions (STG and ITG) and the hippocampus following

Table 3. Regions showing decreased and increased hippocampal connectivity in AD subjects after acupuncture comparing to before acupuncture.

Brain Regions	BA	Cluster size	Coordinates (MNI) x	y	z	T-score
Left hippocampus						
AD after>AD before						
R MFG	8	25	39	30	45	4.04
R MFG	9		39	30	36	3.11
AD before>AD after						
None						
Right hippocampus						
None						

P<0.01 uncorrected, extent threshold=20. BA, Broadman area. MNI, Montreal Neurological Institute; x, y, z, coordinates of primary peak locations in the MNI space. T value represents differences of hippocampal connectivity in AD and normal controls. MFG, middle frontal gyrus.

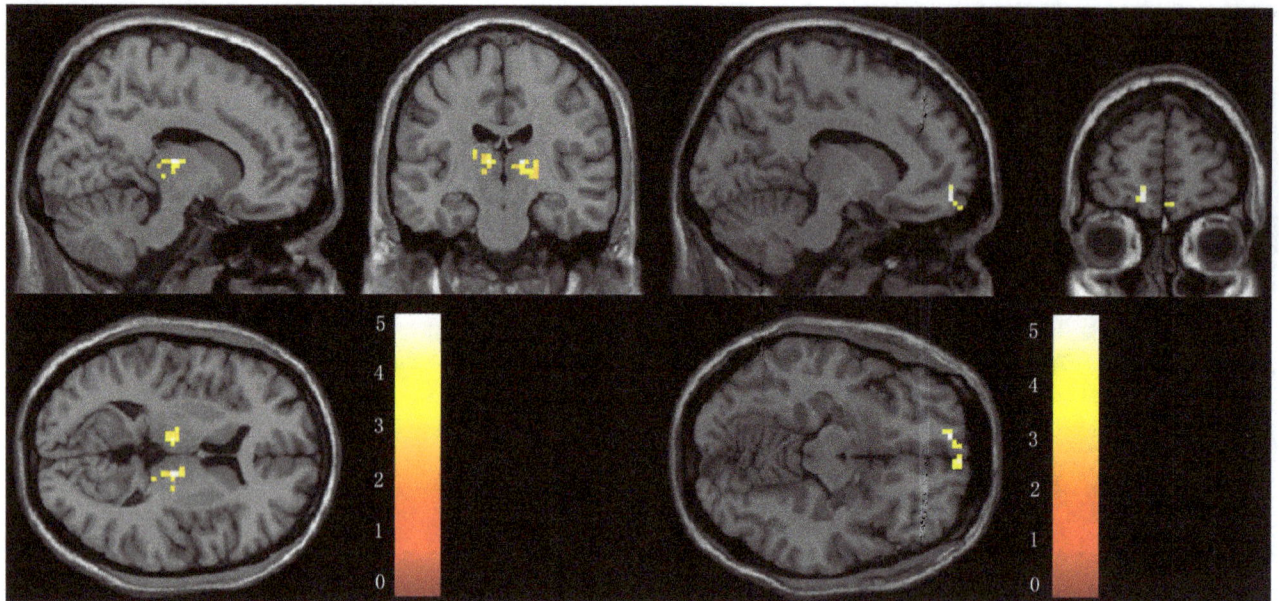

Figure 8. Brain regions showing altered connectivity to left hippocampus in control group after acupuncture comparing to before acupuncture. The thalamus showed increased connectivity while the MPFC showed decreased connectivity to left hippocampus in controls after acupuncture. Left in picture is left in the brain. The color scale represents t values.

acupuncture. Currently, very little is known about how acupuncture affects functional brain connectivity in patients with mild AD. Previous studies suggest that acupuncture can modulate resting state brain connectivity [2–6], and we speculate that enhanced connectivity between the right temporal regions and hippocampus may relate to the specific regulatory effect of acupuncture. Due to the cognitive impairment associated with AD, acupuncture on specific acupoints can modulate the cerebral blood flow and strengthen the hippocampal connectivity in AD patients. In a

recent acupuncture study related to mild cognitive impairment (MCI), increased hippocampal connectivity was detected after acupuncture on acupoint KI3 [34], which was consistent with our study. Our study provides new evidence that acupuncture has a striking, sustained effect on AD patients.

Although no significant differences were found post-acupuncture in the connectivity between the right MPFC and left hippocampus using ROI analysis, whole brain analysis revealed enhanced connectivity between the regions in AD patients.

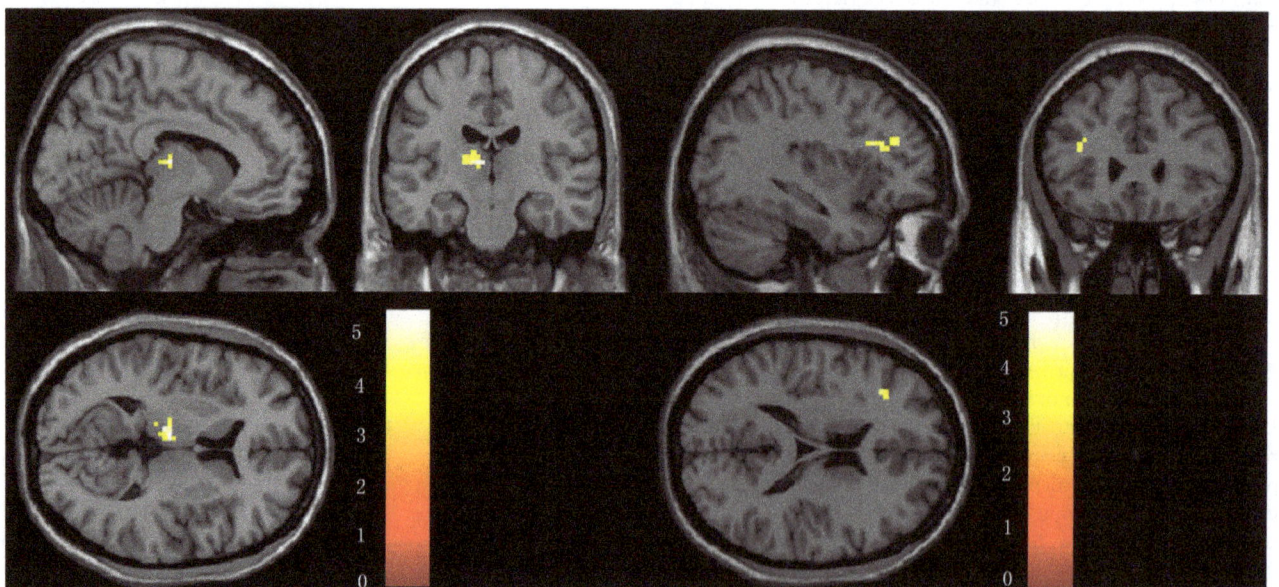

Figure 9. Brain regions showing altered connectivity to right hippocampus in control group after acupuncture comparing to before acupuncture. The left thalamus, MFG and insula showed increased connectivity to right hippocampus in controls after acupuncture. Left in picture is left in the brain. The color scale represents t values.

Table 4. Regions showing decreased and increased hippocampal connectivity in normal controls after acupuncture comparing to before acupuncture.

Brain Regions	BA	Cluster size	Coordinates(MNI) x	y	z	T-score
Left hippocampus						
Controls after>Controls before						
R Thalamus	–	56	12	−18	9	4.69
R Thalamus	–		6	−9	3	4.62
R Thalamus	–		15	−24	3	4.33
L Thalamus	–	23	−18	−21	15	4.23
L Thalamus	–		−9	−18	9	4.14
Controls before>Controls after						
L MPFC	11	27	−12	57	−12	4.33
R MPFC	11		3	63	−12	3.76
Right hippocampus						
Controls after>Controls before						
L Thalamus	–	23	−9	−18	9	4.20
L Thalamus	–		−18	−24	12	3.71
L MFG	46	25	−39	36	24	3.47
L Insula	13		−36	21	21	3.42

P<0.01 uncorrected, extent threshold = 20. BA, Broadman area. MNI, Montreal Neurological Institute; x, y, z, coordinates of primary peak locations in the MNI space. T value represents differences of hippocampal connectivity in normal controls between post-acupuncture and pre-acupuncture. MPFC, medial prefrontal cortex; MFG, middle frontal gyrus.

Previous experiments using task or resting-state fMRI have reported increased activity or connectivity in the frontal region of AD patients compared to healthy controls [15,35–37]. A recent resting fMRI study showed enhanced functional connectivity within the frontal cortex of early-stage MCI patients [38]. These previous studies suggest that AD patients can use additional neural resources to preserve and compensate for losses in memory function attributable to the degenerative effects of the disease. In our study, due to the severe pathological changes in AD patients, the AD group did not have any regions with increased connectivity with the hippocampus during the initial resting state. However, we noticed increased connectivity between the MFG and hippocampus after acupuncture, which suggests that acupuncture may exert modulatory effects on hippocampal connectivity. We speculate that acupuncture activates the compensatory processes in AD patients and strengthens cooperation between brain regions, which is compatible with the theory of dynamic functional reorganization [35,39].

As we all know, hippocampal atrophy correlates significantly with cognitive decline in patients with AD as well as MCI. Thus, assessing and monitoring hippocampal function are very useful for evaluation of AD. Recently, resting state fMRI provided a new promising method for exploring hippocampal function by investigating coherence in the fMRI signal between hippocampus and all other brain regions. In a previous longitudinal study of our group, we explored the correlation between strength of hippocampal connectivity and neuropsychological data to study whether changes in hippocampal connectivity could reflect the cognitive decline in MCI, the early stage of AD. As the result, we found the strength of the ITG-hippocampus connectivity showed significant positive correlation with MMSE scores [18]. This implied that the ITG- hippocampus decreased connectivity may contribute to the cognitive decline in the MCI patients. In another longitudinal MCI study from other group, they also found functional connectivity of hippocampus is associated with MFG, lateral temporal cortex, posterior cingulate cortex and other regions, some of them showed positive correlation with episode memory scores [19]. In addition, some researchers found disruption of hippocampal functional connectivity in AD patients indicating of the cognitive impairment [15,16].Collectively, based on the previous study, we speculated that enhanced hippocampal connectivity, which is induced by acupuncture in the current study, can enhance the information flow and result in improvement of cognitive function in AD patients.

In the current study, we noticed asymmetry between the left and right brain regions during the resting state. The right MPFC, right STG and ITG showed decreased connectivity with the hippocampus in the AD group; after acupuncture, we found enhanced connectivity between the right MFG and left hippocampus in AD patients, which is interesting. We reviewed the literature, and several MRI studies report rightward asymmetry in the volume of the hippocampus in the normal adults, [40,41] and this anatomically rightward asymmetry was diminished in AD patients

[42,43]. Furthermore, in a recent study of AD patients, the authors reported that hippocampal connectivity in normal controls presents with rightward asymmetry, which is diminished in AD patients [15]. In the current study, we found decreased connectivity between the right MPFC, STG and ITG and the hippocampus in AD patients during the resting state, which is consistent with the previous studies. Based on the relationship between the structure and function, we attribute the rightward asymmetry of the hippocampal connectivity to the rightward asymmetry of the hippocampal structure.

There are several limitations of this study. First, an obstacle to imaging the effects of acupuncture is isolating the brain activity related to sensory stimulation from the brain activity associated with any potential therapeutic effects. Even after the needle is withdrawn, the subjects might be influenced by sensory stimulation. Second, the current study would benefit from including a control state that could be compared with real-needle acupuncture, such as sham acupuncture. Third, we didn't show cognitive performances correlations with the functional connectivity and the changes induced by the acupuncture treatments. a longitudinal design will be necessary to determine the impacts of acupuncture on hippocampal connectivity and cognitive performances. In the future, we will trace these subjects using different time points and explore potential hippocampal connectivity changes and their influence on cognitive function in AD patients after acupuncture.

In conclusion, our results revealed the acupuncture at Tai chong and He gu can enhance the hippocampal connectivity in the AD patients. It may provide deep understanding of the therapeutic effect of acupuncture and open a new avenue for the treatment of AD in the future.

Supporting Information

File S1 Supporting Information. Figure S1, Brain regions showing increased connectivity to left hippocampus in acupuncture AD1 group comparing to non-acupuncture AD2 group. These regions include left MTG and FG. **Figure S2, Brain regions showing increased connectivity to right hippocampus in acupuncture AD1 group comparing to non-acupuncture AD2 group.** These regions include left FG, ITG and the right MTG. **Table S1, Characteristics of the acupuncture AD1 patients and non-acupuncture AD2 group. Table S2, Regions showing increased hippocampal connectivity in AD1 group after acupuncture comparing to another non-acupuncture AD2 group.**
(DOC)

Author Contributions

Conceived and designed the experiments: KL JL. Performed the experiments: ZZ ZW JX. Analyzed the data: PL. Contributed reagents/materials/analysis tools: HS YH. Wrote the paper: ZW PL.

References

1. Zhou Y, Jin J (2008) Effect of acupuncture given at the HT 7, ST 36, ST 40 and KI 3 acupoints on various parts of the brains of Alzheimer's disease patients. Acupunct Electrother Res 33: 9–17.
2. Bai L, Qin W, Tian J, Dong M, Pan X, et al. (2009) Acupuncture modulates spontaneous activities in the anticorrelated resting brain networks. Brain Res 1279: 37–49.
3. Dhond RP, Yeh C, Park K, Kettner N, Napadow V (2008) Acupuncture modulates resting state connectivity in default and sensorimotor brain networks. Pain 136: 407–418.

4. Fang J, Jin Z, Wang Y, Li K, Kong J, et al. (2009) The salient characteristics of the central effects of acupuncture needling: limbic-paralimbic-neocortical network modulation. Hum Brain Mapp 30: 1196–1206.
5. Qin W, Tian J, Bai L, Pan X, Yang L, et al. (2008) FMRI connectivity analysis of acupuncture effects on an amygdala-associated brain network. Mol Pain 4: 55.
6. Feng Y, Bai L, Ren Y, Wang H, Liu Z, et al. (2011) Investigation of the large-scale functional brain networks modulated by acupuncture. Magn Reson Imaging 29: 958–965.
7. Wang Z, Nie B, Li D, Zhao Z, Han Y, et al. (2012) Effect of acupuncture in mild cognitive impairment and Alzheimer disease: a functional MRI study. PLoS One 7: e42730.

8. Braak H, Braak E (1995) Staging of Alzheimer's disease-related neurofibrillary changes. Neurobiol Aging 16: 271–278; discussion 278–284.

9. Chetelat G, Baron JC (2003) Early diagnosis of Alzheimer's disease: contribution of structural neuroimaging. Neuroimage 18: 525–541.

10. Pennanen C, Kivipelto M, Tuomainen S, Hartikainen P, Hanninen T, et al. (2004) Hippocampus and entorhinal cortex in mild cognitive impairment and early AD. Neurobiol Aging 25: 303–310.

11. Desikan RS, Cabral HJ, Hess CP, Dillon WP, Glastonbury CM, et al. (2009) Automated MRI measures identify individuals with mild cognitive impairment and Alzheimer's disease. Brain.

12. Buckner RL, Snyder AZ, Shannon BJ, LaRossa G, Sachs R, et al. (2005) Molecular, structural, and functional characterization of Alzheimer's disease: evidence for a relationship between default activity, amyloid, and memory. J Neurosci 25: 7709–7717.

13. Wang Z, Zhao C, Yu L, Zhou W, Li K (2009) Regional metabolic changes in the hippocampus and posterior cingulate area detected with 3-Tesla magnetic resonance spectroscopy in patients with mild cognitive impairment and Alzheimer disease. Acta Radiol 50: 312–319.

14. Li SJ, Li Z, Wu G, Zhang MJ, Franczak M, et al. (2002) Alzheimer Disease: evaluation of a functional MR imaging index as a marker. Radiology 225: 253–259.

15. Wang L, Zang Y, He Y, Liang M, Zhang X, et al. (2006) Changes in hippocampal connectivity in the early stages of Alzheimer's disease: evidence from resting state fMRI. Neuroimage 31: 496–504.

16. Allen G, Barnard H, McColl R, Hester AL, Fields JA, et al. (2007) Reduced hippocampal functional connectivity in Alzheimer disease. Arch Neurol 64: 1482–1487.

17. Bai F, Zhang Z, Watson DR, Yu H, Shi Y, et al. (2009) Abnormal functional connectivity of hippocampus during episodic memory retrieval processing network in amnestic mild cognitive impairment. Biol Psychiatry 65: 951–958.

18. Wang Z, Liang P, Jia X, Qi Z, Yu L, et al. (2011) Baseline and longitudinal patterns of hippocampal connectivity in mild cognitive impairment: evidence from resting state fMRI. J Neurol Sci 309: 79–85.

19. Bai F, Xie C, Watson DR, Shi Y, Yuan Y, et al. (2011) Aberrant hippocampal subregion networks associated with the classifications of aMCI subjects: a longitudinal resting-state study. PLoS One 6: e29288.

20. Goveas JS, Xie C, Ward BD, Wu Z, Li W, et al. (2011) Recovery of hippocampal network connectivity correlates with cognitive improvement in mild Alzheimer's disease patients treated with donepezil assessed by resting-state fMRI. J Magn Reson Imaging 34: 764–773.

21. American Psychiatric Association (1994) DSM-IV:Diagnostic and statistical manual of mental disorders, 4th ed. Washington, DC: Am. Psychiatric Assoc. Press.

22. McKhann G, Drachman D, Folstein M, Katzman R, Price D, et al. (1984) Clinical diagnosis of Alzheimer's disease: report of the NINCDS-ADRDA Work Group under the auspices of Department of Health and Human Services Task Force on Alzheimer's Disease. Neurology 34: 939–944.

23. Morris JC (1993) The Clinical Dementia Rating (CDR): current version and scoring rules. Neurology 43: 2412–2414.

24. Ashburner J, Friston KJ (2005) Unified segmentation. Neuroimage 26: 839–851.

25. Greicius MD, Krasnow B, Reiss AL, Menon V (2003) Functional connectivity in the resting brain: a network analysis of the default mode hypothesis. Proc Natl Acad Sci U S A 100: 253–258.

26. Biswal B, Yetkin FZ, Haughton VM, Hyde JS (1995) Functional connectivity in the motor cortex of resting human brain using echo-planar MRI. Magn Reson Med 34: 537–541.

27. Fox MD, Snyder AZ, Vincent JL, Corbetta M, Van Essen DC, et al. (2005) The human brain is intrinsically organized into dynamic, anticorrelated functional networks. Proc Natl Acad Sci U S A 102: 9673–9678.

28. Maldjian JA, Laurienti PJ, Kraft RA, Burdette JH (2003) An automated method for neuroanatomic and cytoarchitectonic atlas-based interrogation of fMRI data sets. Neuroimage 19: 1233–1239.

29. Tregellas JR, Davalos DB, Rojas DC, Waldo MC, Gibson L, et al. (2007) Increased hemodynamic response in the hippocampus, thalamus and prefrontal cortex during abnormal sensory gating in schizophrenia. Schizophr Res 92: 262–272.

30. Lowe MJ, Mock BJ, Sorenson JA (1998) Functional connectivity in single and multislice echoplanar imaging using resting-state fluctuations. Neuroimage 7: 119–132.

31. Buckner RL, Andrews-Hanna JR, Schacter DL (2008) The brain's default network: anatomy, function, and relevance to disease. Ann N Y Acad Sci 1124: 1–38.

32. Raichle ME, MacLeod AM, Snyder AZ, Powers WJ, Gusnard DA, et al. (2001) A default mode of brain function. Proc Natl Acad Sci U S A 98: 676–682.

33. Greicius MD, Srivastava G, Reiss AL, Menon V (2004) Default-mode network activity distinguishes Alzheimer's disease from healthy aging: evidence from functional MRI. Proc Natl Acad Sci U S A 101: 4637–4642.

34. Feng Y, Bai L, Ren Y, Chen S, Wang H, et al. (2012) FMRI connectivity analysis of acupuncture effects on the whole brain network in mild cognitive impairment patients. Magn Reson Imaging 30: 672–682.

35. Grady CL, McIntosh AR, Beig S, Keightley ML, Burian H, et al. (2003) Evidence from functional neuroimaging of a compensatory prefrontal network in Alzheimer's disease. J Neurosci 23: 986–993.

36. Backman L, Andersson JL, Nyberg L, Winblad B, Nordberg A, et al. (1999) Brain regions associated with episodic retrieval in normal aging and Alzheimer's disease. Neurology 52: 1861–1870.

37. Petrella JR, Coleman RE, Doraiswamy PM (2003) Neuroimaging and early diagnosis of Alzheimer disease: a look to the future. Radiology 226: 315–336.

38. Liang P, Wang Z, Yang Y, Jia X, Li K (2011) Functional disconnection and compensation in mild cognitive impairment: evidence from DLPFC connectivity using resting-state fMRI. PLoS One 6: e22153.

39. Liu Z, Zhang Y, Yan H, Bai L, Dai R, et al. (2012) Altered topological patterns of brain networks in mild cognitive impairment and Alzheimer's disease: a resting-state fMRI study. Psychiatry Res 202: 118–125.

40. Szabo CA, Xiong J, Lancaster JL, Rainey L, Fox P (2001) Amygdalar and hippocampal volumetry in control participants: differences regarding handedness. AJNR Am J Neuroradiol 22: 1342–1345.

41. Pedraza O, Bowers D, Gilmore R (2004) Asymmetry of the hippocampus and amygdala in MRI volumetric measurements of normal adults. J Int Neuropsychol Soc 10: 664–678.

42. Geroldi C, Laakso MP, DeCarli C, Beltramello A, Bianchetti A, et al. (2000) Apolipoprotein E genotype and hippocampal asymmetry in Alzheimer's disease: a volumetric MRI study. J Neurol Neurosurg Psychiatry 68: 93–96.

43. Bigler ED, Tate DF, Miller MJ, Rice SA, Hessel CD, et al. (2002) Dementia, asymmetry of temporal lobe structures, and apolipoprotein E genotype: relationships to cerebral atrophy and neuropsychological impairment. J Int Neuropsychol Soc 8: 925–933.

10

The Antioxidative Effect of Electro-Acupuncture in a Mouse Model of Parkinson's Disease

Haomin Wang[1], Yanli Pan[2], Bing Xue[3], Xinhong Wang[1], Feng Zhao[4], Jun Jia[5], Xibin Liang[6], Xiaomin Wang[1,5]*

1 Neuroscience Research Institute, Peking University, Beijing, People's Republic of China, 2 Science and Education Office, Beijing An Ding Hospital, Beijing, People's Republic of China, 3 Medical Experiment and Test Center, Capital Medical University, Beijing, People's Republic of China, 4 School of Public Health and Family Medicine, Capital Medical University, Beijing, People's Republic of China, 5 Department of Physiology, Capital Medical University, Key Laboratory for Neurodegenerative Disorders of the Ministry of Education, Beijing, People's Republic of China, 6 Department of Neurology and Neurological Sciences, Stanford University, Stanford, California, United States of America

Abstract

Accumulating evidence indicates that oxidative stress plays a critical role in Parkinson's disease (PD). Our previous work has shown that 100 Hz electro-acupuncture (EA) stimulation at ZUSANLI (ST36) and SANYINJIAO (SP6) protects neurons in the substantia nigra pars compacta from 1-methyl-4-phenyl-1,2,3,6-tetrahydropyridine (MPTP) toxicity in male C57BL/6 mice, a model of PD. In the present study we administered 100 Hz EA stimulation at the two acupoints to MPTP-lesioned mice for 12 sessions starting from the day prior to the first MPTP injection. We found that in the striatum of MPTP treated mice 100 Hz EA stimulation effectively inhibited the production of hydrogen peroxide and malonaldehyde, and increased glutathione concentration and total superoxide dismutase activity through biochemical methods. However, it decreased glutathione peroxidase activity via biochemical analysis and did not affect the level of 1-methyl-4-phenylpyridinium in the striatum revealed by high performance liquid chromatography with ultraviolet detection. These data suggest that 100 Hz EA stimulation at ST36 and SP6 has antioxidative effects in the MPTP model of PD. This data, along with our previous work, indicates that 100 Hz EA stimulation at ST36 and SP6 protects the nigrostriatal system by multiple mechanisms including antioxidation and antiapoptosis, and suggests that EA stimulation is a promising therapy for treating PD.

Editor: Huaibin Cai, National Institute of Health, United States of America

Funding: This study was supported by the National Basic Research Program of China (2011CB504100) and the National Natural Science Foundation of China (30472245). The funders had no role in study design, data collection and analysis, decision to publish, or preparation of the manuscript.

Competing Interests: The authors have declared that no competing interests exist.

* E-mail: xmwang@ccmu.edu.cn

Introduction

Parkinson's disease (PD) is a common neurodegenerative disease characterized by motor disorders resulting from the profound loss of dopaminergic neurons in the substantia nigra pars compacta (SNpc) and the subsequent depletion of dopamine (DA) in the striatum. Though significant progress has been made in the treatment of PD, no therapy has been proven to halt or slow disease progression or provide long-term improvement. Numerous investigations have focused on decoding the pathogenesis of PD in an attempt to find a therapeutic strategy. Several postmortem studies show that markers for lipid peroxidation, oxidative DNA and protein damage are significantly increased in the substantia nigra (SN) of PD patients [1–5], indicating that oxidative stress plays an important role in the pathogenesis of PD [6].

Administration of the toxin 1-methyl-4-phenyl-1,2,3,6-tetrahydropyridine (MPTP) causes neurochemical, behavioral, and histopathological alterations in human and nonhuman primates that replicate very closely the clinical symptoms of PD patients, so MPTP is widely used to produce animal models of PD [7]. MPTP is highly lipophilic and crosses the blood-brain barrier soon after systemic administration. In the brain MPTP is metabolized to 1-methyl-4-phenylpyridinium (MPP+), the active toxic compound.

The formation and toxic production process of MPP+ are accompanied by an increased production of free radicals, especially superoxide [8,9], which is poorly reactive but can be turned into hydrogen peroxide (H_2O_2). H_2O_2 participates in MPTP injury through forming hydroxyl radicals [10], the potent oxidants that attack DNA, protein and membrane lipids leading to cell death. Previous studies have suggested that antioxidants could protect DA neurons in the SNpc from MPTP injury [11–13], indicating that antioxidant therapy might be a potential therapeutic choice for PD.

Accumulating clinical evidences have demonstrated that acupuncture helps to improve movement disabilities and reduce the dosage of drugs required by PD patients [14–16]. ZUSANLI (ST36) and SANYINJIAO (SP6) are often used by acupuncturists to treat PD patients at their clinics on the basis of ancient theories of Traditional Chinese Medicine. Modern science research had shown that stimulation in these two acupoints could enhance the immunity and improve the mobility [17–20]. However, the underlying mechanisms are still unclear.

In this study, we hypothesized that the acupuncture stimulation has neuroprotective effect on DA neurons and this effect is stimulation frequency-dependent and is related to the antioxidative effect of acupuncture. We tested this hypothesis by evaluating the DA neuron quantity, the oxidative damage and levels of antioxidants after different frequency EA stimulation at ST36 and SP6 in MPTP treated mice.

Materials and Methods

Ethics statement

All animal experiments were performed by Haomin Wang, whose permit number of License for Performing Animal Experiments of Beijing, which is approved and required by the Ethics Committee of Peking University Health Science Center (a branch committee of the Committee on Animal Care and Usage of Peking University Health Science) before conducting animal experiments in Peking University Health Science Center, is 12928.

Animals

Male C57BL/6 mice weighing 22~25 g were supplied by the Laboratory Animal Center of Peking University, and housed in a temperature-controlled room ($23\pm1°C$) under 12-h on/off light cycle with food and water *ad libitum* in the home cage. Mice were allowed to acclimate to their home environment for 7 days before experiments.

EA stimulation

Mice were randomly divided into five groups: saline (NS), saline plus EA stimulation at 100 Hz (100 Hz + NS), MPTP, MPTP plus EA stimulation at 0 Hz or 100 Hz (0 Hz + MPTP and 100 Hz + MPTP respectively). The EA stimulation was performed from day 1 to day 13 except day 7 (Figure 1) as described before [21] with minor modifications. The mouse was gently restrained in a polyethylene cylinder with its hind limbs and tail outside. Two sterilized stainless-steel needles 0.18 mm in diameter and 3 mm long were inserted in each leg, one at ST36 (2 mm lateral to the anterior tubercle of tibia) and the other at SP6 (2 mm proximal to the upper border of medial melleolus, at the posterior border of the tibia). Bidirectional square wave electrical pulses (0.2 ms duration, 100 Hz) or no electrical pluses (0 Hz), designated as EA, were given for a total of 30 min each day. The intensity of the stimulation at 100 Hz was increased stepwise from 1 to 1.25 mA and then to 1.5 mA, with each step lasting for 10 min. The animals remained relaxed during stimulation, so anesthesia was not performed.

MPTP treatments

Following EA stimulation mice received intraperitoneal (i.p.) injections of MPTP from day 2 to day 6 (Figure 1) (Sigma-Aldrich, St. Louis, MO, USA, 30 mg/kg, dissolved in saline, once a day) or an equivalent volume of saline.

Tissue collection and processing

Three mice from each group were randomly selected on day 14 for tyrosine hydroxylase (TH) immunohistochemistry. They were deeply anesthetized with 400 mg/kg chloral hydrate, and then transcardially perfused with 25 ml saline followed by 75 ml 4%

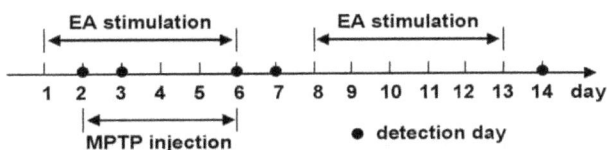

Figure 1. Experimental design of the study. Numbers represent days.

(w/v) paraformaldehyde in phosphate buffer. Brains were removed and post-fixed in the same fixative overnight and then cryoprotected in 30% (w/v) sucrose for 3 ~ 5 days. The brains were frozen on powdered dry ice and then arranged for frontal sectioning according to the mouse brain atlas of Burton M. Slotnick and Christina M. Leonard. Brains were sectioned at 20 μm thickness with a cryostat at $-20°C$ and processed for immunohistochemistry. On day 2 (2 hr. post MPTP injection), 3 (4 hr. post MPTP injection), 6 (2 hr. post MPTP injection), 7 and 14, seven to eight mice from each group were decapitated, and the bilateral striata and the ventral midbrains were dissected quickly and stored at $-80°C$ (Figure 1).

Immunohistochemistry and quantification of TH-ir neuronal profiles

All sections spanning the SN were collected for immunohistochemistry according to the previously described method [22] with minor modifications. Every seventh section was incubated in rabbit anti-TH antibody (1:2000, Chemicon, Temecula, CA, USA) at 4°C overnight. Sections treated with diluted non-immune goat serum instead of primary antibody served as an antibody control. Sections were incubated with biotinylated goat anti-rabbit antibody and then with the avidin–biotin–peroxidase complex for 30 min at 37 °C. The bound complex was visualized by incubating sections in a solution containing 0.1% (w/v) 3,3-diaminobenzidine (Sigma, St. Louis, MO, USA), 1% (v/v) H_2O_2, and 8% (w/v) ammonium nickel sulfate (Fluka Chemie GmbH, Switzerland).

TH-ir neuronal profiles with distinct nuclei were counted in ten sections throughout the entire rostrocaudal extent of the SNpc. All sections were coded and examined blind.

HPLC analysis of dopamine and its metabolites

Striata collected on day 14 were used to detect the levels of DA and its metabolites, dihydroxyphenylacetic acid (DOPAC) and homovanillic acid (HVA), by HPLC with electrochemical detection (HPLC-ECD). In brief, tissues were weighed and then homogenized in 0.4 M ice-cold perchloric acid (150 μl/tissue). All homogenates were kept away from light in an ice bath for 60 min. Centrifuging at 12,000 rpm and 4°C for 20 min, transferring 120 μl supernatant from each sample to a new tube and then adding 60 μl solution (20 mM potassium citrate, 300 mM potassium dihydrogen phosphate, and 2 mM EDTA-2Na). Keeping the mixtures away from light in an ice bath for 60 min, and then centrifuging at 12,000 rpm and 4°C for 20 min. Filtering the supernatant with a 0.22 μm Millipore filter and injecting the filtrate into the HPLC system for analysis. The mobile phase contained 110 mM citrate buffer/100 mM EDTA/70 mM 1-octanesulfonate sodium solution and 20% (v/v) methanol. Flow rate was 1 ml/min. Striata from six to nine animals in each group were used.

H_2O_2, MDA, total SOD, GSH, and GSH-PX assay

On day 3, 7 and 14 mice were sacrificed and the striata as well as the ventral midbrains were dissected as described above. About seven striata and ventral midbrains from each group were homogenized in 30 vol. (wt./vol.) of 0.1 M phosphate buffer solution and centrifuged at 3000 g and 4°C for 15 min. The supernatant was used to determine the level of H_2O_2, malonaldehyde (MDA) and activity of total superoxide dismutase (SOD). The supernatant from the striata and the ventral midbrains diluted in 10 vol. (wt./vol.) buffer was used for glutathione peroxidase (GSH-PX) activity assay. H_2O_2, MDA, SOD and GSH-PX assays were performed according to the procedures provided by the assay kits (Nanjing Jiancheng Bioengineering Institute, Nanjing, PR China). The glutathione (GSH) content was detected by a Total Glutathione Quantification Kit (Dojindo Laboratories, Kumamoto, Japan), following the kits instructions. H_2O_2 content was determined by monitoring at the absorbance at 412 nm of the titanium-peroxide complex [23]. MDA level was analyzed with 2-thiobarbituric acid [24]. SOD activity was analyzed by monitoring the inhibition of the reduction of nitro blue tetrazolium by the sample at 550 nm [25]. GSH-PX activity was detected with 5-5'-dithiobis-p-nitrobenzoic acid [26]. GSH level was measured by DTNB-GSSG reductase recycling assay [27]. All the assays were colorimetric methods based on biochemical reactions, and the absorbance values of the samples were calibrated against that of the standards with known concentration or calibrated to a standard graph generated with known content of the standards.

MPP+ measurement

Striata collected on day 2 and 6 (2 hr. after the first and last injection of MPTP) were used for measuring MPP+ level using HPLC with UV detection (HPLC-UV, wavelength, 293 nm). Samples were weighed, homogenized in 200 μl ice-cold perchloric acid (0.1 M). and then centrifuged at 12,000 rpm at 4°C for 7 min. The supernatant was filtered prior to analysis by HPLC. For HPLC analysis the mobile phase contained 85% (v/v) 0.1 M acetic acid/75 mM triethylamine solution and 15% (v/v) acetonitrile and the flow rate was 1 ml/min.

Statistical analysis

Values are expressed as mean ± SEM. Differences among means were analyzed using one-way ANOVA followed by Newman–Keuls post hoc test of difference between means. A p value <0.05 denoted a statistically significant difference.

Results

100 Hz EA stimulation protects dopaminergic neurons from MPTP toxicity

Profound loss of DA neurons in the SNpc is the main pathological change of PD. Here we assessed whether EA stimulation could rescue DA neurons in the SNpc from MPTP toxicity by TH immunohistochemistry. We found that on day 14, TH positive neurons in MPTP treated mice dramatically decreased ($p<0.05$ vs. NS group; Figure 2, E and F), in comparison with the saline group (Figure 2, A and B). However, TH immunoreactivity could be rescued by 100 Hz EA stimulation ($p<0.05$ vs. MPTP group; Figure 2, I and J). Unlike 100 Hz, EA stimulation at 0 Hz made no difference (Figure 2, G and H). Furthermore, 100 Hz EA stimulation had no effect on saline treated control mice (Figure 2, C and D). These results suggest that 100 Hz EA stimulation can protect DA neurons in the SNpc from MPTP injury.

100 Hz EA stimulation increases the concentration of striatal DA and its metabolites in PD mice

Because the abnormal motor function in PD is mainly caused by subthreshold levels of DA in the striatum, we looked at the concentration of striatal DA and its metabolites, DOPAC and HVA in our different groups. On day 14, MPTP injection caused a significant reduction in the concentration of the three substances ($p<0.001$ vs. NS group, Figure 3). However, 100 Hz EA

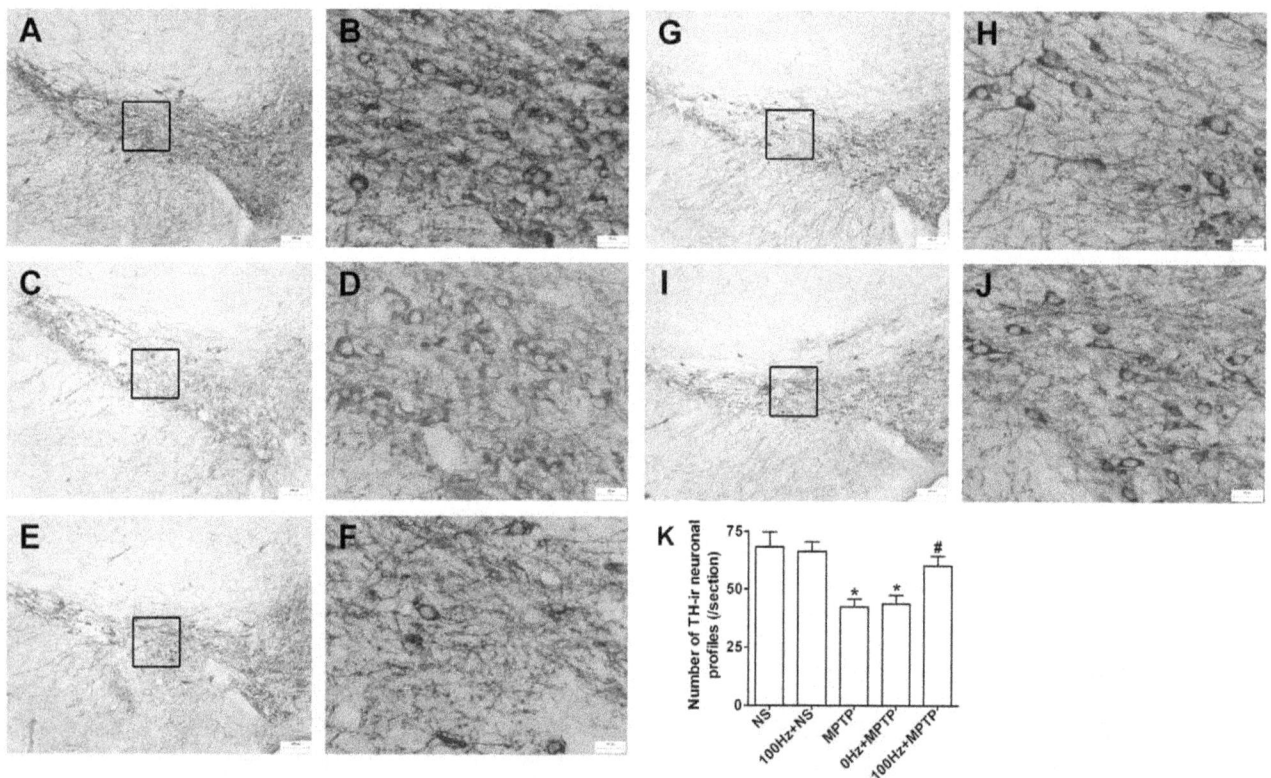

Figure 2. 100 Hz EA stimulation protects dopaminergic neurons from MPTP toxicity. (A and B) NS. (C and D) 100 Hz + NS. (E and F) MPTP. (G and H) 0 Hz + MPTP. (I and J) 100 Hz + MPTP. (K) Quantification of TH positive neuronal profiles in the SNpc. *$p<0.05$, compared with NS group. n = 3. Scale bar, 200 μm (A, C, E, G and I) and 50 μm (B, D, F, H and J).

stimulation elevated DA levels significantly (34% increase, $p < 0.05$ vs. MPTP group, Figure 3A) in the MPTP treated mice, as well as DOPAC and HVA concentrations (19.8% and 22.9% increase respectively, $p < 0.05$ vs. MPTP group; Figure 3, B and C). Consistent with the TH immunohistochemistry results, 0 Hz EA stimulation did not affect the concentrations of DA, DOPAC and HVA in the striatum of the MPTP treated mice.

100 Hz EA stimulation inhibits the elevation of striatal H_2O_2 level in PD model mice

In our model, striatal H_2O_2 content increased significantly at 2 hr. after a single MPTP injection and reached its peak at 4 hr. (Figure S1). Measurement of striatal H_2O_2 level at 4 hr. after every MPTP injection (five injections in total) show that only the first three MPTP injections augment H_2O_2 levels significantly (Figure S1 and S2). Therefore we examined striatal H_2O_2 level on day 3 when mice had been given two MPTP injections. The results show that 100 Hz EA stimulation inhibits the elevation of H_2O_2 in MPTP treated mice ($p < 0.05$ vs. MPTP group, Figure 4), while, 0 Hz EA stimulation has no affects. Additionally, 100 Hz EA stimulation had no effect on normal mice. Moreover, we observed there was no significant change of H_2O_2 contents in the ventral midbrain of the model mice compared with the NS group (Figure S3 and S4).

Since all of our above tests show that 100 Hz EA stimulation had no adverse effect on normal mice and 0 Hz EA stimulation did not have an effect on MPTP treated mice, we abandoned the 100 Hz + NS and 0 Hz + MPTP groups in order to minimize the number of animals used in the following experiments.

Effects of 100 Hz EA stimulation on the concentration/activity of striatal GSH, GSH-PX and SOD

In the brain, major antioxidant defenses consist of antioxidant scavengers such as GSH and enzymes such as GSH-PX and SOD. For the following experiment we measured striatal concentration and activity of GSH, GSH-PX and total SOD on day 3, 7 and 14.

On day 3 EA stimulation enhanced GSH content significantly ($p < 0.001$ vs. NS and $p < 0.001$ vs. MPTP group on day 3, Figure 5A), but the effect disappeared on day 7 and 14. MPTP injection did not affect GSH content in the striatum.

GSH-PX activity was significantly increased on day 3 in the MPTP group ($p < 0.01$ vs. NS, Figure 5B). 100 Hz EA stimulation significantly decreased GSH-PX activity at that time point ($p < 0.01$ vs. NS group). On day 7, high levels of GSH-PX activity were still seen in the MPTP treated mice (13.3% increase compared to NS group, Figure 5B) but EA stimulation normalized GSH-PX activity in model mice. On day 14, MPTP and EA stimulation had no effect on GSH-PX activity.

SOD activity was decreased in the striatum of MPTP treated mice on all of the three time points, i.e., day 3, day 7 and day 14 (6.0% ~ 8.3% compared to NS group, Figure 5C). 100 Hz EA stimulation increased the SOD activity in a time dependent manner, i.e., 3 sessions (day 3) of treatment did not affect SOD activity, 6 sessions (day 7) significantly increased SOD activity (8.8% increase compared to EA group on day 3, $p < 0.01$ vs. MPTP group on day 7, Figure 5C) and 12 sessions (day 14) of treatment also increased SOD activity too.

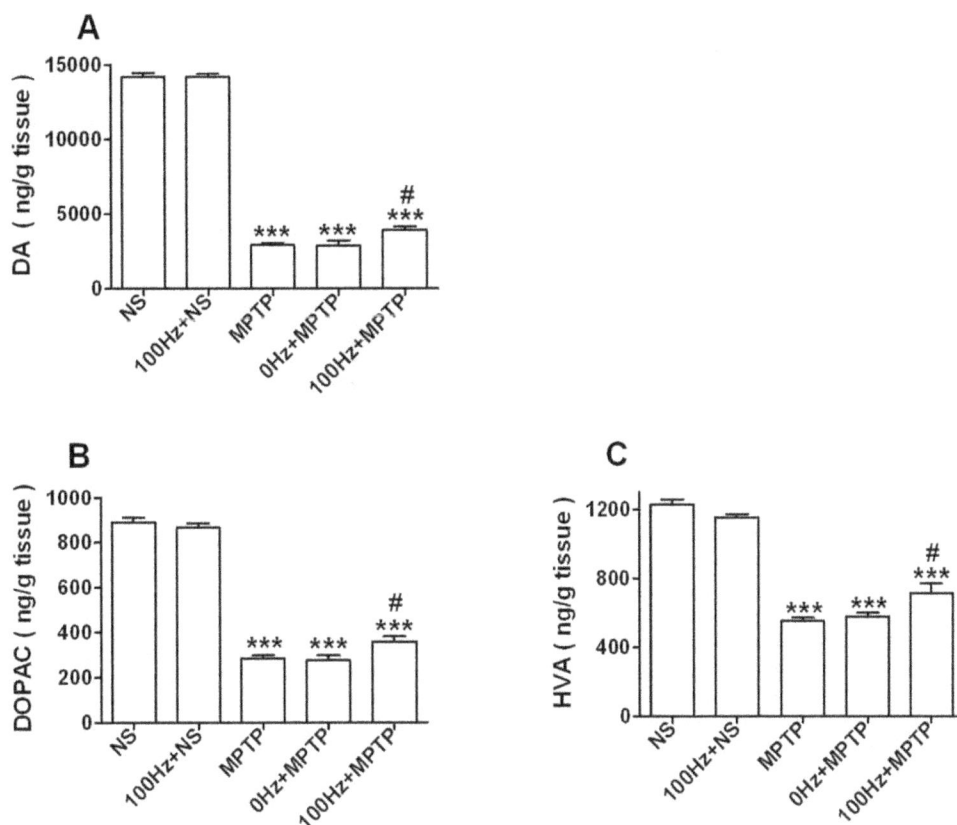

Figure 3. 100 Hz EA stimulation increases the contents of striatal DA and its metabolites in MPTP-treated mice. (A) DA. (B) DOPAC. (C) HVA. ***$p < 0.001$, compared with NS group; #$p < 0.05$, compared with MPTP group. n = 6~9.

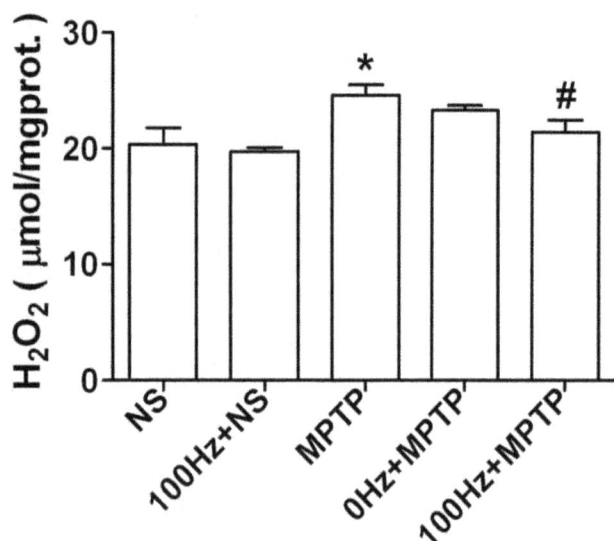

Figure 4. 100 Hz EA stimulation inhibits the elevation of striatal H_2O_2 level in MPTP-treated mice. *$p<0.05$, compared with NS group; #$p<0.05$, compared with MPTP group. n = 5~8.

100 Hz EA stimulation depresses the elevation of striatal MDA content

MDA is one of the final products of polyunsaturated fatty acid peroxidation in cells. An increase in free radicals causes overproduction of MDA. Therefore, it is used as a lipid peroxidation marker. We detected striatal MDA content on day 7 and 14, the 1st and 8th day after the last MPTP injection respectively. On day 7, MDA levels were significantly increased in MPTP treated mice (155% increase, $p<0.001$ vs. NS group, Figure 5D) but EA stimulation reduced this increase (38% decrease, $p<0.01$ vs. MPTP group on day 7). On day 14 there were no statistic differences among the three groups. Moreover, we found there was no significant change of MDA levels in the ventral midbrain of the model mice compared with the NS group (Figure S5).

100 Hz EA stimulation does not affect MPP^+ metabolism

In the brain the toxicity of MPTP is due to its toxic form, MPP^+, which is selectively toxic to dopaminergic neurons. We evaluated if the antioxidative effect of EA stimulation was related to the formation or degradation of MPP^+. On day 2 and day 6 when the 1st and 5th MPTP injections were performed, mice were killed for the analysis of striatal MPP^+ content by HPLC-UV. Our data shows that EA stimulation does not influence the concentration of MPP^+ in the striatum of the MPTP treated mice (Figure 6), suggesting that the target of EA stimulation at 100 Hz does not involve in the MPP^+ metabolic pathway.

Discussion

More and more people turn to acupuncture for the treatment of Parkinson's disease and clinical evidence has proven the effectiveness of acupuncture in the management of this dread disease. But the underlying mechanism still needs to be clarified. In this study we found that 100 Hz, but not 0 Hz of EA stimulation at ST36 and SP6 can protect dopaminergic neurons in the substantia nigra from MPTP insult, suggesting that the response of the body to EA stimulation is frequency-dependent. Although multiple mechanisms may be involved in this process, our findings highlight the possibility that the antioxidative effect of

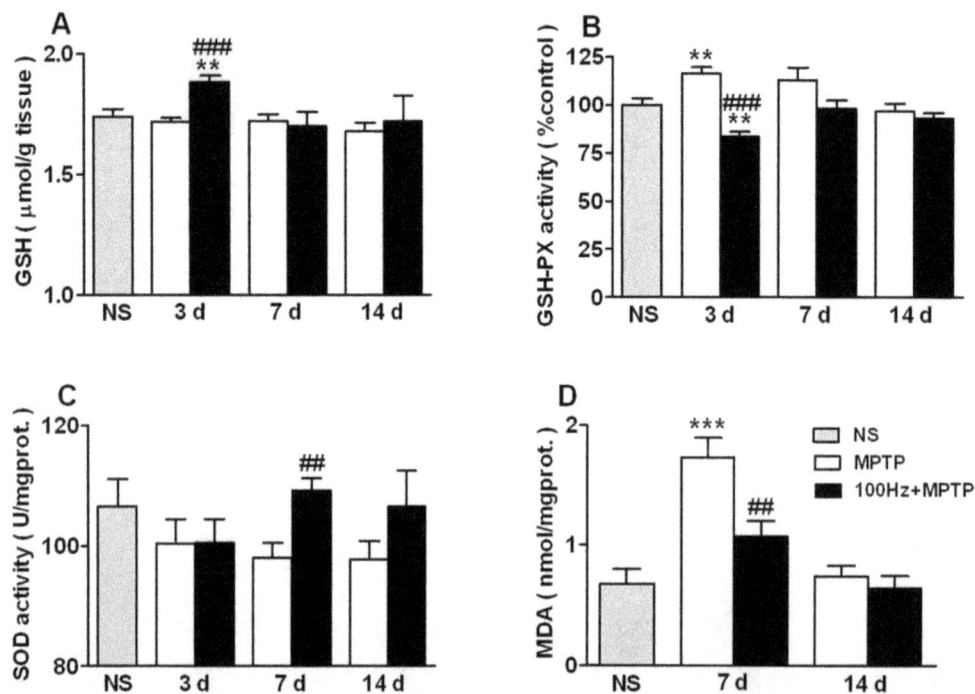

Figure 5. 100 Hz EA stimulation effects on the content/activity of GSH, GSH-PX, SOD and MDA in the striatum. Saline group (gray bar), MPTP group (white bar) and 100 Hz + MPTP group (black bar). (A) GSH content. (B) GSH-PX activity. (C) SOD activity. (D) MDA content. **$p<0.01$, ***$p<0.001$, compared with NS group; ##$p<0.01$, ###$p<0.001$, compared with MPTP group on the same day. n = 6~7 (A and B) or n = 5~7 (C and D).

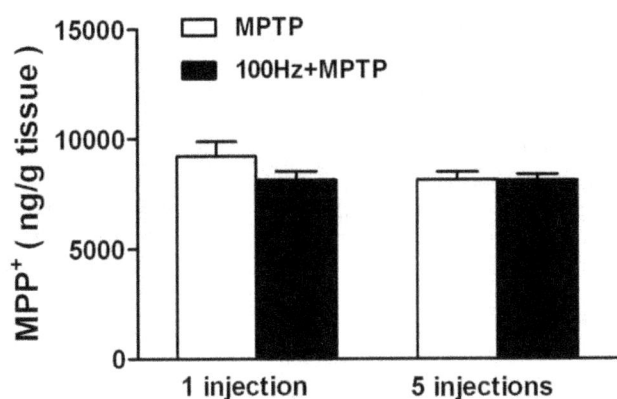

Figure 6. 100 Hz EA stimulation does not affect MPP$^+$ formation. MPTP group (white bar) and 100 Hz + MPTP group (black bar). n = 6~8.

EA stimulation may be a leading mechanism. Oxidative stress is involved in dopaminergic neuronal injury in MPTP-lesioned mice. EA at 100 Hz reverses the elevation of striatal MDA concentration in PD model mice. This antioxidative activity of EA partially relies on its ability to reduce H_2O_2 content and elevate GSH level and total SOD activity. This activity also depends on frequency because 0 Hz EA stimulation did not benefit PD mice. In addition, 100 Hz EA stimulation did not adversely affect normal mice.

In tissues obtained at autopsy from PD patients the activity of SOD is increased, while GSH-PX activity and GSH content are decreased [28-30]. SOD is often regarded as the first line of defense against an upswing of reactive oxygen species (ROS) and responsible for the conversion of superoxide to H_2O_2 in the cytoplasm and mitochondria. Enhanced SOD activity may be neuroprotective since transgenic mice with increased SOD activity are resistant to MPTP injury [31,32], while mice with decreased SOD activity are more susceptible to MPTP toxicity [10,33]. GSH is considered to be a major antioxidant in the brain, capable of attenuating oxidative damage [34]. Impairment of the GSH system may trigger a cascade of events leading to oxidative stress and destruction of the nigrostriatal pathway as well as render the pathway susceptible to a toxic insult [35]. GSH depletion is a primary event in incidental Lewy body disease which is thought to be presymptomatic Parkinson's disease. GSH-PX is an enzyme of major importance in the detoxification of peroxides such as H_2O_2. Deficiency of GSH-PX activity leads to aggravating MPTP lesions [10]. Ebselen, an antioxidant drug with GSH-PX-like activity, prevents both neuronal loss and clinical symptoms in a primate MPTP model of PD [13].

Our findings reveal that 100 Hz EA stimulation at ST36 and SP6 can prevent the decrease of striatal total SOD activity, elevate striatal GSH concentration, and consequently inhibit the increase of striatal H_2O_2 and MDA level caused by MPTP. On day 3 (3 sessions of EA) the decrease of striatal GSH-PX activity in the EA group might relate to the augmented striatal GSH content, which helps to consume the excessive H_2O_2.

Recently, Yu et al. claimed that acupuncture mitigated oxidative stress in the SN of 6-hydroxydopamine lesioned rats [36]. Compared with their study we used MPTP mice model, which is the best available and the most popular animal model of PD at present [7,9,37-41]. Furthermore, we detected the oxidative indicators in a time-course manner (on day 3, 7 and 14), and illustrated a picture on the oxidative changes in MPTP mice model. In our model the rapid elevation of H_2O_2 content

and GSH-PX activity suggests that the production of ROS is an early event in MPTP toxicity, consistent with the observations in other experiments [42,43]. Also, our study suggested that oxidative stress could be more profound in the striatum than that in the ventral midbrain, which might be due to the fact that the DA neuron loss induced by MPTP results from molecular events initiated in the striatum [44-46]. Thus, the antioxidative effect of EA at these two acupoints on the striatum could be significant to rescue the DA neurons in the SN. Kim et al. found that 100 Hz EA normalized the elevation of glyoxalase II, which plays a pro-survival role in the metabolic stress response through detoxifying methylglyoxal in MPTP mice, and they assumed that it could be due to the relief of oxidative stress in the striatum by increasing antioxidant enzyme activities, thereby precluding methylglyoxal accumulation [47].

Motor behavioral abnormality is the cardinal characteristics of human PD. Therefore, therapies that can improve the abnormal behavior will significantly help PD patients in their daily life. In this study we found that 100 Hz EA stimulation normalized the motor disorders of the model mice. We think that the mechanism is due to the regulatory effect of EA on other nuclei in the basal ganglia, such as the globus pallidus, but not the neuroprotective effect of EA on the dopaminergic neurons in the nigrostriatal system (Wang HM et al. unpublished). It is in accordance with previous studies in our lab [48-50].

MPP$^+$ activates microglia which exaggerates its toxicity via ROS dependent and independent mechanisms [51]. Our previous work revealed that 100 Hz EA stimulation can suppress the activation of microglia and up-regulate BDNF and GDNF expression in medial forebrain bundle-transected PD rats [22,50,52]. Therefore, 100 Hz EA stimulation might rescue DA neurons through multiple ways besides mitigating oxidative stress in MPTP mice. Indeed, we have discovered that 100 Hz EA stimulation at ST36 and SP6 has an anti-apoptotic effect by elevating the Bcl-2/Bax ratio in this model (Pan YL et al., unpublished).

In its late stage PD destroys multiple regions of the brain except for the nigrostriatal system, which leads to complex clinical symptoms such as pain and insomnia. A clinical report demonstrated that acupuncture benefited the sleep of PD patients and eased the patients' subjective sufferings from pain [53] suggesting that acupuncture stimulation produces extensive neuroprotective and regulative effects. Therefore, it is highly possible that the integration of several activated signal pathways during acupuncture stimulation plays a role in alleviating the pathological changes in the brain of PD patients.

Supporting Information

Figure S1   Time course of striatal H_2O_2 levels after a single injection of MPTP. ** $p < 0.01$, *** $p < 0.001$, compared with NS group. n = 5~7.
(TIF)

Figure S2   Time course of H_2O_2 contents in the striatum of the subacute MPTP mouse model. * $p < 0.05$, ** $p < 0.01$, compared with NS group. n = 6.
(TIF)

Figure S3   Time course of H_2O_2 levels in the ventral midbrain after a single injection of MPTP. Animals were sacrificed at 2, 4, 6, 8, 10 and 12 hours post one MPTP injection (30 mg/kg, i.p.). H_2O_2 contents of the ventral midbrains were detected. n = 5~7.
(TIF)

Figure S4 Time course of H₂O₂ contents in the ventral midbrain of the subacute MPTP mouse model. At 4 hours after the 2nd, 3rd, 4th and 5th MPTP injection (30 mg/kg, i.p.), animals were decapitated. Contents of H_2O_2 in the ventral midbrains were detected. n = 6.
(TIF)

Figure S5 Time course of MDA contents in the ventral midbrain of the subacute MPTP mouse model. After the 2nd, 3rd, 4th and 5th MPTP injection (30 mg/kg, i.p.), animals were decapitated. Contents of MDA in the ventral midbrains were detected. n = 6.
(TIF)

Acknowledgments

We express sincere thanks to Dr. Kristian Doyle (Stanford University) for the critical reading of the manuscript.

Author Contributions

Conceived and designed the experiments: XMW HMW XBL FZ. Performed the experiments: HMW XHW. Analyzed the data: HMW YLP. Contributed reagents/materials/analysis tools: XMW BX JJ. Wrote the paper: HMW. Final approval of the version to be published: WXM LXB.

References

1. Dexter DT, Carter CJ, Wells FR, Javoy-Agid F, Agid Y, et al. (1989) Basal lipid peroxidation in substantia nigra is increased in Parkinson's disease. J Neurochem 52: 381–389.
2. Floor E, Wetzel MG (1998) Increased protein oxidation in human substantia nigra pars compacta in comparison with basal ganglia and prefrontal cortex measured with an improved dinitrophenylhydrazine assay. J Neurochem 70: 268–275.
3. Alam ZI, Daniel SE, Lees AJ, Marsden DC, Jenner P, et al. (1997) A generalised increase in protein carbonyls in the brain in Parkinson's but not incidental Lewy body disease. J Neurochem 69: 1326–1329.
4. Yoritaka A, Hattori N, Uchida K, Tanaka M, Stadtman ER, et al. (1996) Immunohistochemical detection of 4-hydroxynonenal protein adducts in Parkinson disease. Proc Natl Acad Sci U S A 93: 2696–2701.
5. Shigenaga MK, Ames BN (1991) Assays for 8-hydroxy-2′-deoxyguanosine: a biomarker of in vivo oxidative DNA damage. Free Radic Biol Med 10: 211–216.
6. Greenamyre JT, Hastings TG (2004) Biomedicine. Parkinson's–divergent causes, convergent mechanisms. Science 304: 1120–1122.
7. Beal MF (2001) Experimental models of Parkinson's disease. Nat Rev Neurosci 2: 325–334.
8. Przedborski S, Jackson-Lewis V, Djaldetti R, Liberatore G, Vila M, et al. (2000) The parkinsonian toxin MPTP: action and mechanism. Restor Neurol Neurosci 16: 135–142.
9. Przedborski S, Vila M (2003) The 1-methyl-4-phenyl-1,2,3,6-tetrahydropyridine mouse model: a tool to explore the pathogenesis of Parkinson's disease. Ann N Y Acad Sci 991: 189–198.
10. Zhang J, Graham DG, Montine TJ, Ho YS (2000) Enhanced N-methyl-4-phenyl-1,2,3,6-tetrahydropyridine toxicity in mice deficient in CuZn-superoxide dismutase or glutathione peroxidase. J Neuropathol Exp Neurol 59: 53–61.
11. Liang LP, Huang J, Fulton R, Day BJ, Patel M (2007) An orally active catalytic metalloporphyrin protects against 1-methyl-4-phenyl-1,2,3,6-tetrahydropyridine neurotoxicity in vivo. J Neurosci 27: 4326–4333.
12. Luo D, Zhang Q, Wang H, Cui Y, Sun Z, et al. (2009) Fucoidan protects against dopaminergic neuron death in vivo and in vitro. Eur J Pharmacol 617: 33–40.
13. Moussaoui S, Obinu MC, Daniel N, Reibaud M, Blanchard V, et al. (2000) The antioxidant ebselen prevents neurotoxicity and clinical symptoms in a primate model of Parkinson's disease. Exp Neurol 166: 235–245.
14. Ren XM (2008) Fifty cases of Parkinson's disease treated by acupuncture combined with madopar. J Tradit Chin Med 28: 255–257.
15. Zhuang X, Wang L (2000) Acupuncture treatment of Parkinson's disease–a report of 29 cases. J Tradit Chin Med 20: 265–267.
16. Chen L (1998) Clinical observations on forty cases of paralysis agitans treated by acupuncture. J Tradit Chin Med 18: 23–26.
17. Dos SJG, Jr., Kawano F, Nishida MM, Yamamura Y, Mello LE, et al. (2008) Antidepressive-like effects of electroacupuncture in rats. Physiol Behav 93: 155–159.
18. Lee SH, Chung SH, Lee JS, Kim SS, Shin HD, et al. (2002) Effects of acupuncture on the 5-hydroxytryptamine synthesis and tryptophan hydroxylase expression in the dorsal raphe of exercised rats. Neurosci Lett 332: 17–20.
19. Rho SW, Choi GS, Ko EJ, Kim SK, Lee YS, et al. (2008) Molecular changes in remote tissues induced by electro-acupuncture stimulation at acupoint ST36. Mol Cells 25: 178–183.
20. Kung YY, Chen FP, Hwang SJ (2006) The different immunomodulation of indirect moxibustion on normal subjects and patients with systemic lupus erythematosus. Am J Chin Med 34: 47–56.
21. Huang C, Wang Y, Chang JK, Han JS (2000) Endomorphin and mu-opioid receptors in mouse brain mediate the analgesic effect induced by 2 Hz but not 100 Hz electroacupuncture stimulation. Neurosci Lett 294: 159–162.
22. Liang XB, Liu XY, Li FQ, Luo Y, Lu J, et al. (2002) Long-term high-frequency electro-acupuncture stimulation prevents neuronal degeneration and up-regulates BDNF mRNA in the substantia nigra and ventral tegmental area following medial forebrain bundle axotomy. Brain Res Mol Brain Res 108: 51–59.

23. Zhao LC, Shi LG (2009) Metabolism of hydrogen peroxide in univoltine and polyvoltine strains of silkworm (Bombyx mori). Comp Biochem Physiol B 152: 339–345.
24. Placer ZA, Cushman LL, Johnson BC (1966) Estimation of product of lipid peroxidation (malonyl dialdehyde) in biochemical systems. Anal Biochem 16: 359–364.
25. Winterbourn CC, Hawkins RE, Brian M, Carrell RW (1975) The estimation of red cell superoxide dismutase activity. J Lab Clin Med 85: 337–341.
26. Hafemen DG (1974) Effect of dietary selenium on erythrocyte and liver glutathione peroxidase in the rats. J Nutr 104: 580–587.
27. Anderson ME (1985) Determination of glutathione and glutathione disulfide in biological samples. Methods Enzymol 113: 548–555.
28. Kish SJ, Morito C, Hornykiewicz O (1985) Glutathione peroxidase activity in Parkinson's disease brain. Neurosci Lett 58: 343–346.
29. Saggu H, Cooksey J, Dexter D, Wells FR, Lees A, et al. (1989) A selective increase in particulate superoxide dismutase activity in parkinsonian substantia nigra. J Neurochem 53: 692–697.
30. Sian J, Dexter DT, Lees AJ, Daniel S, Agid Y, et al. (1994) Alterations in glutathione levels in Parkinson's disease and other neurodegenerative disorders affecting basal ganglia. Ann Neurol 36: 348–355.
31. Przedborski S, Kostic V, Jackson-Lewis V, Naini AB, Simonetti S, et al. (1992) Transgenic mice with increased Cu/Zn-superoxide dismutase activity are resistant to N-methyl-4-phenyl-1,2,3,6-tetrahydropyridine-induced neurotoxicity. J Neurosci 12: 1658–1667.
32. Klivenyi P, St Clair D, Wermer M, Yen HC, Oberley T, et al. (1998) Manganese superoxide dismutase overexpression attenuates MPTP toxicity. Neurobiol Dis 5: 253–258.
33. Andreassen OA, Ferrante RJ, Dedeoglu A, Albers DW, Klivenyi P, et al. (2001) Mice with a partial deficiency of manganese superoxide dismutase show increased vulnerability to the mitochondrial toxins malonate, 3-nitropropionic acid, and MPTP. Exp Neurol 167: 189–195.
34. Rabinovic AD, Hastings TG (1998) Role of endogenous glutathione in the oxidation of dopamine. J Neurochem 71: 2071–2078.
35. Jha N, Jurma O, Lalli G, Liu Y, Pettus EH, et al. (2000) Glutathione depletion in PC12 results in selective inhibition of mitochondrial complex I activity. Implications for Parkinson's disease. J Biol Chem 275: 26096–26101.
36. Yu YP, Ju WP, Li ZG, Wang DZ, Wang YC, et al. (2010) Acupuncture inhibits oxidative stress and rotational behavior in 6-hydroxydopamine lesioned rat. Brain Res 1336: 58–65.
37. Betarbet R, Sherer TB, Greenamyre JT (2002) Animal models of Parkinson's disease. Bioessays 24: 308–318.
38. Dauer W, Przedborski S (2003) Parkinson's disease: mechanisms and models. Neuron 39: 889–909.
39. Hirsch EC, Hoglinger G, Rousselet E, Breidert T, Parain K, et al. (2003) Animal models of Parkinson's disease in rodents induced by toxins: an update. J Neural Transm Suppl. pp 89–100.
40. Schmidt N, Ferger B (2001) Neurochemical findings in the MPTP model of Parkinson's disease. J Neural Transm 108: 1263–1282.
41. Orth M, Tabrizi SJ (2003) Models of Parkinson's disease. Mov Disord 18: 729–737.
42. Ara J, Przedborski S, Naini AB, Jackson-Lewis V, Trifiletti RR, et al. (1998) Inactivation of tyrosine hydroxylase by nitration following exposure to peroxynitrite and 1-methyl-4-phenyl-1,2,3,6-tetrahydropyridine (MPTP). Proc Natl Acad Sci U S A 95: 7659–7663.
43. Mandir AS, Przedborski S, Jackson-Lewis V, Wang ZQ, Simbulan-Rosenthal CM, et al. (1999) Poly(ADP-ribose) polymerase activation mediates 1-methyl-4-phenyl-1, 2,3,6-tetrahydropyridine (MPTP)-induced parkinsonism. Proc Natl Acad Sci U S A 96: 5774–5779.
44. Herkenham M, Little MD, Bankiewicz K, Yang SC, Markey SP, et al. (1991) Selective retention of MPP+ within the monoaminergic systems of the primate brain following MPTP administration: an vivo autoradiographic study. Neuroscience 40: 133–158.

45. Bradbury AJ, Costall B, Jenner PG, Kelly ME, Marsden CD, et al. (1986) MPP+ can disrupt the nigrostriatal dopamine system by acting in the terminal area. Neuropharmacology 25: 939–941.
46. Nirenberg MJ, Vaughan RA, Uhl GR, Kuhar MJ, Pickel VM (1996) The dopamine transporter is localized to dendritic and axonal plasma membranes of nigrostriatal dopaminergic neurons. J Neurosci 16: 436–447.
47. Kim ST, Moon W, Chae Y, Kim YJ, Lee H, et al. (2010) The effect of electroaucpuncture for 1-methyl-4-phenyl-1,2,3,6-tetrahydropyridine-induced proteomic changes in the mouse striatum. J Physiol Sci 60: 27–34.
48. Jia J, Sun Z, Li B, Pan Y, Wang H, et al. (2009) Electro-acupuncture stimulation improves motor disorders in Parkinsonian rats. Behav Brain Res 205: 214–218.
49. Jia J, Li B, Sun ZL, Yu F, Wang X, et al. (2010) Electro-acupuncture stimulation acts on the basal ganglia output pathway to ameliorate motor impairment in Parkinsonian model rats. Behav Neurosci 124: 305–310.
50. Liang XB, Luo Y, Liu XY, Lu J, Li FQ, et al. (2003) Electro-acupuncture improves behavior and upregulates GDNF mRNA in MFB transected rats. Neuroreport 14: 1177–1181.
51. Drechsel DA, Patel M (2008) Role of reactive oxygen species in the neurotoxicity of environmental agents implicated in Parkinson's disease. Free Radic Biol Med 44: 1873–1886.
52. Liu XY, Zhou HF, Pan YL, Liang XB, Niu DB, et al. (2004) Electro-acupuncture stimulation protects dopaminergic neurons from inflammation-mediated damage in medial forebrain bundle-transected rats. Exp Neurol 189: 189–196.
53. Shulman LM, Wen X, Weiner WJ, Bateman D, Minagar A, et al. (2002) Acupuncture therapy for the symptoms of Parkinson's disease. Mov Disord 17: 799–802.

11

Exploring the Patterns of Acupuncture on Mild Cognitive Impairment Patients Using Regional Homogeneity

Zhenyu Liu[1], Wenjuan Wei[1], Lijun Bai[1]*, Ruwei Dai[1], Youbo You[1], Shangjie Chen[2], Jie Tian[1,3]*

1 Key Laboratory of Molecular Imaging and Functional Imaging, Institute of Automation, Chinese Academy of Sciences, Beijing, China, **2** Department of Acupuncture and Massage, Bao'an Hospital, Southern Medical University, Shenzhen, China, **3** Life Sciences Research Center, School of Life Sciences and Technology, Xidian University, Xi'an, Shaanxi, China

Abstract

Purpose: To investigate the different responses to acupuncture in MCI patients and age-matched healthy subjects reflected by the Regional Homogeneity (ReHo) indices.

Methods: The experiment was performed at the acupoint KI3 in 12 MCI patients and 12 healthy controls, respectively. A novel non-repeated event-related (NRER) fMRI design paradigm was applied to separately detect neural activities related to different stages of acupuncture (pre-acupuncture resting state, needling manipulation and post-acupuncture resting state). ReHo values were calculated for MCI patients and healthy controls in pre- and post-acupuncture resting state. Then, a two-way ANCOVA with repeated measures with post-hoc two sample t-tests was performed to explore the different responses to acupuncture in the two groups.

Results: The ANCOVA revealed a significant main effect of group, but no significant main effect of acupuncture and interactions between group and acupuncture. During the pre-acupuncture resting state, ReHo values increased in the precentral gyrus (PCG), superior frontal gyrus (SFG), and insula (INS) and decreased mainly in middle temporal gyrus (MTG), parahippocampal (PHIP) and cingulate cortex in MCI patients compared with healthy controls. Furthermore, we found that the regions including precuneus (PCUN), and cingulate cortex showed increased ReHo values for MCI patients following acupuncture. For healthy controls, the medial frontal gyrus, PCG, anterior cingulate cortex (ACC) and INS showed enhanced ReHo values following acupuncture. During the post-acupuncture resting state, MCI patients showed increased ReHo values mainly in the MTG, superior parietal lobule (SPL), middle frontal gyrus (MFG), supramarginal (SMG), and PCG, and decreased ReHo values mainly in the frontal regions, PHIP, and posterior cingulated cortex (PCC) compared to healthy controls.

Conclusion: Though we found some ReHo changes between MCI patients and healthy controls, the two-way ANCOVA results showed no significant effects after multiple corrections. Further study is needed to reveal the real acupuncture effects on MCI patients.

Editor: Hengyi Rao, University of Pennsylvania, United States of America

Funding: This paper is supported by the National Basic Research Program of China (973 Program) under grant 2011CB707700 (http://www.973.gov.cn/Default_3.aspx), the National Natural Science Foundation of China under grant no. 81227901, 61231004, 30970771, 81000640, 81171314, 30970769, 81071217 (http://www.nsfc.gov.cn/Portal0/default152.htm), the Fundamental Research Funds for the Central Universities (2011JBM226) and NIH (R01HD046526 & R01HD060595), the Beijing Nova program (grant number Z111101054511116), and Beijing Natural Science Foundation (grant number 4122082), the Fellowship for Young International Scientists of the Chinese Academy of Sciences under grant no. 2010Y2GA03, the Chinese Academy of Sciences Visiting Professorship for Senior International Scientists under grant no. 2012T1G0036, 2010T2G36, 2012T1G0039. The funders had no role in study design, data collection and analysis, decision to publish, or preparation of the manuscript.

Competing Interests: The authors have declared that no competing interests exist.

* Email: tian@ieee.org (JT); bailj4152615@gmail.com (LB)

Introduction

Alzheimer's disease (AD), the most common form of dementia, is characterized by significant impairments in multiple cognitive domains including memory, attention, reasoning, language and executive-functions. There is currently little effective disease-modifying treatment, and many potential treatments being tested may have significant side-effects. Given that pathological changes begin well before the appearance of clinical symptoms [1], earlier interventions could improve disease prognosis. As an intermediate state between normal aging and dementia, the most prominent feature of mild cognitive impairment (MCI) is an isolated mild

decline in memory, whereas other cognitive functions remain intact [2]. MCI patients would turn into AD at a high rate of approximately 10% to 15% per year [3]. MCI has become a hot topic of dementia researchers in recent years. The increased risk for the elderly that suffer from MCI to progress to AD makes it an appropriate condition for investigation.

The use of acupuncture as a complementary therapeutic method for treating a variety of neurologic diseases, including MCI, AD and dementia, is popular in certain parts of the world [4]. Previous study suggested that acupuncture had significant therapeutic effects and well tolerated in ameliorate the key clinical symptoms of vascular dementia [5]. Luijpen et al. [6] explored the effects of transcutaneous electrical nerve stimulation on self-efficacy and mood in MCI patients by measuring four outcomes including a Dutch translation of the General Self-Efficacy Scale (Algemene Competentie Schaal), the Groninger Activity Restriction Scale, the Philadelphia Geriatric Center Morale Scale, and the Geriatric Depression Scale. The results indicated that the transcutaneous electrical nerve stimulation could improve the outcomes compared with placebo. In spite of its public acceptance, the neural mechanism underlying is still elusive. In the past decades, noninvasive fMRI technique has provided new insights into the central physiological function involving acupuncture. Neuroimaging studies of acupuncture have indicated that primary acupuncture effects are mediated by the central nervous system [7–20]. Previous neuroimaging studies [7–11] on acupuncture at commonly used acupoints have demonstrated significant modulatory effects involving widespread cerebrocerebellar brain regions including the limbic, hippocampus, somatosensory cortices, hypothalamic, insula and brainstem neural nuclei. However, the majority of these studies were performed on healthy subjects. It is generally agreed that acupuncture plays a homeostatic role and thus may have a greater effect on patients with a pathological imbalance, compared with healthy controls [21,22]. Therefore, exploring the effects of acupuncture on the central nervous system in patients may further help to elucidate its mechanism. One previous study adopts fMRI to explore the acupuncture effects in 26 AD patients [23]. The results showed that acupuncture could activate the temporal lobe (such as the hippocampus, and insula), some regions of the parietal lobe and cerebellum in AD patients. The regions activated by acupuncture are consistent with impaired brain areas in AD patients. Meanwhile, these regions are also closely correlated with the cognitive function (memory, reasoning, language, executive, and etc.). This study provides preliminary neurophysiological evidence for the potential efficacy effect of acupuncture on AD. Another recent study [24] investigating the acupuncture effects on the functional connectivity in MCI patients using deep and superficial acupuncture found significantly increased correlations related with the temporal regions following deep acupuncture. However, few fMRI studies focused on the modulatory effects of acupuncture on brain regions in MCI patients. Hence, imaging the regions mainly affected in MCI patients may help to unravel the mechanisms how acupuncture achieves its therapeutic effects.

According to the theory of the Traditional Chinese Medicine, acupuncture can induce long-lasting effects even after the needling manipulation being terminated [25]. Recently, several studies demonstrated the existence of various function-guided brain networks even after the needling manipulation, which underlay the prolonged effects of acupuncture [12,15,16], and the block

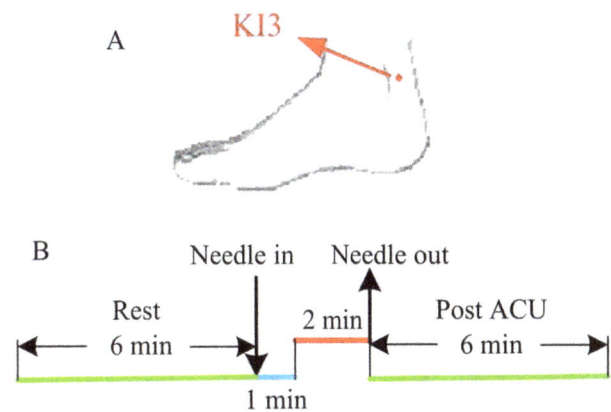

Figure 1. Experimental paradigm. A: The location of the acupoint used in the experiment. B: The paradigm of the experiment: the resting state run lasted for 6 minutes; acupuncture run totally lasted for 9.0 minutes.

design may be not fit for the acupuncture study. Therefore, the sustained effects of acupuncture should be taken into account for which the actual effects of acupuncture can be appropriately studied. In the present study, we adopted the newly non-repeated event-related (NRER) fMRI design [13]. This new design could be used to explore the sustained effect of acupuncture (the modulatory patterns during the resting state following acupuncture). In the present study, we used the NRER design to investigate whether the effects of acupuncture on ReHo are different for MCI patients and healthy controls during the resting state following acupuncture.

Regional Homogeneity (ReHo) [26], evaluating the similarity between the time series of a given voxel and its nearest neighbors by calculating Kendall's coefficient of concordance (KCC) [27], can effectively evaluate the resting-state brain activity. On the other hand, ReHo is a reliable method with its test-retest reliability established recently by Zuo et al [28]. Therefore, ReHo can rapidly map the level of regional activity of every voxel across the whole brain of individuals [29]. A previous study [30] found that in amnestic MCI patients, the ReHo indices were decreased in regions that included the PCC, the right anterior cingulate cortex (ACC), the right inferior frontal regions, the right STG and the bilateral cuneus, and were increased in the right IPL, the right fusiform gyrus and the bilateral putamen. In a recent study [31], differences in the ReHo indices between MCI and healthy controls were mainly found in the medial prefrontal cortex (mPFC), bilateral PCC and left IPL. By calculating ReHo indices, we may

Table 1. Subject characteristics.

	Patients	Controls
N	12	12
Age (mean ± SD)	59.3±3.3	60.6±5.8
Sex(M/F)	1/11	4/8
Education (year)	10.5±1.81	10.6±2.06
MMSE score * (mean ± SD)	26.4±0.9	29.8±0.4
CDR	0.5	0

MMSE: Mini-Mental State Examination, CDR: Clinical Dementia Rating.
* $p<0.0001$ (two sample two tailed t test).

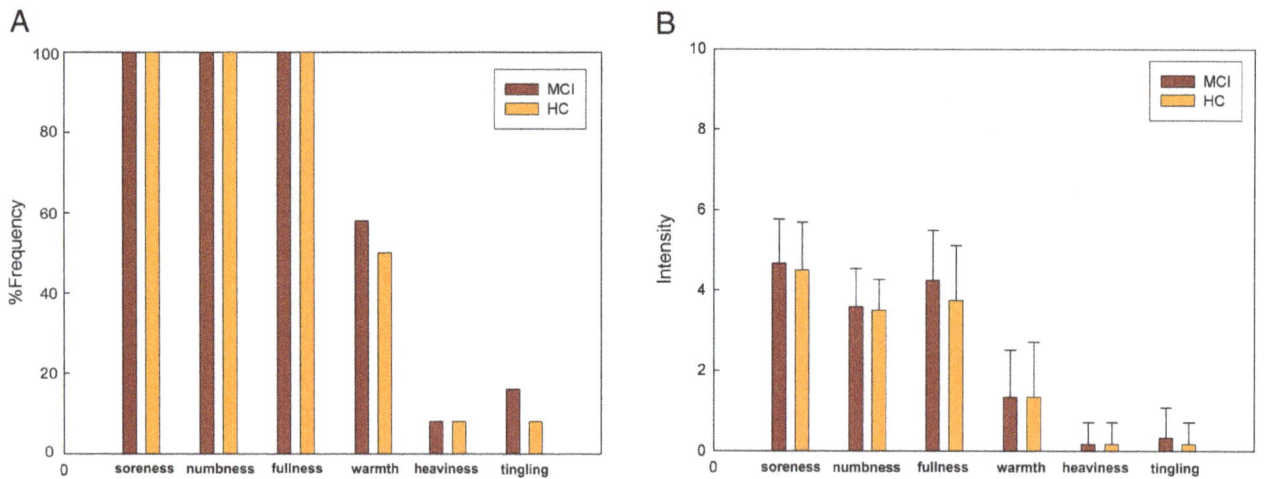

Figure 2. Averaged psychophysical response (N = 12) in MCI and HC groups. A: The percentage of subjects who reported having experienced the given sensation (at least one subject experienced the six sensations listed). B: The intensity of reported sensations measured by an average score (with standard error bars) on a scale from 0 denoting no sensation to 10 denoting an unbearable sensation.

evaluate the different responses to acupuncture in MCI patients during the following acupuncture resting state. Studying ReHo indices provides us a new way to exploring the mechanisms of acupuncture and will be helpful for a better understanding of acupuncture effects on MCI.

In the present study, we sought to investigate the different responses of MCI patients and healthy controls to acupuncture at the same acupoint reflected by the ReHo indices. The fMRI experiment was performed at an acupoint KI3. We first performed a two-way ANCOVA with repeated measures (two factors: group, acupuncture; repeated factor: acupuncture; covariates: gender, head motion) to test the main effect of group and acupuncture, and the interaction of the two factors. Then we identified regions

showing abnormal ReHo indices in MCI group compared with the HC during the resting state. Subsequently, we tested the effects of acupuncture on MCI patients and healthy controls, respectively. Finally, we made the comparison between MCI patients and healthy controls to test whether there were any specific modulatory patterns during post-acupuncture resting state. We hypothesized that the specific effects of acupuncture on MCI patients may be reflected by the ReHo indices.

Materials and Methods

All research procedures were approved by the Bao'an People's Hospital Subcommittee on human studies and conducted in accordance with the Declaration of Helsinki.

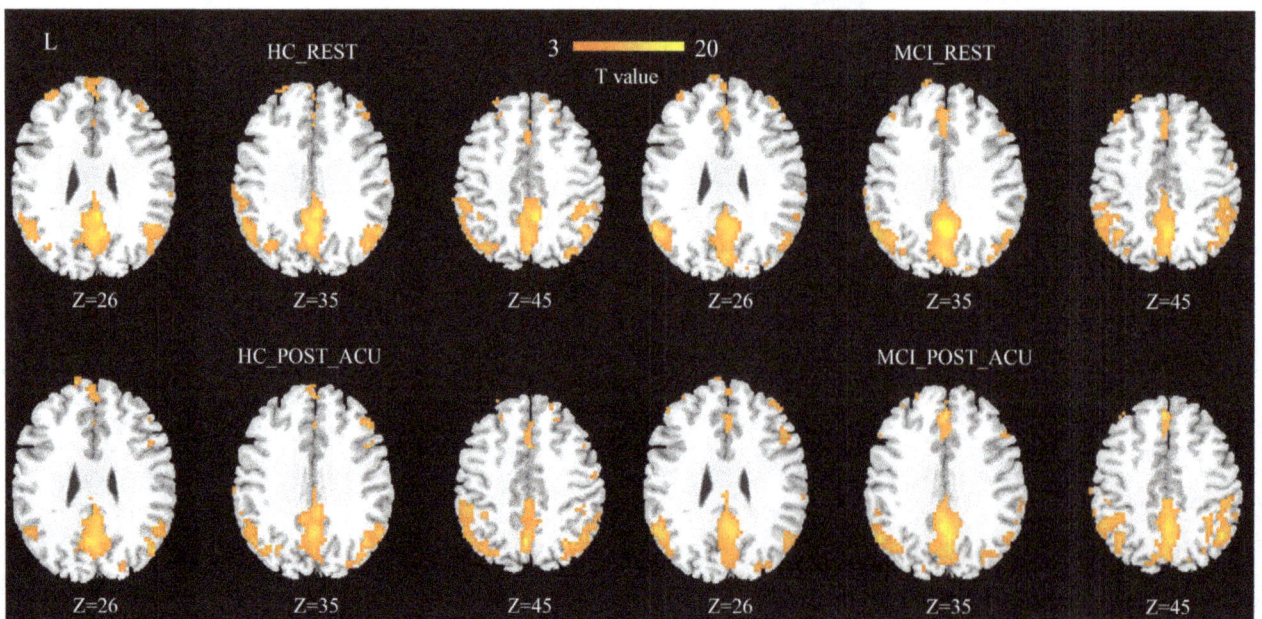

Figure 3. Results of regional homogeneity (ReHo) shown as a Kendall's coefficient of concordance (KCC) map across all subjects for MCI patients and healthy controls during resting state and post-acupuncture resting state (p<0.05, FDR correction).

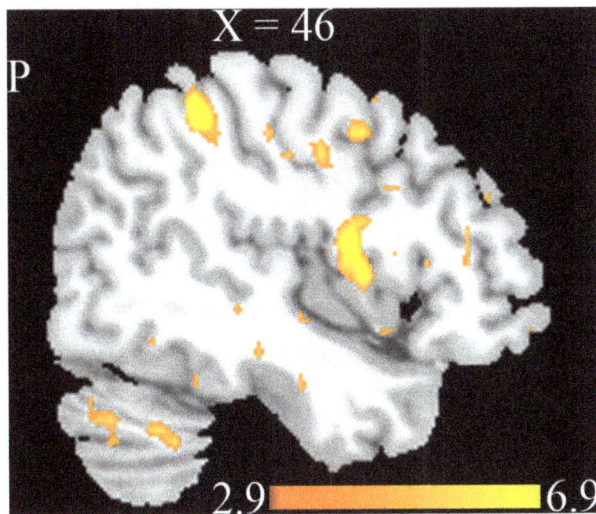

Figure 4. Brain areas showed significant main effect of group at p<0.001 (uncorrected, cluster size >30 voxels) with increased ReHo values in MCI patients compared with normal controls. Warm colors indicate the significantly increased ReHo values.

Experimental Paradigm

In this study, we adopted a new experimental paradigm, namely the NRER fMRI design to investigate the prolonged effects after acupuncture administration [13]. For each group, the experiment consisted of two functional runs. For a baseline control, a resting state (REST) scan was conducted for 6 minutes without any stimulation (Fig. 1A). We then employed the new experimental paradigm, in which acupuncture was conducted and only one stimulation period was given (Fig. 1B). For acupuncture run, an acupuncture needle was inserted from the beginning, and after resting for 1 min, the needle was manipulated for 2 minutes; then, another resting state scan was conducted for 6 minutes without any stimulation. All participants were asked to keep their eyes closed and remain relaxed without engaging in any mental tasks. According to participants' reports after the scanning, they affirmed keeping awake during the whole process. At the end of acupuncture scan, the subjects adopted a 10-point scale to self-rate the intensities about the deqi sensations they had felt during the stimulation (0 = no sensation, 1–3 = mild, 4–6 = moderate, 7–8 = strong, 9 = severe and 10 = unbearable sensation) [39].

Acupuncture was performed at an acupoint KI3 (Taixi, located in a depression between medial malleolus and heel tendon) on the right leg. This is one of the most frequently used acupoints and proved to have various efficacies in the treatments of dementia [23]. Acupuncture stimulation was delivered using a sterile disposable 38 gauge stainless steel acupuncture needle, 0.2 mm in diameter and 40 mm in length. The needle was inserted vertically to a depth of 1–2 cm, and administration was delivered by a balanced "tonifying and reducing" technique [7]. Stimulation consisted of rotating the needle clockwise and counterclockwise for 1 min at a rate of 60 times per min. The procedure was performed by the same experienced and licensed acupuncturist on all participants.

Subjects

12 MCI patients and 12 age-matched healthy control subjects were included in this study (see Table 1 for subjects' characteristics). MCI patients were recruited at the rehabilitation department of the Bao'an People's Hospital of Shenzhen. MCI patients were diagnosed using criteria for amnestic MCI [32], with Mini-Mental State Examination (MMSE) scores between 25 and 27 [33], and Clinical Dementia Rating (CDR) scale scores of 0.5 [34]. Healthy control subjects were recruited from a community. All subjects were right-handed according to the Edinburgh Handedness Inventory [35]. In addition, all subjects were acupuncture naive as several previous studies [17,36,37] did, because previous experience of acupuncture is believed to affect people's expectation of future treatments. Using non-naïve subjects may account for placebo effects in acupuncture study [38]. Subjects were excluded if they had any significant medical, neurological, or psychiatric illness, or if they were taking medication or other substances known to influence cerebral function. After given a complete description of the study, all subjects signed the informed consent form. All protocols were approved by the Bao'an People's Hospital Subcommittee on human studies.

Data Acquisition and Preprocessing

Magnetic resonance imaging data were acquired using a 3.0 Tesla Signa (GE) MR scanner. Head movements were prevented by a custom-built head holder. The images were parallel to the AC-PC line and covered the whole brain. Thirty axial slices were obtained using a T2*-weighted single-shot, gradient-recalled echo planar imaging sequence (FOV = 220 mm×220 mm, matrix = 64×64, thickness = 4 mm, TR = 2000 ms, TE = 30 ms, flip angle = 77°). After the functional run, high-resolution structural information on each subject was also acquired using 3D MRI sequences with a voxel size of 1 mm3 for anatomical localization (TR = 2.1 s, TE = 4.6 ms, matrix = 256×256, FOV = 230 mm× 230 mm, flip angle = 8°, slice thickness = 1 mm).

For REST run, the data were preprocessed by removing the first 5 time points to eliminate nonequilibrium effects of

Table 2. Brain areas with significant main effect of group at $P<0.001$ (uncorrected, 30 voxels).

Brain regions	BA	Hemisphere	MNI			Maximal Z-score	Volume (voxels)
			x	y	z		
Precentral Gyrus	6	L	−39	−12	66	6.44	32
Superior Parietal Lobule	7	L	−24	−63	57	5.98	73
Insula	13	L	−30	−24	21	5.92	36
Superior Temporal Gyrus	39	R	39	−51	27	5.58	111
Inferior Temporal Gyrus	20	L	−51	0	−36	5.52	72

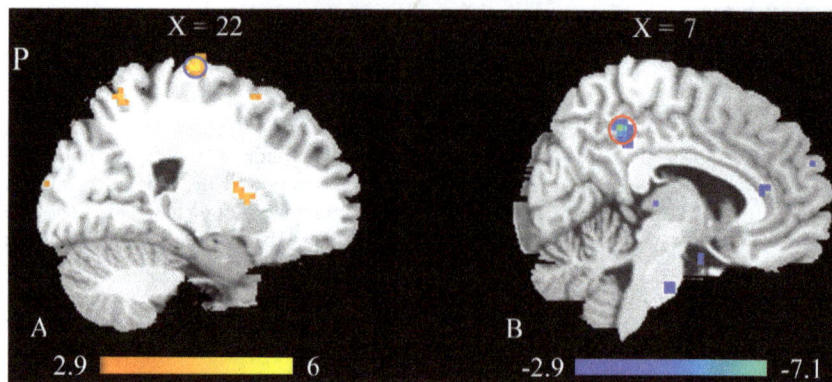

Figure 5. Brain areas with significant different ReHo values between MCI and HC groups during the resting state are shown. Warm and cool colors indicate the significantly increased and decreased ReHo values in MCI patients compared with healthy controls at P<0.01 (Alphasim corrected, p<0.01, 30 voxels). (Abbreviation: PCG- Precentral Gyrus).

magnetization. For acupuncture run, only the datasets after manipulation were selected (labeled by green-color in Fig. 1, total of 180 time points, the same time points as in REST run), and the first 5 time points were discarded in order to obtain a stable resting state. The remaining time points were used for following analysis. All of data preprocessing procedures were performed in Statistical Parametric Mapping 5 (SPM5) (http://www.fil.ion.ucl.ac.uk/ spm). All the remaining volumes were firstly realigned to correct for head motions using the least-squares minimization. The images were corrected for the acquisition delay between slices, aligned to the first image of each session for motion correction, and spatially normalized to standard MNI template in SPM5 [40]. No subjects had head motions exceeding 1 mm movement or 1° rotation in any direction. Finally, A band-pass filter (0.01 Hz<f<0.08 Hz) was applied to remove physiological and high frequency noise [41].

Data Processing and Statistical Analysis

Kendall's coefficient concordance (KCC) [27] was used to evaluate regional homogeneity [26], which was performed using the Resting-State fMRI Data Analysis Toolkit (REST, by SONG Xiao-Wei et al. [42], http://www.restfmri.net). Individual ReHo maps were generated by assigning each voxel a value corresponding to the KCC of its time series with its nearest 26 neighboring

voxels [26]. A whole brain mask was used to remove non-brain tissues. Only the voxels within the mask were further analyzed. The individual ReHo maps were standardized by their own mean KCC within the mask [43,44]. In this step, KCC value of each voxel was divided by the mean KCC within the mask in each individual ReHo map. To test if there were any changes of global mean ReHo across groups as well as acupuncture, we performed a two way ANCOVA with repeated measures (two factors: group, acupuncture; repeated factor: acupuncture; covariates: gender, head motion). Then, a Gaussian kernel of 4 mm full width at half-maximum (FWHM) [45–47] was used to smooth the images for the aim to reduce noise and residual differences.

Statistical analysis was using SPM5 (http://www.fil.ion.ucl.ac. uk/spm). A one-sample t test (p<0.05, false discovery rate (FDR) correction) was performed to extract the ReHo results across the subjects within each group for both conditions. We first performed a two-way ANCOVA with repeated measures in the present study to test the main effect of group and acupuncture, and the interaction of the two factors. Then we performed two-sample t-test to test the differences between HC and MCI patients in both rest condition and post acupuncture resting state. We also compared the ReHo results between post-acupuncture and rest by performing paired t-test in each group.

Table 3. Brain areas with significant different ReHo values between MCI patients and healthy controls during the resting state at P<0.01 (Alphasim corrected, p<0.01, 30 voxels).

Brain regions	BA	Hemisphere	MNI			Maximal Z-score	Volume (voxels)
			x	y	z		
Precentral Gyrus	6	L	−21	−24	72	5.44	86
Superior Frontal Gyrus	6	−	0	2	51	4.28	30
Cuneus	18	−	0	−99	0	4.66	35
Insula	13	R	33	9	15	3.74	31
Cingulate Gyrus	31	L	−6	−48	42	−7.11	62
ParaHippocampal	20	R	33	−15	−39	−4.71	37
	37	L	−30	−45	−15	−5.27	39
Middle Temporal Gyrus	21	L	−51	0	−33	−4.82	66

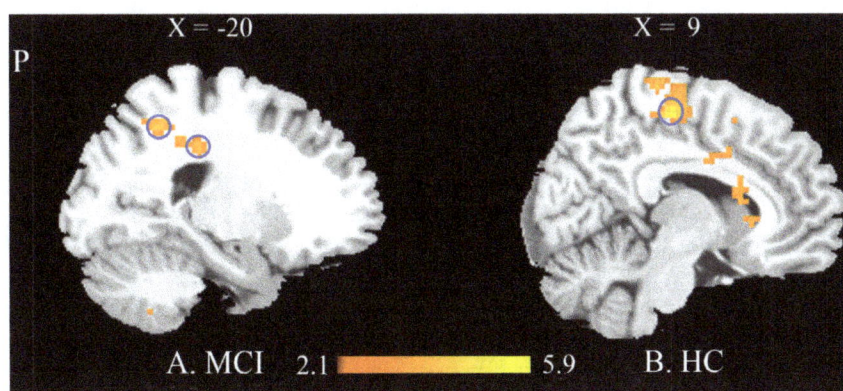

Figure 6. Brain areas with significant different ReHo values following acupuncture compared with the resting state in MCI (A) and HC (B) groups. Warm colors indicate the significantly increased ReHo values in the two groups following acupuncture at $P<0.01$ (Alphasim corrected, $p<0.01$, 30 voxels). (Abbreviation: MFG- Medial Frontal Gyrus).

Results

Psychophysical Response

The prevalence of subjective "deqi" sensations was expressed as the percentage of individuals in the group that reported the given sensations (Fig. 2A). For both conditions, no statistically significant changes were found with regard to the prevalence of the listed sensations between MCI and HC (paired t-test, $P>0.05$). However, differences did exist with respect to the type of sensations. Warmth (MCI: 58%, HC: 50%), tingling (MCI: 16%, HC: 8%) were found greater in MCI group. The intensity of sensations was expressed as the average score $\pm$ SE (Fig. 2B). The averaged intensities were approximately similar in MCI and HC groups (paired t-test, $P>0.05$). Considering a little difference in psychophysical response between MCI and HC, the neuroimaging findings were likely not the results of differences induced by the sensations.

ReHo Results of each Condition in the Two Groups

ReHo results across all subjects of the two groups during the two conditions are shown in Figure 3 ($p<0.05$, FDR correction). The major regions of DMN exhibited significant higher ReHo values than other brain regions during the resting state (Fig. 3 A, B), i.e. the MTL, PCC, mPFC, and IPL.

Results of Two-way ANCOVA

We found no changes of global mean ReHo values across groups as well as acupuncture using the two way ANCOVA with repeated measures ($P<0.05$).

We performed a two-way ANCOVA with repeated measures to test the main effect of group and acupuncture, and the interaction of the two factors. The analysis revealed a significant main effect of

group at $p<0.001$ (uncorrected, 30 voxels) with the regions including the PCG, SPL, INS, STG, and Inferior Temporal Gyrus (ITG) showing increased ReHo values in MCI patients (Fig. 4 and Table 2). The results suggested that the brain spontaneous activity differs between MCI patients and healthy controls during resting state and post acupuncture resting state. We found no significant main effect of acupuncture and interaction of the two factors at $p<0.001$ (uncorrected, 30 voxels) from the two-way ANCOVA. Then, we performed post hoc two sample t-tests to characterize the statistical differences between MCI patients and healthy controls before and after acupuncture respectively.

Comparisons for MCI vs. HC in REST

We first made a comparison between MCI patients and healthy controls to find the regions showing abnormal ReHo values in MCI patients compared with healthy controls during the resting state (Fig. 5 and Table 3). The results of two sample t test revealed that MCI patients showed significantly increased ReHo values at $P<0.01$ (Alphasim corrected, $p<0.01$, 30 voxels) in the regions including the PCG, SFG, cuneus and INS. Meanwhile, MCI patients showed significantly decreased ReHo values at $P<0.01$ (Alphasim corrected, $p<0.01$, 30 voxels) mainly in the MTG, PHIP and cingulate cortex.

Comparisons for Acupuncture Effects in each Group

Then, we performed comparisons in both MCI and HC groups between post acupuncture condition and the resting state to explore the effects of acupuncture on MCI patients and healthy controls, respectively (Fig. 6 and Table 4, 5). For MCI patients, precuneus, and cingulate cortex showed significantly increased ReHo values at $P<0.01$ (Alphasim corrected, $p<0.01$, 30 voxels).

Table 4. Brain areas with significant different ReHo values in the MCI patients after acupuncture at $P<0.01$ (Alphasim corrected, $p<0.01$, 30 voxels).

Brain regions	BA	Hemisphere	MNI			Maximal Z-score	Volume (voxels)
			x	y	z		
Cingulate Gyrus	31	R	21	−33	36	3.31	42
Precuneus	7	R	21	−57	45	3.84	36

Table 5. Brain areas with significant different ReHo values in the healthy controls after acupuncture at $P<0.01$ (Alphasim corrected, $p<0.01$, 30 voxels).

Brain regions	BA	Hemisphere	MNI			Maximal Z-score	Volume (voxels)
			x	y	z		
Medial Frontal Gyrus	6	L	−6	−24	54	5.85	114
	32	R	12	12	48	3.23	40
Precentral Gyrus	6	R	54	−9	54	3.08	49
Anterior Cingulate Cortex	25	L	−3	18	0	3.97	35
Insula	13	R	34	−15	16	3.48	33

While for HC group, significantly increased ReHo values were mainly found in the regions including MFG, PCG, ACC, and INS at $P<0.01$ (Alphasim corrected, $p<0.01$, 30 voxels). No brain regions with significantly decreased ReHo values were found in both groups at $P<0.01$ (Alphasim corrected, $p<0.01$, 30 voxels).

Comparisons for MCI vs. HC for Acupuncture Condition

Finally, we made a comparison between MCI group and HC group to investigate the different effects of acupuncture on MCI patients and healthy controls (Fig. 7 and Table 6). The results of two sample t test demonstrated that the regions including MTG, SPL, MFG, SMG, cuneus and PCG showed significantly increased ReHo values in MCI patients compared with healthy controls at $P<0.01$ (Alphasim corrected, $p<0.01$, 30 voxels). Meanwhile, significantly decreased ReHo values in MCI patients were found in the regions including the frontal regions (IFG, MFG, and SFG), fusiform gyrus, PHIP, ITG and PCC at $P<0.01$ (Alphasim corrected, $p<0.01$, 30 voxels).

Discussion

In the present study, we explored the effects of acupuncture on post-stimulus resting brain of MCI patients by evaluating the ReHo indices. Most resting state fMRI studies adopted functional connectivity to investigate temporal relations between intrinsic fluctuations observed in spatially distinct brain regions. However, functional connectivity provides little local features of spontaneous brain activity observed in specific regions. As a complement of the functional connectivity method, ReHo has been proved to be sufficient to detect regional homogeneity abnormality in the brain during the resting state [44,46,47,48]. ReHo hypothesizes that voxels within a specific functional brain region are more temporally homogeneous when subjects are engaged in a specific condition [26]. Previous studies reported that MCI would result in the abnormal ReHo values in related regions and suggested that this method may be an important factor to improve the understanding of the disease [30,31]. Therefore, changes of ReHo indices during the post-acupuncture resting state may underlie the mechanisms how acupuncture treats MCI. However, few studies investigated the modulatory of acupuncture on MCI patients using ReHo indices. Another advantage of the present study is the use of NRER design. Previous acupuncture studies generally adopted the multi-block design paradigm, which implicitly presumes the temporal intensity profiles of the certain event conforming to the "on - off" specifications [7,8,11]. Due to the sustained effects of acupuncture, the temporal aspects of the blood oxygen level dependent response to acupuncture may violate the assumptions of the block designed estimates [17]. In the present study, we adopted the new experimental paradigm named NRER fMRI design, which has been proved to be more applicable to the acupuncture research proved in several previous studies [13,18,19].

During the resting state, we found the ReHo values significantly increased in the PCG, SFG, cuneus and INS in MCI patients compared with healthy controls. Meanwhile, we found decreased ReHo values mainly in the MTG, PHIP and cingulate cortex in MCI patient compared with healthy controls. These regions are

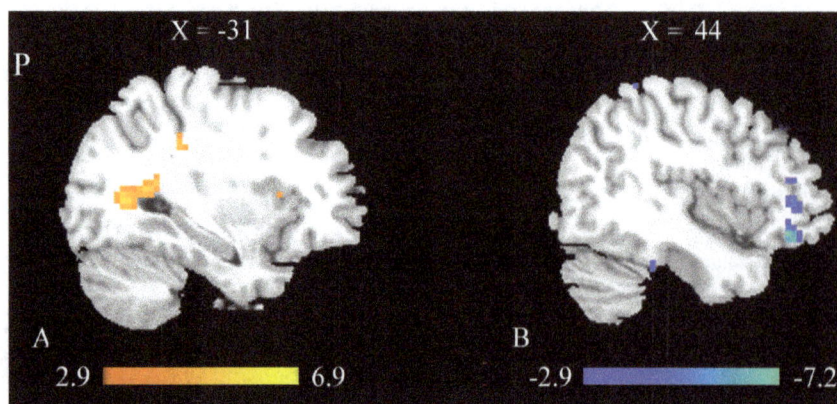

Figure 7. Brain areas with significant different ReHo values between MCI and HC groups during the resting state following acupuncture. Warm and cool colors respectively indicate the significantly increased (A) and decreased (B) ReHo values in MCI patients compared with healthy controls at $P<0.01$ (Alphasim corrected, $p<0.01$, 30 voxels). (Abbreviation: MTG- Middle Temporal Gyrus, MFG- Middle Frontal Gyrus).

Table 6. Brain areas with significant different ReHo values between healthy controls and MCI patients after acupuncture at $P<0.01$ (Alphasim corrected, $p<0.01$, 30 voxels).

Brain regions	BA	Hemisphere	MNI			Maximal Z-score	Volume (voxels)
			x	y	z		
Middle Temporal Gyrus	39	R	39	−54	6	5.11	95
Superior Parietal Lobule	7	L	−27	−63	57	5.27	32
Supramarginal Gyrus	40	L	−39	−51	30	3.85	40
Middle Frontal Gyrus	46	R	45	39	21	4.71	44
Precentral Gyrus	4	L	−24	−24	75	4.61	36
Cuneus	18	–	0	−99	0	4.54	35
Posterior Cingulate Cortex	30	L	−3	−60	−6	−6.68	68
Middle Frontal Gyrus	47	L	−42	36	0	−4.43	31
Superior Frontal Gyrus	9	R	6	54	30	−3.84	32
Fusiform Gyrus	36	L	−39	−39	−30	−4.05	36
Parahippocampal Gyrus	35	L	−24	−15	−30	−4.76	35
Inferior Temporal Gyrus	21	L	−57	−20	−24	−5.11	49
Inferior Frontal Gyrus	47	L	−39	33	−15	−7.21	47

implicated in memory encoding and retrieving. The result is compatible with previous studies that indicated the dysfunctional regions in MCI patients [49–51].

We evaluated the differences between the ReHo indices of the post acupuncture resting state and the ReHo indices of the resting state in both MCI and HC groups to explore the responses of the central nervous system to acupuncture. Though we detected no significant main effect of acupuncture from the two-way ANCOVA, we found changes in ReHo values after acupuncture in MCI patients and healthy controls. We supposed that the small sample size of subjects and no measure of cognitive outcomes may be the reason why we detected no significant main effect of acupuncture. With a large sample size and cognitive outcomes as covariates in ANCOVA, we may detect more precise results of acupuncture effects. In MCI patients, we found that the regions including precuneus, and cingulate cortex showed increased ReHo values during the post acupuncture resting state. The results suggested that acupuncture may enhance the regional connectivity of the abnormal brain regions in MCI patients. Instead of the regions related to cognitive functions, healthy controls showed increased ReHo values in the regions including the MFG, PCG, ACC, and INS during the post stimulus resting state. These different responses to acupuncture between MCI patients and health controls may be related to the different patterns of acupuncture on the two groups.

In order to find out the different effects of acupuncture between MCI patients and healthy controls, we performed a comparison between MCI patients and healthy controls during the post acupuncture resting state. We found that ReHo values of MCI patients increased in the MTG, SPL, MFG, SMG, cuneus and PCG and decreased in the frontal regions (IFG, MFG and SFG), fusiform gyrus, PHIP, ITG and PCC. The results suggested that several regions of DMN showed different ReHo values between MCI patients and HC during the post acupuncture resting state. Different effective connectivity have been reported related with the DMN regions during the post acupuncture resting state in HC in the previous study about the acupuncture specificity [20]. Our results further indicated the effects of acupuncture on the DMN regions in MCI patients and HC. In addition, the results showed that acupuncture increased regional functional connectivity of the abnormal regions related to the disease in MCI patients, aiming to rehabilitate the function of the abnormal regions. In practice, the well-identified physical effects of acupuncture needling and its purported clinical efficacy also suggest that acupuncture acts in maintaining a homeostatic balance of the internal state [52]. We speculated that the different responses to acupuncture between MCI patients and healthy controls reflected the rebalance effects of acupuncture. The rebalance effects of acupuncture may be related to mechanisms of the effects of acupuncture on MCI patients.

There are still some limitations in the study. First, the experience of acupuncture may affect the acupuncture effects. In the present study, we just included acupuncture naïve subjects, the difference in its efficacy between acupuncture naive and experienced may be explored in the future. Second, no clinical outcomes were recorded in the present study. We did not take any cognitive measures in the study for the subjects only received one acupuncture trial. Cognitive measures should be taken in future longitude studies. Third, the sample size in this experiment is small. Although ReHo, the measure we selected in this study, is a widely used measure to characterize local functional homogeneity of resting state fMRI signals with its test-retest reliability established, we should perform further study with more subjects in the future.

Conclusions

In conclusion, we revealed some features of neural responses to acupuncture for MCI patients compared with healthy controls. Firstly, we found several brain regions showing different ReHo values between MCI patients and healthy controls. Furthermore, we found significant ReHo changes related with the previous reported abnormal regions in MCI patients during the post acupuncture resting state. Finally, we explored the different responses to acupuncture in MCI patients and healthy controls. We found some ReHo changes during the post acupuncture resting state between MCI patients and healthy controls. However, the two-way ANCOVA results showed that none of the effects are significant after multiple corrections. The reason why the results showed no statistically significant acupuncture effect may be the small sample size. The results suggested that the modulatory effects of acupuncture on MCI patients should be further investigated with more subjects in the future.

Author Contributions

Conceived and designed the experiments: JT RD. Performed the experiments: SC. Analyzed the data: ZL WW. Contributed reagents/materials/analysis tools: YY LB. Wrote the paper: ZL.

References

1. Ikonomovic MD, Mufson EJ, Wuu J, Cochran EJ, Bennett DA, et al. (2003) Cholinergic plasticity in hippocampus of individuals with mild cognitive impairment: correlation with Alzheimer's neuropathology. J Alzheimers Dis 5: 39–48.

2. Petersen RC, Smith GE, Waring SC, Ivnik RJ, Tangalos EG, et al. (1999) Mild cognitive impairment: clinical characterization and outcome. Arch Neurol 56: 303–308.

3. Grundman M, Petersen RC, Ferris SH, Thomas RG, Aisen PS, et al. (2004) Mild cognitive impairment can be distinguished from Alzheimer disease and normal aging for clinical trials. Archives of Neurology 61: 59–66.

4. NIH (1998) NIH consensus conference statement acupuncture. JAMA.

5. Yu J, Zhang X, Liu C, Meng Y, Han J (2006) Effect of acupuncture treatment on vascular dementia. Neurol Res 28: 97–103.

6. Luijpen MW, Swaab DF, Sergeant JA, Scherder EJ (2004) Effects of transcutaneous electrical nerve stimulation (TENS) on self-efficacy and mood in elderly with mild cognitive impairment. Neurorehabil Neural Repair 18: 166–175.

7. Hui KK, Liu J, Makris N, Gollub RL, Chen AJ, et al. (2000) Acupuncture modulates the limbic system and subcortical gray structures of the human brain: evidence from fMRI studies in normal subjects. Hum Brain Mapp 9: 13–25.

8. Yoo SS, Teh EK, Blinder RA, Jolesz FA (2004) Modulation of cerebellar activities by acupuncture stimulation: evidence from fMRI study. Neuroimage 22: 932–940.

9. Hui KKS, Liu J, Marina O, Napadow V, Haselgrove C, et al. (2005) The integrated response of the human cerebro-cerebellar and limbic systems to acupuncture stimulation at ST 36 as evidenced by fMRI. Neuroimage 27: 479–496.

10. Napadow V, Makris N, Liu J, Kettner NW, Kwong KK, et al. (2005) Effects of electroacupuncture versus manual acupuncture on the human brain as measured by fMRI. Human Brain Mapping 24: 193–205.

11. Fang J, Jin Z, Wang Y, Li K, Kong J, et al. (2009) The salient characteristics of the central effects of acupuncture needling: limbic-paralimbic-neocortical network modulation. Hum Brain Mapp 30: 1196–1206.

12. Dhond RP, Yeh C, Park K, Kettner N, Napadow V (2008) Acupuncture modulates resting state connectivity in default and sensorimotor brain networks. Pain 136: 407–418.

13. Qin W, Tian J, Bai L, Pan X, Yang L, et al. (2008) FMRI connectivity analysis of acupuncture effects on an amygdala-associated brain network. Mol Pain 4: 55.

14. Bai L, Qin W, Liang J, Tian J, Liu Y (2009) Spatiotemporal modulation of central neural pathway underlying acupuncture action: a systematic review. Curr Med Imaging Rev 5: 167–173.

15. Bai L, Qin W, Tian J, Dai J, Yang W (2009) Detection of dynamic brain networks modulated by acupuncture using a graph theory model. Progress in Natural Science 19: 827–835.

16. Bai L, Qin W, Tian J, Dong M, Pan X, et al. (2009) Acupuncture modulates spontaneous activities in the anticorrelated resting brain networks. Brain Res 1279: 37–49.

17. Bai L, Qin W, Tian J, Liu P, Li L, et al. (2009) Time-varied characteristics of acupuncture effects in fMRI studies. Hum Brain Mapp 30: 3445–3460.

18. Bai L, Yan H, Li LL, Qin W, Chen P, et al. (2010) Neural Specificity of Acupuncture Stimulation at Pericardium 6: Evidence From an FMRI Study. Journal of Magnetic Resonance Imaging 31: 71–77.

19. Bai L, Tian J, Zhong CG, Xue T, You YB, et al. (2010) Acupuncture modulates temporal neural responses in wide brain networks: evidence from fMRI study. Molecular Pain 6.

20. Zhong C, Bai L, Dai R, Xue T, Wang H, et al. (2012) Modulatory effects of acupuncture on resting-state networks: a functional MRI study combining independent component analysis and multivariate Granger causality analysis. Journal of Magnetic Resonance Imaging 35: 572–581.

21. Zhu L, editor (1954) New acupuncture (Xin Zhen-jiu Xue). Beijing: Beijing: People's Press.

22. Kaptchuk TJ (2002) Acupuncture: theory, efficacy, and practice. Ann Intern Med 136: 374–383.

23. Zhou Y, Jin J (2008) Effect of acupuncture given at the HT 7, ST 36, ST 40 and KI 3 acupoints on various parts of the brains of Alzheimer's disease patients. Acupunct Electrother Res 33: 9–17.

24. Feng Y, Bai L, Ren Y, Chen S, Wang H, et al. (2012) FMRI connectivity analysis of acupuncture effects on the whole brain network in mild cognitive impairment patients. Magn Reson Imaging 30: 672–682.

25. Beijing Shanghai and Nanjing College of Traditional Chinese Medicine (1980) Essentials of Chinese acupuncture. Beijing: Foreign Languages Press.

26. Zang Y, Jiang T, Lu Y, He Y, Tian L (2004) Regional homogeneity approach to fMRI data analysis. Neuroimage 22: 394–400.

27. Kendall M, Gibbons J, editors (1990) Rank Correlation Methods. Oxford: Oxford Univ. Press.

28. Zuo XN, Xu T, Jiang L, Yang Z, Cao XY, et al. (2013) Toward reliable characterization of functional homogeneity in the human brain: preprocessing, scan duration, imaging resolution and computational space. Neuroimage 65: 374–386.

29. Kiviniemi V (2008) Endogenous brain fluctuations and diagnostic imaging. Hum Brain Mapp 29: 810–817.

30. Bai F, Zhang Z, Yu H, Shi Y, Yuan Y, et al. (2008) Default-mode network activity distinguishes amnestic type mild cognitive impairment from healthy aging: a combined structural and resting-state functional MRI study. Neurosci Lett 438: 111–115.

31. Zhang Z, Liu Y, Jiang T, Zhou B, An N, et al. (2012) Altered spontaneous activity in Alzheimer's disease and mild cognitive impairment revealed by Regional Homogeneity. Neuroimage 59: 1429–1440.

32. Petersen RC, Doody R, Kurz A, Mohs RC, Morris JC, et al. (2001) Current concepts in mild cognitive impairment. Arch Neurol 58: 1985–1992.

33. Forman SD, Cohen JD, Fitzgerald M, Eddy WF, Mintun MA, et al. (1995) Improved assessment of significant activation in functional magnetic resonance imaging (fMRI): use of a cluster-size threshold. Magn Reson Med 33: 636–647.

34. Morris JC (1993) The Clinical Dementia Rating (CDR): current version and scoring rules. Neurology 43: 2412–2414.

35. Oldfield RC (1971) The assessment and analysis of handedness: the Edinburgh inventory. Neuropsychologia 9: 97–113.

36. Molsberger AF, Schneider T, Gotthardt H, Drabik A (2010) German Randomized Acupuncture Trial for chronic shoulder pain (GRASP) - a pragmatic, controlled, patient-blinded, multi-centre trial in an outpatient care environment. Pain 151: 146–154.

37. Goddard G, Shen Y, Steele B, Springer N (2005) A controlled trial of placebo versus real acupuncture. J Pain 6: 237–242.

38. Enck P, Klosterhalfen S, Zipfel S (2010) Acupuncture, psyche and the placebo response. Auton Neurosci 157: 68–73.

39. Kong J, Gollub R, Huang T, Polich G, Napadow V, et al. (2007) Acupuncture de qi, from qualitative history to quantitative measurement. J Altern Complement Med 13: 1059–1070.

40. Ashburner J, Friston KJ (1999) Nonlinear spatial normalization using basis functions. Human Brain Mapping 7: 254–266.

41. Biswal B, Yetkin FZ, Haughton VM, Hyde JS (1995) Functional connectivity in the motor cortex of resting human brain using echo-planar MRI. Magn Reson Med 34: 537–541.

42. Song XW, Dong ZY, Long XY, Li SF, Zuo XN, et al. (2011) REST: a toolkit for resting-state functional magnetic resonance imaging data processing. PLoS One 6: e25031.

43. Yuan Y, Zhang Z, Bai F, Yu H, Shi Y, et al. (2008) Abnormal neural activity in the patients with remitted geriatric depression: a resting-state functional magnetic resonance imaging study. J Affect Disord 111: 145–152.

44. Paakki JJ, Rahko J, Long X, Moilanen I, Tervonen O, et al. (2010) Alterations in regional homogeneity of resting-state brain activity in autism spectrum disorders. Brain Res 1321: 169–179.

45. Liu H, Liu Z, Liang M, Hao Y, Tan L, et al. (2006) Decreased regional homogeneity in schizophrenia: a resting state functional magnetic resonance imaging study. Neuroreport 17: 19–22.

46. He Y, Wang L, Zang Y, Tian L, Zhang X, et al. (2007) Regional coherence changes in the early stages of Alzheimer's disease: a combined structural and resting-state functional MRI study. Neuroimage 35: 488–500.

47. Wu T, Long X, Zang Y, Wang L, Hallett M, et al. (2009) Regional homogeneity changes in patients with Parkinson's disease. Hum Brain Mapp 30: 1502–1510.

48. Yu DH, Yuan K, Zhao L, Zhao LM, Dong MH, et al. (2012) Regional homogeneity abnormalities in patients with interictal migraine without aura: a resting-state study. Nmr in Biomedicine 25: 806–812.

49. Horwitz B, McIntosh AR, Haxby JV, Furey M, Salerno JA, et al. (1995) Network analysis of PET-mapped visual pathways in Alzheimer type dementia. Neuroreport 6: 2287–2292.

50. Grady CL, Furey ML, Pietrini P, Horwitz B, Rapoport SI (2001) Altered brain functional connectivity and impaired short-term memory in Alzheimer's disease. Brain 124: 739–756.

51. Qi Z, Wu X, Wang Z, Zhang N, Dong H, et al. (2010) Impairment and compensation coexist in amnestic MCI default mode network. Neuroimage 50: 48–55.

52. Mayer DJ (2000) Acupuncture: an evidence-based review of the clinical literature. Annu Rev Med 51: 49–63.

12

Influence of Control Group on Effect Size in Trials of Acupuncture for Chronic Pain: A Secondary Analysis of an Individual Patient Data Meta-Analysis

Hugh MacPherson[1]*, Emily Vertosick[2], George Lewith[3], Klaus Linde[4], Karen J. Sherman[5], Claudia M. Witt[6,7], Andrew J. Vickers[2], on behalf of the Acupuncture Trialists' Collaboration[¶]

1 Department of Health Sciences, University of York, York, United Kingdom, 2 Memorial Sloan-Kettering Cancer Center, New York, New York, United States of America, 3 Faculty of Medicine, Primary Care and Population Sciences, University of Southampton, Southampton, United Kingdom, 4 Institute of General Practice, Technische Universität München, Munich, Germany, 5 Group Health Research Institute, Seattle, Washington, United States of America, 6 Center for Complementary and Integrative Medicine, University Hospital Zurich, Zurich, Switzerland, 7 Institute for Social Medicine, Epidemiology and Health Economics, Charité - Universitätsmedizin, Berlin, Germany

Abstract

Background: In a recent individual patient data meta-analysis, acupuncture was found to be superior to both sham and non-sham controls in patients with chronic pain. In this paper we identify variations in types of sham and non-sham controls used and analyze their impact on the effect size of acupuncture.

Methods: Based on literature searches of acupuncture trials involving patients with headache and migraine, osteoarthritis, and back, neck and shoulder pain, 29 trials met inclusion criteria, 20 involving sham controls (n = 5,230) and 18 non-sham controls (n = 14,597). For sham controls, we analysed non-needle sham, penetrating sham needles and non-penetrating sham needles. For non-sham controls, we analysed non-specified routine care and protocol-guided care. Using meta-regression we explored impact of choice of control on effect of acupuncture.

Findings: Acupuncture was significantly superior to all categories of control group. For trials that used penetrating needles for sham control, acupuncture had smaller effect sizes than for trials with non-penetrating sham or sham control without needles. The difference in effect size was -0.45 (95% C.I. -0.78, -0.12; p = 0.007), or -0.19 (95% C.I. -0.39, 0.01; p = 0.058) after exclusion of outlying studies showing very large effects of acupuncture. In trials with non-sham controls, larger effect sizes associated with acupuncture vs. non-specified routine care than vs. protocol-guided care. Although the difference in effect size was large (0.26), it was not significant with a wide confidence interval (95% C.I. -0.05, 0.57, p = 0.1).

Conclusion: Acupuncture is significantly superior to control irrespective of the subtype of control. While the choice of control should be driven by the study question, our findings can help inform study design in acupuncture, particularly with respect to sample size. Penetrating needles appear to have important physiologic activity. We recommend that this type of sham be avoided.

Editor: Yu-Kang Tu, National Taiwan University, Taiwan

Funding: The Acupuncture Trialists' Collaboration is funded by an R21 (AT004189I from the National Center for Complementary and Alternative Medicine (NCCAM) at the National Institutes of Health (NIH) to Dr Vickers) and by a grant from the Samueli Institute. Dr MacPherson's work on this project was funded in part by the National Institute for Health Research (NIHR) under its Programme Grants for Applied Research scheme (RP-PG-0707-10186). Dr. Witt's work has been supported by the Carstens Foundation within the grant for the Chair for Complementary Medicine Research. The views expressed in this publication are those of the author(s) and not necessarily those of the NCCAM, NHS, NIHR or the Department of Health in England. The funders had no role in study design, data collection and analysis, decision to publish, or preparation of the manuscript.

Competing Interests: The authors have declared that no competing interests exist.

* E-mail: hugh.macpherson@york.ac.uk

¶ Membership of the Acupuncture Trialists' Collaboration is provided in the Acknowledgments.

Introduction

One of the challenges of conducting a non-pharmacological clinical trial is choosing an appropriate control intervention. The simplest control arm is to offer patients routine clinical care without the experimental treatment. This controls for the expected course of the disease. However, the control arm can also be designed to control for other factors, for example, the non-specific effects associated with the time and attention that a patient receives from a clinician.

The choice of control is particularly problematic in acupuncture, which has seen a large increase in published trials in recent years [1]. In an individual patient data meta-analysis of high quality trials conducted by the Acupuncture Trialists' Collaboration [2], acupuncture reduced pain scores by 0.15 to 0.23 standard deviations in comparison to sham (placebo) acupuncture. When the control group did not involve sham, effect sizes ranged from 0.42 to 0.57 [2]. Yet within the general categories of control - those with sham and those without sham - there were marked differences in the exact nature of the intervention received in the control group. For example, trials with sham control included those with acupuncture needles inserted at points not thought to be active, needles that did not penetrate the skin, and non-needle approaches, such as detuned electrical devices. For trials without sham control, the control group in some were simply advised to "avoid acupuncture"; in other trials, both acupuncture and control groups were offered additional treatment, such as physical therapy for back pain.

In this paper, we aim to conduct an analysis of the Acupuncture Trialists' Collaboration dataset to determine how trial results vary by type of control. Specifically, we sought to determine the extent that effect sizes varied depending on whether needles were used for sham acupuncture, whether they penetrated the skin, and whether they were placed at or away from true acupuncture points. We also sought to determine whether there was variation in the effects of acupuncture associated with controls that did not involve sham, comparing "routine care", such as rescue medication made available to patients in both arms of the trial, with "protocolled care" where the control treatment was a standard care specified in the study protocol. Establishing effect sizes associated with commonly used types of controls will be of value in informing future clinical trial design for acupuncture, as well as helping the interpretation of published trial results.

Methods

Included Trials

Trials included in these analyses were identified through a systematic literature review that has been previously described [2]. The initial search was to November 2008, followed by a subsequent one conducted in December 2010. The searches included trials of acupuncture in four specified chronic pain conditions – non-specific musculoskeletal pain, shoulder pain, osteoarthritis, and chronic headache – where allocation concealment was determined unambiguously to be adequate. For trials of musculoskeletal pain, it was additionally specified that the current episode of pain must be of at least four weeks' duration. The search resulted in the identification of 31 trials.

Data Acquisition

Individual patient data were obtained from 29 trials. Data on the trial-level characteristics of the controls were obtained directly from trialists. Twenty trials with 5,230 patients had controls in the form of a sham acupuncture arm (Table 1), and 18 trials with 14,597 patients had non-sham controls (Table 2).

Outcome

The primary outcome used for this analysis was the primary pain endpoint as defined by the study authors. Where multiple criteria were considered in the primary outcome or if the primary outcome was inherently categorical, we used a continuous measure of pain intensity measured at the same time point as the original primary outcome. To make the various outcome measurements comparable between different trials, the primary endpoint of each was standardized by dividing by pooled standard deviation.

Types of Sham Acupuncture Controls

The characteristics we aimed to study in those trials with a sham acupuncture control group included whether or not a needle was used, whether a needle that penetrated the skin was used, whether sham was performed on true acupuncture points or non-acupuncture points, and whether needle insertion was deep or superficial. Information on acupuncture characteristics was obtained from the trial manuscript supplemented by a questionnaire sent to trialists.

Trials were classified as "needle sham" if it was reported that either a penetrating or non-penetrating needle was used for sham acupuncture. A non-penetrating needle is a device specially developed for acupuncture research in which the needle retracts into the handle rather than penetrating the skin; however, the pressure of the needle against the skin is a very similar sensation to insertion. "Non-needle sham" included trials using non-needle methods of sham acupuncture, such as an inactivated laser or transcutaneous electric nerve stimulation (TENS) device. Needle sham trials were further classified as to whether or not the needle used in the sham acupuncture group penetrated the skin. Penetrating needles were almost always inserted at locations away from true acupuncture points (thereby investigating point location) while non-penetrating sham needles were either applied at the same points as in the true acupuncture group (testing exclusively skin penetration and not location) or at non-acupuncture points (investigating penetration and location simultaneously). For example, in the trial of Linde et al [3], needles were inserted superficially away from true acupuncture points; in contrast, the sham technique in the Kleinhenz et al [4] trial consisted of a special needle that retracted into the handle rather than penetrating through the skin at true acupuncture points.

We initially planned to investigate two other features of sham control: whether the depth of insertion for penetration was categorized by trialists as superficial or deep and whether sham was applied at or away from true acupuncture points. However, as shown in Table 1, only one trial reported using deep insertion in sham acupuncture [5]. For point location, there was strong collinearity with sham technique, with only techniques avoiding skin penetration using true acupuncture points.

As a sensitivity analysis, we re-analyzed the data excluding four trials which were determined by consensus among external reviewers as having an "intermediate likelihood of unblinding" [6][7][8][9]. However, after excluding these trials, only one remaining trial used non-needle sham acupuncture, limiting our ability to use meta-regression.

Types of Non-sham Controls

Trials that included controls without sham were categorized into two types: "routine care" and "protocolled care." Trials were identified as "routine care" if patients in both treatment and control groups had access to non-specified care as needed, such as rescue medications or other conventional care, but the use of such treatment was at the discretion of patients and doctors, with no specification in the protocol as to what treatments patients could receive. If protocols proscribed some treatments, such as surgery, but did not make specific recommendations as to allowable treatments, trials were defined as "routine care". Control groups where treatment consisted of information or education given to a patient ("attention control") were also considered to be routine care control groups. Trials were considered to be "protocolled care" if the care in the control group was specified in the study protocol. This was typically when the acupuncture group and the usual care control group both received an additional non-acupuncture treatment that was specifically indicated as part of the trial protocol. For example, trials that studied the effect of acupuncture and physical therapy compared to physical therapy alone were categorized as protocolled care.

Table 1. Sham Acupuncture-Controlled Trials, by Types of Sham Control.

Needle Used?	Penetrating?	True Acupuncture Points?	Depth of Insertion?	Trials
Yes	Yes	No	Superficial	Linde (2005) [3], Melchart (2005) [25], Diener (2006) [6], Scharf (2006) [26], Haake (2007) [11], Endres (2007) [27], Witt (2005) [28], Brinkhaus (2006) [29]
Yes	Yes	No	Deep	Berman (2004) [5] *
Yes	No	No	N/A	Vas (2008) [14]
Yes	No	Yes	N/A	Foster (2007) [24], Guerra (2004) [30], Kennedy (2008) [31], Kleinhenz (1999) [4], Vas (2004) [12], Vas (2006) [13]
No	No	No	N/A	Carlsson (2001) [9], Kerr (2003) [8]
No	No	Yes	N/A	Irnich (2001) [7], White (2004) [32]

*In this trial, penetrating needles were used on non-acupuncture points and non-penetrating needles were used on true acupuncture points. For the main analysis, we considered this trial as penetrating-needle sham used on non-acupuncture points.

In two trials there was a disagreement about whether the close specification of medication and other treatment in the control group constituted "protocolled care" or an active control group, which are excluded from analyses as per the review protocol [10]. The trial of acupuncture for migraine by Diener et al. [6] had a control group in which patients received standard pharmacological therapy for migraine prophylaxis. However, acupuncture and sham acupuncture groups did not receive prophylactic medication. The trial of acupuncture for lower back pain by Haake et al. [11] offered "routine management" up to and including physiotherapy, drugs and exercise to control group patients. Acupuncture and sham acupuncture patients had the same access to rescue medication as the "routine management" group, but did not have access to the same physiotherapy sessions or exercise consultations with physicians.

Statistical Methods

We used random-effects meta-regression to test the effect of each characteristic of sham acupuncture on the main effect estimate using the Stata command *metareg*. This command was also used to run a random-effects meta-regression to test the effect of routine versus protocolled care on the main effect estimate for usual care control groups. The main effect estimate of each trial was determined using linear regression, and the coefficient and standard error for each trial were entered as the dependent variable in the random-effects meta-regression.

A sensitivity analysis was performed excluding three trials by Vas et al. [12][13][14]. In our initial publication on effect size [2], we reported that these trials have very much larger effect sizes than average and that their exclusion resulted in heterogeneity becoming non-significant in the comparisons between acupuncture and sham. The trial of acupuncture for knee osteoarthritis by Berman et al. [5] used a combined insertion and non-insertion method for sham acupuncture. As a sensitivity analysis, we performed the analysis with this trial reclassified as using non-penetrating needles on true acupuncture points as well. We also excluded trials where the risk of bias from unblinding was not classed as being low. As a final sensitivity analysis of non-sham controlled trials, we excluded the trials by Haake et al. [11] and Diener et al. [6] for which there was disagreement as whether the control arm constituted active control, which is not eligible for analysis [10]. All analyses were conducted using Stata 12 (Stata Corp., College Station, TX).

Results

Sham acupuncture controls

Trial-level characteristics for sham-controlled trials are described in Table 3. The majority of sham-controlled trials (80%) used needle-based sham acupuncture. The number of trials using penetrating or non-penetrating needles was similar: seven trials used non-penetrating needles and nine trials used penetrating needles. All trials using penetrating needles placed these outside true acupuncture points, while only one of seven trials using non-penetrating needles did so.

Table 4 shows the effect sizes of sham-controlled acupuncture trials categorized by the type of sham. Acupuncture is significantly superior to sham irrespective of the type of sham control, both in the main analysis and in a sensitivity analysis excluding outlying studies. Table 4 also includes the results of the primary sensitivity analyses that excluded the Vas trials, which we had previously found to be outliers [2].For example, not only was the effect size of the Vas trial for neck pain [13] about five times greater than the meta-analytic estimate, but between-trial heterogeneity was no longer statistically significant after excluding the Vas trials. Using the same rationale for exclusions, overall we found larger effect sizes were associated with acupuncture vs. non-penetrating sham needles (0.43; 95%CI: 0.01, 0.85) than vs. penetrating sham needles (0.17; 95%CI: 0.11, 0.23) although the difference between groups did not reach conventional levels of statistical significance.

Statistical comparisons between types of sham are given in Table 5, which shows the results of the random-effects meta-regression for sham-controlled trials. While trials that used needles as sham did not differ significantly from trials with non-needle sham (p≥0.2 for all comparisons), there is clear evidence of a greater effect size when acupuncture is compared against non-penetrating sham than when compared to penetrating sham. Trials using a penetrating needle had an effect size of −0.21 (95% C.I. −0.41, −0.01) standard deviations lower than trials that did not use a needle sham (p = 0.036). Trials that used penetrating needles for sham control had smaller effect sizes than those with non-penetrating sham or sham control without needles. The difference in effect size was −0.45 (95% C.I. −0.78, −0.12; p = 0.007). For the sensitivity analysis that excluded the Vas trials, this effect size reduced to −0.19 (95% C.I. −0.39, 0.01; p = 0.058). There were no significant differences between non-penetrating needles and sham techniques that did not involve needling.

In further sensitivity analyses, reclassification of the Berman trial had little effect on our results. For example, the comparison of

Table 2. Types of non-sham control group by trial: categorised as "protocolled care" or "routine care".

Trial	Control Group	Type of Control Group
Foster (2007) [24]	Advice and exercise: All three arms of the trial received advice and exercise. Patients received leaflet with information on knee osteoarthritis. Patients on NSAID therapy were allowed to continue with stable dose. Individualized exercises of progressive intensity for lower limb stretching, strengthening and balance (up to six 30-minute sessions over six weeks). Patients in the control arm did not receive verum or sham acupuncture.	Protocolled
Linde (2005) [3], Melchart (2005) [25]	Waiting list control: Control patients were not permitted to have prophylactic treatment for 12 weeks. All patients were allowed to treat acute headache as necessary (following current guidelines).	Routine
Thomas (2006) [33], Salter (2006) [34], Vickers (2004) [23]	General practitioner care: All patients received NHS treatment according to general practitioner's assessment and recommendation. Control patients did not receive acupuncture or any other specified interventions.	Routine
Berman (2004) [5]	Education-attention control: Patients in this arm attended six two-hour group sessions based for arthritis self-management, and received periodic educational materials by mail. Patients in the acupuncture and sham acupuncture arms did not participate in this intervention.	Routine
Cherkin (2001) [35]	Self-care education: Patients in this group received a book with information about back pain, treatment, improving quality of life and coping with emotional and interpersonal issues surrounding back pain. Patients also received two professionally-produced videos which addressed self-management of back pain and demonstrated exercises. Patients in the acupuncture and massage groups did not receive this educational material.	Routine
Scharf (2006) [26]	Conservative therapy: Patients in the conservative therapy group had 10 visits with physicians and received prescriptions for either diclofenac (up to 150 mg/day) or rofecoxib (25 mg/day) up to week 23. Patients in this group who had "partially successful" results were offered the choice of attending an additional five visits. Patients in the verum acupuncture and sham acupuncture groups were permitted to take up to 150 mg/day of diclofenac for the first two weeks and a total of 1 g of diclofenac during the rest of the study. Patients in both acupuncture groups and in the conservative management group received up to six sessions of physiotherapy. All patients were prohibited from taking any analgesics other than diclofenac and rofecoxib and any corticosteroids.	Protocolled
Diener (2006) [6]	Standard migraine treatment: Control group patients were treated according to the guidelines of the German Migraine and Headache Society. Patients had six to seven visits in which standard treatment was established. First choice of treatment was beta blockers, followed by flunarizine, and then valproic acid. Acute medication use was permitted in all groups.	Protocolled
Haake (2007) [11]	Conventional therapy: Patients in the conventional therapy group were treated according to German guidelines. Conventional therapy patients had 10 visits with physician or physiotherapist where physiotherapy, exercise and/or similar treatments were offered. Patients in all three arms were permitted to take NSAIDs up to the maximum daily dose.	Protocolled
Williamson (2007) [36]	Education and exercise: Patients in the control group were told they were in the "home exercise" group and received an exercise and advice leaflet.	Routine
Witt (2005) [28], Brinkhaus (2006) [29]	Waiting list control: Patients in the waiting list control group received no acupuncture treatment for eight weeks after randomization. All patients were allowed oral NSAIDs for pain as rescue medication. All patients were prohibited from taking corticosteroids or pain medication that acted on the central nervous system.	Routine
Witt (2006 – OA) [37], Witt (2006 – LBP) [38]	Conventional treatment: Patients in the control group were not allowed to use any kind of acupuncture during the first three months. All patients were allowed to use additional conventional treatments as needed.	Routine
Jena (2008) [39], Witt (2006 – Neck Pain) [40]	Conventional treatment: Patients in the control group were not allowed to use any kind of acupuncture during the first three months. All patients were allowed to use additional conventional treatments as needed.	Routine

penetrating needle vs. non-needle or non-penetrating needle gave a difference in effect size of 0.18 rather than 0.19 and a p value of 0.057 rather than 0.058. Excluding the four trials that were classified as "intermediate risk of unblinding" did not significantly change the effect sizes or p-values for most analyses. For example, the difference in effect size and 95% confidence interval when comparing penetrating needle sham to non-penetrating needle sham was −0.57 (−0.96, −0.18) in the main analysis, while the difference in effect size and 95% confidence for the same comparison was −0.57 (−0.98, −0.15) after excluding these four trials. However, the comparison with non-needle-based sham acupuncture included only one trial using non-needle sham. As a result, the standard error becomes much larger, and the p value

non-significant. Excluding the trials at intermediate risk of unblinding and the outlying Vas trials gave very similar results to the analyses excluding the outlying Vas trials alone. For example, the central estimate for the comparison of penetrating needle with non-needle sham changes from −0.21 to −0.18. Statistical significance was lost, presumably because of the limited number of trials remaining in the analysis (see Table S1, Supporting Information).

Non-sham controls

Trial-level characteristics for trials without sham controls are described in Table 2. The majority of these trials (72%) were

Table 3. Trial-level Characteristics for Trials with Sham Acupuncture Control Groups, N = 20.

Needle Used	
Yes	16 (80%)
No	4 (20%)
Penetrating Needle Used	
Yes	9 (45%)
No	7 (35%)
Non-needle	4 (20%)
True Acupuncture Points Used	
Yes	8 (40%)
No	12 (60%)
Superficial or Deep Sham	
Superficial	8 (40%)
Deep	1 (5%)
Non-penetrating sham	11 (55%)
Pain Type	
Low Back Pain	5 (25%)
Migraine	2 (10%)
Neck	3 (15%)
Osteoarthritis	5 (25%)
Shoulder	3 (15%)
Tension-type Headache	2 (10%)

Frequency (%).

classified as routine care. Table 6 provides further details of the control groups, separately by pain type.

The effect size for acupuncture in trials with routine care control (0.55, 95% CI 0.40, 0.70) was larger than when acupuncture was compared against protocolled care (0.29, 95% CI 0.01, 0.58). Although the difference in effect size was large, it was not significant (difference in effect size = 0.26, 95% CI -0.05, 0.57, p = 0.1). Removing the two studies [6] [11] in the sensitivity analysis had little effect on the effect size estimate (0.25, 95% CI -0.26, 0.76) for the comparison with protocolled care. The difference in effect size between trials utilizing protocolled vs. routine care was also similar (0.29, 95% CI -0.13, 0.72).

Discussion

Principal findings

Acupuncture was significantly superior to sham irrespective of the type of sham control and superior to non-sham control irrespective of whether that constituted routine or protocolled care. That said, there were differences in effect sizes between trials with different control conditions. With regard to the types of sham control, we found that sham controls involving penetrating needles had smaller effect sizes than trials that did not use a needle control or where the needles in the control group did not penetrate the skin. An important implication is that the central estimates from our meta-analysis [2] may have underestimated the effects of acupuncture compared to sham. With regard to non-acupuncture controls, we found evidence that the effect size of acupuncture when compared to protocolled care is smaller than when compared to the less intensive routine care, although differences did not reach statistical significance.

There are two possible explanations for the differences in effect size by type of sham control: bias from unblinding and physiologic activity. It is plausible that penetrating needles are more credible to patients than non-penetrating approaches, such that patients are less likely to give biased responses on pain questionnaires. That said, there is no evidence in favor of such a hypothesis and considerable evidence against. In particular, the most common form of non-penetrating needle used was the "Streitberger" needle that has been carefully validated as a credible placebo in an empirical study. Indeed, study participants were unable to distinguish between the Streitberger needle and true acupuncture even when subject to both in crossover fashion [15]. The other explanation for our findings is that penetrating needles have important physiologic activity, that is, inserting an acupuncture needle superficially away from an acupuncture point may be less effective than deep insertion at a correct location, but nonetheless has some therapeutic activity against pain [16][17].

Relationship to the literature

There has been considerable interest in the literature regarding the appropriate choice of placebo controls for non-pharmacological therapies. One approach has been to investigate trials that included a placebo arm and a no-treatment arm, and then compare outcomes between these two, and in this way explore variations in the impact of the different types of placebo. An example of this is a Cochrane review of placebo controls covering a wide range of trials for different conditions, including some acupuncture trials [18]. In a sub-group analysis the authors found that trials using "physical placebos" (including sham acupuncture) were associated with greater placebo effects than trials with

Table 4. Effect size of acupuncture compared to type of sham acupuncture control.

	Main Analysis		Excluding Vas et al. trials [12] [13] [14]	
	Number of Trials	Effect Size	Number of Trials	Effect Size
Needle sham	16	0.42 (0.19, 0.66)	13	0.22 (0.11, 0.33)
Non-needle sham	4	0.38 (0.19, 0.57)	4	0.38 (0.19, 0.57)
Non-penetrating needle	7	0.76 (0.31, 1.21)	4	0.43 (0.01, 0.85)
Penetrating needle	9	0.17 (0.11, 0.23)	9	0.17 (0.11, 0.23)
Non-needle and non-penetrating needle	11	0.63 (0.33, 0.94)	8	0.40 (0.18, 0.62)

Estimates obtained using meta-regression.

Table 5. Difference in effect sizes between types of sham control. Estimates obtained using meta-regression.

	Main Analysis			Excluding Vas et al. trials [12] [13] [14]		
	No. of Trials*	Change in Effect Size	p value	No. of Trials*	Change in Effect Size	p value
Needle vs. Non-needle sham	16 vs. 4	0.02 (−0.49, 0.53)	0.9	13 vs. 4	−0.17 (−0.43, 0.09)	0.2
Non-penetrating needle vs. Non-needle sham	7 vs. 4	0.35 (−0.28, 0.99)	0.3	4 vs. 4	0.01 (−0.45, 0.47)	1
Penetrating needle vs. Non-penetrating needle	9 vs. 7	−0.57 (−0.96, −0.18)	0.004	9 vs. 4	−0.19 (−0.47, 0.08)	0.2
Penetrating needle vs. Non-needle sham	9 vs. 4	−0.21 (−0.41, −0.01)	0.036	9 vs. 4	−0.21 (−0.41, −0.01)	0.036
Penetrating needle vs. Non-needle or Non-penetrating needle	9 vs. 11	−0.45 (−0.78, −0.12)	0.007	9 vs. 8	−0.19 (−0.39, 0.01)	0.058

*The number listed in the top row is the number of trials in the first comparison group. The number of trials listed in the bottom row is the number of trials in the second comparison group. For example, there were 16 needle sham-controlled trials and 4 non-needle sham-controlled in the main analysis.

pharmacological placebos [18]. This finding is consistent with the results of a trial that was specifically designed to compare a sham device (sham acupuncture) with an inert pill, the sham device being associated with a greater reduction of self-reported pain [19]. These results provide supportive evidence for our finding that different types of sham control lead to different estimates of treatment effects.

The data from the above Cochrane review of placebo controls were re-analysed by a different group of authors who observed that sham acupuncture interventions vs. no treatment have larger effects than other "physical placebos" vs. no treatment [20]. In a sub-analysis that is similar to what we report in this paper, they found that the standardised effect for acupuncture versus sham was similar for trials using penetrating sham needling (−0.43; 95%CI: −0.59, 0.28) compared to trials using non-penetrating sham (−0.37; 95%CI: −0.70, 0.04) [20]. By contrast, we found significantly smaller effect sizes when acupuncture was compared to sham acupuncture with penetrating needles (0.17; 95%CI: 0.11, 0.23) than when compared to non-penetrating needles (0.43; 95%CI: 0.01, 0.85). The differences might be explained by differences in the trials included - our data involved only chronic pain trials of methodologically high quality – and the greater precision afforded by individual patient data meta-analysis: note that the wide confidence intervals in the Cochrane data are consistent with the main estimates from the current analysis.

Table 6. Trial-level Characteristics for Trials with Non-sham Control Groups, N = 18.

Pain Type	Routine Care	Protocolled Care	Total
Headache	2	0	2
Migraine	1	1	2
Tension-Type Headache	1	0	1
Osteoarthritis	4	2	6
Lower Back Pain	3	2	5
Neck Pain	2	0	2
Total	13 (72%)	5 (28%)	18 (100%)

Frequency (%).

Study strengths and limitations

Combining patient data from 29 high-quality trials in a single database provides us for the first time with sufficient power to explore the role of controls in trials of acupuncture for chronic pain, because the power of meta-regression is strongly influenced by the number of trials and their variation. We were unable to address questions as to the depth and location of sham needle placement as only one trial used deep sham needle insertion and all sham-controlled trials that used true acupuncture points avoided penetrating needles. While the difference in effect size between routine and protocolled care is large and in the direction expected, it is associated with wide confidence intervals. Partially, this is due to the wide variety of non-sham controls, and the difficulty we had in categorizing them.

Even with this large dataset we do not have a full understanding of the different physiologic and psychologic effects of sham acupuncture. One limitation within the field generally is that the mechanisms for a persistent effect of acupuncture on chronic pain are incompletely understood and therefore we have no clear idea of whether a sham control inadvertently activates these mechanisms or not. This lack of understanding about the physiological mechanisms of acupuncture limits any firm conclusions we can draw regarding the extent that any of the sham controls discussed above can be considered as a true 'placebo'. Moreover when implementing sham acupuncture trials, the outcome may also be influenced by factors not included in our analysis, such as the believability of the control, prior knowledge of patients about acupuncture, whether the true acupuncture group was treated identically, the extent that practitioners were able to maintain equipoise, and practical implementation issues, such as how carefully the ring that comes with the Streitberger needle [15] was taped in place.

Implications for research

The research question remains the primary determinant on choice of control. In a strategy document developed with a range of collaborators using consensus methods, a useful distinction has been drawn between efficacy trials that seek to determine whether there are specific effects beyond the placebo in an ideal treatment environment, and effectiveness trials that seek to determine the overall impact of acupuncture in which specific and non-specific effects are combined [21]. Moreover research questions investigating the value of specific point location need to have sham needles located away from true acupuncture points while research questions testing skin penetration require non-penetrating sham needle controls applied at the same points as in the true acupuncture group.

The choice of a sham acupuncture control needs to be informed by consideration of the likely impact of the sham intervention. In the past, judgments on this have often used expert opinion on putative physiological activity of a sham control, even though we have yet to understand the mechanism(s) of the action of acupuncture [17]. A number of commentators have speculated that penetrating sham needling may be physiologically active and thus be an inappropriate sham control [16]. Our results provide support for this contention, suggesting that needle penetration should be avoided as a sham technique to control for non-specific effects associated with acupuncture in trials involving chronic pain patients. However sham acupuncture involving penetrating needles may well have a place when addressing questions of point specificity in explanatory trials. We are more cautious with regard to recommending the use of non-penetrating needles. Many forms of Japanese acupuncture use shallow insertion or non-insertion (the *toya hari* method) [22]. Using non-penetrating needles in controlled trials is not without its challenges: although apparently less active than other types of sham, we cannot assume that non-penetrating needles have complete physiologic inactivity; furthermore, there are practical questions regarding whether to enroll only acupuncture-naïve patients and whether practitioners can maintain equipoise in large trials over reasonable periods of time.

When sham acupuncture is not used, the choice of control is clearly driven by the research question. For instance, in the UK National Health Service (NHS) trial of acupuncture for chronic headache, the study question of Vickers et al was related to the effects of making acupuncture more widely available in primary care, a pragmatic comparison of "use acupuncture" and "avoid acupuncture" [23]. On the other hand, Foster et al. were interested in the impact of acupuncture when added to an existing rehabilitation program [24]. Yet our findings have clear implications for sample size calculations, with larger sample sizes needed in trials where care in the control arm is carefully specified.

Conclusion

From a large database of individual patient data from high-quality randomized trials, we found acupuncture to be significantly superior to control irrespective of the subtype of control. When compared against sham, trials with penetrating needles reported lower effect sizes for acupuncture than trials with non-penetrating needles or those that used non-needle sham. This suggests that penetrating needles have important physiologic activity, even when inserted superficially away from true acupuncture points. Accordingly, we recommend that this type of sham be avoided. In trials without sham control, we found that the effect size likely depends on the intensity of treatment in the control group, with smaller differences between acupuncture and protocol guided programs of treatment than between acupuncture and routine care. While the choice of control should be driven by the study question, these findings can help inform study design in acupuncture, particularly with respect to sample size.

Supporting Information

Table S1 Sensitivity analyses.
(DOCX)

Acknowledgments

This is a study from the Acupuncture Trialists' Collaboration, which includes physicians, clinical trialists, biostatisticians, practicing acupunc-

turists and others. The collaborators within the Acupuncture Trialists' Collaboration are:

Claire Allen, BS, Cochrane Collaboration Secretariat, Oxford, England;

Mac Beckner, MIS, Information Technology and Data Management Center, Samueli Institute, Alexandria, Virginia;

Brian Berman, MD, University of Maryland School of Medicine and Center for Integrative Medicine, College Park; Maryland;

Benno Brinkhaus, MD, Institute for Social Medicine, Epidemiology and Health Economics, Charité University Medical Center, Berlin, Germany;

Remy Coeytaux, MD, PhD, Department of Community and Family Medicine, Duke University, Durham, North Carolina;

Angel M. Cronin, MS, Dana-Farber Cancer Institute, Boston, Massachusetts;

Hans-Christoph Diener, MD, PhD, Department of Neurology, University of Duisburg-Essen, Germany;

Heinz G. Endres, MD, Ruhr–University Bochum, Bochum, Germany;

Nadine Foster, DPhil, BSc(Hons), Arthritis Research UK Primary Care Centre, Keele University, Newcastle-under-Lyme, Staffordshire, England;

Juan Antonio Guerra de Hoyos, MD, Andalusian Integral Plan for Pain Management, and Andalusian Health Service Project for Improving Primary Care Research, Sevilla, Spain;

Michael Haake, MD, PhD, Department of Orthopedics and Traumatology, SLK Hospitals, Heilbronn, Germany;

Richard Hammerschlag, PhD, Oregon College of Oriental Medicine, Portland, Oregon;

Dominik Irnich, MD, Interdisciplinary Pain Centre, University of Munich, Munich, Germany;

Wayne B. Jonas, MD, Samueli Institute, Alexandria, Virginia;

Kai Kronfeld, PhD, Interdisciplinary Centre for Clinical Trials (IZKS Mainz), University Medical Centre Mainz, Mainz, Germany;

Lixing Lao, PhD, University of Maryland and Center for Integrative Medicine, College Park, Maryland;

George Lewith, MD, FRCP, Complementary and Integrated Medicine Research Unit, Southampton Medical School, Southampton, England;

Klaus Linde, MD, Institute of General Practice, Technische Universität München, Munich, Germany;

Hugh MacPherson, PhD, Complementary Medicine Evaluation Group, University of York, York, England;

Eric Manheimer, MS, Center for Integrative Medicine, University of Maryland School of Medicine, College Park, Maryland;

Alexandra Maschino, BS, Memorial Sloan-Kettering Cancer Center, New York, New York;

Dieter Melchart, MD, PhD, Centre for Complementary Medicine Research (Znf), Technische Universität München, Munich, Germany;

Albrecht Molsberger, MD, PhD, German Acupuncture Research Group, Duesseldorf, Germany;

Karen J. Sherman, PhD, MPH, Group Health Research Institute, Seattle, Washington;

Hans Trampisch, PhD, Department of Medical Statistics and Epidemiology, Ruhr–University Bochum, Germany;

Jorge Vas, MD, PhD, Pain Treatment Unit, Dos Hermanas Primary Care Health Center (Andalusia Public Health System), Dos Hermanas, Spain;

Andrew J. Vickers (collaboration chair), DPhil, Memorial Sloan-Kettering Cancer Center, New York, New York;

Norbert Victor, PhD (deceased), Institute of Medical Biometrics and Informatics, University of Heidelberg, Heidelberg, Germany;

Peter White, PhD, School of Health Sciences, University of Southampton, England;

Lyn Williamson, MD, MA (Oxon), MRCGP, FRCP, Great Western Hospital, Swindon, and Oxford University, Oxford, England;

Stefan N. Willich, MD, MPH, MBA, Institute for Social Medicine, Epidemiology, and Health Economics, Charité University Medical Center, Berlin, Germany;

Claudia M. Witt, MD, MBA, University Medical Center Charité and Institute for Social Medicine, Epidemiology and Health Economics, Berlin, Germany.

Data sharing policy:

The Acupuncture Trialists' Collaboration obtained some data that cannot be publicly deposited as this was a condition of us receiving the data from third parties. All summary data for the trial-level analyses will immediately be made available to investigators on request; requests for individual patient data will be considered on a case-by-case basis depending on the trials involved for the analysis concerned. Such data are fully de-identified.

Author Contributions

Analyzed the data: AV EV. Wrote the paper: HM AV EV. Co-ordinated the development and conduct of the study: HM. Designed the study: AV.

Gave input on the design of the study: HM CW GL KL KS. Wrote first draft of the Methods and Results sections: AV EV. Wrote first draft of the manuscript as a whole: HM. Gave comments on early drafts and approved the final version of the manuscript: HM EV GL KL KS CW AV. Had full access to all of the data in the study, takes responsibility for the integrity of the data and the accuracy of the data analysis: AV.

References

1. Han JS, Ho YS (2011) Global trends and performances of acupuncture research. Neurosci.Biobehav.Rev. 35(1873–7528):680–7.
2. Vickers AJ, Cronin AM, Maschino AC, Lewith G, MacPherson H, et al. (2012) Acupuncture for Chronic Pain: Individual Patient Data Meta-analysis.x Neurosci.Biobehav.Rev. 172(19):1444–53.
3. Linde K, Streng A, Jurgens S, Hoppe A, Brinkhaus B, et al. (2005) Acupuncture for patients with migraine: a randomized controlled trial. JAMA. 293:2118–25.
4. Kleinhenz J, Streitberger K, Windeler J, Gussbacher A, Mavridis G, et al. (1999) Randomised clinical trial comparing the effects of acupuncture and a newly designed placebo needle in rotator cuff tendinitis. Pain. 83:235–41.
5. BM, Lao L, Langenberg P, Lee WL, Gilpin AMK, et al. (2004) Effectiveness of acupuncture as adjunctive therapy in osteoarthritis of the knee: a randomized, controlled trial. Ann Intern Med. 141:901–10.
6. Diener HC, Kronfeld K, Boewing G, Lungenhausen M, Maier C, et al. (2006) Efficacy of acupuncture for the prophylaxis of migraine: a multicentre randomised controlled clinical trial. Lancet Neurol. 5:310–6.
7. D, Behrens N, Molzen H, Konig A, Gleditsch J, et al. (2001) Randomised trial of acupuncture compared with conventional massage and "sham" laser acupuncture for treatment of chronic neck pain. BMJ. 322(322(7302)):1574–8.
8. DP, Walsh DM, Baxter D (2003) Acupuncture in the management of chronic low back pain: a blinded randomized controlled trial. Clin J Pain. 19(6):364–70.
9. Carlsson CP, Sjölund BH (2001) Acupuncture for chronic low back pain: a randomized placebo-controlled study with long-term follow-up. Clin J Pain. 17(4):296–305.
10. Vickers AJ, Cronin AM, Maschino AC, Lewith G, MacPherson H, et al. (2010) Individual patient data meta-analysis of acupuncture for chronic pain: protocol of the Acupuncture Trialists' Collaboration. Trials. 11:90.
11. Haake M, Muller HH, Schade-Brittinger C, Basler HD, Schafer H, et al. (2007) German Acupuncture Trials (GERAC) for chronic low back pain: randomized, multicenter, blinded, parallel-group trial with 3 groups. Arch Intern Med. 167:1892–8.
12. Vas J, Mendez C, Perea-Milla E, Vega E, Panadero MD, et al. (2004) Acupuncture as a complementary therapy to the pharmacological treatment of osteoarthritis of the knee: randomised controlled trial. Br.Med.J. 329(1468-5833):1216.
13. Vas J, Perea-Milla E, Méndez C, Sánchez Navarro C, León Rubio JM, et al. (2006) Efficacy and safety of acupuncture for chronic uncomplicated neck pain: a randomised controlled study. Pain. 126(1–3):245–55.
14. Vas J, Ortega C, Olmo V, Perez-Fernandez F, Hernandez L, et al. (2008) Single-point acupuncture and physiotherapy for the treatment of painful shoulder: a multicentre randomized controlled trial. Rheumatology (Oxford). 47(6):887–93.
15. Streitberger K, Kleinhenz J (1998) Introducing a placebo needle into acupuncture research. Lancet. 352(0140–6736):364–5.
16. Lund I, Lundeberg T (2006) Are minimal, superficial or sham acupuncture procedures acceptable as inert placebo controls? Acupuncture in Medicine. 24(1):13–5.
17. Birch S (2006) A review and analysis of placebo treatments, placebo effects, and placebo controls in trials of medical procedures when sham is not inert. J Alternat Complement Med. 12:303–10.
18. Hróbjartsson A, Gøtzsche PC (2010) Placebo interventions for all clinical conditions. Cochrane Database Syst Rev. CD003974.
19. Kaptchuk TJ, Stason WB, Davis RB, Legedza ATR, Schnyer RN, et al. (2006) Sham device vs. inert pill: randomised controlled trial of two placebo treatments. BMJ. 332:391–7.
20. Linde K, Niemann K, Meissner K (2010) Are sham acupuncture interventions more effective than (other) placebos? A re-analysis of data from the Cochrane review on placebo effects. Forsch Komplementrmed. 17:259–64.
21. Witt CM, Aickin M, Baca T, Cherkin D, Haan MN, et al. (2012) Effectiveness guidance document (EGD) for acupuncture research - a consensus document for conducting trials. BMC Complementary and Alternative Medicine. 12(1):148.
22. Birch S, Felt R (1999) Understanding Acupuncture. Edinburgh: Churchill Livingstone.
23. Vickers AJ, Rees RW, Zollman CE, McCarney R, Smith CM, et al. (2004) Acupuncture for chronic headache in primary care: large, pragmatic, randomised trial. Br.Med.J. 328(1468-5833):744.
24. Foster NE, Thomas E, Barlas P, Hill JC, Young J, et al. (2007) Acupuncture as an adjunct to exercise based physiotherapy for osteoarthritis of the knee: randomised controlled trial. BMJ. 335:436.
25. Melchart D, Streng A, Hoppe A, Brinkhaus B, Witt C, et al. (2005) Acupuncture in patients with tension-type headache: randomised controlled trial. BMJ. 331:376–82.
26. Scharf H, Mansmann U, Streitberger K, Witte S, Kramer J, et al. (2006) Acupuncture and Knee Osteoarthritis: a three-armed randomized trial. Ann Intern Med. 145:12–20.
27. Endres HG, Böwing G, Diener H-C, Lange S, Maier C, et al. (2007) Acupuncture for tension-type headache: a multicentre, sham-controlled, patient- and observer-blinded, randomised trial. J Headache Pain. 8(5):306–14.
28. Witt C, Brinkhaus B, Jena S, Linde K, Streng A, et al. (2005) Acupuncture in patients with osteoarthritis of the knee: a randomised trial. Lancet. 366:136–43.
29. Brinkhaus B, Witt CM, Jena S, Linde K, Streng A, et al. (2006) Acupuncture in patients with chronic low back pain: a randomized trial. Arch Intern Med. 166:450–7.
30. Guerra de Hoyos JA, Andres Martin MdC, Bassas y Baena de Leon E, Vigára Lopez M, Molina López T, et al. (2004) Randomised trial of long term effect of acupuncture for shoulder pain. Pain. 112(3):289–98.
31. Kennedy S, Baxter GD, Kerr DP, Bradbury I, Park J, et al. (2008) Acupuncture for acute non-specific low back pain: a pilot randomised non-penetrating sham controlled trial. Complement Ther Med. 16(3):139–46.
32. White P, Lewith G, Prescott P, Conway J (2004) Acupuncture versus placebo for the treatment of chronic mechanical neck pain: a randomized, controlled trial. Ann.Intern.Med. 141(1539-3704):911–9.
33. Thomas KJ, MacPherson H, Thorpe L, Brazier J, Fitter M, et al. (2006) Randomised controlled trial of a short course of traditional acupuncture compared with usual care for persistent non-specific low back pain. BMJ. 333:623–6.
34. Salter GC, Roman M, Bland MJ, MacPherson H (2006) Acupuncture for chronic neck pain: a pilot for a randomised controlled trial. BMC Musculoskelet Disord. 7:99.
35. Cherkin DC, Eisenberg D, Sherman KJ, Barlow W, Kaptchuk TJ, et al. (2001) Randomized trial comparing traditional Chinese medical acupuncture, therapeutic massage, and self-care education for chronic low back pain. Arch. Intern. Med. 161(8):1081–8.
36. Williamson L, Wyatt MR, Yein K, Melton JT (2007) Severe knee osteoarthritis: a randomized controlled trial of acupuncture, physiotherapy (supervised exercise) and standard management for patients awaiting knee replacement. Rheumatology (Oxford). 46(9):1445–9.
37. Witt CM, Jena S, Brinkhaus B, Liecker B, Wegscheider K, et al. (2006) Acupuncture in patients with osteoarthritis of the knee or hip: a randomized, controlled trial with an additional nonrandomized arm. Arthritis Rheum. 54:3485–93.
38. Witt CM, Jena S, Selim D, Brinkhaus B, Reinhold T, et al. (2006) Pragmatic randomized trial evaluating the clinical and economic effectiveness of acupuncture for chronic low back pain. Am.J.Epidemiol. 164:487–96.
39. Jena S, Witt CM, Brinkhaus B, Willich SN (2008) Acupuncture in patients with headache. Cephalalgia. 28(9):969–79.
40. Witt CM, Jena S, Brinkhaus B, Liecker B, Wegscheider K, et al. (2006) Acupuncture for patients with chronic neck pain. Pain. 125:98–106.

13

Dense Cranial Electroacupuncture Stimulation for Major Depressive Disorder—A Single-Blind, Randomized, Controlled Study

Zhang-Jin Zhang[1]*, Roger Ng[1], Sui Cheung Man[1], Tsui Yin Jade Li[1], Wendy Wong[1], Qing-Rong Tan[3], Hei Kiu Wong[1], Ka-Fai Chung[4], Man-Tak Wong[2], Wai-Kiu Alfert Tsang[2], Ka-chee Yip[2], Eric Ziea[5], Vivian Taam Wong[5]

1 School of Chinese Medicine, LKS Faculty of Medicine, The University of Hong Kong, Hong Kong, China, 2 Department of Psychiatry, Kowloon Hospital, Hong Kong, China, 3 Department of Psychiatry, Fourth Military Medical University, Xi'an, Shaanxi, China, 4 Department of Psychiatry, LKS Faculty of Medicine, The University of Hong Kong, Hong Kong, China, 5 Chinese Medicine Section, Hospital Authority, Hong Kong, China

Abstract

Background: Previous studies suggest that electroacupuncture possesses therapeutic benefits for depressive disorders. The purpose of this study was to determine whether dense cranial electroacupuncture stimulation (DCEAS) could enhance the antidepressant efficacy in the early phase of selective serotonin reuptake inhibitor (SSRI) treatment of major depressive disorder (MDD).

Methods: In this single-blind, randomized, controlled study, patients with MDD were randomly assigned to 9-session DCEAS or noninvasive electroacupuncture (n-EA) control procedure in combination with fluoxetine (FLX) for 3 weeks. Clinical outcomes were measured using the 17-item Hamilton Depression Rating Scale (HAMD-17), Clinical Global Impression-severity (CGI-S), and Self-rating Depression Scale (SDS) as well as the response and remission rates.

Results: Seventy-three patients were randomly assigned to n-EA (n = 35) and DCEAS (n = 38), of whom 34 in n-EA and 36 in DCEAS group were analyzed. DCEAS-treated patients displayed a significantly greater reduction from baseline in HAMD-17 scores at Day 3 through Day 21 and in SDS scores at Day 3 and Day 21 compared to patients receiving n-EA. DCEAS intervention also produced a higher rate of clinically significant response compared to n-EA procedure (19.4% (7/36) vs. 8.8% (3/34)). The incidence of adverse events was similar in the two groups.

Conclusions: DCEAS is a safe and effective intervention that augments the antidepressant efficacy. It can be considered as an additional therapy in the early phase of SSRI treatment of depressed patients.

Trial Registration: Controlled-Trials.com ISRCTN88008690

Editor: Kenji Hashimoto, Chiba University Center for Forensic Mental Health, Japan

Funding: This study was supported by Health and Health Services Research Fund (HHSRF) from Food and Health Bureau of Hong Kong (ref. No.: 06070831). The funders had no role in study design, data collection and analysis, decision to publish, or preparation of the manuscript.

Competing Interests: The authors have declared that no competing interests exist.

* E-mail: zhangzj@hku.hk

Introduction

Although selective serotonin reuptake inhibitors (SSRIs) are the mainstay in the treatment of depressive disorders, the treatment outcomes are unsatisfactory [1]. There remains a large portion of depressed patients who cannot obtain a full remission and experience relapse and functional impairment [1,2]. Moreover, the delay in the onset of the action of SSRIs prolongs patients' suffering and exposes them to great risk of suicide [3]. These shortcomings have led to a high demand for seeking alternative strategies that can enhance the antidepressant efficacy of SSRIs particularly in the early phase of the treatment [4].

Numerous studies and recent meta-analyses have shown that acupuncture is efficacious for various types of depressive disorders

[5–7]. Although most acupuncture protocols used were developed from the doctrine of traditional Chinese medicine and empiricism rather than modern scientific rationale, experimental and clinical observations have found that electroacupuncture has robust immediate and short-term effects in alleviating pain, autonomic dysfunction, sleep, and mood symptoms [8–10]. This rapid effect is thought to be associated with the fast and direct modulation of multiple central neurochemical systems, especially the brainstem adrenalinergic (NA), serotonergic (5-HT) neuronal and hypothalamic neuroendocrine systems [10], which play the principal role in the pathophysiology of major depression [11]. These are the reasons to hypothesize that electroacupuncture can serve to enhance the antidepressant action in the early phase of SSRI treatment.

Dense cranial electroacupuncture stimulation (DCEAS) is a novel stimulation mode in which electrical stimulation is delivered on dense acupoints located on the forehead mainly innervated by the trigeminal nerve, efficiently modulating multiple central transmitter systems via the trigeminal sensory-brainstem NA and 5-HT neuronal pathways [12]. Several pilot studies have shown that DCEAS and similar approaches are effective in improving refractory obsessive-compulsive disorder (OCD) [12], major depressive disorder (MDD) [13], post-stroke depression [14], and MDD-associated residual insomnia [15].

Fluoxetine (FLX) is one of the most prescribed SSRIs for major depression worldwide [16]. This single-blind, randomized, controlled trial was designed to determine whether DCEAS intervention could produce greater clinical improvement compared to noninvasive electroacupuncture (n-EA) control procedure in the early phase of FLX treatment of patients with MDD.

Methods

Subjects

This single-blind, randomized, sham-acupuncture controlled trial was conducted in Department of Psychiatry at Kowloon Hospital of Hong Kong between August 2009 and March 2011. The study protocol was approved by Institutional Review Board (IRB) of the University of Hong Kong/Hospital Authority Hong Kong West Cluster and registered in www.controlled-trials.com (ISRCTN88008690). The protocol for this trial and supporting CONSORT checklist are available as supporting information (see Checklist S1 and Protocol S1).

Psychiatrists referred outpatients to the study. The inclusion criteria were: (1) age 25–65 years; (2) DSM-IV diagnosis of MDD [17]; (3) 17-item Hamilton Rating Scale for Depression (HAMD-17) score ≥ 18 [18]; and (4) Clinical Global Impression-Severity (CGI-S) score ≥ 4 [19]. Subjects were excluded if they had: (1) unstable medical conditions; (2) suicidal attempts or aggressive behavior; (3) a history of manic, hypomanic, or mixed episode; (4) a family history of bipolar or psychotic disorders; (5) a history of substance abuse within the previous 12 months; (6) investigational drug treatment in the previous 6 months; (7) current psychotropic treatment exceed one week; or (8) needle phobia. All participants gave voluntary, written and informed consent before entering the trial.

Randomization and blinding

Patients were randomly assigned to either n-EA or DCEAS treatment at a ratio of 1:1, using a random block scheme from an automatic computer program (SPSS version II). The assignment was done in a single-blind manner, in which the random codes were only known by the acupuncturists (W.W. and M. S.C.). The validity of the subject-blind design was ensured by sham acupuncture procedure performed on the forehead acupoints, which were outside the visual field of the subjects (see below). In order to minimize the expected effects, patients were not told about the potential response of control and DCEAS procedure during random assignment.

Fluoxetine treatment

Unmedicated patients in both groups received orally administered FLX for 3 weeks in an open manner. FLX dose was initiated at 10 mg/day and escalated to an optimal dose within one week based on individual patients' response, with a maximum dose of 40 mg/day. Attaining a balance of efficacy and side effects, this FLX dosing regimen has been widely used in previous studies of major depression in the Chinese population [20,21]. Those who

were currently treated with FLX for no more than one week continued their FLX treatment with the same dose. Those who were currently treated with other psychotropic medications for no more than one week were required to be switched to the FLX regimen by gradually withdrawing the drugs within one week in order to wash out potential "carryover" effects. The information about the equivalent efficacy of FLX was offered to the patients. Concomitant use of other psychotropic drugs was not allowed. Medication compliance was determined by pill count at each study visit. Patients who required concomitant medications and those having less than 80% FLX compliance were advised to withdraw from the study.

DCEAS and n-EA procedure

The patients received 9 sessions of n-EA or DCEAS intervention (3 sessions per week) during FLX treatment. Electrical stimulation was delivered on the following 6 matches of forehead acupoints that are innervated by the trigeminal nerve via inserted or non-inserted needles (Fig. 1): Baihui (Du-20) and Yintang (EX-HN3), left Sishencong (EX-HN1) and Toulinqi (GB15), right Sishencong (EX-HN1) and Toulinqi (GB15), bilateral Shuaigu (GB8), bilateral Taiyang (EX-HN5), and bilateral Touwei (ST8). For DCEAS, disposable acupuncture needles (0.30 mm in diameter and 25–40 mm in length) were inserted into acupoints for a depth of 10–30 mm in a direction oblique or parallel to the surface. To ensure allocation concealment, the inserted needles were affixed with adhesive tapes so that DCEAS procedure was identical to control acupuncture procedure. Electrical stimulation with continuous waves at 2 Hz and constant current and voltage (9 V) was delivered via an acupuncture stimulation instrument (Hwarto, SDZ-II) for 30 min (the pulse width could not be determined in this model instrument). The choice of this stimulation mode was based on the fact that low frequency could exert broader effects on central neurochemical systems compared to high frequency and has been widely introduced into the treatment of neuropsychiatric disorders [10,22]. The intensity of stimulation was adjusted to a level at which the patients felt most comfortable. For n-EA procedure, Streitberger's noninvasive acupuncture needles were used [23,24]. Its validity and credibility have been well demonstrated [23,24]. The needles with blunt tips were quickly put onto the same acupoints used in DCEAS without inserting into the skin. The needles were then affixed with plastic O-rings and adhesive tapes. Electrical stimulation was delivered with the same parameters as DCEAS. Patients felt the stimulation via blunt tips touched on the skin.

To ensure consistency in acupuncture procedure, the principal investigator (Z.J.Z.) provided a training workshop of acupuncture protocol. Acupuncture intervention was performed by registered acupuncturists (W.W. and S.C.M.) who had received 5-year undergraduate training in Chinese medicine and had practiced Chinese medicine over three years.

Assessment

Treatment outcomes were changes from baseline in the total score on HAMD-17 [18], CGI-S [19], and the Chinese-version Self-rating Depression Scale (SDS) [25] at baseline and at day 3, 7, 14, and 21. The secondary outcome measures included treatment response, defined as $\geq 50\%$ reduction at endpoint from baseline on HAMD-17, and remission, defined as an endpoint HAMD-17 score of ≤ 7. Safety and tolerability were assessed using the Treatment Emergent Symptom Scale (TESS) [19], in which adverse events were recorded at each visit, including their date and time of onset, duration, severity, relationship to intervention, and the action taken.

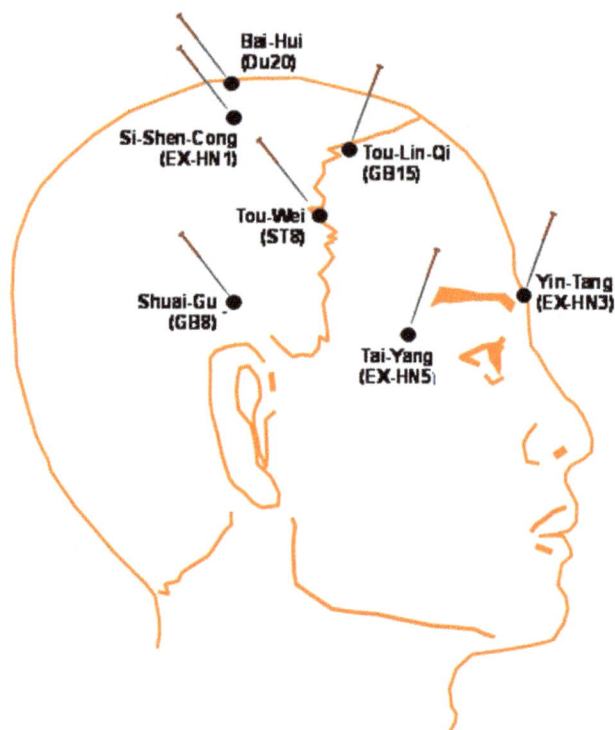

Figure 1. Acupoints used in dense cranial electroacupuncture stimulation (DCEAS).

Both patients and raters were blind to the treatment allocation. A training workshop with video materials was conducted for raters who might be involved in clinical assessments. An interrater reliability coefficient (κ value) of >0.80 was achieved after the completion of training workshop. In this study, all assessments were completed by the same rater (J.L.).

The credibility of n-EA and DCEAS procedure was evaluated based on Fink et al. method [26] by asking the patients: "As we informed you that you had an equal chance of receiving sham or active acupuncture treatment, which do you think you had received?"

Statistical analysis

Based on our recent meta-analysis, a sample size of 70 patients (n = 35 per group) could provide approximately 80% power to detect an estimated difference in HAMD-17 score of 3 points, with α set at 0.05 and an estimated standard deviation of 4.5 at the endpoint of 3-week treatment [5].

Efficacy analyses were performed on the intention-to-treat population, defined as participants who completed baseline and at least one evaluation after treatment. Since measure time points were not balanced, a linear mixed-effects model was preferably applied to compare treatment outcomes (HAMD-17, CGI-S and SDS) over time between the two groups. The model was established using time and group for categorical fixed factors and random intercepts with scaled identity covariance matrix. Subject's age, gender, duration of the illness, number of relapse, baseline HAMD-17, tolerability and credibility for acupuncture procedure were treated as covariates. Between-group differences at each measure time point were examined using Student t-test. The data was expressed as mean with 95% confidence interval (95% CI). Student t test was used to compare continuous baseline variables between the two groups. Categorical variables, including categorical baseline variables, response and remission rates, incidence of adverse events, treatment compliance, and credibility, were analyzed using Chi-square (χ^2) test or Fisher exact test if one or more expected frequencies were less than 5. Statistical significance was defined as a two-sided $P<0.05$. The analyses were performed with SPSS version 16 software (Chicago, IL, USA).

Results

Disposition and characteristics of patients

Of 188 outpatients referred by psychiatrists for screening, 73 eligible patients were randomly assigned to n-EA (n = 35) and DCEAS (n = 38) group; while 63 (86.3%) of them completed the 3-week assessment. One patient in n-EA group was excluded from analysis, because she was later found to have cocaine use in the past year. Two patients in DCEAS group were excluded from analysis due to a lack of post-baseline assessment. Seventy patients (34 in n-EA and 36 in DCEAS) were included in data analysis (Fig. 2).

Baseline characteristics of patients are summarized in Table 1. The proportion of females assigned to n-EA group was significantly higher than that in DCEAS group (97.1% vs. 69.4%, $P = 0.006$, Chi-square test). Other baseline variables were similar in the two groups. Nearly 93% (65/70) patients had experienced relapses and 66% (46/70) patients had acupuncture treatment previously. There were only 18.6% (13/70) of patients receiving psychotropic medication when entering the study. The compliance with acupuncture and FLX treatment was nearly 95% in the two groups.

Efficacy

Changes from baseline in score on HAMD-17, CGI-S, and SDS over time are illustrated in Table 2 and Fig. 3. The analyses based on linear mixed-effects model revealed highly linear correlations between measure time points and changes from baseline in score on HAMD ($r^2 = 0.497$ in n-EA group and $r^2 = 0.531$ in DCEAS group, $P<0.0001$), CGI ($r^2 = 0.400$ in n-EA group and $r^2 = 0.381$ in DCEAS group, $P<0.0001$), and SDS ($r^2 = 0.192$ in n-EA group and $r^2 = 0.248$ in DCEAS group, $P<0.0001$). There were significant differences in the slope and/or intercept between n-EA and DCEAS groups on HAMD ($F = 5.938$, df = 1,336, $P = 0.015$) and SDS ($F = 5.885$, df = 1,336, $P = 0.016$), but not CGI ($F = 232$, df = 1,336, $P = 0.631$). Between-group comparisons further revealed that DCEAS-treated patients had a significantly greater reduction in scores on HAMD-17 compared to patients receiving n-EA procedure at Day 3 through Day 21 ($P \leq 0.025$). The significantly greater reduction was also observed in SDS scores at day 3 ($P = 0.037$) and day 21 ($P = 0.004$).

The response rate in DCEAS group was not significantly different from that in n-EA group (19.4% (7/36) vs. 8.8% (3/34), $P = 0.308$, Fisher Exact test). The remission rate was also similar in the two groups (2.7% (1/36) vs. 2.9% (1/34), $P = 0.998$, Fisher Exact test).

The average dose of FLX in DCEAS group was similar to that in n-EA group (23.01±3.2 mg/day (mean ± SD) vs. 23.4±2.4 mg/day, $P = 0.599$, t-test).

Safety and tolerability

Adverse events occurred in at least 5% of the patients in either group are listed in Table 3. No significant differences in the incidence of any adverse events were found between the two groups. There were 20.6% (7/34) of patients who felt uncomfortable in n-EA procedure, but not significantly different from 38.9%

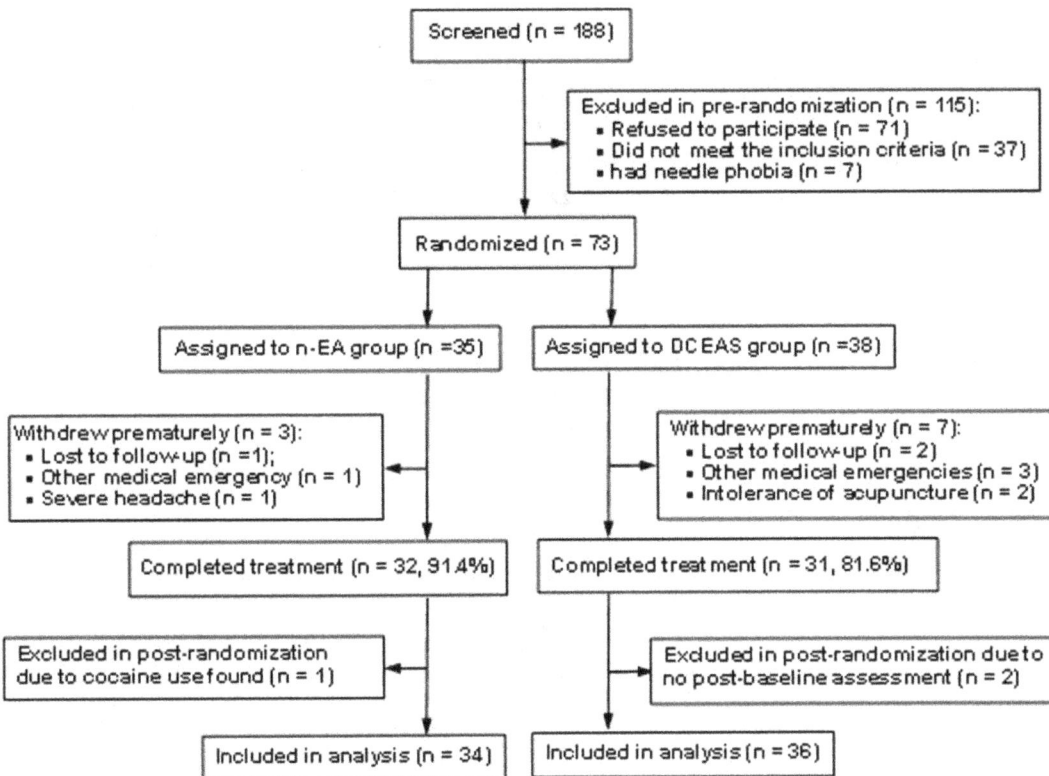

Figure 2. Flowchart of screening and patient recruitment. n-EA, noninvasive electroacupuncture; DCEAS, dense cranial electroacupuncture stimulation.

Table 1. Baseline characteristics of patients.

Variables	n-EA (n = 34)	DCEAS (n = 36)	P values (t or χ^2 test)
Female, n (%)	33 (97.1)	25 (69.4)	0.006
Age (yrs)[a]	48.2±9.8	46.3±9.9	0.414
Duration of MDD (yrs)[a]	7.3±7.1	7.9±8.0	0.744
No. of previous depressive episodes[a]	3.6±4.4	4.9±6.1	0.332
No. (%) of patients with first-onset MDD	3 (8.8)	2 (5.5)	0.669
No. (%) of patients with previous psychiatric admission	8 (23.5)	7 (19.4)	0.901
No. (%) of patients with family members having mental illnesses.	9 (26.5)	13 (36.1)	0.800
No. (%) of patients with previous acupuncture treatment[b]	22 (64.7)	24 (66.7)	0.937
No. (%) of patients receiving psychotropic medications at study entry[c]	6 (17.6)	7 (19.4)	0.909
SSRIs	3	3	
SNRIs	1	1	
Mood stabilizers	1[d]	1	
Benzodiazepines	2	2	
Baseline HAMD-17 score[a]	23.1±3.6	23.9±3.8	0.321
Baseline CGI-S[a]	4.3±0.5	4.4±0.5	0.760
Baseline SDS score[a]	40.6±14.5	41.9±14.0	0.704

[a]Continuous data are expressed as mean ± SD.
[b]Auricular acupuncture was included.
[c]The use of medications did not exceed one week.
[d]One patient received a combination of SNRIs and mood stabilizers.
n-EA, noninvasive electroacupuncture; DCEAS, dense cranial electroacupuncture stimulation; MDD, major depressive disorder; SSRIs, selective serotonin re-uptake inhibitors; SNRIs, Serotonin–norepinephrine reuptake inhibitors; HAMD, 17-item Hamilton Rating Scale for Depression; CGI-S, Clinical Global Impression-Severity; SDS, Self-rating Depression Scale.

Table 2. Changes in score on depression scales from baseline in MDD patients.

Variables	n-EA (n = 34) (95% CI)	DCEAS (n = 36) (95% CI)	Between-group difference (95% CI)	Overall P value[a]	Between-group P value[a]
HAMD-17				0.015	
Day 3	−3.71 (−4.34−−3.06)	−5.97 (−6.71−−5.23)	2.27 (1.29–3.25)		0.000
Day 7	−5.82 (−6.46−−5.18)	−6.97 (−7.71−−6.23)	1.15 (0.17–2.13)		0.025
Day 14	−6.41 (−7.05−−5.77)	−8.44 (−9.18−−7.70)	2.03 (1.05–3.01)		0.000
Day 21	−6.27 (−6.90−−5.62)	−8.66 (−9.39−−7.91)	2.39 (1.41–3.37)		0.000
CGI-S				0.631	
Day 3	−0.32 (−0.42−−0.22)	−0.44 (−0.54−−0.34)	0.12 (−0.03–0.27)		0.116
Day 7	−0.65 (−0.75−−0.55)	−0.53 (−0.63−−0.43)	0.12 (−0.03–0.27)		0.116
Day 14	−0.71 (−0.81−−0.61)	−0.71 (−0.81−−0.61)	0.00 (−0.15–0.15)		1.000
Day 21	−0.74 (−0.84−−0.64)	−0.74 (−0.84−−0.64)	0.00 (−0.15–0.15)		1.000
SDS				0.016	
Day 3	−6.44 (−8.48−−4.40)	−9.76 (−12.03−−7.49)	3.32 (0.26–6.38)		0.037
Day 7	−8.82 (−10.86−−6.78)	−9.12 (−11.39−−6.85)	0.30 (−2.76–3.36)		0.851
Day 14	−11.74 (−13.78−−9.70)	−12.38 (−14.65−−10.11)	0.64 (−2.42–3.70)		0.679
Day 21	−8.38 (−10.42−−6.34)	−13.06 (−15.33−−10.79)	4.68 (1.62–7.74)		0.004

[a]Overall and between-group P values were obtained from linear mixed-effects model analysis and student t-test, respectively.
MDD, major depressive disorder; n-EA, noninvasive electroacupuncture; DCEAS, dense cranial electroacupuncture stimulation; 95% CI, 95% confidence interval; HAMD-17, 17-item Hamilton Rating Scale for Depression; CGI-S, Clinical Global Impression-Severity; SDS, Self-rating Depression Scale.

(14/36) in DCEAS-treated patients ($\chi^2 = 1.985$, df = 1, $P = 0.159$). Two patients in DCEAS group discontinued due to intolerance of acupuncture stimulation.

Credibility of sham and DCEAS procedure

There was no significant difference in the credibility rating between the two groups, with 45.5% (15/33) of patients treated with n-EA perceiving to have received DCEAS, while 23.5% (8/34) of patients in DCEAS believed to have n-EA treatment ($\chi^2 = 2.665$, $P = 0.103$).

Discussion

The present study demonstrated that DCEAS intervention is effective in augmenting the antidepressant efficacy of FLX in the treatment of moderate and severe MDD. While the patients in the two groups had received similar FLX doses during the study, DCEAS-treated patients exhibited greater improvement on depressive symptoms, as indicated with the significant greater reduction of HAMD-17 and SDS score at most measure time points, although the magnitude of the reduction of SGI-S score, the response and remission rates were not different in the two groups. Moreover, the greater reduction of both HAMD-17 and SDS was observed as early as at day 3 after the first session of acupuncture treatment. Similar result was also present at endpoint of three weeks of DCEAS intervention. These data suggest that DCEAS intervention produces a rapid effect in alleviating depressive symptoms in both clinician-rated (HAMD-17) and self-rated (SDS) measures of depression. In addition, there were only two DCEAS-treated patients who discontinued due to intolerance of acupuncture. DCEAS intervention did not increase the incidence of any adverse events compared to n-EA control procedure, suggesting that DCEAS is a tolerable and safe stimulation mode.

While the current study showed the superior antidepressant efficacy of DCEAS over n-EA procedure when combined with FLX, several similar trials failed to demonstrate the superior effects

of active acupuncture regimens in reducing depressive symptoms compared to sham and placebo acupuncture regimens [27–29]. This has raised the argument that the antidepressant benefits of acupuncture observed may be derived from placebo effects rather than physiological mechanisms [28]. Nevertheless, the present study revealed no significant difference in the credibility of the control and DCEAS procedures, with nearly 46% of n-EA-treated patients who perceived to have received active procedure, while 24% of DCEAS-treated patients perceived the control procedure, suggesting that the non-inserted needling stimulation used in the present study for a control procedure was valid and acceptable. In fact, previous studies have well demonstrated the high credibility of the non-inserted needle device [26]. Therefore, it was unlikely that the antidepressant benefits of DCEAS observed in the present study were derived from placebo effects.

There are two possible explanations for negative results in the previous acupuncture studies of major depression [27–29]. Firstly, unlike the present study that used the non-inserted control procedure, the previous studies needled at non-meridian-based acupoints which are located at a certain distances (usually 1–3 cm) from the meridian-based acupoints [27–29]. Although there seems to be some differences in the histological profile between the meridian- and non-meridian-based acupoints [30], it might be difficult to differentiate the physiological responses induced by stimulation at the two types of acupoints. Second, relatively few acupoints were used in the previous studies [27–29]. This may result in inadequacy of acupuncture stimulation which is believed to be an important factor associated with negative results of acupuncture trials [31].

DCEAS was developed mainly based on a neurobiological rationale. It is well documented that the forehead acupoints innervated by the trigeminal sensory pathway have intimate collateral connections with the brainstem reticular formation, in particular the dorsal raphe nucleus (DRN) [32,33] and the locus coeruleus (LC) [34–37]. The latter two brain structures are the major resources of 5-HT and NA neuronal bodies, respectively,

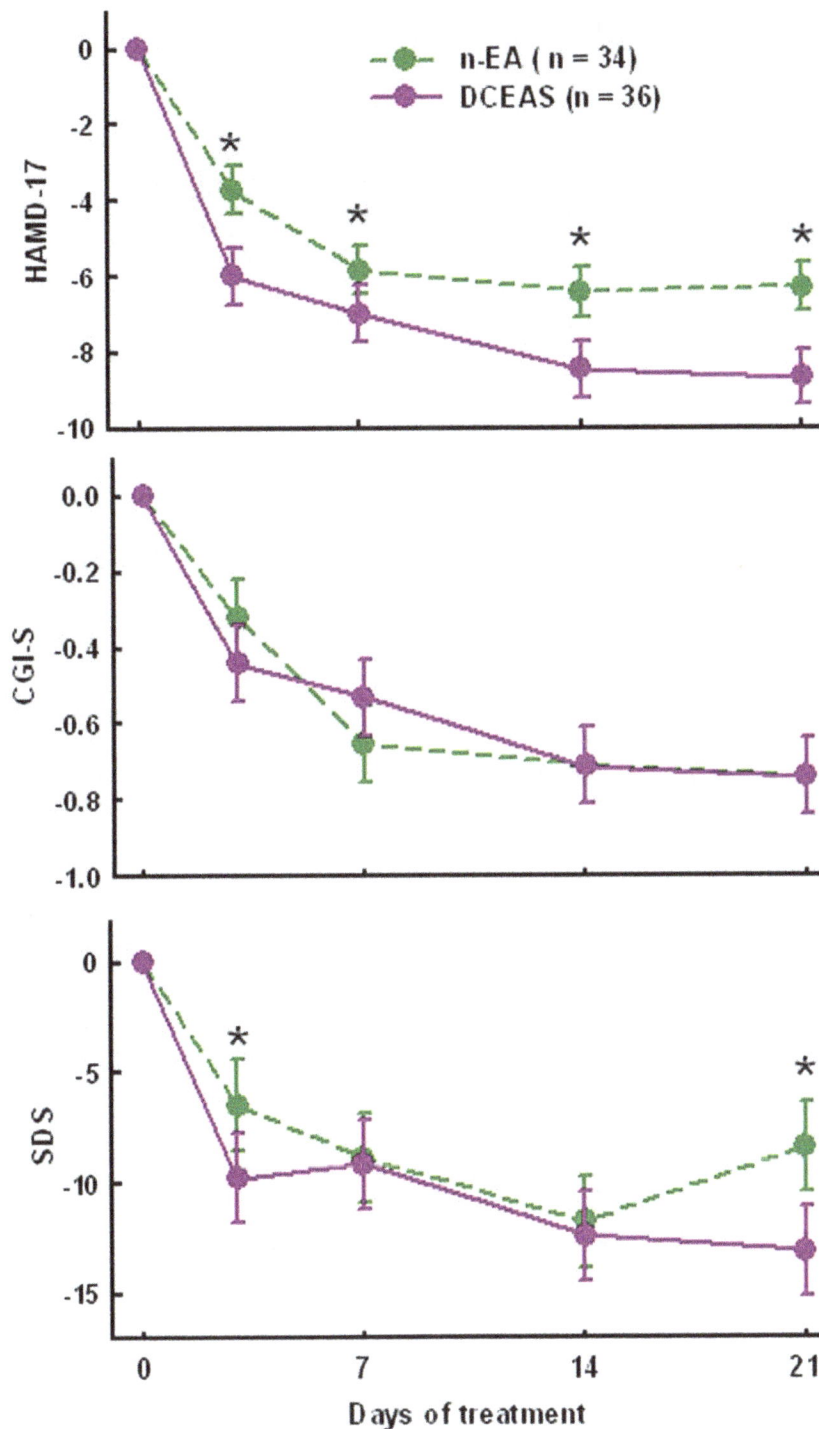

Figure 3. Mean changes from baseline in score on the 17-item Hamilton Rating Scale for Depression (HAMD-17), Clinical Global Impression-Severity (CGI-S) and Self-rating Depression Scale (SDS). Data are expressed as mean with 95% confidence interval (95% CI). * $P \leq 0.037$: between-group comparison using Student t-test.

sending diffuse projections to subcortical and cortical areas, including the prefrontal cortex and the amygdala known to be heavily involved in the pathogenesis of depressive disorders [38]. A large body of evidence confirms that the brainstem 5-HT and NA neuronal systems play a pivotal role in acupuncture modulation of multiple brain functions, including pain, emotion, sleep, and visceral information processing [8–10,39]. Neuroanatomical and

neurophysiological studies have demonstrated that electroacupuncture stimulation increases the expression of 5-HT in the DRN [40] and suppresses the stress-induced increase in neuronal activities of the LC [41,42]. Neuroimaging studies have also shown that electroacupuncture stimulation is capable of directly modulating the activity of the emotion processing-related brain regions [8]. Through the intimate collateral connection from the trigeminal

Table 3. Adverse events occurred in at least 5% of patients in either group.

Event	n-EA (n = 34)	DCEAS (n = 36)	χ^2	P value
Dizziness	15 (44.1)	11 (30.6)	0.858	0.354
Tiredness	10 (29.4)	15 (41.7)	0.672	0.412
Nausea	10 (29.4)	10 (27.8)	0.013	0.910
Excessive sweating	9 (26.5)	6 (16.7)	1.403	0.236
Headache	8 (23.5)	10 (27.8)	0.018	0.894
Transient tachycardia	8 (23.5)	9 (25.0)	0.018	0.892
Insomnia	7 (20.6)	9 (25.0)	0.024	0.877
Uncomfortable for needling sensation	7 (20.6)	14 (38.9)	1.985	0.159
Vomiting	4 (11.8)	3 (8.3)		0.706[a]
Unsteadiness	2 (5.9)	6 (16.7)		0.266[a]
Somnolence	2 (5.9)	6 (16.7)		0.266[a]

[a]P values were calculated from Fisher Exact test.
n-EA, noninvasive electroacupuncture; DCEAS, dense cranial electroacupuncture stimulation.

sensory pathway to the brainstem 5-HT and NA neuronal systems, the needling of the forehead acupoints with subsequent electrical stimulation could robustly elicit afferent acupuncture signals via biophysical and biochemical reactions at local acupoints and, in turn, efficiently modulates central 5-HT and NA neuronal functions [9,10]. On the other hand, like other noninvasive brain stimulation therapies, such as transcutaneous electrical nerve stimulation (TENS), repetitive transcranial magnetic stimulation (rTMS), and electroconvulsive therapy (ECT) [43,44], electrical stimulation was also directly delivered on the scalp in both control and DCEAS procedure. This may elicit a transcutaneous and/or transcranial effect; however, such effect would likely be minimal as the stimulation intensity used in both n-EA control and DCEAS procedures was generally much lower than rTMS, ECT, and most TENS [43,44]. Therefore, we have reason to believe that the antidepressant efficacy of DCEAS observed in the present study should be derived mainly from the biophysical and biochemical effects produced in needling with subsequent electrical stimulation [45]. This also could explain the superior therapeutic efficacy of DCEAS over n-EA control procedure.

Several limitations of the present study should be noticed. First, the study was conducted in a female-dominated sample with a significant difference in the proportion of female subjects between the two groups. Epidemiological evidence suggests that women are more likely to use complementary and alternative medicine (CAM) and have a higher degree of confidence in CAM efficacy and safety [46]. Whether similar therapeutic effects of DCEAS could be achieved in male patients needs to be further investigated. In addition, as the study was conducted in a single-blind manner, effects mediated by non-blinded acupuncturists could not be excluded. Recently, a well-demonstrated control method for single-blind condition has been introduced and could be considered in future studies [47]. Second, although DCEAS achieved a clinically meaningful, over 2-fold difference in the response rate than the control procedure (19.4% vs. 8.8%), the difference did not reach statistical significance level. This may be due to the relatively low response rates in the two groups when compared to other similar trials, with response rates of 22–80% for active acupuncture and 39–78% for sham or placebo-treated groups [27–29]. The relatively low response rate observed in the present study appears to be related to the short-term (3-week) treatment. As long-term effects of DCEAS were not evaluated in this study and a majority of

depressed patients may be required for long-term treatment [48], long-term antidepressant efficacy of DCEAS may deserve to be further investigated. Finally, although we measured patients' platelet 5-HT contents at baseline and posttreatment (data not shown in this report), no significant changes in platelet 5-HT parameters were observed in DCEAS-treated patients compared to patients treated with n-EA, suggesting that acupuncture may have least effects on non-neuronal 5-HT systems. Evaluation of DCEAS effects in the brain 5-HT neuronal system may help gain new insight into central mechanisms responsible for DCEAs effects.

Collectively, the present study demonstrates that DCEAS is a safe and effective intervention in augmenting the antidepressant efficacy in the early phase of SSRI treatment. As patients with moderate and severe major depression have a higher risk of suicide and the worsening of symptoms in the early phase of SSRI treatment, DCEAS can be considered as an additional treatment option. The present study guarantees a larger-scale, multi-site trial to further determine the effectiveness of DCEAS as a viable and safe non-pharmacological augmentation for depressive disorders.

Supporting Information

Checklist S1   CONSORT Checklist.
(PDF)

Protocol S1   Trial Protocol.
(PDF)

Acknowledgments

We thank the following colleagues at Department of Psychiatry of Kowloon Hospital for their assistance in patient recruitment: Ka-Lik Kwan, Chun-Ting Chan, Man-Lui Chan, Chi-Kwan Cheung, Janice Chik, Lung-Kit Hui, Man-Man Kwan, Chee-Kin Lee, Kwok-Chuen Ng, Yin-Ting Ng, Ting-Keung Poon, Fu-Yin Tong, Wai-Ching Yan, Kam-Hing Yeung, Tin-Yan Yeung, Mei-Kuen Frieda Shiu, Cheuk-Kin Tang, Pui-Shan Tse, Ngar-Fong Lam, See-Cheuk Fu, Chui-Lin Carol Ching, Ka-Fai Ho, Sau-Lai Tai, Sau-Ming Chan, Yiu-Kwun Law, and Yuk-Kwan Yvonne Kwong.

Author Contributions

Conceived and designed the experiments: Z-JZ RN Q-RT K-cY. Performed the experiments: SCM TYJL WW M-TW W-KAT. Analyzed the data: Z-JZ HKW. Wrote the paper: Z-JZ RN Q-RT K-FC EZ VTW.

References

1. Arroll B, Macgillivray S, Ogston S, Reid I, Sullivan F, et al. (2005) Efficacy and tolerability of tricyclic antidepressants and SSRIs compared with placebo for treatment of depression in primary care: a meta-analysis. Ann Fam Med 3: 449–456.
2. Blier P, de Montigny C (1994) Current advances and trends in the treatment of depression. Trends Pharmacol Sci 15: 220–226.
3. Blier P (2003) The pharmacology of putative early-onset antidepressant strategies. Eur Neuropsychopharmacol 13: 57–66.
4. Adell A, Castro E, Celada P, Bortolozzi A, Pazos A, et al. (2005) Strategies for producing faster acting antidepressants. Drug Discov Today 10: 578–585.
5. Zhang ZJ, Chen HY, Yip KC, Ng R, Wong VT (2010) The effectiveness and safety of acupuncture therapy in depressive disorders: systematic review and meta-analysis. J Affect Disord 124: 9–21.
6. Smith CA, Hay PP, Macpherson H (2010) Acupuncture for depression. Cochrane Database Syst Rev 20: CD004046.
7. Wang H, Qi H, Wang BS, Cui YY, Zhu L, et al. (2008) Is acupuncture beneficial in depression: a meta-analysis of 8 randomized controlled trials? J Affect Disord 111: 125–134.
8. Dhond RP, Kettner N, Napadow V (2007) Neuroimaging acupuncture effects in the human brain. Altern Complement Med 13: 603–616.
9. Zhao ZQ (2008) Neural mechanism underlying acupuncture analgesia. Prog Neurobiol 85: 355–375.
10. Ulett GA, Han S, Han JS (1998) Electroacupuncture: mechanisms and clinical application. Biol Psychiatry 44: 129–138.
11. Belmaker RH, Agam G (2008) Major depressive disorder. N Engl J Med 358: 55–68.
12. Zhang ZJ, Wang XY, Tan QR, Jin GX, Yao SM (2009) Electroacupuncture for refractory obsessive-compulsive disorder: a pilot waitlist-controlled trial. J Nerv Ment Dis 197: 619–22.
13. Huang Y, Gong W, Zou J, Zhao CH (2004) An SCL-90 analysis of scalp electroacupuncture treatment of major depressive episode. Shanghai Zhen Jiu Za Zhi 23: 5–7. (in Chinese with English abstract).
14. Li HJ, Zhong BL, Fan YP, Hu HT (2011) Acupuncture for post-stroke depression: a randomized controlled trial. Zhongguo Zhen Jiu 31: 3–6. (in Chinese with English abstract).
15. Yeung WF, Chung KF, Tso KC, Zhang SP, Zhang ZJ, et al. (2011) Electroacupuncture for residual insomnia associated with major depressive disorder: a randomized controlled trial. Sleep 34: 807–815.
16. Stark P, Hardison CD (1985) A review of multicenter controlled studies of fluoxetine vs. imipramine and placebo in outpatients with major depressive disorder. J Clin Psychiatry 46: 53–58.
17. American Psychiatric Association (1994) Diagnostic and statistical manual of mental disorders. 4th ed. Washington, DC: American Psychiatric Association Press.
18. Hamilton M (1960) A rating scale for depression. Journal of Neurology Neurosurgery and Psychiatry 23: 56–62.
19. Guy W (1976) ECDEU assessment manual for psychopharmacology. revised. Bethesda, MD: US Department of Health, Education, and Welfare.
20. Hong CJ, Hu WH, Chen CC, Hsiao CC, Tsai SJ, et al. (2003) A double-blind, randomized, group-comparative study of the tolerability and efficacy of 6 weeks' treatment with mirtazapine or fluoxetine in depressed Chinese patients. J Clin Psychiat 64: 921–926.
21. Yu YW, Tsai SJ, Liou YJ, Hong CJ, Chen TJ (2006) Association study of two serotonin 1A receptor gene polymorphisms and fluoxetine treatment response in Chinese major depressive disorders. Eur Neuropsychopharmacol 16: 498–503.
22. Han JS (2003) Acupuncture: neuropeptide release produced by electrical stimulation of different frequencies. Trends Neurosci 26: 17–22.
23. Streitberger K, Kleinhenz J (1998) Introducing a placebo needle into acupuncture research. Lancet 352: 364–365.
24. Enck P, Klosterhalfen S, Zipfel S (2010) Acupuncture, psyche and the placebo response. Auton Neurosci 157: 68–73.
25. Lee HC, Chiu HF, Wing YK, Leung CM, Kwong PK, et al. (1994) The Zung Self-rating Depression Scale: screening for depression among the Hong Kong Chinese elderly. J Geriatr Psychiatry Neurol 7: 216–220.
26. Fink M, Gutenbrunner C, Rollnik J, Karst M (2001) Credibility of a newly designed placebo needle for clinical trials in acupuncture research. Forsch Komplementarmed Klass Naturheilkd 8: 368–372.
27. Allen JJ, Schnyer RN, Chambers AS, Hitt SK, Moreno FA, et al. (2006) Acupuncture for depression: a randomized controlled trial. J Clin Psychiatry 67: 1665–1673.
28. Andreescu C, Glick RM, Emeremni CA, Houck PR, Mulsant BH (2011) Acupuncture for the treatment of major depressive disorder: a randomized controlled trial. J Clin Psychiatry 2011;72: 1129–1135.
29. Zhang WJ, Yang XB, Zhong BL (2009) Combination of acupuncture and fluoxetine for depression: a randomized, double-blind, sham-controlled trial. J Altern Complement Med 15: 837–844.
30. Zhou F, Huang D, Xia Y (2009) Neuroanatomical basis of acupuncture points (Chapter 2). In Xia Y, Wu G, Cao X, Chen J, eds. Acupuncture therapy for neurological diseases: a neurobiological view, Tsinghua University Press, Beijing, and Springer-Verlag Berlin, Heidelberg. pp 32–80.
31. Benham A, Johnson MI (2009) Could acupuncture needle sensation be a predictor of analgesic response? Acupunct Med 27: 65–67.
32. Arbab MA, Delgado T, Wiklund L, Svendgaard NA (1988) Brain stem terminations of the trigeminal and upper spinal ganglia innervation of the cerebrovascular system: WGA-HRP transganglionic study. J Cereb Blood Flow Metab 8: 54–63.
33. Kubota K, Narita N, Ohkubo K, Hosaka K, Nagae K, et al. (1988) Central projection of proprioceptive afferents arising from maxillo-facial regions in some animals studied by HRP-labeling technique. Anat Anz 165: 229–251.
34. Foote SL, Bloom FE, Aston-Jones G (1983) Nucleus locus ceruleus: new evidence of anatomical and physiological specificity. Physiol Rev 63: 844–914.
35. Simpson KL, Altman DW, Wang L, Kirifides ML, Lin RC, et al. (1997) Lateralization and functional organization of the locus coeruleus projection to the trigeminal somatosensory pathway in rat. J Comp Neurol 385: 135–147.
36. Simpson KL, Waterhouse BD, Lin RC (1999) Origin, distribution, and morphology of galaninergic fibers in the rodent trigeminal system. J Comp Neurol 411: 524–534.
37. Takahashi T, Shirasu M, Shirasu M, Kubo KY, Onozuka M, et al. (2010) The locus coeruleus projects to the mesencephalic trigeminal nucleus in rats. Neurosci Res 68: 103–106.
38. Clark L, Chamberlain SR, Sahakian BJ (2009) Neurocognitive mechanisms in depression: implications for treatment. Annu Rev Neurosci 32: 57–74.
39. Takahashi T (2006) Acupuncture for functional gastrointestinal disorders. J Gastroenterol 41: 408–417.
40. Kwon YB, Kang MS, Son SS, Kim JT, Lee YH, et al. (2000) Different frequencies of electroacupuncture modified the cellular activity of serotonergic neurons in brainstem. Am J Chin Med 28: 435–441.
41. Lee HJ, Lee B, Choi SH, Hahm DH, Kim MR, et al. (2004) Electroacupuncture reduces stress-induced expression of c-fos in the brain of the rat. Am J Chin Med 32: 795–806.
42. Li A, Wang Y, Xin J, Lao L, Ren K, et al. (2007) Electroacupuncture suppresses hyperalgesia and spinal Fos expression by activating the descending inhibitory system. Brain Res 1186: 171–179.
43. Kirkcaldie M, Pridmore S, Reid P (1997) Bridging the skull: electroconvulsive therapy (ECT) and repetitive transcranial magnetic stimulation (rTMS) in psychiatry. Convulsive Therapy 13: 83–91.
44. van Dijk KR, Scherder EJ, Scheltens P, Sergeant JA (2002) Effects of transcutaneous electrical nerve stimulation (TENS) on non-pain related cognitive and behavioural functioning. Rev Neurosci 13: 257–270.
45. Zhang ZJ, Wang XM, McAlonan GM (2011) Neural acupuncture unit (NAU): a new concept for interpreting effects and mechanisms of acupuncture. eCAM (accepted, Article ID: 429412).
46. Barnes PM, Powell-Griner E, McFann K, Nahin RL (2004) Complementary and alternative medicine use among adults: United States, Adv Data 27: 1–19.
47. La Marca R, Nedeljkovic M, Yuan L, Maercker A, Ehlert U (2010) Effects of auricular electrical stimulation on vagal activity in healthy men: Evidence from a three-armed randomized trial. Clin Sci (Lond) 118: 537–546.
48. Keller MB, Berndt ER (2002) Depression treatment: a lifelong commitment? Psychopharmacol Bull 36(S2): 133–141.

14

Analysis of 30 Patients with Acupuncture-Induced Primary Inoculation Tuberculosis

Yangbo Liu[1], Jingye Pan[2], Keke Jin[3], Cailong Liu[1], Jing Wang[1], Li Chen[4], Lei Chen[1]*, Jiandong Yuan[1]*

1 Orthopedics, The First Affiliated Hospital of Wenzhou Medical University, Wenzhou, Zhejiang, China, 2 Intensive Care Unit, The First Affiliated Hospital of Wenzhou Medical University, Wenzhou, Zhejiang, China, 3 Pathophysiology, Wenzhou Medical University, Wenzhou, Zhejiang, China, 4 Biomedicine, The University of Melbourne, Melbourne, Victoria, Australia

Abstract

Primary inoculation tuberculosis is a skin condition that develops at the site of inoculation of *Mycobacterium tuberculosis* in tuberculosis-free individuals. This report describes the diagnosis, treatment and >1 year follow-up of 30 patients presenting with acupuncture-induced primary inoculation tuberculosis. Our data provide a deeper insight into this rare route of infection of tuberculosis. We also review effective treatment options.

Editor: Pere-Joan Cardona, Fundació Institut d'Investigació en Ciències de la Salut Germans Trias i Pujol. Universitat Autònoma de Barcelona. CIBERES, Spain

Funding: The authors have no support or funding to report.

Competing Interests: The authors have declared that no competing interests exist.

* Email: chenlei@wzhospital.cn (Lei Chen); liuybwz@me.com (JY)

Introduction

Tuberculosis (TB) has existed in humans for millennia [1]. It is estimated that approximately one third of the world's population is infected with *Mycobacterium tuberculosis* which causes 8.8 million new cases of tuberculosis accounting for approximately 1.1 million deaths each year [2].

Pulmonary tuberculosis is by far the most abundant form: extra-pulmonary tuberculosis accounts for about 20% of cases and tuberculosis of the skeleton-muscular system accounts for 10% of all infections. Interestingly, a low incidence (0.1%) of primary inoculation tuberculosis has also been reported [3–5].

In the United States, extra-pulmonary tuberculosis accounts for 18% of all tuberculosis infection, with cutaneous tuberculosis representing 1.8% of cases [6]. Few case reports of primary inoculation tuberculosis are available, with only 33 cases being described between 1935 to 2012. The largest number of cases described in the literature is five [7].

Given the difference in invasive routes between primary inoculation and pulmonary tuberculosis, no generalization can be made as for incubation period, clinical features, treatment and prognosis of primary inoculation tuberculosis based on lung disease case reports to guide clinical practices. In this study, we described 30 cases with primary inoculation tuberculosis (7 confirmed and 23 suspected) that developed over a short period of time. All subjects were followed up for at least one year to assess the effectiveness of a combination of drug and surgical intervention in treating primary inoculation tuberculosis.

Case Description and Methods

Patients and source of infection

Seven confirmed and 23 suspected, total 30 patients (13 male and 17 female) with primary inoculation tuberculosis were selected from the same clinic in Wenzhou City, China that specialized in treatment of muscle and soft tissue pain and osteoarthritis of the knee. Seven confirmed cases ages ranged from 31 to 67 years (mean: 53.14 years), and total 30 patients ages ranged from 31 to 71 years (mean: 52.3 years).

They had all undergone acupuncture and electrotherapy, administered by the same clinician, once every two days for about two weeks for the treatment of neck, back, elbow, wrist, hip, knee and ankle pain. The procedures took place between May 2011 and August 2011. All the patients were screened by chest X-rays for pulmonary tuberculosis. Only one suspected patient had a history of inactive pulmonary tuberculosis lesions on chest X-rays with negative sputum examination.

Three suspected patients had a medical history of type 2 diabetes. All subjects were negative for HIV.

In most patients the electrotherapy lasted 10–30 min. All injection materials were disposable. A total of four electrotherapeutic pads were used, without disinfection.

Most patients linked the lesion sites to electrotherapy. Therefore, it was speculated that the occurrence of tuberculosis infection might have resulted from the introduction of tubercle bacilli from the electrotherapeutic pads, into soft tissues via small skin wounds. However, culture of samples from the four electrotherapeutic pads appeared negative. Accordingly, it was impossible to determine the source of contamination.

Over the same time period, a total of 58 subjects had undergone invasive treatment at the clinic. There were three cases with unknown condition due to loss of contact, and 25 cases that did not contract infection. 18 patients out of the 55 received triamcinolone acetonide treatment at the acupuncture sites. The same batch of un-used drugs was tested to be qualified and effective. The treatment procedure with triamcinolone acetonide was triamcinolone acetonide + vitamin B12 once every other day for six months prior to the outbreak. On average, they had received 6–8 cycles of the treatment. Within the 18 patients, 12 were infected with TB, six were not. For the 37 of the 55 patients, who did not received triamcinolone acetonide treatment, 18 patients were infected with TB, 19 didn't; there was no significantly statistic difference between triamcinolone acetonide and non-triamcinolone acetonide treatment with chi-square test. The results showed that susceptibility of *Mycobacterium tuberculosis* infection in these patients is not affected by glucocorticoids.

The study was approved by the Ethics Committee of the First Affiliated Hospital of Wenzhou Medical Unversity. Written informed consent was obtained from every participant.

Diagnosis

Purified protein derivative (PPD) skin test was performed in all 30 patients. The PPD tests of all patients were positive.

Quantitative fluorescent PCR assay, rapid identification of *Mycobacterium tuberculosis* Beijing strains, Rifampicin (RFP) susceptibility testing of *M. tuberculosis*, detection of isonicotinylhydrazine (INH)-resistant gene mutation, and variable number tandem repeat (VNTR) genotyping were performed on samples from six patients using Tuberculosis Drug Resistance Detection Array Kit (CapitalBio) and Mycobacteria Identification Array Kit (Capital-Bio). These six patients did not receive any anti-tuberculosis drugs before the PCR assy. The results showed four isolates were caused by RFP and INH sensitive *M. tuberculosis* Beijing strains, and VNTR genotyping revealed that the isolates were of the same genotype, and the other two isolates were negative.

Other eight cases in all 30 patients, biopsied, lesion smears and tubercle bacillus culture from wound saline solution were performed using BacT/ALER MP culture media (BIOMER-IEUX). Acid-fast bacillus was found in all the smears, and positive tubercle bacillus culture was found in three patients (positive rate: 37.5%). The three positive samples were sensitive to INH and RFP in susceptibility testing, no test for other drugs were performed. Prior to the biopsy and culture, these eight patients all had receive a 1-week's quadruple anti-tuberculosis drugs treatment (RFP/INH/PZA/EMB). The results of these eight patients' routine bacterial culture were negative.

In general, there were seven confirmed patients in this cutaneous tuberculosis outbreak while the rest twenty-three were supposed to be suspected patients.

The pathologic examination results are shown in Figure 1.

Clinical manifestations of seven confirmed patients

The incubation period defined as the time between the first invasive treatment and onset of clinical symptoms (subcutaneous mass, local redness, swelling and pain, and fever) ranged from 1.5 to 4 weeks (mean, 2.5 weeks). The lesions were widely distributed at sites of puncture. Figure 2 shows a representative photograph of a typical lesion.

Prior to receiving regular anti-tuberculosis drugs therapy, all seven confirmed cases had ulcerative lesions, which formed sinus tracts. The neighboring lesions developed ulcers or expanded to the neighboring soft tissues to form giant abscesses (Figure 3). Six confirmed patients developed symptoms of severe infection with high fever, including hyperpyrexia (axillary temperature >39.1°C) and shivering. One patient had symptoms commonly associated with tuberculosis, including low-grade fever, night sweats, anorexia and marasmus.

One confirmed patient developed tuberculosis infection of the knee joint, characterized by swelling, positive patellar tap test, limited flexion and extension, ulceration and suppuration of the needle tract. Knee arthroscopy showed hyperplasia of the knee joint synovium, with grey and dark color and soft texture, complicated by necrotic tissues. In addition, knee joint synovium underwent caseous changes, and articular cartilage necrosis and desquamation was observed. Subchondral bone was exposed, and there was evidence of vermiform bone destruction detected on the condyle of femur and the margin of the tibial plateau (Figure 4). Positive joint fluid smear test for acid fast bacilli was detected.

Two severe cases were found with tuberculous meningitis and miliary pulmonary tuberculosis complications (Figure 5), including one case admitted to an intensive care unit (ICU). Tuberculous meningitis was characterized by tuberculous lesions with low-intensity signals on T1-weighted imaging (T1WI), high-intensity signals around T2WI, slightly low-intensity signals on central zone of T2WI. In addition, there were slightly high-intensity signals on DWI of the bilateral frontal and parietal lobes, centrum semiovale, peri-lateral ventricular region, basal ganglia regions, thalamus, brainstem and cerebellum. Enhanced MRI scan showed the appearance of ring-shaped, signal-intensified lesions (Figure 6).

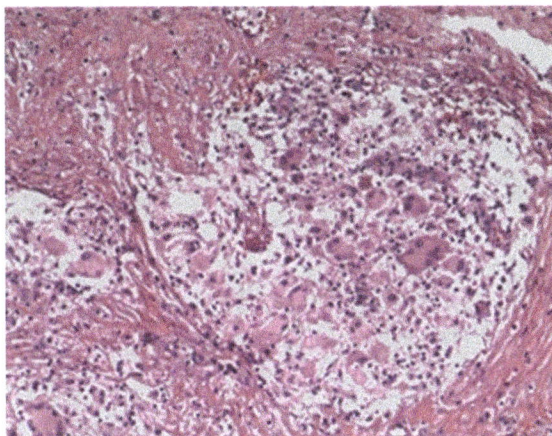

Figure 1. Infiltration of a large number of chronic inflammatory cells among muscle fibers. Many giant cells and epithelioid cells aggregated and formed multiple tubercles. Microabscess was present in the lesion region, and granulomatous inflammatory alteration was detected.

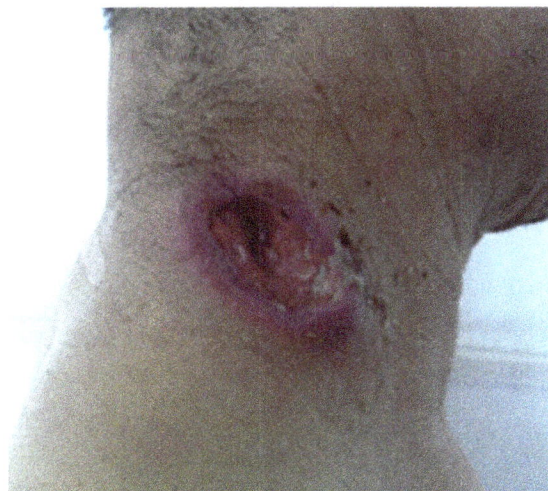

Figure 2. A fresh lesion on the right side of the neck. The ulcer was oval, with the largest diameter of about 5 cm, and a depth of about 2 cm. The basement of the ulcer was thick, with granular protrusions, which bled upon touch. The ulcer was slow to heal, and there was an inflammatory reaction and a small amount of purulent secretions in the surrounding skin.

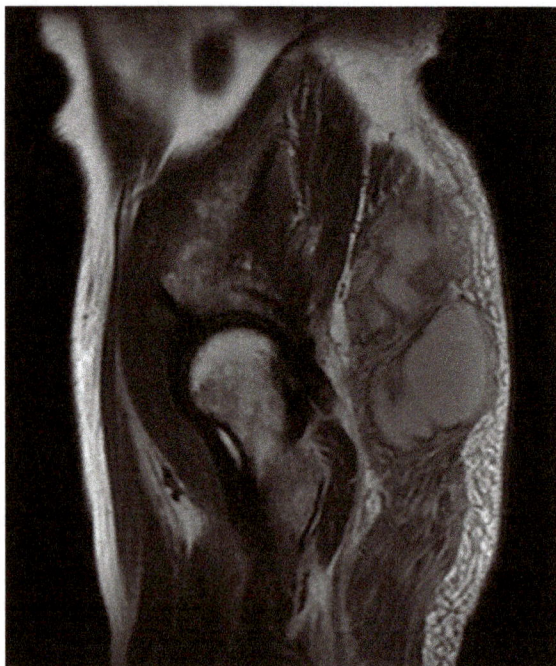

Figure 3. MRI scan of the hip on T1W1 reveals elevated signal intensity on the right gluteus maximus muscle. Massive irregular, homogeneous, mass-like abnormal signal intensity with unclear boundary was observed in the gluteus maximus muscle, measuring about 151 cm×90 cm, and subcutaneous edema-like signal intensities were observed in the right hip.

Clinical manifestations of 23 suspected patients

The incubation period of 23 suspected patients ranged from 1 to 12 weeks (mean, 3.9 weeks). 18 cases had ulcerative lesions, which formed sinus tracts. Among the five patients without sinus tracts, two cases had cold abscesses with normal local skin temperature, and three had an elevated local skin temperature on the lesion together with inflammatory soft tissue reactions, characterized by redness and swelling. Ten patients had high fever, four patients had low-grade fever, night sweats, anorexia and marasmus. The nine remaining cases (30.0%) had local symptoms without systemic manifestations. One patient developed tuberculosis infection of the knee joint, and the clinical manifestation was similar to the confirmed one. One severe case from suspected patients was found with tuberculous meningitis and miliary pulmonary tuberculosis complication.

Treatment options

Since the 30 patients were treated at the identical clinic, developing the similar clinical manifestations, using the close therapeutic program during the short period of time, suspicions were high that the suspected patients were infected by the same tuberculosis as the confirmed patients. Hence the analogous anti-tuberculosis drug treatment protocols were chosen for all the infected patient. Fortunately, the good treatment outcomes, in turn, proved that our speculation was very close to the actual situation.

All 30 patients had onset of primary inoculation tuberculosis within 1 to 3 months of the acupuncture procedure. Prior to definitive diagnosis at our hospital, 25 cases (including seven confirmed cases) had received various treatments at different hospitals or clinics, and the other five late onset cases had not been

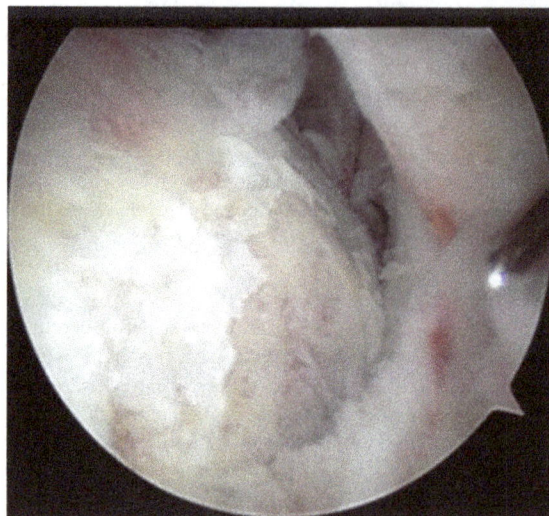

Figure 4. Hyperplasia of the knee joint synovium, grey and dark in color, with a soft texture, complicated by necrotic tissues. Some knee joint synovium underwent caseous changes, and articular cartilage necrosis and desquamation were observed. Subchondral bone was exposed, and vermiform bone destruction was observed on the condyle of femur and the margin of the tibial plateau.

treated. Treatment strategies were classified into surgical treatment alone, treatment with anti-tuberculosis drugs independently, and combination treatment with surgery and anti-tuberculosis drugs.

The anti-tuberculosis drug treatment protocols were developed according to the published guidelines of the American Thoracic Society (2003 version) [8]. The duration of pyrazinamide (PZA) and ethambutol (EMB) treatment was extended in some patients according to the actual therapeutic efficacy and side effects. Other drugs were changed due to side effects or allergy. Therapeutic efficacy was retrospectively evaluated.

Previous treatments

Five confirmed patients underwent surgical debridement procedures prior to definitive diagnosis of primary inoculation tuberculosis. The wound failed to heal after either primary suture

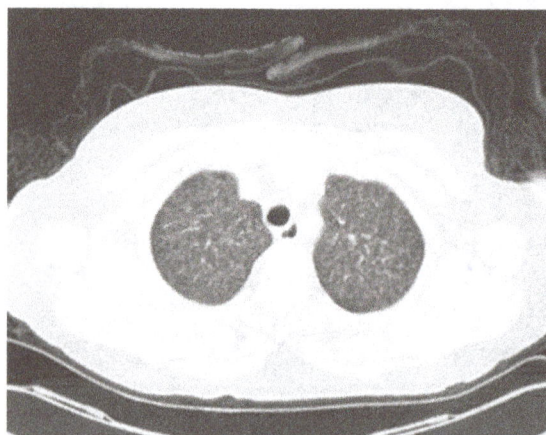

Figure 5. Left and right upper lungs displayed diffuse, ground-glass shadows with increased intensity.

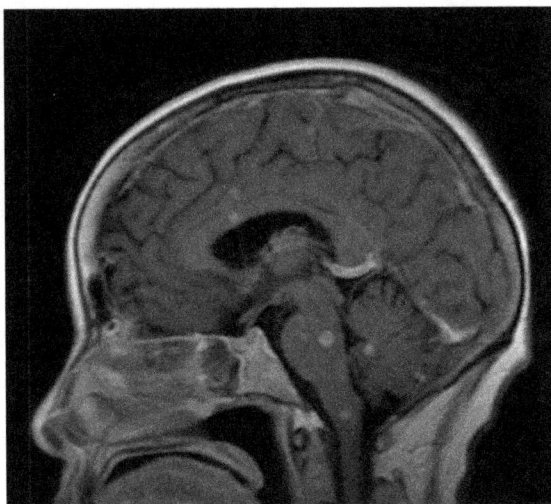

Figure 6. Enhanced MRI scan shows tuberculous, ring-shaped, signal-intensified lesions in bilateral frontal and parietal lobes, centrum semiovale, peri-lateral ventricular region, basal ganglia regions, thalamus, brainstem and cerebellum.

or open dressing without regular administration of anti-tuberculosis drugs. One confirmed and three suspected patients with abscess formation as revealed by imaging, received anti-tuberculosis agents for one week followed by debridement to remove the abscesses. In these subjects, no ulceration was found after primary suture of the wound. One confirmed and eight suspected patients presenting with minor wounds or no ulcerative primary lesions received anti-tuberculosis drugs alone. This achieved gradual reduction and healing of the lesions.

13 suspected patients underwent between two and five surgical debridement procedures before they were told and concentrated to our hospital. Without regular administration of anti-tuberculosis drugs, the wound failed to heal after either primary suture or open dressing. In all cases, the wound healed slowly after the final debridement procedure combined with anti-tuberculosis drugs.

Previous quinolone antibiotics efficacy of total 30 patients

Twenty-five patients underwent antibiotic therapy before anti-tuberculosis drugs administrations, including 17 who received using quinolone antibiotics. Fifteen of the 17 (88.2%) showed a remarkable alleviation of systemic symptoms and redness, as well as reduced swelling of the local lesions. There was also an extended interval before the reemergence of ulceration requiring debridement. No obvious efficacy was achieved in two of the 17 patients using quinolones.

Among eight patients treated with non-quinolone antibiotics, one had alleviation of systemic symptoms, and reduced redness and swelling of focal lesions (this patient received ceftriaxone). Treatment with non-quinolone agents was ineffective in the other seven cases. The 30 patients were divided into quinolone-treatment group and non-quinolone-treatment group. Numbers of relieved and non-relieved were recorded, and analyzed with the Fisher's exact test to compare the difference in relieving rates between the two groups ($P = 0.001$), the result revealed that quinolone antibiotics appeared more effective against tubercle bacillus than non-quinolone non-anti-tuberculosis agents.

Follow Up and Treatment Results

All patients received anti-TB treatment with a combination of four drugs for 2–6 months, depending on the alleviation of systemic symptoms and wound healing. The sequential enhanced treatment with two anti-tuberculosis drugs was ranged from 7 to 12 months. Nine suspected patients with good responses to drug therapies were in group I, their systemic symptoms were completely resolved (or they did not have any symptoms at all from the beginning) and their skin lesions were healed after a 2-month's quadruple anti-tuberculosis drugs (RFP/INH/PZA/EMB), and then this therapy was replaced by two anti-tuberculosis drugs (RFP/INH) for seven months. Due to gout and gastrointestinal reactions, PZA was replaced by Avelox (moxifloxacin hydrochloride and sodium chloride injection) in one suspected patient. PZA was used in the other eight suspected patients in the quadruple anti-tuberculosis drugs therapy. Four confirmed and ten suspected patients with moderate responses to drug therapies were in group II. Their skin lesions were healed between two and four months after the quadruple anti-tuberculosis treatment (RFP/INH/PZA/EMB) started, and then the therapy was replaced by two anti-tuberculosis drugs (RFP/INH) for 8–9 months. In four confirmed and eight suspected patients, the quadruple anti-tuberculosis drugs (RFP/INH/PZA/EMB) were administrated for four months. And two anti-tuberculosis drugs (RFP/INH) were adopted for sequential 8-months. Two suspected patients received a combination of rifapentine, INH, PZA and EMB due to allergy to RFP. Therapy continued with rifapentine-INH combination therapy for nine months.

Seven (3 confirmed and 4 suspected) patients with poor responses to drug therapies were in group III. Their skin lesions were healed between four and six months after the quadruple anti-tuberculosis drugs (RFP/INH/PZA/EMB) were treated, and then this therapy was replaced by two anti-tuberculosis drugs (RFP/INH) for 12 months. Due to liver dysfunction, PZA was stopped in one suspected patient at the 4th month and the three drugs (RFP/INH/EMB) were continued for another two months. PZA was used in the other six patients in the quadruple anti-tuberculosis drugs therapy (RFP/INH/PZA/EMB) for six months. The sequential 12-month's dual anti-tuberculosis drugs therapy (RFP/INH) was adopted in all of the seven patients.

Table 1 specifically lists the information of items of age, gender, diagnostic method, incubation period, sinus, high fever, severe case, operation, anti-tuberculosis drug treatment protocols and efficacy. We found no statistical significance in drug efficacy between the sinus/non-sinus, high fever/non-high fever or operation/non-operation groups. However, significant difference was observed between severe/non-severe patients in drug efficacy.

Group I had one suspected patient and group II had one confirmed patient with tuberculosis of the knee joint. Arthroscopic knee debridement was performed after a 4-week's quadruple anti-tuberculosis drugs therapy (RFP/INH/PZA/EMB) and continuous lavage and drainage using streptomycin saline solution (1 g in 500 ml) was given for one week. Wound of the suspected patient in group I was healed in five weeks. The skin wound was completely healed in the 17th week of the quadruple anti-tuberculosis drugs therapy in the confirmed patient in group II. In the final follow-up, the knee functions of both patients were normal and without obvious sequelae. Two confirmed and one suspected cases in group III complicated by intracranial and pulmonary tuberculosis were treated with four anti-tuberculosis drugs. After four months of treatment, cerebral spinal fluid test was negative, and the chest CT scan displayed no tuberculous lesions. The patients continued

Table 1. Information on clinical features and treatments in 30 patients.

Patient No.	Age/Gender	Diagnostic method	Incubation period (weeks)	Sinus	High fever	Operation	Anti-tuberculosis drug treatment protocols (months)	Efficacy of anti-TB drugs(group)	Follow-up time
Confirmed patients									
01	67,M	PPD+, PCR+	3	+	+	+	4(RFP/INH/PZA/EMB) & 8(RFP/INH)	II	36
02	54,F	PPD+, PCR+	2	+	+	+	6(RFP/INH/PZA/EMB) & 12(RFP/INH)	III	28
03	53,M	PPD+, PCR+	2	+	+	+	4(RFP/INH/PZA/EMB) & 8(RFP/INH)	II	40
04^K	50,M	PPD+, smear+, C+	1.5	+	+	+	4(RFP/INH/PZA/EMB) & 8(RFP/INH)	II	33
05*	50,M	PPD+, smear+, C+	2	+	+	+	6(RFP/INH/PZA/EMB) & 12(RFP/INH)	III	38
06*	67,F	PPD+, smear+, C+	3	+	+	+	6(RFP/INH/PZA/EMB) & 12(RFP/INH)	III	38
07	31,F	PPD+, PCR+	4	+	-^{s}	-	4(RFP/INH/PZA/EMB) & 8(RFP/INH)	II	30
Suspected patients									
01^D	71,F	PPD+	2	+	+	+	6(RFP/INH/PZA/EMB) & 12(RFP/INH)	III	32
02	45,F	PPD+	3	+	-	+	2(RFP/INH/PZA/EMB) & 7(RFP/INH)	I	36
03	40,M	PPD+	4	+	-	+	4(RFP/INH/PZA/EMB) & 8(RFP/INH)	II	30
04	60,F	PPD+, PCR-	3	-	-	-	4(RFP/INH/PZA/EMB) & 8(RFP/INH)	II	38
05	64,M	PPD+	6	-	-	-	4(RFP/INH/PZA/EMB) & 8(RFP/INH)	II	36
06	60,F	PPD+	4.5	+	+	-	2(RFP/INH/PZA/EMB) & 7(RFP/INH)	I	40
07	51,M	PPD+	3	+	+	-	2(RFP/INH/PZA/EMB) & 7(RFP/INH)	I	28
08^D	56,M	PPD+	5	+	-	-	2(RFP/INH/PZA/EMB) & 7(RFP/INH)	I	35
09	54,F	PPD+	3	+	-	+	2(RFP/INH/PZA/EMB) & 7(RFP/INH)	I	33
10	48,F	PPD+	4	+	-^{s}	+	2(RFP/INH/PZA/EMB) & 7(RFP/INH)	I	41
11^D	59,F	PPD+	4	-	+	+	2(RFP/INH/PZA/EMB) & 8(RFP/INH)	II	29
12	50,M	PPD+, smear+, C-	2	+	+^{s}	-	2(RFP/INH/Avelox/EMB) & 7(RFP/INH)	I	39
13	45,F	PPD+, smear+, C-	1.5	+	-^{s}	-	6(RFP/INH/PZA/EMB) & 12(RFP/INH)	III	36
14	48,F	PPD+	4	+	+	+	4(RFP/INH/PZA/EMB) & 8(RFP/INH)	II	35
15^K	48,M	PPD+	3	-	+	+	2(RFP/INH/PZA/EMB) & 7(RFP/INH)	I	36
16*	54,F	PPD+	2	+	+	+	6(RFP/INH/PZA/EMB) & 12(RFP/INH)	III	35
17	44,F	PPD+	1	-	+	+	2(RFP/INH/PZA/EMB) & 7(RFP/INH)	I	34
18	40,M	PPD+, smear+, C-	12	+	-	+	4(RFP/INH/PZA/EMB) & 8(RFP/INH)	II	28
19	50,M	PPD+, smear+, C-	2	+	-^{s}	+	4(RFP/INH/PZA/EMB) & 8(RFP/INH)	II	29
20	36,F	PPD+, PCR-	4	+	+	+	4(Rifapentine/INH/PZA/EMB) & 9(Rifapentine/INH)	III	40
21	60,F	PPD+, smear+, C-	2	+	+	+	4(Rifapentine/INH/PZA/EMB) & 9(Rifapentine/INH)	II	38
22	55,F	PPD+	6	+	-^{s}	+	4(RFP/INH/PZA/EMB) & 2(RFP/INH/EMB) & 12(RFP/INH)	III	32
23	60,M	PPD+	8	+	-	+	4(RFP/INH/PZA/EMB) & 8(RFP/INH)	II	27

+: positive;
-: negative;
*: severe case,
K: knee TB,
D: type 2 diabetes,
s: symptoms commonly associated with tuberculosis, including low-grade fever, night sweats, anorexia and marasmus.
Good efficacy of drug treatment in nine suspected patients named group I; moderate efficacy of drug treatment in four confirmed and ten suspected patients named group II; poor efficacy of drug treatment in three confirmed and four suspected patients named group III.

treatment with four anti-tuberculosis drugs for two months and two drugs for 12 months (total of 18 months).

Seven confirmed patients and the seven confirmatory tests negative ones were compared. No significantly statistics difference was found in the incidence of sinus ($P=1.000$) and high fever ($P=0.559$) with Fisher's exact test. Incubation period and efficacy of anti-tuberculosis drugs also had no statistical difference between the confirmatory tests positive patients and negative ones with chi-square test ($P=0.134$) and Student's t test ($P=0.121$) respectively.

In cases where liver injury occurred, treatment was interrupted for three weeks during which liver-protective therapy was administered, before resuming with the anti-tuberculosis drug regimen.

After a mean follow-up of 34.33 weeks (range: 27–42 weeks), all lesions were healed. Two suspected patients still presented with subcutaneous nodules, but without newly formed lesions. The three cases with intracranial and pulmonary tuberculosis complications were negative for cerebral spinal fluid test as well as chest CT scan. No cases of recurrent tuberculosis were detected.

Discussion

Again, on account of the similar epidemiological history, clinical manifestation and treatment effects, along with the four coincident VNTR genotyping results, the authors still considered the 30 cases as one outbreak of infection caused by the identical pathogen and discuss them together.

Primary inoculation tuberculosis is an infection of *Mycobacterium tuberculosis*, which usually results from direct introduction of the bacterium into the skin of a tuberculosis-free person. In most cases, minor injuries are found on skin [9]. The typical histological features of primary inoculation tuberculosis involve granulomatous nodules with infiltration of epithelioid cells, Langerhans' cells and mononuclear macrophages. However, these characteristics are not specific to tuberculosis, and other infectious lesions, e.g. from mycoses may present similar manifestations.

Since Laennec's description of the "prosector's wart" in 1826, science has made great strides forward. The cutaneous forms of the infection with *Mycobacterium tuberculosis* are various [10]. Such cutaneous infection is general via single superficial skin hurt, time and frequency of the contact with *Mycobacterium tuberculosis* are very short. The use of Chinese acupuncture needles which are able to deeply penetrate into the tissues surrounding tendons and nerves provide an ideal route for the inoculation of tuberculosis. The patients in our outbreak underwent acupuncture twice daily for two weeks. This high degree of potential exposure may explain why there were no cases of spontaneous healing. It was also possible that patients with self-healing of skin lesions had ignored their short-lasting symptoms and became the so called 'non-incident' patients.

PPD results of 30 patients were positive, indicating that PPD test was sensitive to primary inoculation tuberculosis. Due to factors of funding and patient compliance, we were unable to perform diagnosing experiments of biopsy, culture and PCR for each patient. We thought PPD trial could serve as a key diagnosing, since these patients were treated at the same clinic, with the parallel therapeutic program and during the short period of time. However, PPD is only a screening measure for sporadic cases. Nevertheless, if it were combined with clinical symptoms, its diagnostic reliability would greatly increase, particularly when the diagnosed specimens are hard to obtain. Goette, D. K., et al. thought a transition from a negative result to positive one in PPD trial could serve as a diagnostic criterion for primary inoculation

tuberculosis [3], but it is difficult to get a result of PPD trial in the real clinical atmosphere before onset.

Previous literatures have reported that quantitative fluorescent PCR assay has a high sensitivity and specificity, but there continues to be no more than 25% of the false-negative rate [11–13]. Improper operation can cause *Mycobacterium tuberculosis* lost and specimen contamination. On the other hand, no tissue fluid around the lesions will also reduce the detection rate, and affect the authenticity of the results. Of course, we cannot ignore the possibility that there was no *Mycobacterium tuberculosis* exist in those samples at all. Negative tubercle bacillus culture rate was up to 62.5%. The most likely cause may be the effects of the anti-tuberculosis drug treatment which low the bacterial activity. Other possibilities include L-form conversion of *Mycobacterium tuberculosis* and technical error caused by improper operation. There was no statistical difference in incubation period, incidence of sinus, incidence of high fever and efficacy of anti-tuberculosis drugs between the patients of positive confirmatory tests and their negative counterparts. Therefore, we believe that the possibility of false-negatives is very big.

Only one patient (in suspected group) in our study had a medical history of tuberculosis. This patient was not admitted to the acupuncture clinic earlier than the other cases. In addition, three sputum smear examinations were all negative, and the pulmonary lesions did not indicate active tuberculosis. Therefore, the case was not considered as the source of infection. Despite the unsuccessful identification of the source of contamination, it is apparent that these infections were linked to acupuncture and moxibustion, because the 30 patients had the same epidemiological characteristics. Several previous studies have demonstrated that tuberculosis can occur as a result of tattoo or acupuncture treatments [14–16].

Most of the 30 patients had multiple skin infections, but the lesions were located to the sites of acupuncture and electrotherapy. Lesion severity and drug reactions in individual patient were similar, but we did not know whether these multiple lesions were independent or the result of the inoculation infections in the wounds via hemo-disseminated *Mycobacterium tuberculosis*. Although, occurrence of the three patients with meningeal and pulmonary tuberculosis and two patients with knee tuberculosis had confirmed the hemo-disseminated ability of this primary inoculation *Mycobacterium tuberculosis* to other tissues and the compartments.

To account for possible deviations in patients remembering the exact dates, the incubation period was recorded in weeks instead of days. In this study, the incubation period ranged from 1 to 12 weeks, in good accordance with similar studies [14,15].

The lesions in our patients were distributed throughout the body at sites of puncture, indicating that inoculation of tubercle bacilli has no obvious preference for soft tissues. Indeed, tuberculosis can occur at neck (abundant blood supply) and muscle-tendon tissues (relatively less blood supply) with different characteristics compared with knee-joint tuberculosis that predominantly occurs at weight-bearing sites.

Almost all patients had subcutaneous nodules that were not completely inhibited by routine antibiotics including quinolone agents, and the resulting lesions did not readily heal. The lesions sizes ranged in size from a needle tip diameter to a diameter of 8 cm. They were characterized by the presence of a thick basement, and granular protrusions with bleeding upon touch. Ulcers surrounded by scarring and pigmentation were very slow to heal. Examination of the lesion smears showed positive acid-fast stained bacillus. Most lesions were relatively independent, although one patient presented with large cold abscesses on hip and waist. These findings indicate that primary inoculation tuberculosis lesions occur relatively independently, seldom with a local distribution.

There were three cases of tuberculous meningitis and military pulmonary tuberculosis complications. Our data suggest that 10% primary inoculation tuberculosis may develop hematogenous dissemination, which is rarely described in previous case reports. The occurrence of knee-joint tuberculosis demonstrated that invasive tubercle bacilli can be inoculated into a limited space, and we showed that satisfactory knee-joint function could be achieved through arthroscopic synovial debridement and lavage with streptomycin.

It is well recognized that debridement without anti-tuberculosis agents does not control tuberculosis, and that multiple debridements may cause deeper and wider local infections. In our series, surgical debridement was undertaken 2–4 weeks after administration of anti-tuberculosis agents to remove abscesses. Local lesions were lavaged with streptomycin, and the wound could heal with primary suture. Following surgery, more effusion fluid was released than in a normal wound. However, the wound was closed after at least two weeks. Two patients presented subcutaneous nodules after non-surgical drug therapy, no recurrence was observed after follow-up completion, and these patients rejected surgical removal of the nodules. But, the final outcomes required longer follow-up periods. Lesions without abscess were all healed following anti-tuberculosis drugs therapy. Therefore, treatment with anti-tuberculosis is sufficient to achieve satisfactory therapeutic efficacy, while the option of surgical treatment depends on abscess formation.

Our treatment plans with a combination of four or two anti-tuberculosis drugs for 6–9 or 9–12 months are recommended for treatment of tuberculosis. This is in accordance with the guidelines for treatment of tuberculosis as proposed by the American Thoracic Society [8]. To optimize the treatment regimen, patients were followed up every month, and the treatment regimen was adjusted as clinically indicated. Treatment with a four drug combination for two months, followed by a two drug combination for seven months (total of nine months) provided a satisfactory response for small primary lesions. However, treatment with a four drug regimen should be extended to six months, with total treatment duration of 18 months for patients without obvious improvement in wounds after four months of therapy, and for cases with intracranial and pulmonary tuberculosis complications.

Due to safety and ethical considerations, it was impossible to compare the relative therapeutic efficacy of treatments with various drugs at different cycles. Some patients stopped drug intake due to side effects. Nevertheless, all patients were treated for at least nine months, and all wounds were healed with no resistant strains detected. These findings show that drug sensitivity testing in combination with regular anti-tuberculosis drugs therapy achieves efficacy in the treatment of primary inoculation tuberculosis without recurrence.

Drug resistance is the predominant factor affecting efficacy but this was not seen in this outbreak. The bacteria counts and immune state are also important factors affecting symptoms and efficacy [10].

Based on the description of symptoms by patients, we simply divide the local symptoms into sinus and non-sinus groups and the systemic symptoms into high fever and non-high fever groups (since low fever and normal state were hard to recall and identify. High fever was easier to identify, and was, therefore, chosen as the

parameter). The presence of sinus and high fever did not affect drug efficacy or antimicrobial sensitivity to the drug. Surgical treatment did not influence the sensitivity of the drug. In fact, efficacy was inferior in patients with severe conditions than in those with milder lesions.

There were only three severe patients who had meningeal or pulmonary tuberculosis. The efficacy of drug therapy in these patients was undoubtedly poor, which might be the result of the large amount of Mycobacterium tuberculosis entering into the cerebrospinal fluid where drugs were hard to reach.

Interestingly, glucocorticoids has been used in combination with electroacupuncture for the treatment of tuberculosis [17,18]. Based on cytological findings, Rook, G., et al. reported that glucocorticoids play an important role in the process of tuberculosis infection. They suggested that a local increase in glucocorticoids will raise susceptibility to tuberculosis [19,20]. However, our findings, which were contrary to previous experimental results, show that no statistical significance was found, and glucocorticoids did not affect the susceptibility of primary inoculation tuberculosis. The causes may be that the earlier results were just confined to animal experiments and cytological studies. In vitro and animal experiments cannot completely simulate the real human Mycobacterium tuberculosis infection. Another reason may be that glucocorticoids do affect the incidence of primary inoculation tuberculosis, but because of small sample size of this study and the lost to follow-up for 3 patients we didn't get the positive result. Anyway, the risk of Mycobacterium tuberculosis infection should be given high priority when invasive procedures are involved, and glucocorticoids should not be used blindly, frequently nor excessively.

Conclusions

Based on our findings we make the following recommendations: Mycobacterium can easily spread without proper microbiological control of these procedures. To this end, it was recently suggested that herbal medicine and acupuncture professions should also develop a system of statutory regulation [21] which should help prevent these issues.

Diverse symptoms (from subcutaneous induration to systemic dissemination or even intracranial infection) may appear after Mycobacterium tuberculosis infection. Therefore, infection of Mycobacterium tuberculosis should be excluded in patients with a history of invasive treatment, repeated symptoms or poor antibiotic efficacy. This would avoid large-scale outbreaks, similar to the one studied here.

For lesions with abscesses, surgical removal should be adopted in combination with anti-tuberculosis drugs, since operative removal alone is ineffective and may even make the condition worse. Different drug reactions may appear even among patients infected by the same Mycobacterium tuberculosis spp.

Classical anti-tuberculosis drug treatment programs are effective against lesions of the primary inoculation tuberculosis and with continued treatment, all patients can be cured.

Author Contributions

Conceived and designed the experiments: YL Lei Chen JY. Performed the experiments: YL JP KJ CL JW. Analyzed the data: YL Lei Chen JY. Contributed reagents/materials/analysis tools: JP KJ CL JW Li Chen. Wrote the paper: YL.

References

1. Luca S, Mihaescu T (2013) History of BCG Vaccine. Maedica (Buchar) 8: 53–58.
2. Organization WH (2011) Global tuberculosis control 2011: WHO report 2011. Geneva: WHO.
3. Goette DK, Jacobson KW, Doty RD (1978) Primary inoculation tuberculosis of the skin. Prosector's paronychia. Arch Dermatol 114: 567–569.
4. Ho CK, Ho MH, Chong LY (2006) Cutaneous tuberculosis in Hong Kong: an update. Hong Kong Med J 12: 272–277.
5. Centers for Disease Control and Prevention. Mantoux TB skintest facilitator guide, at. Appendix D: Mantouxtuberculin skin test interpretation table.
6. Bloch AB, Rieder HL, Kelly GD, Cauthen GM, Hayden CH, et al. (1989) The epidemiology of tuberculosis in the United States. Implications for diagnosis and treatment. Clin Chest Med 10: 297–313.
7. Haim S, Friedman-Birnbaum R (1978) Cutaneous tuberculosis and malignancy. Cutis 21: 643–647.
8. American Thoracic Society C, and Infectious Diseases Society of America, (2003) MMWR Recommendations and Reports.
9. Tappeiner G (2008) Fitzpatrick's dermatology in general medicine. 7th ed. New York: McGraw-Hill.
10. Tigoulet F, Fournier V, Caumes E (2003) Clinical forms of the cutaneous tuberculosis. Bull Soc Pathol Exot 96: 362–367.
11. Saitoh H, Yamane N (2000) Comparative evaluation of BACTEC MGIT 960 system with MB/BacT and egg-based media for recovery of mycobacteria. Rinsho Biseibutshu Jinsoku Shindan Kenkyukai Shi 11: 19–26.
12. Lee JJ, Suo J, Lin CB, Wang JD, Lin TY, et al. (2003) Comparative evaluation of the BACTEC MGIT 960 system with solid medium for isolation of mycobacteria. Int J Tuberc Lung Dis 7: 569–574.
13. Otu J, Antonio M, Cheung YB, Donkor S, De Jong BC, et al. (2008) Comparative evaluation of BACTEC MGIT 960 with BACTEC 9000 MB and LJ for isolation of mycobacteria in The Gambia. J Infect Dev Ctries 2: 200–205.
14. Kim JK, Kim TY, Kim DH, Yoon MS (2010) Three cases of primary inoculation tuberculosis as a result of illegal acupuncture. Ann Dermatol 22: 341–345.
15. Wong HW, Tay YK, Sim CS (2005) Papular eruption on a tattoo: a case of primary inoculation tuberculosis. Australas J Dermatol 46: 84–87.
16. Da Mata Jardin O, Hernandez-Perez R, Corrales H, Cardoso-Leao S, de Waard JH (2010) Follow-up on an outbreak in Venezuela of soft-tissue infection due to Mycobacterium abscessus associated with Mesotherapy. Enferm Infecc Microbiol Clin 28: 596–601.
17. Lu HQ (2012) Thirty-three cases of tuberculous intestinal obstruction treated by moxibustion on garlic combined with electroacupuncture. Zhongguo Zhen Jiu 32: 570.
18. Zhao XP, Chen RX, Lu HQ (2009) Influence of garlic moxibustion on the therapeutic effect in re-treatment patients of tuberculosis. Zhongguo Zhen Jiu 29: 10–12.
19. Rook GA, Hernandez-Pando R (1997) Pathogenetic role, in human and murine tuberculosis, of changes in the peripheral metabolism of glucocorticoids and antiglucocorticoids. Psychoneuroendocrinology 22 Suppl 1: S109–113.
20. Rook G, Baker R, Walker B, Honour J, Jessop D, et al. (2000) Local regulation of glucocorticoid activity in sites of inflammation. Insights from the study of tuberculosis. Ann N Y Acad Sci 917: 913–922.
21. Walker LA, Budd S (2002) UK: the current state of regulation of complementary and alternative medicine. Complement Ther Med 10: 8–13.

15

Acupuncture for the Treatment of Dry Eye: A Multicenter Randomised Controlled Trial with Active Comparison Intervention (Artificial Teardrops)

Tae-Hun Kim[1,2], Jung Won Kang[1,3], Kun Hyung Kim[1,4], Kyung-Won Kang[1], Mi-Suk Shin[1], So-Young Jung[1], Ae-Ran Kim[1], Hee-Jung Jung[1], Jin-Bong Choi[5], Kwon Eui Hong[6], Seung-Deok Lee[7], Sun-Mi Choi[1]*

1 Acupuncture, Moxibustion & Meridian Research Centre, Korea Institute of Oriental Medicine, Daejeon, South Korea, 2 Department of Cardiovascular and Neurologic Diseases, College of Oriental Medicine, Graduate School, Kyung Hee University, Seoul, South Korea, 3 Department of Acupuncture and Moxibustion, College of Oriental Medicine, Kyung Hee University, Seoul, South Korea, 4 Division of Clinical Medicine, School of Korean Medicine, Pusan National University, Gyeongsangnam-do, South Korea, 5 Department of Oriental Rehabilitation Medicine, Dongshin University, Gwangju, South Korea, 6 Department of Acupuncture and Moxibustion, Daejeon University, Daejeon, South Korea, 7 Department of Acupuncture and Moxibustion, Dongguk University, Goyang, South Korea

Abstract

Purpose: To evaluate the effects of acupuncture compared to a control group using artificial tears.

Methods: Setting & design: multicenter randomised controlled trial (three local research hospitals of South Korea). *Study Population:* 150 patients with moderate to severe dry eye. *Intervention:* Participants were randomly allocated into four weeks of acupuncture treatment (bilateral BL2, GB14, TE 23, Ex1, ST1, GB20, LI4, LI11 and single GV23) or to the artificial tears group (sodium carboxymethylcellulose). *Main Outcome Measure(s):* The ocular surface disease index (OSDI), tear film break-up time (TFBUT), Schirmer I test, visual analogue scale (VAS) for self-assessment of ocular discomfort, general assessment (by both acupuncture practitioners and participants) and quality of life (QOL) through the Measure Yourself Medical Outcome Profile-2 (MYMOP-2).

Results: There was no statistically significant difference between two groups for the improvement of dry eye symptoms as measured by OSDI (MD −16.11, 95% CI [−20.91, −11.32] with acupuncture and −15.37, 95% CI [−19.57, −11.16] with artificial tears; P = 0.419), VAS (acupuncture: −23.84 [−29.59, −18.09]; artificial tears: −22.2 [−27.24, −17.16], P = 0.530) or quality of life (acupuncture: −1.32 [−1.65, −0.99]; artificial tears: −0.96 [−1.32, −0.6], P = 0.42) immediately after treatment. However, compared with artificial tears group, the OSDI (acupuncture: −16.15 [−21.38, −10.92]; artificial tears: −10.76 [−15.25, −6.27], P = 0.030) and VAS (acupuncture: −23.88 [−30.9, −16.86]; artificial tears: −14.71 [−20.86, −8.55], P = 0.018) were significantly improved in the acupuncture group at 8 weeks after the end of acupuncture treatment. TFBUT measurements increased significantly in the acupuncture group after treatment.

Conclusions: Acupuncture may have benefits on the mid-term outcomes related to dry eye syndrome compared with artificial tears.

Trial registration: ClinicalTrials.gov NCT01105221 http://clinicaltrials.gov/ct2/show/NCT01105221?term = NCT01105221.

Editor: James T. Rosenbaum, Oregon Health & Science University, United States of America

Funding: This study was supported by the Development of Acupuncture, Moxibustion and Meridian Standard Health Technology Project (K11010) of the Korea Institute of Oriental Medicine. The funders had no role in study design, data collection and analysis, decision to publish, or preparation of the manuscript.

Competing Interests: The authors have declared that no competing interests exist.

* E-mail: smchoi@kiom.re.kr

Introduction

Dry eye syndrome is a common ophthalmologic disorder causing ocular discomfort in daily life. An increased knowledge of dry eye pathology has changed the definition of dry eye syndrome from describing a trivial ocular disorder related to secretion deficiency or excess tear evaporation to detailing a multi-factorial disease, which may involve chronic inflammation or tear film instability [1]. According to previously published literature, the overall prevalence of dry eye syndrome is estimated to be 5 to 35 percent in various populations [2]. Moreover, the incidence is now increasing, which may be related to changes in life style and working environments, increased average life expectancies and usage of medical interventions that can cause dry eye syndrome, including laser-assisted in situ keratomileusis (LASIK) surgery, radiation therapy, contact lenses and medications such as antihistamines or diuretics [1].

Recent studies have suggested that dry eye syndrome may pose a considerable economic burden on the patient and on society [3,4]. Patients with dry eye syndrome not only have ocular discomfort but also visual disturbances; therefore, the impact is significant, affecting individual daily activities such as driving and reading as well as social functioning and productivity [4]. Many treatment options have been suggested, but artificial tears are the most widely chosen as lubricants or supplements for tear deficiency [5].

Acupuncture is one of the oldest interventions in East Asian countries. However, clinical evidence for the effectiveness of acupuncture has been provided for only a small number of diseases [6]. In the ophthalmologic field, recent studies have suggested that acupuncture may be helpful for several conditions including glaucoma [7] and amblyopia [8]. The efficacy and effectiveness of acupuncture for dry eye syndrome has also been explored in recent decades, but rigorous clinical trials have been needed to confirm the effectiveness of this intervention [9]. In this context, we tested the effectiveness of acupuncture compared to artificial tears as a control, an active treatment for dry eyes with high methodological rigor. A cost-effectiveness study and qualitative research were conducted simultaneously [10].

Methods

The protocol for this trial and supporting CONSORT checklist are available as supporting information; see Checklist S1 and Protocol S1. This was a randomised, active controlled, parallel designed trial. The study protocol has been previously published [10]. This multicentre trial was conducted in three clinical research centres of South Korea from June to November 2010: Korea Institute of Oriental Medicine (Daejeon University Hospital), DongGuk University Ilsan Oriental Hospital and Dongshin University Gwangju Oriental Hospital. The research protocol was approved before study onset by the institutional review board (IRB) of each participating hospital. Participants were independently recruited by each centre through advertisements in local newspapers. The protocol was registered with ClinicalTrials.gov (Identifier: NCT01105221) before participant enrolment. Written informed consent was obtained from all of the participants.

Patients aged nineteen to sixty five years old with aggravating dry eye symptoms in a single eye or in both eyes were recruited [1]. Physicians and ophthalmologists assessed participant eligibility [11]. Inclusion criteria were based on the following ophthalmologic tests: a tear film break-up time (TFBUT) below 10 seconds and a Schirmer I test (with application of alcaine, a local anaesthetic) value below 10 mm/5 minutes [12]. These ophthalmologic tests were performed by the ophthalmologists who did not know the allocation results. Participants with several conditions were excluded: pathological changes of the eye, Stevens-Johnson syndrome, external injuries and eye-surgery history affecting dry eye. Participants who had been taking or needed active treatment for dry eyes were also excluded, as were patients with punctal occlusion history or current usage of anti-inflammatory eye drops. Contact lens use was prohibited throughout the participation period.

Participants were allocated into either acupuncture or artificial tears evenly. Random numbers were generated through computerised block-randomisation with the SAS package (SAS® Version 9.1, SAS Institute, Inc., Cary, NC) by separate statistician. Opaque assignment envelopes with consecutive numbers for each centre were used for allocation concealment. The necessary sample size was calculated from the results of previous studies regarding the effects of acupuncture [11,13] and artificial tears [14]. The mean difference (standard deviation) of ocular surface disease index (OSDI) after acupuncture treatment was 17.61 (15.61), and after artificial tears (sodium carboxymethylcellulose), it was 11.3 (6.3) [13,14]. Anticipating a 20% dropout rate, a total

of 150 participants was recruited and was evenly assigned to each centre (50 participants in each centre).

Interventions

Acupuncture Treatment Group. Acupuncture was administered according to the theory of traditional Korean medicine (TKM) without using lubricants. An expert committee composed of clinical experts and researchers working on acupuncture research or ophthalmologic practice of TKM decided on acupuncture points and needling methods based on published literature and textbooks about acupuncture for ophthalmologic diseases or dry eye syndrome [9,15]. Certified practitioners with at least 7 years of TKM education and 3 years of clinical experience performed the acupuncture treatment. To reduce non-specific effects originating from the close relationship between patients and practitioners, interactions were strictly limited [16].

Seventeen acupuncture points (bilateral BL2, GB14, TE 23, Ex1, ST1, GB20, LI4, and LI11 and single GV23), located according to the WHO Standard Acupuncture Point Locations in the Western Pacific Region, were treated with 0.20×30-mm disposable acupuncture needles (Dongbang Co., Korea) [17]. The depths of inserted needles differed but were approximately 0.6 to 3 cm for the acupuncture points at the face and head (BL2:1.5 to 3 cm; GB14:0.9 to 1.5 cm; TE23:1.5 to 3 cm; Ex1:1.5 to 3 cm; ST1:0.6 to 0.9 cm; GV 16:0.9 to 1.5 cm) and 3 to 4.5 cm for points of hand (LI4) and arm (LI11). Each acupuncture needle was twisted until patient felt a 'deqi' sensation and retained for 20 minutes before removal. Participants had acupuncture treatments three times per week for four weeks (a total of 12 treatments).

Artificial Tears Group. Preservative-free single-use artificial teardrops (0.5% sodium carboxymethylcellulose) were provided, and participants were advised to use them as needed (at least once per day) for four weeks. A diary of both the frequency and quantity of drops used was collected at every visit. In both groups, other treatments for dry eyes were forbidden during the four weeks of treatment. However, during the follow-up period, participants were allowed to use any kind of treatment for dry eyes, and participant reports on treatment usage were requested at every visit.

Outcome Assessment. Outcome assessment included two aspects, subjective ophthalmologic tests and objective questionnaires for both ocular symptoms and quality of life related to dry eyes. The primary outcome was the difference in OSDI changes between the two groups. The secondary outcomes were the differences in 100 mm VAS for the ocular discomfort, quality of life questionnaire using the Measure Yourself Medical Outcome Profile-2 (MYMOP-2), TFBUT, Schirmer I test (with anaesthesia) score and adverse event rate of acupuncture treatment and artificial tears usage. Both eyes were assessed for the evaluation of TFBUT and Schirmer I test, respectively. Outcomes were assessed 13 weeks after the first visit.

OSDI is a validated questionnaire consisting of twelve questions for evaluating ocular symptoms and worsening conditions related to dry eyes [18]. Each question has a score between zero and four, where zero indicates "none of the time" and four indicates "all of the time". The OSDI score was calculated according to the following formula: OSDI = [(sum of scores for all questions answered)*100]/[(total number of questions answered)*4]. The score ranges from 0 to 100, and higher scores represent a more severe dry eye state. The minimal clinically important difference (MCID) of OSDI for dry eye syndrome is suggested to be 7.3 to 13.4 points in severe dry-eye patients [19]. A version translated into the Korean language was used [20].

A 100 mm VAS for self-assessment of ocular discomfort was reported by participants. Ocular symptoms related to dry eye (e.g., ocular itching, foreign body sensation, burning, pain and dryness, blurred vision, sensation of photophobia, ocular redness, and sensations of tearing) were quantified and summarised in a standard 100 mm VAS scale.

The QOL section of the MYMOP-2 was adopted for assessing dry eye-related QOL [21,22]. A seven-point Likert scale (from zero as 'excellent' to six as 'worst') was used for the assessment of QOL grade. The question was "During last week, how would you express your quality of life related to dry eyes, overall?".

Tear film break-up time (TFBUT) is a test for assessing tear film stability [23,24]. Sodium fluorescein (2.5%) was applied to both eyes, and the interval between the blink of eyes and the first appearance of a dry spot or disruption in the tear film was measured. If TFBUT is below 10 sec, it suggests at least a moderate severity of dry eyes [1,12].

The Schirmer I test (with anaesthesia) is a diagnostic method to measure the basic quantity of tear secretion [12]. After application of local anaesthesia, Schirmer test paper (Color Bar, Eagle Vision, USA) was placed in the lateral third of the lower eyelids for 5 minutes with closed eyes. If the Schirmer test result is below 10 mm/5 min, it also suggests at least a moderate severity of dry eyes [1,12].

General improvements of dry eye-related symptoms were assessed by practitioners and participants using a five-grade Likert scale: excellent, good, fair, poor and aggravation.

For the evaluation of safety issues, we assessed adverse events rates of acupuncture and artificial tears. If unexpected responses happened, the type and frequency were collected. The type and frequency of adverse events were reported for each group. According to the criteria of the WHO Toxicity Grading Scale for Determining The Severity of Adverse Events, the severity of the adverse event was evaluated by practitioners as grade 1 (mild) to grade 4 (life threatening) [25]. OSDI, VAS and quality of life were assessed by separate outcome assessors who did not perform acupuncture treatment. TFBUT and Schrmir I test were evaluated by ophthalmologists.

Statistics. To determine the differences between the acupuncture and artificial tears groups, the changes in values from baseline were compared at each visit on an intention-to-treat basis at a 95% significant level. Missing data of dropped-out participants were assigned by the last observation carried forward (LOCF) method. Participant expectations of acupuncture treatment for dry eye symptoms were collected with a nine-point Likert scale and were compared between the two groups [26]. Key baseline characteristics including risk factors for dry eyes such as computer use, age, occupational environment, contact lens usage, etc. were evaluated for the difference between two groups. ANCOVA (Analysis of Covariance) were used for continuous outcomes such as OSDI score, TFBUT, Schirmer test result, QOL and VAS for self-assessment of ocular discomfort, adjusted for baseline values and research centres as covariates. Adjusted differences, which were calculated from the ANCOVA model, were reported at each visit to estimate the effect size. Chi-squared tests were used for dichotomous outcomes such as general improvements of dry eye-related symptoms and differences in the usage of additional treatment during follow-up period. As suggested in the study protocol, repeated measures of analysis of variance for OSDI were performed to show trend changes. Statistical analyses were conducted using the SAS statistical package.

Results

A total of 214 participants were assessed for eligibility at the three research centres. There were 150 dry-eye patients who met the inclusion criteria and were equally allocated into the acupuncture and artificial tears groups. Nine participants from the acupuncture group and 8 from the artificial tears group dropped out during the study (figure 1). In acupuncture treatment group, 2 participants were lost to follow up and 7 participants discontinued treatment because of acute keratitis (1), protocol violation (3), usage of prohibited treatments such as acupuncture in other clinic, application of steroid or anti-inflammatory drug (3), pain related to the acupuncture (1) and unknown reason (1). In the control group, 3 participants were lost to follow up and 5 discontinued participation because of protocol violation i.e. infringement of visiting schedule (2) and refusal of artificial tear usage due to inconvenience (3).

The baseline characteristics did not show important imbalances between the two groups, with similar risk factors for dry eyes such as time watching television and computer use, age, occupational environment, contact lens use and smoking [1]. Many participants had used artificial tears for controlling dry eye symptoms before study participation (table 1). Patient expectations for the effectiveness of acupuncture treatment for dry eyes did not differ between the two groups (Wilcoxon rank summed test, P = 0.8817).

During the 4-week treatment period, the control participants applied artificial tears an average of 2.79 times per day (95% CI [2.50, 3.08]) and used a total of 38.87 [36.24, 31.50] units of artificial teardrops.

OSDI

Changes in OSDI from baseline values did not show significant differences between the two groups after 2 weeks of treatment, with the acupuncture group showing a change of -16.38 (95% CI [−20.7, −12.06]) and the artificial tears group showing a change of −13.1 (95% CI −[17.68, −8.52]), as tested by ANCOVA, P = 0.058. After 4 weeks of treatment, the change in OSDI was −16.11, [−20.91, −11.32] and −15.37 [−19.57, −11.16] for the acupuncture and artificial tears groups, respectively (P = 0.419). At 4 weeks after the end of acupuncture, the change in OSDI was −15.35 [−19.82, −10.88] and −14.38 [−18.84, −9.92] for the acupuncture and artificial tears groups, respectively (P = 0.416). However, significant improvement in OSDI in the acupuncture group was reported at the 8-week after acupuncture treatment (acupuncture: −16.15 [−21.38, −10.92]; artificial tears: −10.76 [−15.25, −6.27], P = 0.030). As the MCID for severe dry eyes is estimated to be 7.3 to 13.4 [19], these results can be interpreted to show that both acupuncture and artificial tears improved the symptoms of dry eyes during the treatment period, but the therapeutic effect was maintained longer in the acupuncture group (figure 2). The adjusted difference of OSDI was −0.75 [−4.22, 2.72] after 4 weeks of acupuncture treatment, and it increased in favour of acupuncture to −0.98 [−4.08, 2.14] at 4 weeks and to −5.39 [−8.62, −2.16] at 8 weeks after the end of treatment (table 2). From the result of repeated measure analysis of variance, no significant differences in the trends of changes in OSDI value were observed between the two groups (p = 0.31).

VAS

Changes in VAS showed a pattern similar to that of OSDI. Statistically significant improvements did not appear at 2 weeks (−17.89 [−23.27, −12.51] in the acupuncture group and −21.29

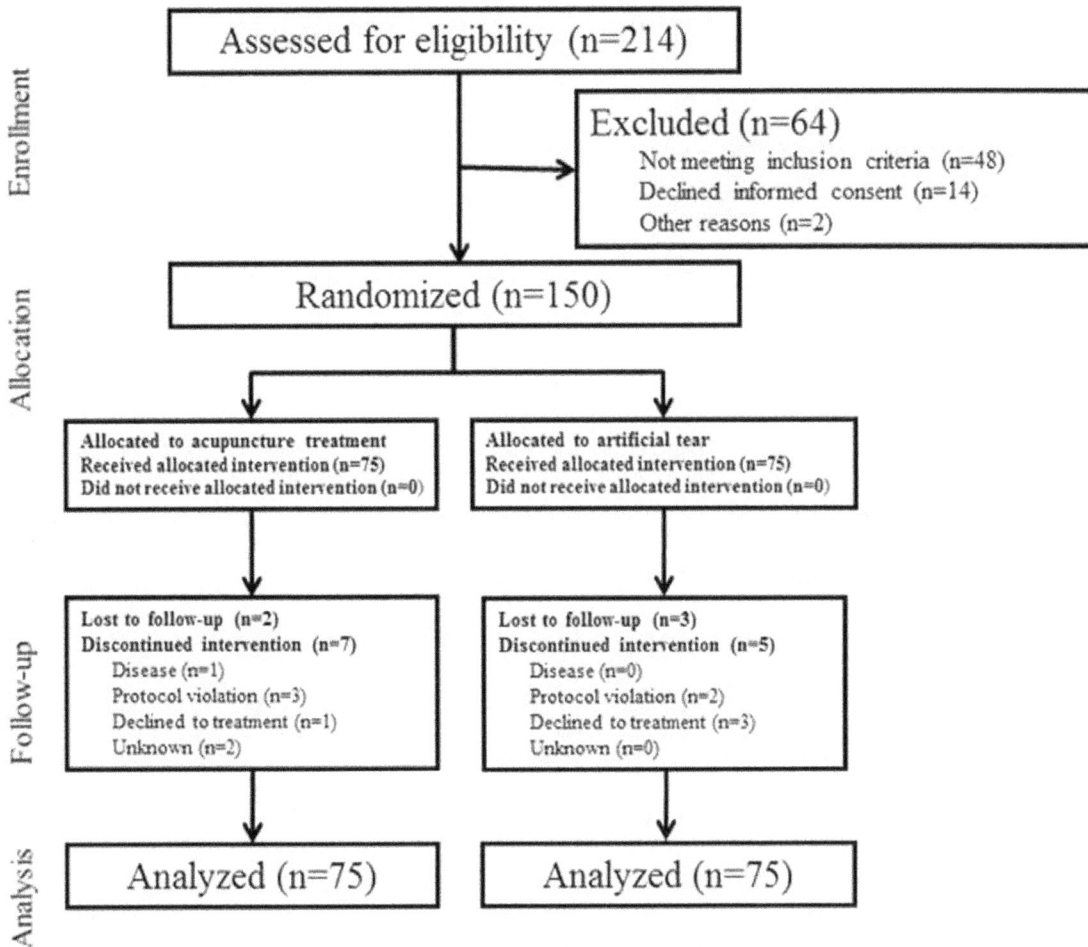

Figure 1. Study flow chart.

[−26.19, −16.4] in the artificial tears group, P = 0.359) or 4 weeks of treatment (acupuncture: −23.84 [−29.59, −18.09]; artificial tears −22.2 [−27.24, −17.16], P = 0.530) or at 4 weeks after treatment (acupuncture: −19.37 [−25.51, −13.24]; artificial tears: −14.71 [−20.86, −8.55], P = 0.327). However, significant changes were reported in the acupuncture group at 8 weeks after acupuncture treatment compared with control group (acupuncture: −23.88 [−30.9, −16.86]; artificial tears: −14.71 [−20.86, −8.55], P = 0.018). The adjusted difference of VAS was −1.64 [−5.17, 1.89] for the acupuncture group after 4 weeks of treatment, and it increased to −2.92 [−7.99, 2.15] at 4 weeks and to −9.17 at 8 weeks after treatment (table 2, figure 3).

QOL

Changes in QOL from baseline values did not show significant differences between the two groups after 2 weeks of treatment (−1.03 [−1.34, −0.71] in the acupuncture group and −1.2 [−1.53, −0.87] in the artificial tears group, as tested by ANCOVA, P = 0.63), after 4 weeks of treatment (acupuncture: −1.32 [−1.65, −0.99]; artificial tears: −0.96 [−1.32, −0.6], P = 0.42), at 4 weeks after treatment (acupuncture: −1.09 [−1.47, −0.72]; artificial tears: −0.96 [−1.32, −0.6], P = 0.47) or at 8 weeks after treatment (acupuncture: −1.09 [−1.47, −0.72]; artificial tears: −0.76 [−1.1, −0.42], P = 0.11, table 2).

TFBUT

TFBUT increased significantly in the acupuncture group after 4 weeks of treatment compared to the artificial tears group (figure 4). The change from the baseline of TFBUT in the left eye was 0.46 [−0.04, 0.96] in the acupuncture group and −0.37 [−0.95, 0.21] in the artificial tears group (P = 0.005), and that in the right eye was 0.59 [0.05, 1.14] and −0.09 [−0.63, 0.44] (P = 0.017), respectively. At 8 weeks after acupuncture, TFBUT in the right eye showed a significant increase in the acupuncture group (acupuncture: 0.72, [0, 1.43]; artificial tears: −0.23 [−0.76, 0.31], P = 0.017) but TFBUT in the left eye did not (acupuncture: 0.3 [−0.38, 0.97]; artificial tears: −0.21 [−0.81, 0.39], P = 0.151). Adjusted differences between the two groups (calculated using representative values from the eye with the higher baseline value) were 0.73 [0.32, 1.14] after 4 weeks (P = 0.007, tested by ANCOVA) and 0.61 [0.14, 1.07] at 8 weeks after acupuncture (P = 0.054).

Schirmer I Test Scores

There were no statistically significant differences in the Schirmer I test score changes of both eyes between the two groups after 4 weeks of treatment (left eye: 0.59 [−0.22, 1.4] in the acupuncture group and 0.55 [−0.64, 1.73] in the artificial tears group, tested by ANCOVA, P = 0.997; right eye, acupuncture: 0.59 [0.05, 1.14] and artificial tears: −0.09

Table 1. Baseline characteristics (intention-to-treat population).

Characteristics	Acupuncture group (n = 75)	Artificial tears group (n = 75)
Age (year, mean (SD))	47.95 (11.11)	46.05 (13.10)
Sex M/F (frequency)	22/53	19/56
Menopause (frequency)	26	25
Symptom duration (frequency, mean (SD))	6.00 (5.69)	5.91 (4.97)
Computer or TV use (hour/week, mean (SD))	16.87 (15.53)	18.61 (16.80)
Contact lens wearer (frequency)	7	6
Smoker (frequency)	7	7
Full time-outdoor workers/full time-indoor workers (frequency)	36/4	27/3
>10 years of school education (frequency)	65	67
Previous treatment (frequency)		
Artificial tears use	33	44
Other treatment use	5	3
No-treatment	37	28
Past history related to dry eye (frequency)		
Sjogren syndrome	0	0
Keratitis	7	10
Cataract	2	3
Glaucoma	2	1
LASIK surgery	1	6
Blepharitis	2	3

[−0.63, 0.44], P = 0.904) or after 8 weeks after treatment (left eye, acupuncture: 1.77 [0.4, 3.13] and artificial tears: 0.61 [−0.54, 1.76], P = 0.192; right eye, acupuncture: 1.45 [0.13, 2.77] and artificial tears: 1.4 [0.11, 2.69], P = 0.857, figure 5).

General Improvements of Dry Eye-related Symptoms

More participants in the acupuncture group experienced general improvements than did those in the artificial tears group; however, there were no significant differences between the two groups (P = 0.060). In contrast, a statistically significant difference was reported between the two groups in the general improvements assessed by physicians (P = 0.001, table 3).

Use of Additional Treatment During the Follow-up Period

During the follow-up period, 9 participants in the artificial tears group treated dry eyes continuously; 3 participants visited ophthalmic clinics and used prescribed lubricants or eye drops, and 6 participants applied over-the-counter artificial teardrops. In addition, 4 participants in the acupuncture group used artificial tears after acupuncture treatment; 1 participant visited an ophthalmic clinic, and the other 3 applied over-the-counter artificial tears.

Adverse Events

Three cases of hematoma were reported in the acupuncture treatment group; 1 patient had moderate severity, and the others had mild severity. Among them, one participant declined further acupuncture treatment because of the hematoma and pain. In the other two cases, the hematomas completely disappeared in several weeks. Adverse events related to artificial tear usage was not reported.

Discussion

This clinical trial assessed the effectiveness of a 4-week standard acupuncture treatment on the subjective and objective outcomes

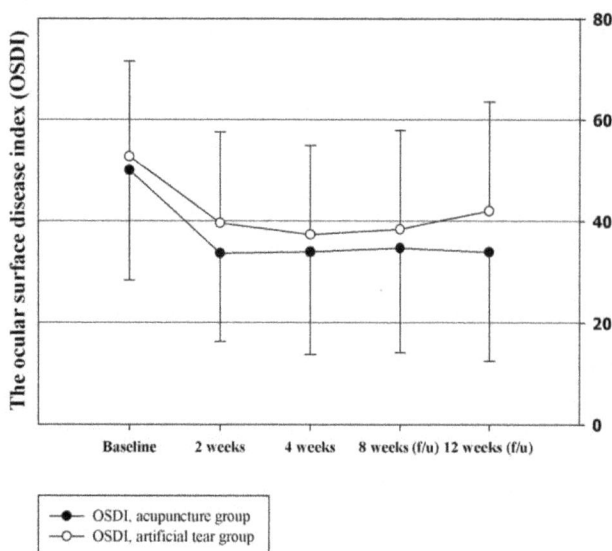

Figure 2. Ocular surface disease index (OSDI).

Table 2. Primary and secondary outcomes at each visit.

| | Acupuncture group (n=75) Mean (SD) | | | | | Artificial tears group (n=75) Mean (SD) | | | | | Adjusted difference† (95% CI) | | | |
| | Baseline | During treatment | | | Follow up | Baseline | During treatment | | | Follow up | During treatment | | | Follow up |
		2 weeks	4 weeks	8 weeks	12 weeks		2 weeks	4 weeks	8 weeks	12 weeks	2 weeks	4 weeks	8 weeks	12 weeks
OSDI	50.05 (21.63)	33.67 (17.35)	33.94 (20.16)	34.70 (20.57)	33.90 (21.42)	52.75 (18.79)	39.65 (17.94)	37.38 (17.61)	38.37 (19.51)	41.99 (21.54)	−3.28 (−7.06, 0.50)	−0.75 (−4.22, 2.72)	−0.98 (−4.08, 2.14)	−5.39* (−8.62, −2.16)
VAS	66.67 (19.18)	48.77 (21.44)	42.83 (23.74)	47.29 (22.90)	42.79 (26.88)	67.52 (17.31)	46.23 (17.92)	45.32 (20.24)	51.07 (23.07)	52.81 (24.12)	3.40 (−0.52, 7.32)	−1.64 (−5.17, 1.89)	−2.92 (−7.99, 2.15)	−9.17* (−13.70, −4.65)
QOL	4.04 (1.20)	3.01 (1.34)	2.72 (1.22)	2.96 (1.31)	2.95 (1.47)	4.08 (1.21)	3.12 (1.11)	2.88 (1.15)	3.12 (1.30)	3.32 (1.37)	−0.07 (−0.31, 0.18)	−0.12 (−0.40, 0.15)	−0.12 (−0.37, 0.13)	−0.34 (−0.58, −0.09)
BUT	6.19 (2.18)		6.80 (2.25)		6.68 (2.85)	6.01 (1.98)		5.89 (2.02)		5.89 (1.99)		0.73* (0.32, 1.14)		0.61* (0.14, 1.07)
Schirmer	4.49 (2.56)		4.88 (3.70)		5.95 (5.02)	4.16 (2.66)		4.95 (4.34)		5.28 (4.07)		−0.40 (−0.75, −0.05)		0.33 (0.02, 0.64)

ANCOVA was used for the statistical analysis of changes from baseline in each outcome between two groups. *P<0.05.
†All the outcomes were adjusted for baseline values and clinical research centres. Negative values of adjusted difference in OSDI, VAS and QOL (positive difference in BUT and Schirmer) are in favour of acupuncture group.

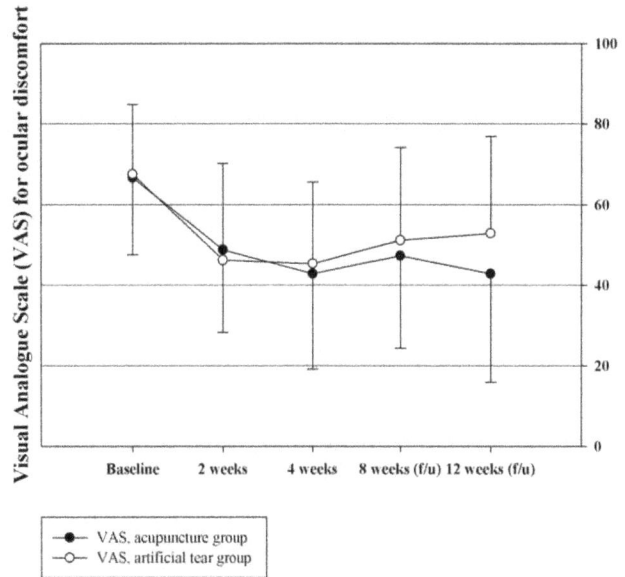

Figure 3. Visual analogue scale (VAS) for self-assessment of ocular discomfort.

of dry eye syndrome. Although overall improvement was observed in both groups, there was no statistically significant difference in favour of acupuncture treatment for OSDI, VAS or quality of life during the treatment period or immediately after treatment. Improved OSDI and VAS scores, however, were sustained for 8 weeks in the acupuncture group, but not in the artificial tears group. Among the ophthalmologic tests, TFBUT increased significantly in the acupuncture group, but the Schirmer test results did not.

Strength and Weakness

Previous research on dry eye syndrome has provided limited evidence of the effectiveness of acupuncture due to poor methodological quality and insufficient statistical power [9]. We previously conducted a case study to test the validity and

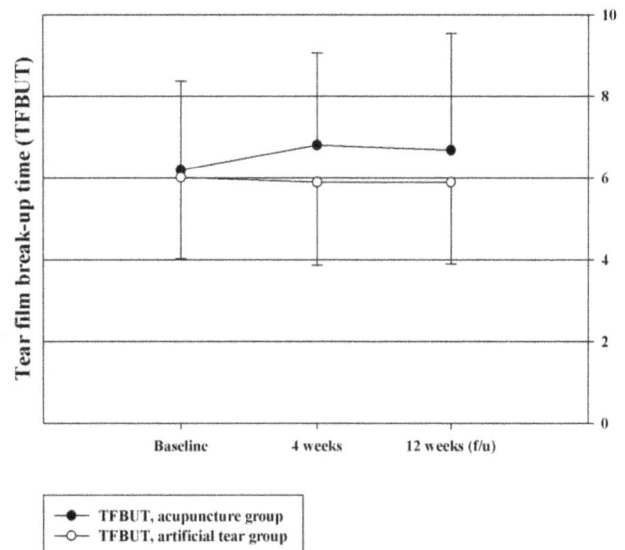

Figure 4. Tear film break-up time (TFBUT).

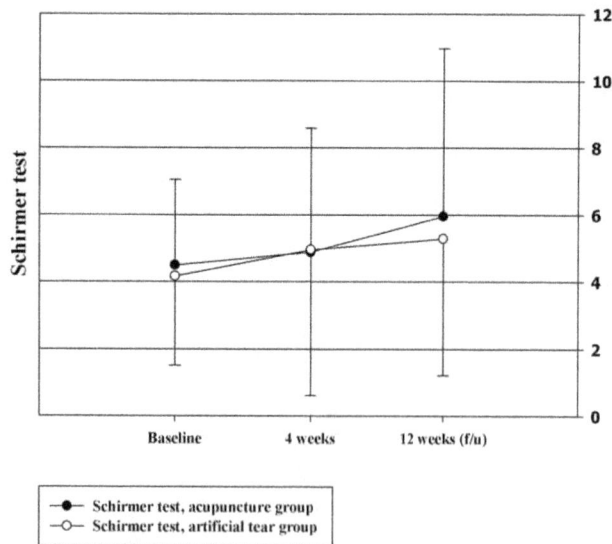

Figure 5. Schirmer I test.

availability of acupuncture [27] and an RCT using sham acupuncture as a control to evaluate the efficacy of acupuncture for dry eye syndrome [13]. From the results of these studies, we designed a clinical trial adopting an active control for assessing the effectiveness of acupuncture with a sufficient number of subjects for statistical analyses [10]. To increase the universality of the study results (i.e., external validity), three research hospitals located in different areas conducted this trial simultaneously. To the best of our knowledge, this is the first study that had the statistical power (calculated from previous studies) and methodological rigor to allow strong conclusions regarding the effectiveness of acupuncture for the treatment of dry eye syndrome.

Along with subjective outcomes, it has recently been suggested that objective outcomes should also be tested for the interventions that involve large non-specific effects such as acupuncture [28]. Therefore, we assessed both subjective and objective outcome measures simultaneously. To reduce detection bias, separate outcome assessors evaluated treatment effects, and practitioners were instructed to not have active interaction with their patients in the process of acupuncture treatment. However, despite these attempts, it is possible that the non-specific effects of acupuncture could not be completely avoided.

This study has several weaknesses. First, because the main outcomes showed the effectiveness of the acupuncture group 8 weeks after treatment, the follow-up period should have been longer to evaluate the sustained effects of acupuncture treatment. Considering the average symptom duration of dry eye syndrome,

evaluating the long term effects would be necessary in future trials. Second, this study result may not completely reflect actual clinical practice situations. There are multiple variations of acupuncture treatment including the style of acupuncture, needling methods, point selection and treatment sessions [9]. We adopted a standardised acupuncture modality based on TKM theory, which differs from previous researchers in the style of acupuncture and treatment regimen [29–31]. We believe that different acupuncture methods result in different effects. To optimise acupuncture effects, the styles, needling details and other components involved in this intervention should be compared in future research. Third, the use of a control intervention might be considered a controversial issue. Our previous study comparing actual and sham acupunctures [13] did not prove the specific effects of acupuncture, which is the general anticipated outcome of acupuncture trials [32]. Literature review has suggested that sham acupuncture interventions might have larger effects than placebo drugs, and they are usually associated with a comparatively large non-specific effect, which is one of the major obstacles in evaluating the efficacy of acupuncture [33]. In this sense, comparative effectiveness trials have emerged as alternatives for evaluating the clinical value of acupuncture treatment in the real world [34,35]. As an active treatment for dry eyes, artificial tears are generally recommended as a first-line therapy [36]. According to a survey report of ophthalmologists, preservative-free artificial tears were most frequently used for moderate to severe dry-eye patients among various treatment modalities in Korea [37]. From this perspective, comparing acupuncture and artificial tears is a basic step for establishing the effectiveness of acupuncture treatment for dry eyes, as we originally intended in this trial. Additionally, if there may be any confirmed benefit in favour of acupuncture and no evidence of harm, we suggest that acupuncture can be given to patients who want acupuncture or who did not show a good response to conventional treatment on the basis of these results [38]. Fourth, the frequency of the average usage of artificial tear was below four times a day which is suggested to be the standard dose of sodium carboxymethylcellulose, so participants in the control group used artificial tear relatively infrequently. However, participants were allowed to apply artificial tear freely for easing their dry eye symptoms without frequency limit. As a result, there was one participant who used tears 15 times a day at most. Suggesting that artificial tear is generally accepted for alleviating bothering symptoms related to dry eye, allowing different frequency of usage in accordance with dry eye severity might not contribute the effectiveness of artificial tear drop in this trial. Finally, although we adopted the results of objective ophthalmologic tests as screening criteria for moderate to severe dry eye syndrome, there is a possibility that false-positive or false-negative dry eye patients might have been included in this study. Recent studies about TFBUT and Schirmer test suggested that

Table 3. General improvements of dry eye-related symptoms.

Grade	Assessed by participants (n = 137)*					Assessed by physicians (n = 136)[†]				
	E	G	F	P	A	E	G	F	P	A
Acupuncture	2 (2.99%)	27 (40.30%)	28 (41.79%)	10 (14.93%)	0 (0%)	4 (5.97%)	28 (41.79%)	25 (37.31%)	10 (14.93%)	0 (0%)
Artificial tears	2 (2.86%)	17 (24.29%)	26 (37.14%)	24 (34.29%)	1 (1.43%)	0 (0%)	17 (24.64%)	22 (31.88%)	27 (39.13%)	3 (4.35%)

Tested by Chi-squared test; *P = 0.060, [†]P = 0.001; E: excellent, G: good, F: fair, P: poor, A: aggravation.

very limited utility of these tests might introduce bias for identifying patients with mild to moderate dry eye [39,40]. However, considering that tear osmolarity, which is accepted as a good marker for dry eye, was not available because of the required laboratory instruments and the participants' discomforts over collecting large amount of tear specimens, TFBUT and Schirmer test were the second best policy for this study [39].

Meaning of the Study

This study indicates that acupuncture is not more effective than artificial tears for the treatment of dry eyes in the improvement of subjective ocular symptoms such as OSDI during the treatment period. However, this does not mean that acupuncture is not a good intervention for dry eye syndrome. Acupuncture may have benefits on the mid-term outcomes related to dry eye syndrome. Although statistically significant differences were not observed in the assessment of dry eye symptoms after 4 weeks of treatment, both treatments showed improvements in symptoms greater than the MCID for OSDI [19]. In addition, the improvement of OSDI was sustained until 8 weeks after treatment in the acupuncture group, but not in the artificial tears group. Furthermore, fewer patients visited ophthalmic clinics to manage dry eye symptoms in the acupuncture treatment group during the follow-up period. Apart from these subjective outcomes, TFBUT (which objectively reflects the stability of pre-corneal tear film) showed significant improvement in the acupuncture group. A comprehensive discussion about the effectiveness of acupuncture (including the results of the cost-effectiveness analysis and qualitative study) will be necessary to conclusively judge the benefits of this intervention.

Unanswered Questions and Suggestions for the Future Research

Contrary to the temporal effect of artificial tear which works as a lubricant, acupuncture may act in other ways to improve dry eye syndrome. Acupuncture may reduce chronic inflammation of the ocular surface or accessory organs through the cholinergic anti-inflammatory pathway by enhancing vagus nerve activity [41]. Dry eye patients treated with acupuncture showed prolonged improvement in this trial and it might be explained by the effect of acupuncture of relieving pathologic cause of dry eye. In addition, ocular irritation, one of the disturbing symptoms of dry eye, can be decreased through the analgesic effects of acupuncture as well [42].

Previous research on dry eye syndrome has shown the benefits of acupuncture on the improvement of both objective (TFBUT, Schirmer and cornea fluorescent staining) and subjective (response rate) outcomes [29–31]. However, the results of this study indicate that there was no significant difference between the acupuncture and artificial tears groups after 4 weeks of treatment, and only TFBUT measurements improved significantly. This might be partially due to the heterogeneity in treatment durations and acupuncture treatment methods (including acupuncture points) utilised in the previous studies. However, the effect of acupuncture might be overestimated in these studies because of methodological flaws and inappropriate statistical power [43]. Generally, less rigorous trials are prone to exaggerate treatment effects [44] and studies with small sample sizes may underestimate it [45].

As with other medical interventions, acupuncture-related adverse events have been reported, but acupuncture is typically regarded as safe when applied by well-trained practitioners [46]. Recent observational studies have suggested that the frequency of adverse events related to acupuncture in trials and clinical practices ranges from 3.2% to 7.4% according to the population and treatment modalities [47–49]. Although serious adverse events did not occur in this study, 3 participants (4%) in the acupuncture group experienced adverse events related to their treatment in agreement with the general risk rate accompanying usual acupuncture practice. Because adverse events affect patient compliance to acupuncture, patients should be informed before treatment, and practitioners should adhere to safety guidelines on acupuncture use to avoid preventable errors.

Supporting Information

Checklist S1   CONSORT Checklist.
(PDF)

Protocol S1   Trial Protocol. (published at open assess journal, Trials 2010)
(DOC)

Author Contributions

Conceived and designed the experiments: THK. Performed the experiments: THK JWK KHK JBC KEH SDL SMC. Analyzed the data: KWK. Contributed reagents/materials/analysis tools: KWK. Wrote the paper: THK. Revised the design of this trial and revised the paper: MSS. Revised the paper: SYJ ARK. Monitored data collection: HJJ.

References

1. Lemp MA, Baudouin C, Baum J, Dogru M, Foulks GN, et al. (2007) The definition and classification of dry eye disease: report of the Definition and Classification Subcommittee of the International Dry Eye WorkShop (2007). Ocul Surf 5: 75–92.
2. Epidemiology Subcommittee of the International Dry Eye WorkShop (2007) The epidemiology of dry eye disease: report of the Epidemiology Subcommittee of the International Dry Eye WorkShop (2007). Ocul Surf 5: 93–107.
3. Yu J, Asche CV, Fairchild CJ (2011) The economic burden of dry eye disease in the United States: a decision tree analysis. Cornea 30: 379–387.
4. Pflugfelder SC (2008) Prevalence, burden, and pharmacoeconomics of dry eye disease. Am J Manag Care 14: S102–106.
5. Lemp MA (2008) Management of dry eye disease. Am J Manag Care 14: S88–101.
6. NIH Consensus Conference (1998) Acupuncture. JAMA 280: 1518–1524.
7. Law SK, Li T (2007) Acupuncture for glaucoma. Cochrane Database Syst Rev. CD006030 p.
8. Lam DS, Zhao J, Chen LJ, Wang Y, Zheng C, et al. (2011) Adjunctive Effect of Acupuncture to Refractive Correction on Anisometropic Amblyopia One-Year Results of a Randomized Crossover Trial. Ophthalmology.
9. Lee MS, Shin BC, Choi TY, Ernst E (2011) Acupuncture for treating dry eye: a systematic review. Acta Ophthalmol 89: 101–106.
10. Kim TH, Kang JW, Kim KH, Kang KW, Shin MS, et al. (2010) Acupuncture for dry eye: a multicentre randomised controlled trial with active comparison

intervention (artificial tear drop) using a mixed method approach protocol. Trials 11: 107.
11. Kim TH, Kim JI, Shin MS, Lee MS, Choi JY, et al. (2009) Acupuncture for dry eye: a randomised controlled trial protocol. Trials 10: 112.
12. Behrens A, Doyle JJ, Stern L, Chuck RS, McDonnell PJ, et al. (2006) Dysfunctional tear syndrome: a Delphi approach to treatment recommendations. Cornea 25: 900–907.
13. Shin MS, Kim JI, Lee MS, Kim KH, Choi JY, et al. (2010) Acupuncture for treating dry eye: a randomized placebo-controlled trial. Acta Ophthalmol 88: e328–333.
14. Hardten DR, Brown MJ, Pham-Vang S (2007) Evaluation of an isotonic tear in combination with topical cyclosporine for the treatment of ocular surface disease. Curr Med Res Opin 23: 2083–2091.
15. Kwon D-H, Kim Y-S, Choi D-Y (2009) Book research into acupuncture treatment for dry eye. The Journal of Korean Acupuncture & Moxibustion society 27: 10–24.
16. So DW (2002) Acupuncture outcomes, expectations, patient-provider relationship, and the placebo effect: implications for health promotion. American Journal Of Public Health 92: 1662–1667.
17. WHO Reginoal Office for the Western Pacific (2008) WHO Standard Acupuncture Point Locations in the Western Pacific Region. Manila: World Health Organization.

18. Schiffman RM, Christianson MD, Jacobsen G, Hirsch JD, Reis BL (2000) Reliability and validity of the Ocular Surface Disease Index. Arch Ophthalmol 118: 615–621.

19. Miller KL, Walt JG, Mink DR, Satram-Hoang S, Wilson SE, et al. (2010) Minimal clinically important difference for the ocular surface disease index. Arch Ophthalmol 128: 94–101.

20. Her J, Yu S, Seo S (2006) Clinical Effects of Various Antiinflammatory Therapies in Dry Eye Syndrome. J Korean Opthalmol Soc 47: 1901–1910.

21. Paterson C (1996) Measuring outcomes in primary care: a patient generated measure, MYMOP, compared with the SF-36 health survey. Br Med J 312: 1016–1020.

22. Yuan J, Purepong N, Hunter RF, Kerr DP, Park J, et al. (2009) Different frequencies of acupuncture treatment for chronic low back pain: an assessor-blinded pilot randomised controlled trial. Complement Ther Med 17: 131–140.

23. Bron AJ, Abelson MB, Ousler G, Pearce E, Tomlinson A, et al. (2007) Methodologies to diagnose and monitor dry eye disease: report of the Diagnostic Methodology Subcommittee of the International Dry Eye WorkShop. Ocul Surf 5: 108–152.

24. Foulks GN, Bron AJ (2003) Meibomian gland dysfunction: a clinical scheme for description, diagnosis, classification, and grading. Ocul Surf 1: 107–126.

25. Anonymous WHO toxicity grading scale for determining the severity of adverse events. Available: http://www.icssc.org/Documents/Resources/AEManual2003AppendicesFebruary_06_2003%20final.pdf. Accessed: 13 May 2011.

26. Linde K, Witt CM, Streng A, Weidenhammer W, Wagenpfeil S, et al. (2007) The impact of patient expectations on outcomes in four randomized controlled trials of acupuncture in patients with chronic pain. Pain 128: 264–271.

27. Jeon JH, Shin MS, Lee MS, Jeong SY, Kang KW, et al. (2010) Acupuncture reduces symptoms of dry eye syndrome: a preliminary observational study. J Altern Complement Med 16: 1291–1294.

28. Wechsler ME, Kelley JM, Boyd IO, Dutile S, Marigowda G, et al. (2011) Active albuterol or placebo, sham acupuncture, or no intervention in asthma. N Engl J Med 365: 119–126.

29. He HQ, Wang ZL, Hu HL, Liu R (2004) Effect of acupuncture on lacerimal film of xeroma patients. J Nanjing TCM University 20: 158–159.

30. Pang YJ, Jia GQ, Feng JL (2003) The effect of acupuncture on the tear production in patients with Sjogren's syndrome. J Tradit Chin Opahtalmol 13: 18–20.

31. Wang ZL, He HQ, Huang D, Shi CG (2005) Effect of integral syndrome differentiation acupuncture on the tear film stability in the patient of xerophthalmia. Zhongguo Zhen Jiu 25: 460–463.

32. Moffet HH (2009) Sham acupuncture may be as efficacious as true acupuncture: a systematic review of clinical trials. J Altern Complement Med 15: 213–216.

33. Witt CM (2011) Clinical research on acupuncture - Concepts and guidance on efficacy and effectiveness research. Chin J Integr Med 17: 166–172.

34. Witt CM, Brinkhaus B (2010) Efficacy, effectiveness and cost-effectiveness of acupuncture for allergic rhinitis - An overview about previous and ongoing studies. Auton Neurosci 157: 42–45.

35. Garber AM, Tunis SR (2009) Does comparative-effectiveness research threaten personalized medicine? N Engl J Med 360: 1925–1927.

36. Anonymous (2007) Management and therapy of dry eye disease: report of the Management and Therapy Subcommittee of the International Dry Eye WorkShop (2007). Ocul Surf 5: 163–178.

37. Kim WJ, Kim HS, Kim MS (2007) Current Trends in the Recognition and Treatment of Dry Eye: A Survey of Ophthalmologists. J Korean Ophthalmol Soc 48: 1614–1622.

38. Berman BM, Langevin HM, Witt CM, Dubner R (2010) Acupuncture for chronic low back pain. N Engl J Med 363: 454–461.

39. Lemp MA, Bron AJ, Baudouin C, Benitez Del Castillo JM, Geffen D, et al. (2011) Tear osmolarity in the diagnosis and management of dry eye disease. Am J Ophthalmol 151: 792–798 e791.

40. Sullivan BD, Whitmer D, Nichols KK, Tomlinson A, Foulks GN, et al. (2010) An objective approach to dry eye disease severity. Invest Ophthalmol Vis Sci 51: 6125–6130.

41. Oke SL, Tracey KJ (2009) The inflammatory reflex and the role of complementary and alternative medical therapies. Ann N Y Acad Sci 1172: 172–180.

42. Nepp J, Jandrasits K, Schauersberger J, Schild G, Wedrich A, et al. (2002) Is acupuncture an useful tool for pain-treatment in ophthalmology? Acupunct Electrother Res 27: 171–182.

43. Detsky AS, Naylor CD, O'Rourke K, McGeer AJ, L'Abbe KA (1992) Incorporating variations in the quality of individual randomized trials into meta-analysis. J Clin Epidemiol 45: 255–265.

44. Egger M, Juni P, Bartlett C, Holenstein F, Sterne J (2003) How important are comprehensive literature searches and the assessment of trial quality in systematic reviews? Empirical study. Health Technol Assess 7: 1–76.

45. Altman DG (1980) Statistics and ethics in medical research: III How large a sample? Br Med J 281: 1336–1338.

46. White A, Cummings TM, Filshie J (2008) An introduction to Western medical acupuncture. Edinburgh: Churchill Livingstone/Elsevier. xviii: 240.

47. Park JE, Lee MS, Choi JY, Kim BY, Choi SM (2010) Adverse events associated with acupuncture: a prospective survey. J Altern Complement Med 16: 959–963.

48. Zhao L, Zhang FW, Li Y, Wu X, Zheng H, et al. (2011) Adverse events associated with acupuncture: three multicentre randomized controlled trials of 1968 cases in China. Trials 12: 87.

49. Witt CM, Pach D, Reinhold T, Wruck K, Brinkhaus B, et al. (2011) Treatment of the adverse effects from acupuncture and their economic impact: a prospective study in 73,406 patients with low back or neck pain. Eur J Pain 15: 193–197.

16

Getting the Grip on Nonspecific Treatment Effects: Emesis in Patients Randomized to Acupuncture or Sham Compared to Patients Receiving Standard Care

Anna Enblom[1,2,3]*, **Mats Lekander**[3,4], **Mats Hammar**[5], **Anna Johnsson**[6], **Erik Onelöv**[7], **Martin Ingvar**[3], **Gunnar Steineck**[7,8], **Sussanne Börjeson**[1,9]

1 Division of Nursing Science, Department of Medical and Health Sciences, Linköping University, Linköping, Sweden, **2** The Vårdal Institute, Lund, Sweden, **3** Department of Clinical Neuroscience, Osher Centre for Integrative Medicine, Karolinska Institute, Stockholm, Sweden, **4** Stress Research Institute, Stockholm University, Stockholm, Sweden, **5** Department of Clinical and Experimental Medicine, Obstetrics and Gynecology, Linköping University, Linköping, Sweden, **6** Division of Physiotherapy, Department of Oncology, University Hospital, Lund, Sweden, **7** Division of Clinical Cancer Epidemiology, Department of Oncology, Karolinska Institute, Stockholm, Sweden, **8** Division of Clinical Cancer Epidemiology, Department of Oncology, Sahlgrenska Academy, Gothenburg, Sweden, **9** Centre of Surgery and Oncology, Linköping University Hospital, Linköping, Sweden

Abstract

Background: It is not known whether or not delivering acupuncture triggers mechanisms cited as placebo and if acupuncture or sham reduces radiotherapy-induced emesis more than standard care.

Methodology/Principal Findings: Cancer patients receiving radiotherapy over abdominal/pelvic regions were randomized to verum (penetrating) acupuncture (n = 109; 99 provided data) in the alleged antiemetic acupuncture point PC6 or sham acupuncture (n = 106; 101 provided data) performed with a telescopic non-penetrating needle at a sham point 2–3 times/ week during the whole radiotherapy period. The acupuncture cohort was compared to a reference cohort receiving standard care (n = 62; 62 provided data). The occurrence of emesis in each group was compared after a mean dose of 27 Gray. Nausea and vomiting were experienced during the preceding week by 37 and 8% in the verum acupuncture group, 38 and 7% in the sham acupuncture group and 63 and 15% in the standard care group, respectively. The lower occurrence of nausea in the acupuncture cohort (verum and sham) compared to patients receiving standard care (37% versus 63%, relative risk (RR) 0.6, 95 % confidence interval (CI) 0.5–0.8) was also true after adjustment for potential confounding factors for nausea (RR 0.8, CI 0.6 to 0.9). Nausea intensity was lower in the acupuncture cohort (78% no nausea, 13% a little, 8% moderate, 1% much) compared to the standard care cohort (52% no nausea, 32% a little, 15% moderate, 2% much) (p = 0.002). The acupuncture cohort expected antiemetic effects from their treatment (95%). Patients who expected nausea had increased risk for nausea compared to patients who expected low risk for nausea (RR 1.6; CI 1.2–2.4).

Conclusions/Significance: Patients treated with verum or sham acupuncture experienced less nausea and vomiting compared to patients receiving standard care, possibly through a general care effect or due to the high level of patient expectancy.

Trial Registration: ClinicalTrials.gov NCT00621660

Editor: Pedro R Lowenstein, Cedars-Sinai Medical Center and University of California Los Angeles, United States of America

Funding: This study was supported by The Swedish Cancer Society, The Vardal Institute, The County Council of Ostergotland, The University of Linköping, Cancer and Traffic Injury Fund and The Vardal Foundation for Health Care Sciences and Allergy Research. Mats Lekander and Martin Ingvar are members of Stockholm Brain Institute funded by Vinnova and The Swedish Strategic Research Foundation. The funders had no role in study design, data collection and analysis, decision to publish, or preparation of the manuscript.

Competing Interests: The authors have declared that no competing interests exist.

* E-mail: anna.enblom@ki.se

Introduction

Many cancer patients express interest in acupuncture for nausea [1-2] but it is not known if acupuncture is more effective for emesis (nausea and vomiting) than standard care during radiotherapy. Approximately 60% of patients irradiated over abdominal and/or pelvic fields experienced emesis during radiotherapy [1,3–4]. Antiemetics are effective, especially serotonin-receptor antagonists combined with corticosteroids [5]. However, some patients at risk

for nausea do not receive potent antiemetics, do not respond satisfactorily [1,3,5], or experience side-effects [5]. In a previous study we found that of 145 nauseous patients irradiated over a variety of regions, one third asked for more treatment against nausea while 40% rejected antiemetics [1].

Between two and 31% of patients undergoing cancer treatment use acupuncture for various kinds of symptoms [2]. In chemotherapy-induced nausea, acupuncture and acupressure reduced nausea more than antiemetics, but those studies did not include any sham treated control groups [6–11]. In a study of 80 chemotherapy patients, penetrating acupuncture did not reduce nausea more than telescopic non-penetrating sham needles [12]. In our study of radiotherapy-induced nausea, 70% of patients randomized to penetrating acupuncture and 62% of patients treated with telescopic sham needles experienced nausea during the radiotherapy period [13]. Apparently there was a lack of effects that could be related to the specific characteristics of verum (genuine) acupuncture; i.e. stimulation of skin penetrating needles in traditional acupuncture points resulting in a "deqi" sensation. However, as many as 95% of patients in *both* groups considered the treatment to be effective, and 89% were interested in receiving the treatments in the future [13]. In the light of the apparent conflict between lack of specific effects from verum acupuncture and large subjectively experienced positive effects it seems interesting to evaluate if acupuncture has antiemetic effects related to nonspecific mechanisms.

The aims of the study were to compare nausea and vomiting experienced by a cohort treated with verum or sham acupuncture with that experienced by a cohort receiving standard care during radiotherapy, and to evaluate if expectations of nausea and of acupuncture effects were related to the actual occurrence of nausea.

Materials and Methods

The protocol for this trial and supporting CONSORT checklist are available as supporting information; see Protocol S1 and Checklist S1.

Inclusion

Two cohorts of patients treated for cancer in three Swedish oncology departments were included: one a standard care and the other an acupuncture cohort, see figure 1. The standard care cohort was created by a cross-sectional selection in four different days at two oncology departments in 1999 and 2003 [1] (n = 62). The acupuncture cohort was created from consecutively included patients in 2004 to 2006 at one of the two oncology departments referred to above and also in another oncology department [13]. Members of this cohort were randomized to verum acupuncture (n = 109) or sham acupuncture (n = 106). Inclusion criteria for both cohorts were that patients were at least 18 years of age, had radiotherapy over abdominal or pelvic fields and were able to take part in the study procedure. Exclusion criteria for the acupuncture cohort only were radiotherapy of less than 800 cm^3 volume and 25 Gray dose, antiemetic treatment or persistent nausea within 24 hours prior to the start of radiotherapy and acupuncture treatment during the past year for any indication or ever for nausea.

All patients gave their informed written consent and the Regional Ethical Review Board in Linköping, Sweden, approved the study. The informed consent form used in the acupuncture cohort contained the information: "You will receive an ordinary acupuncture treatment with needles penetrating the skin or another treatment with needles placed just against the skin". The study-evaluator and all health-care professionals, with the exception of the acupuncture-providing therapists, were blind to the acupuncture allocation. The standard care group knew, of course, that no acupuncture was given. They had been informed that the aim of the data collection was to evaluate the prevalence of nausea during radiotherapy.

Treatment regimens

The acupuncture and the standard care cohort were, except for study participation, treated according to clinical routines,

including the use of rescue antiemetics. The standard care cohort received no acupuncture therapy. One physiotherapist at each hospital (performing 1412 and 607 treatments) performed both verum and sham acupuncture and they had five deputy physiotherapists (performing 228, 75, 54, 32 and 6 treatments). Treatments started on the first day of radiotherapy, continued 30 minutes per session three times/week for two weeks, and then twice/week, until the end of radiotherapy according to a standardised treatment protocol. The patients were in a hotel, ward unit or at the radiotherapy department during the treatments, received either in a sitting or a supine position. The physiotherapists treated one to three patients simultaneously and maintained an everyday conversation, but avoided the subject of nausea.

Verum acupuncture was administered bilaterally to the traditional antiemetic point pericardium six (PC6) [14] between the tendons of palmaris longus and flexor carpii radialis at two body-inches proximal of the wrist crease. Sharp needles, diameter 0.30 × length 40 millimetres, were inserted into a depth of a half body-inch. One body-inch (or a "cun": approximate 1.5 cm) is equivalent to the greatest width of the individual patient's thumb at the distal phalanx. The needles were manipulated three times/ treatment by twirling and lifting until "deqi" occurred. "Deqi" is the specific sensation of verum acupuncture, involving heaviness, numbness, soreness and a minimal muscular contraction around the needle [15].

Sham acupuncture was administered bilaterally to a sham point located two body-inches proximal to PC6, outside traditional acupuncture points. "Park's sham devise" [16], 0.30×40 millimetres (extended length) was used. The credible [13] blunt telescopic needle glides upwards into its handle instead of penetrating the skin, and thus gives the illusion of penetration. Double-sticky marking tubes, used in both groups, held the sham needles in place. The therapists manipulated the sham needles three times/ session until the needles touched the skin, but no "deqi" occurred. The duration of needle pressure to the skin was approximately ten seconds/session.

Data collection

Background data. Clinical data, listed in table 1, were extracted from the patients' medical records. Other background variables, listed in table 2, were collected in a written questionnaire.

Nausea, vomiting and use of antiemetics. Type/dose of antiemetics and emesis during the previous 24-hours were measured by written established emesis questions [1,17]: "Have you experienced nausea?", answered on a four-level category scale: "No, not at all" or "Yes, a little/moderate/much" and "Have you been vomiting?" answered by "No" or "Yes". In the acupuncture cohort the questions were asked daily during the whole radiotherapy period. In the standard care cohort, the questions were asked only once (after a mean dose of 27 Gray of radiotherapy) and at that time the questions were asked regarding the previous 24 hours and also within the time frame of the preceding week. Every patient who had experienced nausea at least once within the preceding seven days (irrespective of intensity) or vomiting was assigned to the groups "Experiencing nausea" or "Experiencing vomiting". The emesis questions showed in pilot studies satisfactory face-validity (n = 9), construct validity (Spearman's correlation coefficient (r) 1.0; n = 456 paired observations) and test-retest reliability (r 0.98–1.0; n = 36).

Expectations of treatment effects and on nausea. At the end of the first, the sixth and the last verum or sham treatment the physiotherapists asked the patients: "Do you believe that the

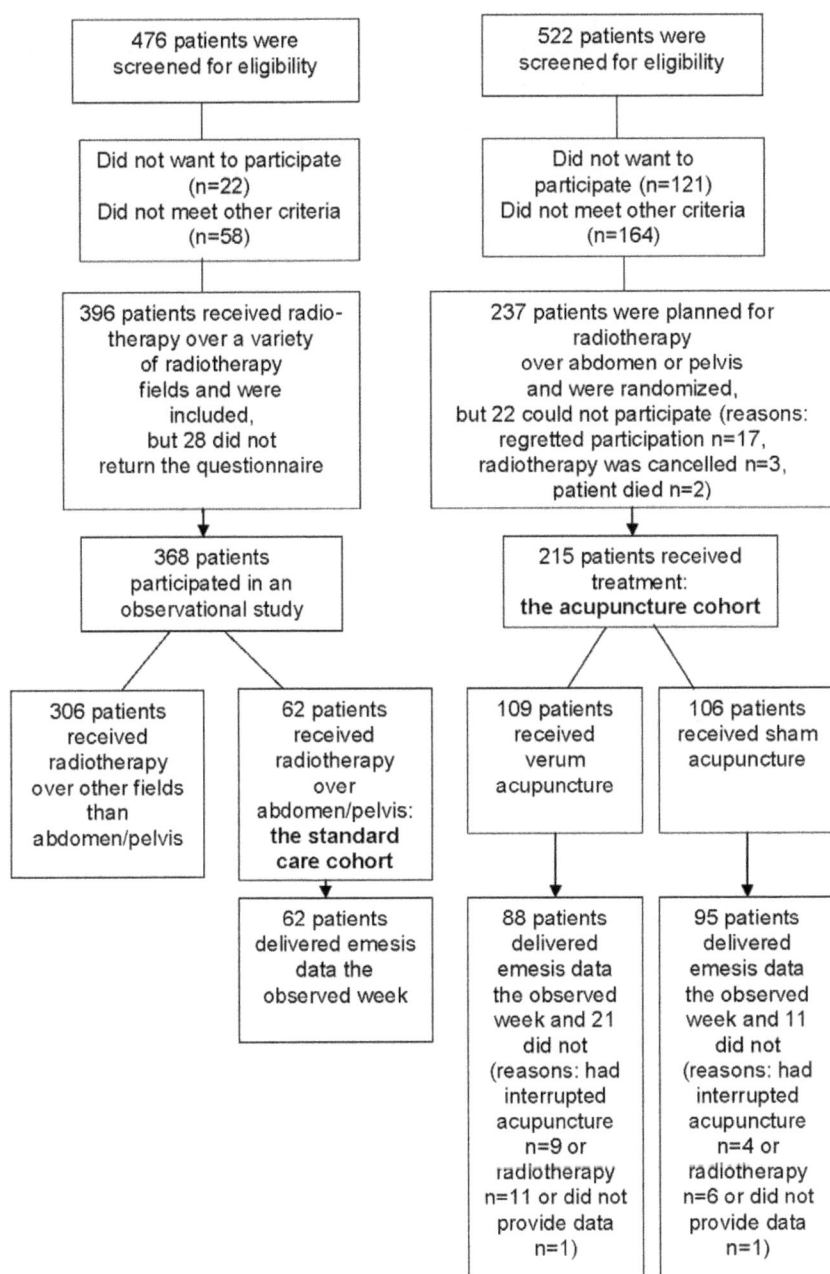

Figure 1. Selection of the patients in the standard care and the acupuncture cohort.

treatment that you have just received is effective in preventing or reducing nausea?" The four answer categories were "No, I do not think the treatment is effective" and "Yes, I believe a little/ moderately/much that the treatment is effective". Before treatment was started, the verum and sham treated patients answered the written question: "In relation to others, how do you estimate your own risk for becoming nauseous during the radiotherapy period?" to be answered on a five-grade category scale from "Much lower risk" to "Much higher risk".

Statistical analysis

The acupuncture cohort was compared with the standard care cohort using Student's t-test regarding continuous data, Mann Whitney U-test regarding ordinal or continuous, not normally distributed, data and by Fisher's exact (two categories), or Chi2-test (three categories or more), regarding category data. Relative risk (RR) for nausea with 95% confidence intervals (CI) was calculated for each of the different subgroups shown in table 1 and table 2 as compared to a reference group (RR 1.0), defined as the subgroup with the lowest prevalence of nausea. One exception was made; the subgroup of patients believing "little" in antiemetic effects of verum/sham treatment was not chosen as a reference group, because it consisted of only ten patients. A multivariable logistic regression model was constructed to determine the relative importance of the different characteristics seen in and table 2 1 for explaining the occurrence of nausea (Logistic procedure, forward selection) and the RR for nausea was adjusted in proc Genmod, with a log link and binomial error distribution. At the time that

Table 1. Clinical characteristics of the patients in the verum acupuncture, sham acupuncture or standard care group.

Characteristics	Acupuncture cohort n = 215		Standard care cohort n = 62	Experiencing nausea n = 172/total n providing data = 267[1]	Univariable relative risk (95 % confidence interval)	Multivariable[2] relative risk, (95 % confidence interval) adjusted for three groups
	Verum acupuncture n = 109	Sham acupuncture n = 106				
Tumor diagnose, n (%)	n = 109	n = 106	n = 62	n = 267		
Gynecological-	72 (66)	75 (71)	37 (60)	111/178 (62)	1.0 (Ref.)	1.0 (Ref.)
Colon-/rectal-	31 (28)	29 (27)	11 (18)	43/67 (64)	1.0 (0.8–1.3)	1.0 (0.8–1.3)
Testicular-	2 (2)	0 (0)	6 (10)	7/8 (88)	1.4 (1.1–1.8)	1.5 (1.0–2.2)
Pancreas, stomach or gallbladder-tumor	4 (4)	2 (2)	8 (13)	11/14 (79)	1.3 (0.9–1.7)	1.3 (0.9–1.9)
Total radiotherapy dose (Gray) mean ± SD	47.9 ±10.7	50.3 ± 10.3	41.8 ± 10.0	47.3 ± 10.5		
Concomitant chemotherapy, n (%)	n = 100	n = 99	n = 61	n = 260		
Yes	28 (28)	29 (29)	15 (25)	57/72 (79)	1.3 (1.1–1.6)	1.3 (1.1–1.6)
No	72 (72)	70 (71)	46 (75)	112/188 (60)	1.0 (Ref.)	1.0 (Ref.)
Consumption of antiemetics at least once, n (%)	n = 100	n = 101	n = 62	n = 263		
No	67 (67)	69 (68)	36 (58)	74/162 (46)	1.0 (Ref)	1.0 (Ref)
Any type	42 (42)	37 (37)	26 (42)	98/105 (93)	2.1 (1.7–2.4)	2.0 (1.7–2.4)
Serotonin-receptor antagonists	21 (21)	23 (23)	7 (11)	48/51 (94)	2.1 (1.7–2.5)	1.6 (1.2–2.0)
Dopamine-receptor antagonists	24 (24)	21 (21)	6 (10)	48/51 (94)	2.1 (1.7–2.5)	2.1 (1.7–2.6)
Corticosteroids	13 (13)	25 (25)	1 (2)	34/39 (87)	1.9 (1.6–2.3)	1.9 (1.5–2.3)
Antihistamines or neuroleptics	12 (12)	9 (9)	18 (29)	37/39 (95)	2.1 (1.7–2.5)	1.6 (1.3–2.0)
Medication for any other illness/symptom, n (%)	n = 99	n = 100	n = 62	n = 261		
Yes	80 (80)	88 (88)	40 (65)	140/208 (67)	1.2 (0.9–1.5)	1.2 (0.9–1.6)
No	19 (19)	12 (12)	22 (35)	30/53 (57)	1.0 (Ref.)	1.0 (Ref.)

Numbers (n) of patients answering the questions are presented, [1]267 of 277 patients provided data regarding nausea. Experiencing nausea was defined as any day within the radiotherapy period in the acupuncture cohort and within the past week in the standard care cohort. [2]Including the variables seen in table 1 and 2. SD = Standard Deviation.

both cohorts received a mean radiotherapy dose of 27 Gray the standard care cohort was compared with the acupuncture cohort regarding occurrence of nausea and vomiting. SPSS for Windows (version 15.0.0) was used, except for calculating adjusted RR risks for nausea where we used SAS (version 9.1.3.). The significance level was set as p<0.05.

Results

Participants

Compared to the acupuncture cohort the standard care cohort comprised more men (p = 0.02), more patients with a testicular tumour (p = 0.001) and fewer patients consuming potent antiemetics; serotonin-receptor antagonists (p = 0.09) or corticosteroids (p<0.001) (table 1). According to the univariable analysis, nausea was not related to gender (table 2) but was more frequent in patients with testicular tumours and in patients treated with serotonin-receptor antagonists or corticosteroids (table 1). In the

multivariable analysis, concomitant chemotherapy (p = 0.01, table 1), age less than 40 years (p<0.001), previous nausea in any situation (p<0.001) and a self estimated risk for nausea as higher than others during radiotherapy (p = 0.01) all indicated a significantly increased risk for nausea (table 2).

Emesis in the verum, sham and standard care group

The patients in the acupuncture cohort the past week and the past 24 hours experienced significantly less occurrence of nausea and vomiting than those in the standard care cohort. The lower occurrence of nausea in the acupuncture cohort (37%) compared to the standard care cohort (63%) the past week (RR 0.6, CI 0.45–0.77) was also true when patients taking serotonin-receptor antagonists and corticosteroids were excluded (figure 2) and after adjustment for confounding factors for nausea (table 3).

The intensity of nausea was lower in the acupuncture cohort (n 140; 78% experienced no nausea, n = 24; 13% a little nausea, n = 14; 8% moderate nausea and n = 2; 1% much nausea) than in

Table 2. Personal characteristics of the patients in the verum acupuncture, sham acupuncture or standard care group.

Characteristics	Acupuncture cohort n = 215		Standard care cohort n = 62	Experiencing nausea n = 172/ total n providing data = 267[1]	Univariable relative risk (95 % confidence interval)	Multivariable[2] relative risk, (95 % confidence interval) adjusted for three groups
	Verum acupuncture n = 109	Sham acupuncture n = 106				
Sex, n (%)	n = 109	n = 106	n = 62	n = 267		
Man	20 (18)	15 (14)	19 (31)	35/53 (66)	1.0 (0.8–1.3)	1.0 (0.8 1.3)
Woman	89 (82)	91 (86)	43 (69)	137/214 (64)	1.0 (Ref.)	1.0 (Ref.)
Age in years: mean ± SD	64 ± 13.8	63 ±13.9	63 ± 14.5	62 ± 14.8		
19–40	7 (6)	6 (6)	6 (10)	17/19 (89)	1.5 (1.2–1.8)	1.5 (1.2–2.0)
41–60	34 (31)	34 (32)	17 (27)	55/82 (67)	1.1 (0.9–1.4)	1.1 (0.9–1.3)
61–89	68 (62)	66 (62)	39 (63)	98/164 (60)	1.0 (Ref.)	1.0 (Ref.)
Labor status, n (%)	n = 106	n = 104	n = 62	n = 257		
Employed	35 (33)	41 (38)	21 (34)	65/94 (69)	1.2 (1.0–1.0)	1.2 (1.0–1.4)
Retired/Sickness pension	69 (65)	59 (57)	26 (42)	82/142 (58)	1.0 (Ref.)	1.0 (Ref.)
Other	2 (2)	4 (4)	15 (24)	18/21 (86)	1.5 (1.2–1.9)	1.6 (1.1–2.1)
Previous nausea, n (%)						
During previous chemotherapy	n = 96	n = 97	n = 62	n = 256		
Not relevant	55 (57)	58 (60)	43 (69)	95/155 (61)	1.0 (0.8–1.4)	1.0 (0.8–1.4)
No	11 (11)	12 (12)	15 (24)	23/39 (59)	1.0 (Ref.)	1.0 (Ref.)
Yes	30 (31)	28 (29)	4 (6)	47/62 (76)	1.3 (1.0–1.7)	1.3 (0.9–1.7)
During pregnancy	n = 89	n = 92	n = 61	n = 242		
Not relevant	26 (29)	28 (30)	33 (54)	56/87 (64)	1.3 (0.9–1.7)	1.3 (1.1–1.9)
No	19 (21)	24 (26)	6 (10)	25/49 (51)	1.0 (Ref.)	1.0 (Ref.)
Yes	44 (49)	40 (43)	22 (36)	78/106 (74)	1.4 (1.1–1.9)	1.4 (1.1–1.9)
In any previous situation[3]	n = 96	n = 98	n = 61	n = 256		
No	22 (23)	29 (30)	17 (27)	30/74 (41)	1.0 (Ref.)	1.0 (Ref.)
Yes	74 (77)	69 (70)	44 (72)	134/182 (74)	1.8 (1.4–2–4)	2.0 (1.3–3.3)
N of previous nausea situations[3], md (25th–75th percentile)	n = 97 2 (1–3)	n = 98 2 (1–3)	n = 61 2 (0–3)	n = 257 2 (1–3)		
0–2 situations	68 (70)	67 (68)	44 (71)	110/179 (61)	1.0 (Ref.)	1.0 (Rcf.)
3–5 situations	29 (30)	31 (32)	18 (29)	56/78 (72)	1.2 (1.0–1.4)	1.2 (1.0–1.4)
Patients' estimation of risk for nausea, n (%)	n = 89	n = 94	not mea-sured	n = 183		not relevant
Lower than others	19 (21)	25 (27)		22/44 (50)	1.0 (Ref.)	
Similar to others	57 (64)	55 (59)		73/112 (65)	1.3 (1.0–1.9)	
Higher than others	13 (15)	14 (15)		22/27 (81)	1.6 (1.2–2.4)	
Expectation of antiemetic treatment effects, n (%)	n = 105	n = 105	not mea-sured	n = 201		not relevant
Do not believe	0 (0)	0 (0)		0/0 (0)		
Believe little	5 (5)	6 (6)		4/10 (40)	0.64 (0.3–1.4)	
Believe moderately	50 (46)	57 (54)		70/102 (68)	1.1 (0.9–1.3)	
Believe much	50 (46)	42 (40)		56/89 (62)	1.0 (Ref)	
Previous experience of acupuncture[4], n (%)	n = 109	n = 101	not mea-sured	n = 209		not relevant
Yes	36 (33)	36 (34)		47/72 (65)	1.1 (0.6–1.3)	
No	73 (66)	65 (62)		82/137 (60)	1.0 (Ref)	

Numbers (n) of patients answering the questions are presented, [1]267 of 277 patients provided data regarding nausea. Experiencing nausea was defined as any day within the radiotherapy period in the acupuncture cohort and within the past week in the standard care cohort. [2]Including the variables seen in table 1 and 2. [3]In travelling, unpleasant smells/sights, anxiety, chemotherapy or pregnancy. [4]For other conditions than emesis. SD = Standard Deviation. Md = Median.

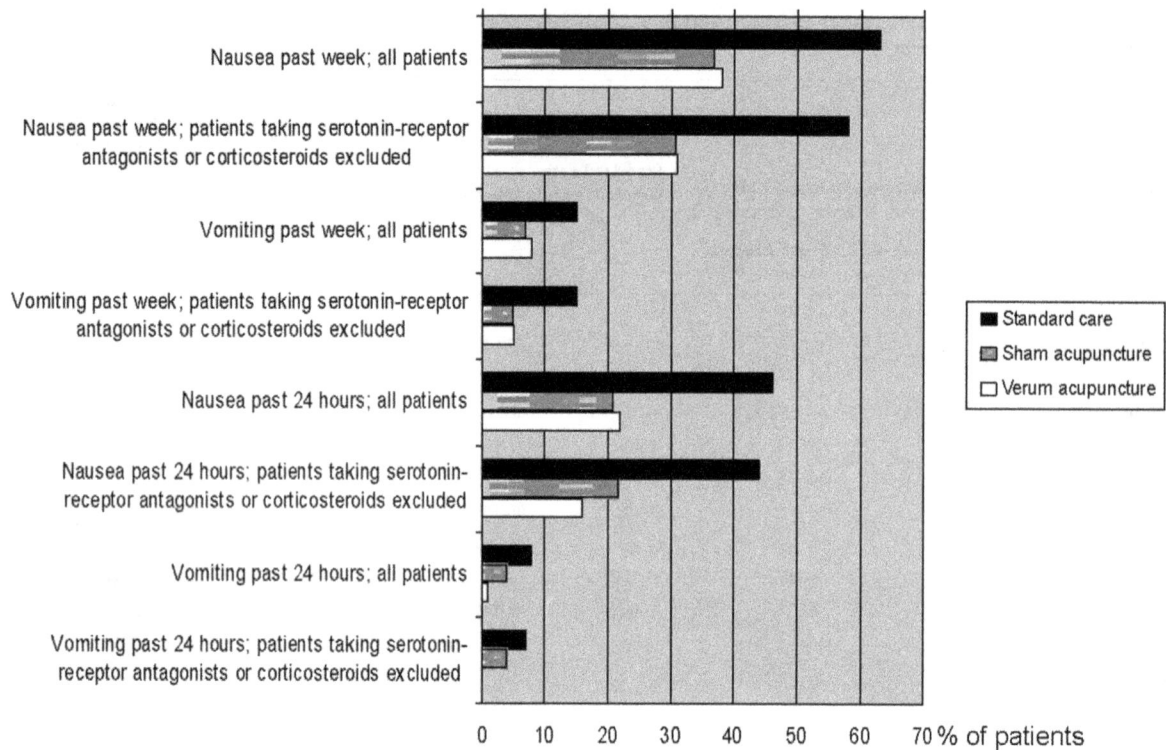

Figure 2. Nausea and vomiting within the past 24 hours and the past week. Emesis was measured at that time the radiotherapy dose was 27 Gray (mean) in the verum, sham and standard care groups. Measured in all patients and in patients not receiving potent antiemetics in the verum (n = 88 and n = 77), sham (n = 95 and n = 78) and standard care group (n = 62 and n = 55).

the standard care cohort (n = 32; 52% no nausea, n = 20; 32% a little, n 9; 15% moderate and n 1; 2% much) (p = 0.002). Within the acupuncture cohort, no statistically significant differences between the verum and the sham group were seen regarding

Table 3. Comparison of nausea occurrence between the standard care cohort and the acupuncture cohort, adjusted for confounding factors for nausea.

	Nausea occurrence the past week
Acupuncture cohort[1], number (%) n = 183	68 (37)
Standard care cohort, number (%) n = 62	39 (63)
Relative Risk, unadjusted (95 % Confidence Interval)	0.6 (0.5–0.8)
Relative Risk, adjusted for concomitant chemotherapy (95 % Confidence Interval)	0.3 (−0.7–0.7)
Relative Risk, adjusted for age (95 % Confidence Interval)	0.4 (−0.1–0.8)
Relative Risk, adjusted for nausea in previous situations (95 % Confidence Interval)	0.3 (−0.2–0.7)
Relative Risk, overall adjustment[2] (95 % Confidence Interval)	0.8 (0.6–0.9)

Relative risks for nausea (prevalence acupuncture cohort/ standard care cohort) during a cross sectional week of radiotherapy (mean dose 27 Gray in both cohorts). [1]Verum and sham treated patients. [2]Overall adjustment included adjustment for concomitant chemotherapy, age and nausea in any previous situation.

nausea occurrence or intensity, vomiting or antiemetic consumption the past 24 hours or the past week.

Expectations of nausea and the effects of treatment in the verum and sham acupuncture groups

The 27 patients in the acupuncture cohort who estimated their own risk for becoming nauseous during the radiotherapy as higher than other patients had an increased risk for nausea compared to the 44 patients who estimated that they had a lower risk for nausea than others (table 2). No statistically significant differences in baseline expectations of antiemetic treatment effects were seen between the patients who experienced nausea and the patients who stayed free from nausea during the radiotherapy period (table 2). The patients who experienced nausea between the sixth and last treatments either retained or decreased their original belief in the antiemetic effects of the received treatment. The patients who stayed free from nausea either retained their original belief that the treatment would help or even reported an increase in the extent to which they trusted this treatment (figure 3). Of the patients mostly treated by therapist A (performing 1412 of 1700 treatments, 83%), 20 of 69 (29%) in the verum acupuncture group and 25 of 76 (33%) in the sham acupuncture group experienced nausea the past week. In the patients mostly treated by therapist B (performing 607 of 693 treatments, 87%), corresponding figures were 13 of 41 (32%) and 10 of 29 (35%), respectively.

Discussion

We found lower occurrence of nausea and vomiting in patients treated with penetrating "deqi"-creating acupuncture or sham acupuncture compared to patients who had received standard

Patients free from nausea *both* before and after the sixth verum/sham treatment:

*Level of trust in beneficial effects of treatment
at the last verum/sham treatment*

Level of trust in beneficial effects of treatment at the sixth verum /sham treatment		No	Little	Moderate	Much	Totals
	No					0
	Little			3	1	4
	Moderate		1	14	12	27
	Much			4	49	53
	Totals	0	1	21	62	84

Patients free from nausea *until* the sixth verum/sham treatment that *after* then became nauseous:

*Level of trust in beneficial effects of treatment at
the last verum/sham treatment*

Level of trust in beneficial effects of treatment at the sixth verum /sham treatment		No	Little	Moderate	Much	Totals
	No		1			1
	Little	1	2	3		6
	Moderate		2	25	11	38
	Much		2	13	39	54
	Totals	1	7	41	50	99

Figure 3. Trust in the effect of the received treatment for preventing and reducing nausea. The trust was stated at the sixth and the last verum or sham treatment in patients free from nausea and patients experiencing nausea after the sixth verum or sham treatment. Number of patients rating trust in antiemetic effects of received treatment at both the sixth and the last session was 183.

care. Almost all patients in the acupuncture cohort highly expected antiemetic effects from the treatment. Patients who expected nausea had increased risk for nausea compared to patients who expected low risk for nausea.

There are many, not sham-controlled studies, reporting emesis-reducing effects of acupuncture compared to standard care in chemotherapy-induced nausea [14]. Our results indicate that nonspecific factors such as the extra care or the high expectations of positive treatment effects, not the specific characteristics of verum acupuncture, reduced emesis. Alternatively, the findings could result from flaws in our non-randomized design. Since the patients were not randomized to standard care, we investigated if an imbalance of confounding factors possibly contributing to emesis may have explained the higher prevalence of emesis in the standard care group, according to the hierarchical step model [18]. The higher risk for nausea in the standard care cohort was valid also after adjusting for possible confounding factors for emesis and after omitting patients taking serotonin-receptor antagonists and corticosteroids, indicating that our findings are valid. We have not identified any previous study of the effect of verum or sham acupuncture compared to standard care on radiotherapy-induced emesis (Pubmed, http://www.ncbi.nlm.nih.

gov/ pubmed/accessed 10/11/10, using the combined search terms acupuncture, radiotherapy, nausea and vomiting). A Cochrane review of acupuncture for chemotherapy-induced nausea included eleven studies [14]. Only two sham-controlled studies were reported, one positive (n = 104) [19] and one negative (n = 80) [12], except for a pilot study including only 10 patients [20]. As concerns conditions in general, there exist positive sham controlled studies, but there are also indications that the effect of acupuncture may not be related to the specific characters of verum acupuncture. In line with our results, Haake and co-workers [21] found substantial improvement of back pain in 48% of 387 patients treated by verum acupuncture, in 44% of 387 patients treated with sham and in 27% of 388 patients receiving standard care. In other studies sham acupuncture reduced musculoskeletal arm pain significantly more than verum acupuncture [22].

The verum and the sham group received extra care compared to the standard care group, which may have reduced emesis: patient-therapist communication, the knowledge that continuous contact with one single therapist would continue during the whole radiotherapy period, the tactile stimulation from the therapists' hands, the extra time for rest and relaxation and the extra attention to the patient's symptoms through the daily emesis questions all are important elements of this extra care. The verum and sham performing therapists in our study might have had a supportive attitude. Arving and co-workers [23] found that chemotherapy patients who received supportive conversations reported higher quality of life and less nausea than did patients receiving standard care. Börjeson and co-workers [24] also found that chemotherapy patients who received extra care comprising information and relaxation training increased their well-being compared to patients receiving antiemetics only, despite the fact that the extra-care group received a less optimal antiemetic treatment.

Both verum acupuncture and sham-acupuncture like tactile stimulation have been seen to activate the limbic system [15]; did the low dose of sensory stimulation at the non-acupuncture point reduce emesis? Kaptchuk and co-workers [25] implied that the patient-therapist meeting was more important than the needle stimulation. Of 87 patients who received sham acupuncture from an emphatic committed therapist 62% reported adequate symptom relief of irritable bowel symptoms, compared to 44% of 88 patients receiving sham acupuncture from a non-communicating therapist and 28% of 87 patients on waiting list. The verum and sham treated patients in our study received extra time for rest and relaxation and slightly more body-contact than the standard care patients, which may have reduced distress. Psychological distress has been seen as a predictor for emesis [26] and studies indicate that relaxation [27] as well as body-contact (tactile stimulation, massage) [28] may reduce nausea in cancer patients.

Since almost all patients in the acupuncture cohort expected positive antiemetic effects of the treatment, the positive expectation may be another factor that reduced emesis. Expectations are known to influence intervention outcomes in general [29]. Indeed, Pariente and co-workers [30] found with the use of positron emission tomography (PET) that when individuals were informed that the blunt sham needle they were treated with was ineffective, no activity in the pain modulating areas in the mid-brain was seen. When a credible telescopic sham needle was used that the individuals believed was effective, a large pain-modulating activity was seen. Likewise, Linde and co-workers [31] found that acupuncture and sham treated patients with headache, chronic low back pain or osteoarthritis who had high expectations on pain-reduction reported better effects than patients with low expectations. In our study there were no differences in the occurrence of nausea between the patients who believed in the antiemetic effects of treatment and those who had a lesser belief in the antiemetic effects of treatment. Either expectations about the treatment effect were not important for nausea, or the category scale used was not sufficiently sensitive, thus resulting in a "roof effect". The patients' trust in the antiemetic effect of verum or sham acupuncture decreased if nausea occurred and increased if nausea did not occur. This finding is in concordance with results from experiments indicating that the placebo response is a short-time effect; for example if a noxious stimulation is performed after taking a placebo pill, the study subject no longer believes in the effect of the placebo pill [29]. In our study, patients who expected nausea apparently had an increased risk for nausea, in concordance with findings regarding chemotherapy-induced nausea [32]. Thus, patients are either capable of judging their own risk for nausea or the negative expectations per se produce nausea. This finding implies that health care professionals might well consider asking the patients about their expectations about experiencing nausea and might consider the information to decide on appropriate antiemetic treatment.

Since nausea was prevalent in the standard care group and nausea may be associated with a reduced quality of life [1,33] treatment using verum or sham acupuncture may be valuable and cost-effective since positive effects do occur. A crude calculation of the cost for providing the median number of 11 verum or sham sessions lasting 30 minutes each results in a mean cost per patient of $69 USD. Two patients (median) were treated at the same time, meaning that one patient consumed three therapist hours*. In comparison, the approximate costs of the recommended dose [6] of 8 mg of a serotonin-receptor antagonists once per day during the radiotherapy period is $98 USD**.

Emesis was measured using a well-established method [17]. The standard care cohort rated emesis only once, covering the preceding week. Some patients in the standard care cohort may, by forgetfulness, have underreported emesis, compared to the acupuncture cohort, who rated emesis daily. The acupuncture cohort was compared with a reference group, not to a third randomized arm. That design requires for a thorough investigation of potential imbalance of confounding factors between groups, as discussed above, but the design may have the benefit of avoiding the impact of the data collection per se on reported emesis. Repeated measurement of emesis per se may reduce (through the so called Hawthorne effect) or increase emesis experience [34]. Young and co-workers found that emesis questions per se increased self-reported occurrence of nausea [34]. To pay extra attention to emesis through daily data collection, without performing any extra emesis-reducing treatment in this frail patient cohort, was therefore evaluated as being unethical. We presented a cross sectional comparison at the time when the mean radiotherapy dose was the same in the acupuncture and the standard care cohorts. If we instead had observed another week of the radiotherapy period, it would not have changed the conclusions of this study; the weekly proportion of patients experiencing nausea was lower in the acupuncture cohort all radiotherapy weeks (varied 22 to 44% as described previously [13]) compared to the standard care cohort. The patients who were treated by verum or sham experienced close to 50% lower occurrence of emesis compared to the patients receiving standard care. If the extra care caused the emesis reduction, this indicates that as long as the best available antiemetic treatment is offered, patients who believe that acupuncture has beneficial effects may be satisfied with treatment with verum acupuncture or non-penetrating needles, either of which produces a moment of relaxation and attention from the therapist. A next obvious step is to further study what components in the acupuncture procedures are of importance for this dramatically positive but as yet not fully understood effect, in an effort to make possible the use of those components to further increase quality of care.

* A public hospital employing a physiotherapist for three hours spends $68 USD (408 SEK to provide the mean salary value for that service according to Swedish Association of Registered Physiotherapists 2007, www.valuta.se, date 080404). Costs for needles may be approximately $0.72 USD (24 needles consumed during 12 sessions, at six US cents according to prices at www.acuprime.com, date 101109).

** Consuming one tablet at a cost of 16.25 SEK (www.fass.se) during the mean value of 36 radiotherapy days in treatment costs $98 USD (based on cost in Sweden of 850 SEK www.valuta.se, date 101109).

Supporting Information

Protocol S1 Trial Protocol.
Found at: doi:10.1371/journal.pone.0014766.s001 (0.05 MB DOC)

Checklist S1 CONSORT Checklist.
Found at: doi:10.1371/journal.pone.0014766.s002 (0.22 MB DOC)

Acknowledgments

We are thankful to the participating patients, to Boel Lindberg and Ingrid Tillgren for coordinating, to Marianne Frid, Annica Tomasson, Clary Skoglund, Eva Ahlner and Lotta Robert for acupuncture treatments and to the health-care professionals at the radiotherapy-departments for cooperation.

Author Contributions

Conceived and designed the experiments: AE MH GS SB. Performed the experiments: AE AJ. Analyzed the data: AE EO SB. Contributed reagents/materials/analysis tools: AE MH AJ GS SB. Wrote the paper: AE ML MH AJ EO MI GS SB.

References

1. Enblom A, Bergius Axelsson B, Steineck G, Hammar M, Börjeson S (2009) One third of patients with radiotherapy-induced nausea consider their antiemetic treatment insufficient. Support Care Cancer 17: 23–32.
2. Lu W (2005) Acupuncture for side effects of chemoradiation therapy in cancer patients. Seminars in oncology nursing 21: 190–195.
3. IGARR (the Italian Group for Antiemetic Research in Radiotherapy) (1999) Radiation-induced emesis: a prospective observational multicenter Italian trial. Int J Radiat Oncol Biol Phys 44: 619–625.
4. Mystakidou K, Katsouda E, Linou A, Parpa E, Kouloulias V, et al. (2006) Prophylactic tropisetron versus rescue tropisetron in fractionated radiotherapy to moderate or high emetogenic areas: a prospective randomized open label study in cancer patients. Med Oncol 23: 251–262.
5. Feyer PC, Maranzano E, Molassiotis A, Roila F, Clark-Snow RA, et al. Radiotherapy-induced nausea and vomiting (RINV): MASCC/ESMO guideline for antiemetics in radiotherapy: update 2009. Support Care Cancer. In press. Available: http://www.ncbi.nlm.nih.gov/pubmed/20697746. Accessed 2010 Aug 10.
6. Aglietti L, Roila F, Tonato M, Basurto C, Bracarda S, et al. (1990) A Pilot Study of Metoclopramide, Dexamethasone, Diphenhydramine and Acupuncture in Women Treated with Cisplatin. Cancer Chemotherapy and Pharmacology 26: 239–240.
7. Xia YS, Wang JH, Shan LJ (2000) Acupuncture Plus Ear-Point Press in Preventing Vomiting Induced by Chemotherapy with Cisplatin. International Journal of Clinical Acupuncture 11: 145–154.
8. Dibble SL, Chapman J, Mack KA, Shih A (2000) Acupressure for Nausea: Results of a Pilot Study. Oncology Nursing Forum 27: 41–45.
9. Roscoe JA, Morrow GR, Hickok JT, Bushunow P, Pierce I, et al. (2003) The Efficacy of Acupressure and Acustimulation Wrist Bands for the Relief of Chemotherapy-Induced Nausea and Vomiting: A University of Rochester Cancer Center Community Clinical Oncology Programme Multicenter Study. Journal of Pain and Symptom Management 26: 731–742.
10. Shin YH, Kim TI, Shin MS, Juon HS (2004) Effect of Acupressure on Nausea and Vomiting during Chemotherapy Cycle for Korean Postoperative Stomach Cancer Patient. Cancer Nursing 27: 267–274.
11. Molassiotis A, Helin AM, Dabbour R, Hummerston S (2007) The effects of P6 acupressure in the prophylaxis of chemotherapy-related nausea and vomiting in breast cancer patients. Complement Ther Med 15: 3–12.
12. Streitberger K, Friedrich-Rust M, Bardenheuer H, Unnebrink K, Windeler J, et al. (2003) Effect of acupuncture compared with placebo-acupuncture at P6 as additional antiemetic prophylaxis in high-dose chemotherapy and autologous peripheral blood stem cell transplantation: a randomized controlled single-blind trial. Clin Cancer Res 9: 2538–2544.
13. Enblom A, Johnsson A, Hammar M, Onelöv E, Steineck G, et al. (2008) Acupuncture compared to placebo acupuncture in radiotherapy-induced nausea – a randomized controlled study. In: Enblom A. Nausea and vomiting in patients receiving acupuncture, sham acupuncture or standard care during radiotherapy. Linköping University Medical Dissertations No. 1088. Paper 3 pp 1–12. Available at http://liu.diva-portal.org/smash/record.jsf?searchId=2&pid= diva2:207705. Accessed 2009 March 13.
14. Ezzo JM, Richardson MA, Vickers A, Allen C, Dibble SL, et al. (2006) Acupuncture-point stimulation for chemotherapy-induced nausea or vomiting. Cochrane Database Syst Rev 19: CD002285.
15. Hui KK, Liu J, Marina O, Napadow V, Haselgrove C, et al. (2005) The integrated response of the human cerebro-cerebellar and limbic systems to acupuncture stimulation at ST 36 as evidenced by fMRI. Neuroimage 27: 479–496.
16. Park J, White A, Lee H, Ernst E (1999) Development of a new sham needle. Acupunct Med 17: 110–112.
17. Börjeson S, Hursti TJ, Peterson C, Fredrikson M, Fürst CJ, et al. (1997) Similarities and differences in assessing nausea on a verbal category scale and a visual analogue scale. Cancer Nurs 20: 260–266.
18. Steineck G, Hunt H, Adolfsson J (2006) A hierarchical step-model for causation of bias-evaluating cancer treatment with epidemiological methods. Acta Oncol 45: 421–429.
19. Shen J, Wenger N, Glaspy J, Hays RD, Albert PS, et al. (2000) Electroacupuncture for control of myeloablative chemotherapy-induced emesis: A randomized controlled trial. JAMA 284: 2755–2761.
20. Dundee JW, Ghaly RG, Fitzpatrick KT, Abram WP, Lynch GA (1989) Acupuncture prophylaxis of cancer chemotherapy-induced sickness. J R Soc Med 82: 268–271.
21. Haake M, Müller HH, Schade-Brittinger C, Basler HD, Schäfer H, et al. (2007) German Acupuncture Trials (GERAC) for chronic low back pain: randomized, multicenter, blinded, parallel-group trial with 3 groups. Arch Intern Med 167: 1892–1898.
22. Goldman RH, Stason WB, Park SK, Kim R, Schnyer RN, et al. (2008) Acupuncture for treatment of persistent arm pain due to repetitive use: a randomized controlled clinical trial. Clin J Pain 24: 211–218.
23. Arving C, Sjödén PO, Bergh J, Hellbom M, Johansson B, et al. (2007) Individual psychosocial support for breast cancer patients: a randomized study of nurse versus psychologist interventions and standard care. Cancer Nurs. 30: E10–19.
24. Börjeson S, Hursti TJ, Tishelman C, Peterson C, Steineck G (2002) Treatment of nausea and emesis during cancer chemotherapy. Discrepancies between antiemetic effect and well-being. J Pain Symptom Manage 24: 345–358.
25. Kaptchuk TJ, Kelley JM, Conboy LA, Davis RB, Kerr CE, et al. (2008) Components of placebo effect: randomised controlled trial in patients with irritable bowel syndrome. BMJ 336: 999–1003.
26. Zachariae R, Paulsen K, Mehlsen M, Jensen AB, Johansson A, et al. (2007) Chemotherapy-induced nausea, vomiting, and fatigue–the role of individual differences related to sensory perception and autonomic reactivity. Psychother Psychosom 76: 376–384.
27. Luebbert K, Dahme B, Hasenbring M (2001) The effectiveness of relaxation training in reducing treatment-related symptoms and improving emotional adjustment in acute non-surgical cancer treatment: a meta-analytical review. Psychooncology 10: 490–502.
28. Myers CD, Walton T, Bratsman L, Wilson J, Small B (2008) Massage modalities and symptoms reported by cancer patients: narrative review. J Soc Integr Oncol 6: 19–28.
29. Price DD, Finniss DG, Benedetti F (2008) A comprehensive review of the placebo effect: recent advances and current thought. Annu Rev Psychol 59: 565–590.
30. Pariente J, White P, Frackowiak RS, Lewith G (2005) Expectancy and belief modulate the neuronal substrates of pain treated by acupuncture. Neuroimage 25: 1161–1167.
31. Linde K, Witt CM, Streng A, Weidenhammer W, Wagenpfeil S, et al. (2007) The impact of patient expectations on outcomes in four randomized controlled trials of acupuncture in patients with chronic pain. Pain 128: 264–271.
32. Higgins SC, Montgomery GH, Bovbjerg DH (2007) Distress before chemotherapy predicts delayed but not acute nausea. Support Care Cancer 15: 171–177.
33. Shun SC, Chiou JF, Lai YH, Yu PJ, Wei LL, et al. (2008) Changes in quality of life and its related factors in liver cancer patients receiving stereotactic radiation therapy. Support Care Cancer 16: 1059–1065.
34. Young SD, Adelstein BD, Ellis SR (2007) Demand characteristics in assessing motion sickness in a virtual environment: or does taking a motion sickness questionnaire make you sick? IEEE Trans Vis Comput Graph 13: 422–428.

17

Assessing the Quality of Reports about Randomized Controlled Trials of Acupuncture Treatment on Diabetic Peripheral Neuropathy

Chen Bo[1,9], Zhao Xue[1,9], Guo Yi[1]*, Chen Zelin[1], Bai Yang[1], Wang Zixu[1], Wang Yajun[2]

1 College of Acupuncture and Moxibustion, Tianjin University of Traditional Chinese Medicine, Tianjin, China, **2** Department of Acupuncture and Massage, Gansu College of Traditional Chinese Medicine, Gansu Province, China

Abstract

Background: To evaluate the reports' qualities which are about randomized controlled trials (RCTs) of acupuncture treatment on Diabetic Peripheral Neuropathy (DPN).

Methodology/Principal Findings: Eight databases including The Cochrane Library(1993–Sept.,2011), PubMed (1980–Sept., 2011), EMbase (1980–Sept.,2011), SCI Expanded (1998–Sept.,2011), China Biomedicine Database Disc (CBMdisc, 1978–Sept., 2011), China National Knowledge Infrastructure (CNKI, 1979–Sept., 2011), VIP (a full text issues database of China, 1989–Sept., 2011), Wan Fang (another full text issues database of China 1998–Sept., 2011) were searched systematically. Hand search for further references was conducted. Language was limited to Chinese and English. We identified 75 RCTs that used acupuncture as an intervention and assessed the quality of these reports with the Consolidated Standards for Reporting of Trials statement 2010 (CONSORT2010) and Standards for Reporting Interventions Controlled Trials of Acupuncture 2010(STRICTA2010). 24 articles (32%) applied the method of random allocation of sequences. No article gave the description of the mechanism of allocation concealment, no experiment applied the method of blinding. Only one article (1.47%) could be identified directly from its title as about the Randomized Controlled Trials, and only 4 articles gave description of the experimental design. No article mentioned the number of cases lost or eliminated. During one experiment, acupuncture syncope led to temporal interruption of the therapy. Two articles (2.94%) recorded the number of needles, and 8 articles (11.76%) mentioned the depth of needle insertion. None of articles reported the base of calculation of sample size, or has any analysis about the metaphase of an experiment or an explanation of its interruption. One (1.47%) mentioned intentional analysis (ITT).

Conclusions/Significance: The quality of the reports on RCTs of acupuncture for Diabetic Peripheral Neuropathy is moderate to low. The CONSORT2010 and STRICTA2010 should be used to standardize the reporting of RCTs of acupuncture in future.

Editor: Massimo Pietropaolo, University of Michigan Medical School, United States of America

Funding: This work was financially supported by the National Natural Science Foundation of China (No. 81072881 and 81173204) and the Doctoral Program of Higher Education the Special Research Funded Issues (No 20101210110007). The funders had no role in study design, data collection and analysis, decision to publish or preparation of the manuscript.

Competing Interests: The authors have declared that no competing interests exist.

* E-mail: guoyi_168@163.com

9 These authors contributed equally to this work

Introduction

Diabetic Peripheral Neuropathy is a common complication of diabetic, which may lead to diabetic foot ulcers, even foot or limb amputations. The first step in the treatment of diabetic peripheral neuropathy is prevention. Diabetic peripheral neuropathy cannot be cured and the damage done to the nerves cannot be repaired, so it is vital that people with diabetes prevent its occurrence. Treatment may include medications to help minimize pain and other uncomfortable sensations. Alternative or complementary treatments that may be helpful for some symptoms include acupuncture. Diabetic peripheral neuropathy is one of the syndromes commonly treated with acupuncture. Earlier in 1987, The WHO proposed 43 kinds of acupunctural indications, in which peripheral neuropathy was included.

Many cases reports of acupuncture treatment on Diabetic Peripheral Neuropathy (DPN) have been published, which declare the effectiveness of acupuncture treatment on DPN. However, it is necessary to find out a much more reliable scientific method to test the effectiveness. Some researchers adopt the randomized controlled trials (RCTs) to test the efficacy and effectiveness of acupuncture treatment on DPN, which is generally considered as the best design plan to verify the efficacy of intervention measures at present.

The CONSORT (Consolidated Standards of Reporting Trials) Statement [1], has been recommended as the reporting guideline of RCT by International Committee of Medical Journal Editors.

The 2010 STRICTA (Standards for Reporting Interventions in Clinical Trials of Acupuncture) [2] have been extending the CONSORT statement. According to previous studies, it has been shown that the quality of reports about RCT for TCM on the mainland of China has been gradually improved but the actual state of current studies is not yet satisfactory [3]. How about the quality of reports on RCT of acupuncture, and the application of CONSORT and STRICTA to these reports? With a view to answering these questions, this paper evaluates the application of the standards using diabetic peripheral neuropathy as an example to analyze and evaluate the reports on the RCT of acupuncture for diabetic peripheral neuropathy and the degree to which CONSORT and STRICTA had been applied to these reports, with the objective to help designing future clinical research studies.

Methods

Literature Inclusion Criteria

We have chosen all the RCTs of acupuncture treatment for diabetic peripheral neuropathy. Among the selected, the intervention groups were treated with acupuncture therapy or with some other standard therapies accompanied by acupuncture, such as taking oral hypoglycemic agents, having diabetic diet and so on. Chinese and English have been limited as the searching languages.

Literature Collecting Methods

We have searched 8 databases, namely, The Cochrane library(1993–Sept.,2011), PubMed (1980–Sept., 2011), EMbase (1980–Sept., 2011), SCI Expanded (1998–Sept., 2011), China Biomedicine Database disc (CBMdisc,1978–Sept., 2011), China National Knowledge Infrastructure (CNKI, 1979–Sept., 2011), VIP (a full text issues database of China, 1989–Sept., 2011), Wan Fang (another full text issues database of China 1998–Sept., 2011), with searching languages limited to Chinese and English. We selected all references to the RTCs of acupuncture for diabetic peripheral neuropathy and decided on the finial bibliographies mentioned above.

Chinese Key Words

"zhen jiu"(acupuncture and moxibustion), "zhen ci"(acupuncture), "dian zhen"(electric acupuncture), "jing pi dian ci ji" (transcetaneous electrical stimulation), "xue wei mai xian"(catgut implantation at acupoint), "xue wei zhu she"(acupoint injection of drugs), "shui zhen"(hydro-acupuncture therapy), "wan huai zhen"(wrist and ankle acupuncture), "tou zhen"(scalp acupuncture), " mei hua zhen"(plum-blossom needle)," edged needle "(three-edged needle),"ci xue "(blood-letting method), "fang xue"(blood-letting method), "pricking "(blood-letting method)," ba guan" (acupuncture cupping), "tang niao bing shen jing bing bian" (diabetic neuropathy), " tang niao bing zhou wei shen jing bing bian " (diabetic peripheral neuropathy).

English Key Words

"Acupuncture", "acupuncture and moxibustion", "needling ","acupuncture therapy", "Diabetic Neuropathy", "diabetic peripheral neuropathy", "DPN". The deadline of searching dates was ended in September, 2011.

Methods of Quality Assessment for the References

This paper evaluates the reports on the references selected based on 25 standards of CONSORT, 2010 and six standards from STRICTA 2010 [1–2]. We responded with "yes" or "no" to each standard to judge whether the authors had reported, or had recorded concrete details of the reports accomplished in accor-dance with the requirement of each standard. Before assessment, two evaluators had a full understanding of these standards, held discussion, and made consultation if disagreement occurred. Finally, we counted the number of reports which met the standards of CONSORT2010 and STRICTA2010, and calculated the percentage of application of each standard.

Results

We gleaned 399 references in total to acupuncture treatment for diabetic peripheral neuropathy, from which we found out 179 reports of clinical value by collecting and selecting all the references from different database and then eliminating the duplicates. Moreover, after eliminating the case reports and non-randomized controlled trials among 179 reports, we got 88 potential reports on RCTs. After further reading, however, we excluded 9 references [4–12] published in duplicate and 4 references [6,13,14,15] having two or more control groups. Finally, we adopted 75 eligible references, among which 73 references are in Chinese version and the other two in English [16,17]. All were published between the year 1995 and 2011. (See Figure S1).

The Results of evaluation of 75 RCTs shown in Table S1 and Table S2 are assessed respectively based on 25 standards of CONSORT2010 and 6 standards of STRICTA2010.We have found there were no report followed either all the items of the CONSORT checklist or all the STRICTA items. Above all, the primary problems we found occurred at the following aspects:lack of sample size estimation, allocation concealment, information about implementation, method of blinding, participant flow and recruitment, analysis, harms, interpretation consistent with results, registration, details of needling, details of other interventions, practitioner background and so on.

Basic information of the reports:only one article (1.47%) could be identified directly from its title as the report of Randomized Controlled Trials, 4 articles gave description of the experimental design [16–19]. No article mentioned the number of cases lost or eliminated, or the process of recruitment or follow-up studies. During one experiment [20], acupuncture syncope led to temporal interruption of the therapy, which was continued later without results being affected. 2 articles (2.94%) analyzed the limitations of experiments and 29 articles (38.67%) analyzed the possibility of the popularization of the experiments' results. 2 articles (2.94%)recorded the number of needles, and 8 articles (11.76%) mentioned the depth of needle insertion. 20 articles (29.41%) mentioned the type of needle. 3 articles (4.41%) described the acupuncturists who participated in these researches, and only 3 articles (4.41%) quoted data to explain the rationality of contrasting and comparing similar experiments.

Methods in the reports: As for the acupuncture treatment group, there were various kinds of interventions, such as needling with acupoint injection [21], scalp acupuncture with acupoint injection [22] and other comprehensive methods.24 articles (32%) applied the method of random allocation of sequences. Among all 24 articles, 9 applied random number tables, 3 used stratified random, 2 employed random table of Doll's clinical cases, and 11 adopted treatment and the order of admission. No article gave the description of the mechanism of allocation concealment, nor the concrete implementation of random method. Besides, no experiment applied the method of blinding. No article refers to (mentions) the sample size evaluation, or has any analysis about the metaphase of an experiment or an explanation of its interruption. 50 articles (66.67%) referred to the statistics, and one (1.47%) mentioned intentional analysis (ITT). Only one article applied the 95% of the confidence interval to describe the estimated value of an effect and its veracity. There was one article that has neither P value nor 95% of the confidence interval, and 74 articles applied P value for replacement.(See Table S1 and Table S2).

Discussion

We have chosen diabetic peripheral neuropathy as the disease that acupuncture widely treat. Our researchers are well-trained. We searched a total of eight databases for involving all the related reports. Besides, the CONSORT and STRICTA statement are the most widely accepted standards for reporting quality assessment in acupuncture studies. All of these are the main strength of our study.

Limitations: Although we have assessed the 75 reports comprehensively and systematically, which are more than Xiao Lu's paper [23], there are still some limitations. First, we limited searching languages, only including Chinese and English, which may lost either non-Chinese or non-English reports like Japanese, Korean and so on. However, a majority of papers on acupuncture are published in these two languages. Second, it was easy to get the Chinese full texts through the four Chinese data bases. But it was a little bit difficult to get the full texts of all these papers and fortunately we have found these full texts of papers we needed. Third, even if the searching time was limited as wide as possible, from the year 1995 to 2001, it still covered a narrow time span. That may bring the limitation to the value of our study. Nevertheless, RCTs were conducted on TCM to test the efficacy of acupuncture treatment just in the recent two decades, so there were rarely no RCTs before 1990s on acupuncture. Last, We have excluded four articles with two or more than two control groups, it may lead to selection bias. That is because the database we designed for analyzing data can only input the information of two groups: the control group and treatment group. Moreover, it is difficult for us to analyzing data of two or more than two control groups for it hard to calculate the percentage of each item. But according to our preliminary analysis, even if we included these four articles, the result won't be impacted. Therefore, to do this will not affect our study result.

Therefore, we recommend that clinical trials of acupuncture should be improved in the following aspects: At first, it is necessary to modify clinical designs and explore suitable approaches of Chinese characteristics to improve the general quality of the research. Then, pre-tests, along with precisely estimated sample sizes, are needed before carrying out the experiment. Moreover, the well-known "Golden Standards" should be applied as the standard for diagnosis in order to minimize possible bias. By applying the proper random methods and random allocation methods, selecting bias can also be avoided. Measurement bias can also be eliminated by suitable methods of blinding. In addition, in order to reduce the impact of uncertain factors, ways to limit errors in I type and II type should be designed; matching and stratifying analysis should be used to clearly define any confusing syndrome terminology in TCM. Furthermore, statistics should be thoroughly traced in scientific exactitude. At last, the rules of CONSORT and STRICTA should be taken as standards in the whole experimental process.

Conclusion

The general quality of the reports on RCTs of acupuncture for Diabetic Peripheral Neuropathy assessed by CONSORT2010 and STRICTA2010 is moderate to low. The low quality of existing reports on acupuncture treatment for pathological changes of diabetic peripheral neuropathy has created difficulty for the reader to realize the value in its designs, the veracity in its implementation, and the validity of its results. And, it also slows down the process of a widespread application of acupuncture to clinical treatment. The CONSORT and STRICTA are reporting guideline, but not about design. However, the reporting can reflects how about the design, progress of the trial. This paper aims to apply the international CONSORT2010 and STRICTA2010 assessing the related reports and experiments so as to contribute to the future application of acupunctural treatment.

Supporting Information

Figure S1 Flow chart of reports selection. This figure shows the process of the selection. The researchers applied the search method to find out 399 reports related to the topic, among which 45 reports of duplicates, 86 reports of non-acupuncture therapy, 89 reports of animal experiments, reviews and comments are excluded. 179 reports obtained for further evaluation. Then researchers viewed the full text of all potentially eligible reports obtained and picked out 16 case reports, 40 case series reports and 35 non-randomized controlled reports. Then 88 RCTs preliminarily were adopted. After carefully reselecting, we pick out 8 duplicated publishing reports and 4 reports with two or more control groups. At last, 75 reports are included for final analysis. (DOC)

Table S1 Results of evaluation of 75 RCTs based on 25 standards of CONSORT2010. We have found there were no report followed all the items of the CONSORT checklist. They were lacking in sample size estimation, allocation concealment, information about implementation, method of blinding, participant flow and recruitment, analyses, harms, Interpretation consistent with results, registration and so on. (DOC)

Table S2 Results of evaluation of 75 RCTs based on 6 standards of STRICTA 2010. We have found there were no report followed all the items of the STRICTA 2010 checklist. They were lacking in details of needling, details of other interventions, practitioner background and so on. (DOC)

Checklist S1 (DOC)

Acknowledgments

Give our thanks to Wang Zixu and Lu Shijia for translation.

Author Contributions

Conceived and designed the experiments: CB ZX GY. Performed the experiments: CB WZ BY. Analyzed the data: BY CZL. Contributed reagents/materials/analysis tools: WZ GY. Wrote the paper: GY CZL WY CB ZX.

References

1. Kenneth F, Douglas G, David M, and the CONSORT Group (2010) CONSORT 2010 Statement: updated guidelines for reporting parallel group randomised trials. J Chin Integer Med 8(7): 604–612.
2. MacPherson H, Altman DG, Hammerschlag R, Youping L, Taixiang W, et al. (2010)Revised Standards for Reporting Interventions in Clinical Trials of Acupuncture (STRICTA): Extending the CONSORT Statement. PLoS Med 7(6): e1000261.
3. Mao B, Wang G, Fan T,Chen XD,Liu J, et al. (2007)Assessing the Quality of Reporting of Randomized Controlled Trials in Traditional Chinese Medicine. Chinese Journal of Evidence-Based Medicine 7(12): 880–887.

4. Chen JF, Ding P, Shen J,Liang HR (2002)Effect of Acupuncture on Hormones of the Pituitary-Adrenal-Axis, Immunocytokines and Blood Coagulational Parameters in the Patients of Diabe tic Peripheral Neuropathy. Chinese Acuponcture & Moxibustion 22(04): 255–258.

5. Xu LB, Long SJ, Chen XL(2003)Clinical observation on treatment of diabetic peripheral neuropathies by tapping collaterals with skin needles. Chinese Acupuncture & Moxibustion 23(06): 329–331.

6. Zhen HT, Li YF, Yuan SX, Zhang CG, Chen GM, et al. (2000)Clinical observations on the treatment of diabetic peripheral neuropathy by combined acupuncture and medicament. Shanghai Journal Of Acupuncture And Moxibusition 19(1): 8–9.

7. Cui ZC, Yu JF (2000)Changes of Hemorheology Indexes of the Patients with Diabetic Peripheral Neuropathy. Journal Of Nantong Medical 20(02): 162.

8. Yu JF, Cui ZC (2000)Clinical Observations on the Treatment of Diabetic Peripheral Neuropathy by Acupuncture. Chinese Acupuncture & Moxibustion 4(4): 203–204.

9. YU JF, Chen GS, Li JX,Cui ZC (2000)Analysis of Physicochemical Indices in Patients with Diabetic Neuropathy Treated with Acupuncture. Shanghai Journal of Acupuncture and Moxibustion 19(06): 12–13.

10. Cui ZC, Chen GS, Yu JF (2000)Analysis on Physiochemical Indexes Before and After Treatment for the Patients with Diabetic Peripheral Neuropathy [J]. Medical Journal of Communications 14(06): 588–589.

11. Zhang P, Zhang S (2009) Efficacy Analysis on 50 Cases of Diabetic Peripheral Neuropathy Treated by Acupuncture. Shenzhen Journal of Integrated Traditional Chinese and Western Medicine 25(5): 73–74.

12. Jin Z,Zhang BF,Shang LX (2011)Clinical observation on diabetic peripheral neuropathy treated with electroacupuncture and acupoint injection.Chinese Acupuncture and Moxibustion 31(07): 613–616.

13. Sun YZ, Liu TT (2005)Observations on the Efficacy of Acupuncture, Point Injection and Plum-blossom Needle Tapping for Treating Diabetic Peripheral Neuropathy. Shanghai Journal of Acupuncture and Moxibustion 24(06): 3–6.

14. Yu LQ, Sun YZ, Liu TT (2005) Efficacy Observations on Three Kinds of Acupunctural and Moxbustion Therapies for Diabetic Peripheral Neuropathy[J]. Chinese Journal of Modern Integrated Medicine 3(10): 918–919.

15. Lei SH, Fan JY, Zhang L Lai XY (2007)Clinical Control Study on Photoimpact Acupoint Stimulation for Diabetic Neuropathy. Practical Clinical Medicine 8(11): 15–18.

16. Ahn AC, Ennani T, Freeman R (2007)Two styles of acupuncture for treating painful diabetic neuropathy–a pilot randomised control trial. Acupuncture in medicine : Journal of the British Medical Acupuncture Society 25(1): 11–17.

17. Hamza MA, White PF, Craig WF (2000)Percutaneous electrical nerve stimulation: a novel analgesic therapy for diabetic neuropathic pain. Diabetes care 23(3): 67–70.

18. Han BX, Zhou L (2009)Acupuncture and Chinese Herbal Medicine Treatment of Diabetic Peripheral Neuropathy Clinical Observation. Guangming Journal of Chinese Medicine 24(08):1521–1522.

19. Zhang P, Ji XQ, Yu SG, Xie L (2005)Clinical observations on 32 cases of the treatment of diabetic peripheral neuropathy by combined acupuncture and medicament. Jiangxi Journal of Traditional Chinese Medicine 36(06): 56–57.

20. Dong YM Zhou J (2003)Clinical Observation on Treatment of Diabetes Peripheral Neuropathy by Acupuncture Based on the Method of Nourishing Qi and Blood and Smoothing the Meridian. Medical Reasearch 32(11): 54–55.

21. Su YW (2009)Efficacy Observation on Treatment of 30 Diabetes Peripheral Neuropathy Cases by Methylcobalamin point injection. Tianjin Pharmacy 21(03): 48–49.

22. Chen TY (2001)Treatment of Scalp Needling with Point Injection for limb Numbness Caused by Diabetic. Chinese Acuponcture & Moxibustion 21(04): 207–208.

23. Lu X, Hongcai S, Jiaying W, Jing H, Jun X (2011) Assessing the Quality of Reports about Randomized Controlled Trials of Acupuncture Treatment on Mild Cognitive Impairment. PLoS ONE 6(2): e16922.

18

Registration Quality Assessment of Acupuncture Clinical Trials

Jing Gu[1,2], Ye Zhao[1], Xiaogang Wang[1], Jianjun Jiang[3], Jinhui Tian[1], Kehu Yang[1]*

1 Evidence-Based Medicine Center, Institute of Integrated Traditional Chinese and Western Medicine, School of Basic Medical Sciences, Lanzhou University, Lanzhou, Gansu, China, 2 Institute of Integrated Traditional Chinese and Western Medicine, Gansu University of Traditional Chinese Medicine, Lanzhou, Gansu, China, 3 Second School of Clinical Medicine of Lanzhou University, Lanzhou, Gansu, China

Abstract

Background: Registration can help with transparency of acupuncture clinical trials (ACTs) by making protocol information and results available to the public. Recently, the number of registered ACTs has increased greatly, but only a few researchers have focused on the quality of ACTs registration. This review provides the first assessment of the registration quality of ACTs and the baseline information for future development.

Methods: All records of ACTs registered in the World Health Organization (WHO) International Clinical Trials Registry Platform (ICTRP) were collected. Data was extracted and input to Excel spreadsheets. The current 20 items of the WHO Trial Registration Data Set (TRDS) and the special prepared items for acupuncture intervention details were used to assess the registration quality of ACTs.

Results: A total of 740 records, found in 11 registries, were examined. The number of registered ACTs increased rapidly and involved a number of different diseases. The completeness of 20 items was not too poor due to 16 of them had a higher reported percentage (>85%). The completeness of the 20 items was different among registries. For example, the average registration percentage of 20 items in Clinicaltrials.gov, ChiCTR, ISRCTN and ANZCTR were 89.6%, 92.2%, 82.4% and 91.6% respectively. Detailed information regarding acupuncture intervention was seriously insufficient. Among the 740 registration records, 89.2% lacked information on the style of acupuncture, 80.8% did not contain details regarding the needles used, 53.5% lacked information on the treatment regimen and 76.2% did not give details of other interventions administered with acupuncture.

Conclusions: The overall registration quality of ACTs is not high enough due to the serious lack of information on the specifics of acupuncture intervention. It is vital that a number of special items be set regarding acupuncture in order to develop a suitable system for the registration of ACTs.

Editor: Lamberto Manzoli, University of Chieti, Italy

Funding: The authors have no support or funding to report.

Competing Interests: The authors have declared that no competing interests exist.

* E-mail: yangkhebm2006@126.com

Introduction

As an alternative medicine methodology, acupuncture has proved effective for the treatment of many diseases and symptoms of disease, such as chronic pain, drug addiction, stroke rehabilitation, asthma and chemotherapy-induced nausea and vomiting [1,2]. Acupuncture has been shown to provide definite curative effects and to cause fewer adverse reactions than some other treatment modalities and has been approved by the WHO and by many other medical and health institutions in some western countries [3–6], and is now practiced widely around the world.

Due to the availability of increased research funding, acupuncture clinical trials (ACTs) have been extensively conducted in many countries in recent decades. As a result, the number of papers related to acupuncture is growing rapidly. Many researchers have not only summarized the clinical efficacy and safety of acupuncture, but have also expressed concern regarding the quality of ACTs. These studies revealed that ACTs had many

problems, such as poor methodological quality, unscientific research protocols, and repeated trials of acupuncture [7]. Moreover, the report quality of ACTs was low [8]. Information regarding acupuncturists' qualifications, adverse reactions and follow-up was missing [9]. Problems with publication bias had also extended to ACTs. Vickers reported that all ACTs from mainland China, Hong Kong, Taiwan and Japan were reported to be effective [10]. Additionally, all acupuncture treatments reported in China and Russia (or the former Soviet Union) were reported to be valid. Obviously, the high proportion of positive results reported in these countries was unusual, which could be attributed to publication and selective reporting bias [11]. Based on the above findings, the results of acupuncture trails were found to be unconvincing and unreliable.

The protocol of study is a predefined written document to state the structure of a research project and guide the implementation. A typical protocol has the following elements: background information and scientific rationale, objectives, study design, study population, study procedure, statistical consideration, subject confidentiality, informed consent process, literature references and supplements/appendices. WHO International Clinical Trials Registry Platform (ICTPR) has put key protocol information about each trial in public domain. These information make us learn about general characteristics of trails before it is reported. The registration of clinical trial required that soon after the trial was completed, its salient data be entered onto registries. This would bring negative data to light. Recently, the number of registered ACTs has been greatly increasing. According to a single web portal provided by the WHO International Clinical Trials Registry Platform (ICTPR), the number of registered ACTs has climbed to 740 [12], 520 of which were registered after 2008.

Thus far researchers have focused mainly on the quality of trial registration [13–15], however, to our knowledge, no study has yet examined the registration quality of ACTs. It has also been unclear whether existing general registered items reflect the characteristics of acupuncture intervention and are suitable for ACTs. Therefore, the objective of this study is to summarize and evaluate the quality of ACTs registration with the current 20 items of the WHO trial registration data set (TRDS) [16] and the special prepared items for acupuncture intervention details, which will provide the baseline information for the future development of ACTs registration.

Methods

Source of Data

Using the ICTRP Search Portal (http://apps.who.int/trialsearch/Default.aspx), we researched the registration data sets of WHO registries. Registries included the following: Australian New Zealand Clinical Trials Registry (ANZCTR), Chinese Clinical Trial Register (ChiCTR), ClinicalTrials.gov, Clinical Trials Registry-India (CTRI), Cuban Public Registry of Clinical Trials (RPCEC), EU Clinical Trials Register (EU-CTR), German Clinical Trials Register (DRKS), Iranian Registry of Clinical Trials (IRCT), ISRCTN, Japan Primary Registries Network (JPRN), Pan African Clinical Trial Registry (PACTR), Sri Lanka Clinical Trials Registry (SLCTR), the Netherlands National Trial Register (NTR), Clinical Research Information Service (CRiS) public of Korea (KCT), Brazilian Clinical Trials Registry (ReBec).

Search Strategy

WHO ICTRP prodives us with 'standard search' and 'advanced search'. We selected 'standard search' (to input "acupuncture", "needling", "acupressure", "moxibustion", "auriculotherapy" and "acupoint" into the ICTRP Search Portal (http://apps. who.int/trialsearch/Default.aspx)) without any restriction to focus on the sensitivity of retrieval, expand the scope of search results and improve the recall ration. The search was conducted on data sets from the inception of the registries up to 23 July 2012.

Inclusion Criteria

All records of ACTs that were registered in the WHO ICTRP were included. Acupuncture interventions might have been administered singly or with other interventions. For trials with multiple records, data from the record with the earliest registration date was chosen.

Data Extraction and Analysis

Information of registered ACTs was collected from all of the chosen records which imported into the portal and additional information was viewed through a hyperlink to the record in the source registry (i.e. the registry that provided the data) that was

published by ICTRP. A small pilot project designed to test the assessment of framework, and the training and competence of the data extractors, was performed prior to data extraction. Three researchers (Jing GU, Xiaogang WANG and Ye Zhao) extracted the data from 20 random records independently. Results of the pilot were discussed by Kehu Yang and Jing GU and the framework was subsequently adapted.

Two researchers (Jing GU and Ye ZHAO) extracted the data from each record independently. Disagreements were settled through discussion after data extraction. Data was input into a standardized form that was mainly composed of two parts: (1) the minimum 20 items of the WHO TRDS (Text S1) and (2) information related to acupuncture interventions: 1) styles of acupuncture, 2) needling details, 3) treatment regimen, and 4) other interventions administered along with the acupuncture.

Each item was assessed as "yes" (described in records) or "no" (not described in records). Conditions that were studied were classified according to the International Classification of Diseases (ICD-10) by two researchers (Jing GU and Ye Zhao). Discrepancies were resolved by consulting relevant clinical experts.

Descriptive statistics (frequency, percentage) were used to summarize data. Analysis was performed by Microsoft EXCEL software (version Microsoft Excel 2007; http://office.microsoft.com/zh-cn/) and SPSS ware (version 13.0; http://www.spss.com).

Results

A total of 914 registration records were retrieved in the registries. We excluded 174 records and included 740 records of ACTs (Figure 1, Text S2). Information from the registration of 740 trials was collected manually from the registered records.

General Characteristics

1. Year distribution of registration. All of the 740 acupuncture trials were registered during the period of 1999 to 2012. The number of registrations increased from 4 in 1999 to a peak of 149 in 2011. Registration for 2012 was still in process, so the final number was not yet available (Figure 2).

2. The registration quantity of each registry. ACTs were found in the following 11 registries: ClinicalTrials.gov (376), ChiCTR (107), ISRCTN (100), ANZCTR (70), IRCT (46), JPRN (14), KCT (13), EU-CTR (4), DRKS (3), NTR (4) and ReBec (3); No registration records were found in CTRI, RPCEC, PACTR, and SLCTR.

3. Types of diseases. Information was gathered concerning the diseases treated. Of these, 734 (99.2%, 95% CI 98.2–99.6%) records mentioned health condition(s) or problem(s), of which 38 (5.2%, 95% CI 3.8–7.0%) indicated that the participants were otherwise healthy people or did not specify. The most common conditions were "symptoms, signs and abnormal clinical and laboratory findings" (152 (20.7%, 95% CI 17.9–23.8%)). "Diseases of the musculoskeletal system and connective tissue" (100 (13.6%, 95% CI 11.3–16.3%) and "mental and behavioral disorders" (84 (11.4%, 95% CI 9.3–14.0%)) were of special concern (Table 1).

20 Items of WHO TRDS

The completeness of the 20 items of the WHO TRDS was checked. The overall report percentage of these 20 items varied from 38.6% to 100%. Information on the primary register and trial ID, date of registration in primary register and public title, was present in all registration records. Most registration records (>85%) mentioned the following items: source(s) of monetary or material support, primary sponsor, contact for public queries,

Registration records identified through WHO ICTRP searching: n = 914
'acupuncture' = 603; 'acupoint' = 131; 'moxibustion' = 41;
'acupressure' = 85; 'needling' = 48; 'auriculotherapy' = 6

Excluded after screening Main ID: n= 158
Duplication: n = 158

Full text records retrieved: n = 756

Excluded after screening full texts: n = 16
Multiple registration records of
the same trials: n = 4
Non-Acupuncture trials: n = 12

Included registration records: n = 740

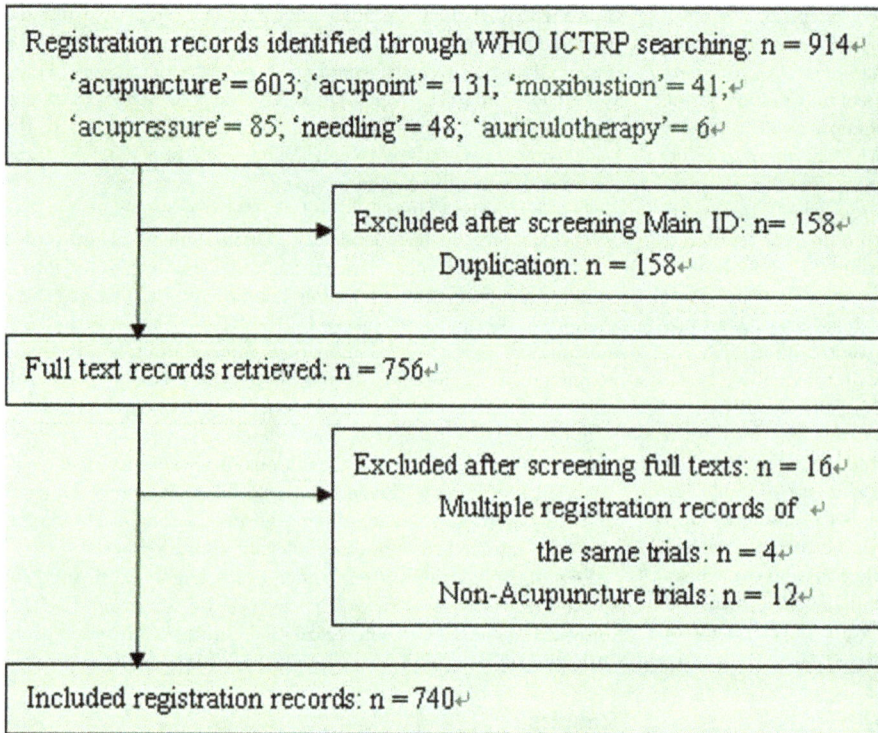

Figure 1. Flow chart of registration records identified, included and excluded.

scientific title, countries of recruitment, health condition(s) or problem(s) studied, intervention(s), key inclusion and exclusion criteria, study type, target sample size, recruitment status, primary outcome(s) and date of first enrollment. More than half of registration records provided items of secondary ID, key secondary outcomes and contact for scientific queries. Less than half of

registration records provided information of secondary sponsor(s) (Table 2).

The four centers that had the largest number of registered ACTs were Clinical Trials.gov, ChiCTR, ISRCTN and ANZCTR, and the average registration rate of 20 items were 89.6%, 92.2%, 82.4%, and 91.6% respectively (Table 2).

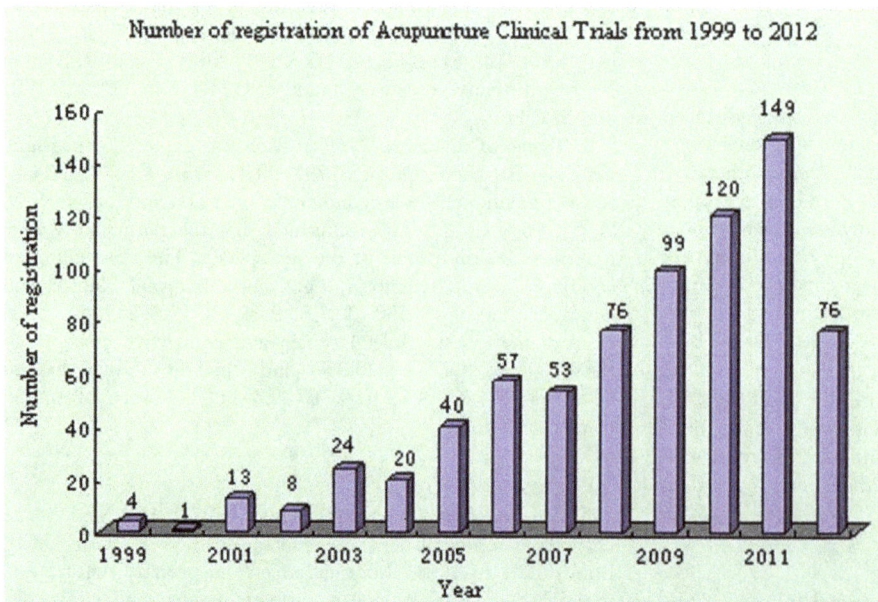

Number of registration of Acupuncture Clinical Trials from 1999 to 2012

Figure 2. Number of registration of acupuncture clinical trials from 1999 to 2012.

Table 1. Types of diseases.

Types of Diseases (Common ICD-10ª)	Number (%) of n = 734, (95% CI)
Symptoms, signs and abnormal clinical and laboratory findings, not classified elsewhere	152 (20.7, 17.9–23.8)
Diseases of the musculoskeletal system and connective tissue	100 (13.6, 11.3–16.3)
Mental and behavioural disorders	84 (11.4, 9.3–14.0)
Diseases of the genitourinary system	50 (6.8, 5.2–8.9)
Diseases of the digestive system	46 (6.3, 4.7–8.3)
Diseases of the nervous system	45 (6.1, 4.6–8.1)
Pregnancy, childbirth and the puerperium	43 (5.9, 4.4–7.8)
Diseases of the circulatory system	41 (5.6, 4.1–7.5)
Diseases of the respiratory system	32 (4.4, 3.1–6.1)
Neoplasms	31 (4.2, 3.0–5.9)
Endocrine, nutritional and metabolic diseases	22 (3.0, 2.0–4.5)
Infectious and parasitic diseases	15 (2.0, 1.2–3.4)
Injury, poisoning and certain other consequences of external causes	14 (1.9, 1.1–3.2)
Diseases of the eye and adnexa	13 (1.8, 1.0–3.0)
Diseases of the skin and subcutaneous tissue	5 (0.7, 0.3–1.6)
Diseases of the ear and mastoid process	3 (0.4, 0.1–1.3)
Not specified or healthy people	38 (5.2, 3.8–7.0)

ªCommon ICD-10: International Classification of Diseases 10.

Information regarding eligibility criteria for participants was also gathered. A total of 615 (83.1%, 95% CI 80.2–85.6%) records mentioned diagnostic criteria, of which 567 were based solely on "western medicine (diseases)", 17 were based solely on "traditional medicine syndrome" and 31 used both "western disease" and "traditional medicine syndrome" diagnostic criteria. Exclusion criteria were reported in 693 (93.6%, 95% CI 91.6–95.2%) records, and most (>90%) provided information regarding the age and sex of participants (Table 3).

Intervention Specifics of ACTs

Quality of registration of acupuncture intervention specifics was also checked. These intervention specifics are shown in Tables 4 and 5.

Style of acupuncture was reported in 80 (10.8%, 95% CI 8.8–13.3%) trials (Table 4). They covered the following seven types: "traditional Chinese medicine acupuncture", "ear acupuncture", "moxibustion", "western style acupuncture" "Japanese medicine acupuncture", "Korean medical acupuncture" and "tongue acupuncture" (Table 5). The lowest reported percentage of this item was 0% from JPRN, EU-CTR, DRKS, ReBec and NTR while the highest was 38.5% from KCT (Table 4).

Details regarding needling could potentially contain seven items: names or location of points used (uni/bilateral), number of needle insertions per subject per session, depth of insertion, response sought (e.g. de qi or muscle twitch response), needle retention time, needle type (diameter, length, and manufacturer or material) and needle stimulation (e.g. manual, electrical). The average report percentage of these seven items was 19.2% and the lowest reported percentage was 0% (Table 4). Regarding needle stimulation, 35.0% had electrical stimulation, 14.9% had manual stimulation and 8.4% had laser stimulation (Table 5).

Treatment regimen, which refers to information of number, frequency and duration of treatment sessions, was present in 344 (46.5%, 95% CI 42.9–50.1%) trials (Table 4). EU-CTR had the

lowest reported percentage (0%) of this item while ReBec, KCT and ANZCTR had the higher reported percentage (>75%) (Table 4).

Details of other interventions administered along with acupuncture were reported in 176 (23.8%, 95% CI 20.9–27.0%) trials (Table 4). They covered the following five types interventions: "western medicine", "traditional Chinese medicine", "exercises rehabilitation, massage, moxibustion, cupping, or similar", "cognitive behavioral therapy, life style advice, or similar", and "other interventions (routine nursing, conventional therapy, etc.)" (Table 5). EU-CTR, ReBec and NTR had the lowest reported percentage (0%) of this item (Table 4).

Discussion

A small number of studies have assessed the registration quality of clinical trials, and only one study was related to ACTs [17]. However, that study only investigated the status quo of the registration for ACTs, but did not report on its quality. In the present study, we retrieved all registered records of ACTs and evaluated the overall quality in order to identify possible deficiencies in ACTs registration and to provide feasible recommendations for development.

We reviewed some of the same variables reported in previous research done by Yang et. al. (2008) [17]. In that study, 206 registration records of ACTs were searched between 1999 and 2008 [17]. In the current study, results retrieved from the WHO ICTRP indicated that the registration number of ACTs has been increasing rapidly in recent years and has reached 740 as of July, 2012. In our research, there are 11 register centers where we can find ACTs while there were only 3 in the Yang study [17]. Similar to previous studies, ClinicalTrials.gov still have the largest number of ACTs while the number of ACTs in ChiCTR has increased from just 5, four years ago [17], to 107, surpassing ISRCTN and ANZCTRN and making it the second biggest registration center. This rapid increase in the number of registration centers that have

Table 2. 20 items of WHO TRDS.

20 Items	Overall	Clinical Trials.gov	ChiCTR	ISRCTN	ANZCTR	IRCT	JPRN	EU-CTR	DRKS	ReBec	KCT	NTR
	N^a (%) of n=740, (95% CI)	N^a (%) of n=376, (95% CI)	N^a (%) of n=107, (95% CI)	N^a (%) of n=100, (95% CI)	N^a (%) of n=70, (95% CI)	N^a (%) of n=46, (95% CI)	N^a (%) of n=14, (95% CI)	N^a (%) of n=4, (95% CI)	N^a (%) of n=3, (95% CI)	N^a (%) of n=3, (95% CI)	N^a (%) of n=13, (95% CI)	N^a (%) of n=4, (95% CI)
Primary Register and Trial ID^b	740 (100.0, 98.9–100.0)	376 (100.0, 97.9–100.0)	107 (100.0, 93.0–100.0)	100 (100.0, 92.6–100.0)	70 (100.0, 89.7–100.0)	46 (100.0, 85.1–100.0)	14 (100.0, 63.4–100.0)	4 (100.0, 32.6–100.0)	3 (100.0, 26.6–100.0)	3 (100.0, 26.6–100.0)	13 (100.0, 61.6–100.0)	4 (100.0, 32.6–100.0)
Date of Registration in Primary Registry	740 (100.0, 98.9–100.0)	376 (100.0, 97.9–100.0)	107 (100.0, 93.0–100.0)	100 (100.0, 92.6–100.0)	70 (100.0, 89.7–100.0)	46 (100.0, 85.1–100.0)	14 (100.0, 63.4–100.0)	4 (100.0, 32.6–100.0)	3 (100.0, 26.6–100.0)	3 (100.0, 26.6–100.0)	13 (100.0, 61.6–100.0)	4 (100.0, 32.6–100.0)
Secondary ID^b	445 (60.1, 56.6–63.6)	345 (91.8, 88.5–94.1)	0 (0.0, 0.0–7.0)	77 (77.0, 67.8–84.2)	10 (14.3, 7.9–24.6)	0 (0.0, 0–14.9)	0 (0.0, 0.0–36.6)	4 (100.0, 32.6–100.0)	3 (100.0, 26.6–100.0)	3 (100.0, 26.6–100.0)	0 (0.0, 0.0–38.4)	3 (75.0, 23.8–96.6)
Source(s) of Monetary or Material Support	730 (98.6, 97.5–99.3)	374 (99.5, 97.9–99.9)	106 (99.1, 93.7–99.9)	100 (100.0, 92.6–100.0)	68 (97.1, 89.3–99.3)	46 (100.0, 85.1–100.0)	14 (100.0, 63.4–100.0)	1 (25.0, 3.4–76.2)	3 (100.0, 26.6–100.0)	3 (100.0, 26.6–100.0)	12 (92.3, 60.9–98.9)	3 (75.0, 23.8–96.6)
Primary Sponsor	737 (99.6, 98.8–99.9)	374 (99.5, 97.9–99.9)	107 (100.0, 93.0–100.0)	100 (100.0, 92.6–100.0)	70 (100.0, 89.7–100.0)	46 (100.0, 85.1–100.0)	14 (100.0, 63.4–100.0)	4 (100.0, 32.6–100.0)	3 (100.0, 26.6–100.0)	3 (100.0, 26.6–100.0)	13 (100.0, 61.6–100.0)	3 (75.0, 23.8–96.6)
Secondary Sponsor(s)	286 (38.6, 35.2–42.2)	144 (38.3, 33.5–43.3)	95 (88.8, 81.3–93.5)	0 (0.0, 0.0–7.4)	27 (38.6, 28.0–50.4)	1 (2.2, 0.3–13.9)	0 (0.0, 0.0–36.6)	0 (0.0, 0.0–67.4)	1 (33.3, 4.3–84.6)	3 (100.0, 26.6–100.0)	13 (100.0, 61.6–100.0)	2 (50.0, 12.3–87.7)
Contact for Public Queries	711 (96.1, 94.4–97.3)	351 (93.4, 90.3–95.5)	107 (100.0, 93.0–100.0)	100 (100.0, 92.6–100.0)	70 (100.0, 89.7–100.0)	46 (100.0, 85.1–100.0)	14 (100.0, 63.4–100.0)	0 (0.0, 0.0–67.4)	3 (100.0, 26.6–100.0)	3 (100.0, 26.6–100.0)	13 (100.0, 61.6–100.0)	4 (100.0, 32.6–100.0)
Contact for Scientific Queries	397 (53.6, 50.0–57.2)	137 (36.4, 31.7–41.4)	107 (100.0, 93.0–100.0)	0 (0.0, 0.0–7.4)	70 (100.0, 89.7–100.0)	46 (100.0, 85.1–100.0)	14 (100.0, 63.4–100.0)	0 (0.0, 0.0–67.4)	3 (100.0, 26.6–100.0)	3 (100.0, 26.6–100.0)	13 (100.0, 61.6–100.0)	4 (100.0, 32.6–100.0)
Public Title	740 (100.0, 98.9–100.0)	376 (100.0, 97.9–100.0)	107 (100.0, 93.0–100.0)	100 (100.0, 92.6–100.0)	70 (100.0, 89.7–100.0)	46 (100.0, 85.1–100.0)	14 (100.0, 63.4–100.0)	4 (100.0, 32.6–100.0)	3 (100.0, 26.6–100.0)	3 (100.0, 26.6–100.0)	13 (100.0, 61.6–100.0)	4 (100.0, 32.6–100.0)
Scientific Title	638 (86.2, 83.5–88.5)	353 (93.9, 91.0–95.9)	106 (99.1, 93.7–99.9)	34 (34.0, 25.4–43.8)	70 (100.0, 89.7–100.0)	46 (100.0, 85.1–100.0)	2 (14.3, 3.6–42.7)	4 (100.0, 32.6–100.0)	3 (100.0, 26.6–100.0)	3 (100.0, 26.6–100.0)	13 (100.0, 61.6–100.0)	4 (100.0, 32.6–100.0)
Countries of Recruitment	723 (97.7, 96.3–98.6)	364 (96.8, 94.5–98.2)	103 (96.3, 90.5–98.6)	100 (100.0, 92.6–100.0)	70 (100.0, 89.7–100.0)	46 (100.0, 85.1–100.0)	14 (100.0, 63.4–100.0)	4 (100.0, 32.6–100.0)	2 (66.7, 15.4–95.7)	3 (100.0, 26.6–100.0)	13 (100.0, 61.6–100.0)	4 (100.0, 32.6–100.0)
Health Condition(s) or Problem(s) Studied	734 (99.2, 98.2–99.6)	374 (99.5, 97.9–99.9)	103 (96.3, 90.5–98.6)	99 (99.0, 93.2–99.9)	70 (100.0, 89.7–100.0)	46 (100.0, 85.1–100.0)	14 (100.0, 63.4–100.0)	4 (100.0, 32.6–100.0)	3 (100.0, 26.6–100.0)	3 (100.0, 26.6–100.0)	13 (100.0, 61.6–100.0)	4 (100.0, 32.6–100.0)
Intervention(s)	737 (99.6, 98.8–99.9)	376 (100.0, 97.9–100.0)	104 (97.2, 91.7–99.1)	100 (100.0, 92.6–100.0)	70 (100.0, 89.7–100.0)	46 (100.0, 85.1–100.0)	14 (100.0, 63.4–100.0)	4 (100.0, 32.6–100.0)	3 (100.0, 26.6–100.0)	3 (100.0, 26.6–100.0)	13 (100.0, 61.6–100.0)	4 (100.0, 32.6–100.0)
Key Inclusion and Exclusion Criteria	720 (97.3, 95.8–98.2)	374 (99.5, 97.9–99.9)	107 (100.0, 93.0–100.0)	82 (82.0, 73.2–88.4)	70 (100.0, 89.7–100.0)	46 (100.0, 85.1–100.0)	14 (100.0, 63.4–100.0)	4 (100.0, 32.6–100.0)	3 (100.0, 26.6–100.0)	3 (100.0, 26.6–100.0)	13 (100.0, 61.6–100.0)	4 (100.0, 32.6–100.0)
Study Type	736 (99.5, 98.6–99.8)	376 (100.0, 97.9–100.0)	107 (100.0, 93.0–100.0)	99 (99.0, 93.2–99.9)	70 (100.0, 89.7–100.0)	46 (100.0, 85.1–100.0)	14 (100.0, 63.4–100.0)	4 (100.0, 32.6–100.0)	3 (100.0, 26.6–100.0)	3 (100.0, 26.6–100.0)	13 (100.0, 61.6–100.0)	4 (100.0, 32.6–100.0)
Date of First Enrollment	739 (99.9, 99.0–100.0)	376 (100.0, 97.9–100.0)	107 (100.0, 93.0–100.0)	100 (100.0, 92.6–100.0)	70 (100.0, 89.7–100.0)	46 (100.0, 85.1–100.0)	14 (100.0, 63.4–100.0)	4 (100.0, 32.6–100.0)	2 (66.7, 15.4–95.7)	3 (100.0, 26.6–100.0)	13 (100.0, 61.6–100.0)	4 (100.0, 32.6–100.0)
Target Sample Size	703 (95.0, 93.2–96.4)	352 (93.6, 90.7–95.7)	103 (96.3, 90.5–98.6)	95 (95.0, 88.5–97.9)	70 (100.0, 89.7–100.0)	46 (100.0, 85.1–100.0)	13 (92.9, 63.0–99.9)	1 (25.0, 3.4–76.2)	3 (100.0, 26.6–100.0)	3 (100.0, 26.6–100.0)	13 (100.0, 61.6–100.0)	4 (100.0, 32.6–100.0)
Recruitment Status	738 (99.7, 98.9–99.9)	376 (100.0, 97.9–100.0)	107 (100.0, 93.0–100.0)	100 (100.0, 92.6–100.0)	70 (100.0, 89.7–100.0)	46 (100.0, 85.1–100.0)	14 (100.0, 63.4–100.0)	4 (100.0, 32.6–100.0)	3 (100.0, 26.6–100.0)	3 (100.0, 26.6–100.0)	13 (100.0, 61.6–100.0)	4 (100.0, 32.6–100.0)
Primary Outcome(s)	677 (91.5, 89.2–93.3)	325 (86.4, 82.6–89.5)	106 (99.1, 93.7–99.9)	91 (91.0, 83.6–95.3)	70 (100.0, 89.7–100.0)	46 (100.0, 85.1–100.0)	13 (92.9, 63.0–99.9)	4 (100.0, 32.6–100.0)	3 (100.0, 26.6–100.0)	3 (100.0, 26.6–100.0)	13 (100.0, 61.6–100.0)	3 (75.0, 23.8–96.6)

Table 2. Cont.

20 Items	Overall	Clinical Trials.gov	ChiCTR	ISRCTN	ANZCTR	IRCT	JPRN	EU-CTR	DRKS	ReBec	KCT	NTR
	N^a (%) of n=740, (95% CI)	N^a (%) of n=376, (95% CI)	N^a (%) of n=107, (95% CI)	N^a (%) of n=100, (95% CI)	N^a (%) of n=70, (95% CI)	N^a (%) of n=46, (95% CI)	N^a (%) of n=14, (95% CI)	N^a (%) of n=4, (95% CI)	N^a (%) of n=3, (95% CI)	N^a (%) of n=3, (95% CI)	N^a (%) of n=13, (95% CI)	N^a (%) of n=4, (95% CI)
Key Secondary Outcomes	495 (66.9, 63.4–70.2)	237 (63.0, 58.0–67.8)	78 (72.9, 63.7–80.5)	72 (72.0, 62.4–79.9)	58 (82.9, 72.2–90.0)	25 (54.3, 40.0–68.0)	4 (28.6, 11.1–56.1)	1 (25.0, 3.4–76.2)	1 (33.3, 4.3–84.6)	3 (100.0, 26.6–100.0)	13 (100.0, 61.6–100.0)	3 (75.0, 23.8–96.6)
Total per Registry (%)	(89.0, 86.5–91.0)	(89.6, 86.1–92.3)	(92.2, 85.4–96.0)	(82.4, 73.7–88.7)	(91.6, 82.5–96.2)	(87.8, 74.9–94.6)	(81.4, 53.3–94.4)	(73.8, 23.2–96.3)	(90.0, 17.2–99.7)	(95.0, 9.6–100.0)	(94.6, 61.3–99.5)	(91.2, 24.5–99.7)

^{a}N = Number.
^{b}ID = Identifying Number.

Table 3. Eligibility criteria for participants.

Category	Number (%) of n = 740, (95% CI)
Diagnostic Criteria	615 (83.1, 80.2–85.6)
Western Medicine (diseases)	567 (76.6, 73.4–79.5)
Traditional Medicine	17 (2.3, 1.4–3.7)
Using both Disease and Syndrome	31 (4.2, 3.0–5.9)
Exclusion Criteria	693 (93.6, 91.6–95.2)
Age	682 (92.2, 90.0–93.9)
Sex	679 (91.8, 89.5–93.5)
Male	14 (2.1^a, 1.2–3.5)
Female	145 (21.4^a, 18.4–24.6)
Both	520 (76.6^a, 73.2–79.6)

^{a}n = 679.

ACTs indicates that ACTs registration has become much more common. Although the number of ACTs in ChiCTR is far less than in ClinicalTrials.gov, the rapid growth is obvious, considering it has only been four years since it was established. Therefore it is possible that ChiCTR will become the principle registration center for ACTs in the future. Previous studies reported that the diseases of registered ACTs were limited [17,18]. In contrast, our study found that the types of diseases studied with ACTs are becoming more varied which will be helpful to better develop acupuncture clinical research.

Each registration record was also analyzed and the quality of ACT registration assessed using the following two guidelines: (1) the completeness of 20 items of WHO TRDS and (2) whether the related information of acupuncture intervention was present in the registration records according to specially preparedspecific items.

The contents of clinical trial registrations should contain the basic information about the trial's implementation. The 20 items of the WHO TRDS [16], regarded as the minimum requirement for trial registration, comprehensively covers this basic information. Therefore, ensuring the completeness of the 20 items is the first step in assessing the quality of ACT registration. Complete registration of 20 items minimizes the chance that relevant information will be omitted. This is of importance since missing or uninformative items required by the WHO TRDS may impair the fulfillment of registration promise. In the current study 20 items of the 740 records were reviewed and appraised for completeness. Our results indicated that most items (16 items) had higher percentages (>85%) of completeness. However, information regarding secondary sponsor(s), contact for scientific queries, secondary ID and key secondary outcomes were insufficient. There are two possible reasons for the omission of relevant information. One is that not every participant is willing to provide all 20 items due to academic or commercial interests [19]; the other is that not every registered trial had all of the 20 items [14]. For example, secondary ID or secondary sponsors do not routinely exist in some clinical trials so that the total percentage of these corresponding entries might be lower.

The completeness of 20 items varied among the 11 registries. Clinicaltrials.gov, the center with the largest number of registered ACTs, did not have the highest registration quality while instead we found that ChiCTR had the highest in the registration quality. The completeness of the 20 items in different register centers may be related to the establishment time of centers. Specifically, the 20 items of the WHO TRDS was announced in 2007 so that those

Table 4. Special items for acupuncture intervention details.

Special Items for Acupuncture Intervention Details	Overall	Clinical Trials.gov	ChiCTR	ISRCTN	ANZCTR	IRCT	JPRN	EU-CTR	DRKS	ReBec	KCT	NTR
	N[a] (%) of n=740, (95% CI)	N[a] (%) of n=376, (95% CI)	N[a] (%) of n=107, (95% CI)	N[a] (%) of n=100, (95% CI)	N[a] (%) of n=70, (95% CI)	N[a] (%) of n=46, (95% CI)	N[a] (%) of n=14, (95% CI)	N[a] (%) of n=4, (95% CI)	N[a] (%) of n=3, (95% CI)	N[a] (%) of n=3, (95% CI)	N[a] (%) of n=13, (95% CI)	N[a] (%) of n=4, (95% CI)
Style of Acupuncture[b]	80 (10.8, 8.8-13.3)	42 (11.2, 8.4-14.8)	12 (11.2, 6.5-18.7)	8 (8.0, 4.1-15.2)	11 (15.7, 8.9-26.2)	4 (8.7, 3.3-21.0)	0 (0.0, 0.0-36.6)	0 (0.0, 0.0-67.4)	0 (0.0, 0.0-73.4)	0 (0.0, 0.0-73.4)	5 (38.5, 17.0-65.6)	0 (0.0, 0.0-67.4)
Needling Details[c]	(19.2, 16.5-22.2)											
Names or Location of Points	216 (29.2, 26.0-32.6)	95 (25.3, 21.1-29.9)	28 (26.2, 18.7-35.3)	16 (16.0, 10.0-24.5)	36 (51.4, 39.9-62.9)	29 (63.0, 48.4-75.6)	5 (35.7, 15.7-62.4)	0 (0.0, 0.0-67.4)	0 (0.0, 0.0-73.4)	1 (33.3, 4.3-84.6)	9 (69.2, 40.9-88.8)	0 (0.0, 0.0-67.4)
Number of Needle Insertions per Session	169 (22.8, 20.0-26.0)	82 (21.8, 17.9-26.3)	17 (15.9, 10.1-24.1)	15 (15.0, 9.2-23.4)	27 (38.6, 28.0-50.4)	19 (41.3, 28.1-55.9)	3 (21.4, 7.1-49.4)	0 (0.0, 0.0-67.4)	0 (0.0, 0.0-73.4)	1 (33.3, 4.3-84.6)	5 (38.5, 17.0-65.6)	0 (0.0, 0.0-67.4)
Depth of Insertion	47 (6.4, 4.8-8.4)	25 (6.6, 4.5-9.7)	3 (2.8, 0.9-8.3)	7 (7.0, 3.4-14.0)	5 (7.1, 3.0-16.0)	2 (4.3, 1.1-15.8)	1 (7.1, 1.0-37.0)	0 (0.0, 0.0-67.4)	0 (0.0, 0.0-73.4)	1 (33.3, 4.3-84.6)	3 (23.1, 7.6-52.2)	0 (0.0, 0.0-67.4)
Response Sought	58 (7.8, 6.1-10.0)	27 (7.2, 5.0-10.3)	6 (5.6, 2.5-11.9)	4 (4.0, 1.5-10.2)	15 (21.4, 13.4-32.6)	2 (4.3, 1.1-15.8)	0 (0.0, 0.0-36.6)	0 (0.0, 0.0-67.4)	0 (0.0, 0.0-73.4)	1 (33.3, 4.3-84.6)	3 (23.1, 7.6-52.2)	0 (0.0, 0.0-67.4)
Needle Retention Time	216 (29.2, 26.0-32.6)	95 (25.3, 21.1-29.9)	21 (19.6, 13.2-28.2)	15 (15.0, 9.2-23.4)	43 (61.4, 49.6-72.0)	28 (60.9, 46.2-73.8)	2 (14.3, 3.6-42.7)	0 (0.0, 0.0-67.4)	0 (0.0, 0.0-73.4)	1 (33.3, 4.3-84.6)	11 (84.6, 54.9-96.1)	0 (0.0, 0.0-67.4)
Needle Type[d]	84 (11.4, 9.3-13.8)	50 (13.3, 10.2-17.1)	3 (2.8, 0.9-8.3)	7 (7.0, 3.4-14.0)	15 (21.4, 13.4-32.6)	1 (2.2, 0.3-13.9)	0 (0.0, 0.0-36.6)	0 (0.0, 0.0-67.4)	0 (0.0, 0.0-73.4)	1 (33.3, 4.3-84.6)	7 (53.8, 28.2-77.6)	0 (0.0, 0.0-67.4)
Needle Stimulation	205 (27.7, 24.6-31.0)	101 (26.9, 22.6-31.6)	30 (28.0, 20.4-37.3)	17 (17.0, 10.8-25.7)	33 (47.1, 35.8-58.8)	10 (21.7, 12.1-35.9)	5 (35.7, 15.7-62.4)	1 (25.0, 3.4-76.2)	0 (0.0, 0.0-73.4)	2 (66.7, 15.4-95.7)	4 (30.8, 12.0-59.1)	0 (0.0, 0.0-67.4)
Treatment Regimen[e]	344 (46.5, 42.9-50.1)	184 (48.9, 43.9-54.0)	18 (16.8, 10.9-25.1)	38 (38.0, 29.0-47.9)	54 (77.1, 65.9-85.5)	30 (65.2, 50.5-77.5)	3 (21.4, 7.1-49.4)	0 (0.0, 0.0-67.4)	1 (33.3, 4.3-84.6)	3 (100.0, 26.6-100)	12 (92.3, 60.9-98.9)	1 (25.0, 3.4-76.2)
Other Interventions[f]	176 (23.8, 20.9-27.0)	80 (21.3, 17.4-25.7)	28 (26.2, 18.7-35.3)	25 (25.0, 17.5-34.4)	21 (30.0, 20.4-41.7)	8 (17.4, 8.9-31.1)	1 (7.1, 1.0-37.0)	0 (0.0, 0.0-67.4)	1 (33.3, 4.3-84.6)	0 (0.0, 0.0-73.4)	4 (30.8, 12.0-59.1)	0 (0.0, 0.0-67.4)

[a]N = Number.
[b]Style of acupuncture (e.g. Traditional Chinese Medicine,Japanese,Korean,Western medical,Five Element,ear acupuncture, etc).
[c]Needling details can contain seven items: names or location of points used (uni/bilateral), number of needle insertions per subject per session, depth of insertion, response sought (e.g. de qi or muscle twitch response), needle retention time, needle type (diameter, length, and manufacturer or material) and needle stimulation (e.g. manual, electrical).The total percentage of the seven items was 19.2%.
[d]Needle Type (e.g. diameter, length, and manufacturer or material).
[e]Treatment regimen, refers to number, frequency and duration of treatment sessions.
[f]Other interventions administered to the acupuncture group (e.g. moxibustion, cupping, herbs, exercises, lifestyle advice).

Table 5. Descriptive information of some acupuncture special items.

Category	Number (%) of n, (95% CI)
Style of Acupuncture	**n = 97**
Traditional Chinese Medicine Acupuncture	33 (34.0, 25.3–44.0)
Ear Acupuncture	28 (28.9, 20.7–38.6)
Moxibustion	14 (14.4, 8.7–22.9)
Western Style Acupuncture	13 (13.4, 7.9–21.7)
Japanese Medicine Acupuncture	5 (5.2, 2.2–11.8)
Korean Medical Acupuncture	2 (2.1, 0.5–7.9)
Tongue Acupuncture	2 (2.1, 0.5–7.9)
Needle Stimulation of the Acupuncture	**n = 309**
Electrical	108 (35.0, 29.8–40.4)
Manual	46 (14.9, 11.3–19.3)
Laser	26 (8.4, 5.8–12.1)
Not specified or other stimulation	129 (41.7, 36.4–47.3)
Details of other Interventions Administered to Acupuncture	**n = 176**
Western Medicine	67 (38.1, 31.2–45.5)
Traditional Chinese Medicine	13 (7.4, 4.3–12.3)
Exercises, Rehabilitation, Massage,Moxibustion, Cupping, etc.	37 (21.0, 15.6–27.7)
Cognitive Behavioural Therapy, Life Style Advice, etc.	9 (5.1, 2.7–9.5)
Other Interventions (Routine nursing, Conventional Therapy, etc.)	50 (28.4, 22.2–35.5)

centers established after this announcement would have set the items according to the WHO TRDS. Thus, the items from those centers would have a higher percentage of registration than the centers established prior to 2007. For example, ChiCTR, which was established after 2007, was found to have better completeness and quality of the 20 items.

In the current study we also have determined that for each register center, there were several items that contained woefully inadequate information. This may have been caused by the absence of related items in that specific center. For instance, ISRCIN has no area for information about 'secondary sponsor(s)' [14], and no record contained relevant information. Similarly, the item 'secondary sponsor' was not found in IRCT [14], and only 2.2% records provided relevant information. This speculation is supported by previous research by Liu's [14]. Liu mentioned that, although the data sets of each registry were based on the 20 items, there were still slight differences among registries due to the increase or reduction of some items so that there are different registration rates in different centers.

Unlike general clinical intervention, acupuncture is a special medical technique that treats patients by inserting thin needles into acupoints. Acupuncture clinical practice is mainly concerned with acupuncture theory, acupoints, unique acupuncture manipulation methods, and acupuncture instruments [20]. The "quality" of an intervention in the sense of "how well made is the intervention" is a preclinical not a clinical issue for drugs, biologics, or devices, but for procedures such as acupuncture, intervention quality is a clinical issue. There are many factors which can influence its curative effect and safety. Arguably more information thoroughly describing the acupuncture intervention should be required in the registration of ACTs, just as in the registration of drug, biological and vaccine trials, information on the dose, frequency, route of administration and duration of treatment are needed [16,21]. As

an open-source, the information of ACTs registration should be detailed enough to make trials as transparent as possible.

Since acupuncture is a unique medical technique, it is not appropriate to evaluate the quality of its intervention specifics with existing evaluation criterion for general intervention measures. As demonstrated by previous studies, special items that describe the intervention details of acupuncture should be added to the registration of item sets [17]. Further assessment on the quality of ACTs registration could potentially be accomplished using these special items. We developed items and evaluation criterion that contain the following four facets: style of acupuncture, needling details, treatment regimen and other interventions administered with acupuncture. We validated these items for quality evaluation of acupuncture intervention details in reference to the Standards for Reporting Interventions in Controlled Trials of Acupuncture (STRICTA) [22]. As is known to all, the intervention details of acupuncture are totally included by STRICTA. However, unlike the trial report, trial registration is a demonstration of the protocol before implementation while the trial report is the demonstration of the process and details about the trial after completion. Therefore, instead of using all of the items published by STRICTA, we integrated the suggestions of intervention from acupuncturists, clinical expert, methodologists and producers of systematic reviews and chose only those items related with intervention that should be included in a protocol of acupuncture research (the protocol without these information will miss the accuracy of the implementation of trails and the results will be unreliable.). However, we found that information on the details of acupuncture intervention is seriously insufficient. Possible reasons for this may be: (1) these special items were not included in 20 items and the registration centers lacked registration requirements for them. Therefore, these items failed to catch the attention of registrants and registrants neglected the description of acupuncture intervention details or (2) the selection of acupoints and acupuncture manipulation takes great skill and heavy reliance on experience, therefore many clinical acupuncture practitioners keep this information private and are reluctant to share technical details. These limitations cause ACTs to be less transparent.

Acupuncture is a part of Traditional Chinese Medicine (TCM). The necessity of acupuncture intervention and selection of acupoints are based on TCM's syndromes. However, most acupuncture researchers focus on 'western disease' for their diagnostic criteria rather than 'TCMs' syndromes'. In the current study, we found that only 6.5% (2.3% + 4.2%) of ACTs registration records provided information about TCM's syndrome in their diagnostic criteria. To comply with the principles of selection of treatment based on the differential diagnosis of TCM, we strongly propose that diagnostic criteria contain information on both western disease and TCM's syndrome in the registration of ACTs.

After the publication of the announcement of International Committee of Medical Journal Editors (ICMJE) [23], the Ottawa Statement and Declaration of Helsinki [24,25], and with the establishment of the WHO ICTRP, the importance of registration has been gradually accepted so that now, clinical trial registration has become a part of the current research paradigm internationally. With increasing numbers and attention in recent years, ACTs should be encouraged to register in order to improve public confidence in clinical effectiveness. Registration could bring the following benefits to the clinical research of acupuncture. First, registration promotes the inspection of study design and provides technical guidance for the clinical trial [26]. Second, whether the key part of clinical trial was reported or not, a registered protocol can be used as a basis for supervision. Registration will also increase the transparency of the clinical trials, so it can be ensured that the reported information from clinical research is complete, true and valid [24,27] while potential biases are reduced as much as possible. Third, registration of ACTs helps to avoid repeating research and/or wasting resources. Fourth, as a precondition of ACTs being published in journals with high impact factors [18], registration could facilitate the communication of the results from ACTs. Therefore, further quantitative and qualitative improvements are needed in ACTs registration.

Although the quality of ACTs registration was fair in regard to the completeness of the 20 items according to our research, the serious lack of information on acupuncture intervention specifics lowered its overall quality greatly, which made trial registration fail to fulfill its promise of promoting research transparency [28–30].

It is very necessary to establish special registration system for ACTs because of the specificity of acupuncture, just like STRICTA – a special version of CONSORT [31] – is made for acupuncture RCTs. Modifying the existing registration system to include criteria (or items) specific to acupuncture could facilitate developing a registration system for ACTs. The first step would be to establish a registration data set suitable for ACTs. We propose that those items used to assess acupuncture intervention details in the current study be added on the basis of the 20 items. The second step would be to establish a special registry center for ACTs.

There were several limitations in the current study. First, assessment of the registration quality of ACTs in different centers according to the completeness of 20 items may be lacking fairness since the 20 items of the WHO TRDS were not announced until 2007. Therefore, those centers established after 2007 may have a higher registration quality since they could more easily meet the standards set by the WHO TRDS. Second, there are likely many clinical trials that are not registered in the WHO ICTRP, so that it would be impossible for our study to include all of the ACTs that are registered throughout the world.

In conclusion, the overall registration quality of ACTs was not high enough due to the serious lack of information on the specifics of acupuncture intervention. Further improvements are needed in this field. This could be achieved by optimizing the WHO TRDS to include those additional items related to acupuncture. It is extremely vital to establish a number of special items regarding acupuncture intervention to develop a suitable system for the registration of ACTs.

Supporting Information

Text S1 The minimum 20 items of the WHO trial registration data set (WHO TRDs).
(DOC)

Text S2 Main ID of all included registration records.
(DOC)

Author Contributions

Conceived and designed the experiments: JG KY X-GW YZ J-HT. Performed the experiments: JG YZ J-JJ. Analyzed the data: X-GW JG YZ J-HT. Contributed reagents/materials/analysis tools: JG KY X-GW YZ J-HT. Wrote the paper: JG X-GW.

References

1. Richardson PH, Vincent CA (1986) Acupuncture for the treatment of pain: a review of evaluative research. Pain 24: 15–40.
2. National Institutes of Health (1998) NIH Consensus Conference. Acupuncture. JAMA 280: 1518–24.
3. NIH Consensus Development Program (1997) Acupuncture–Consensus Development Conference Statement. Available: http://consensus.nih.gov/1997/1997Acupuncture107html.htm. Accessed 2012 Aug 26.
4. World Health Organization (2003) Acupuncture: Review and Analysis of Reports on Controlled Clinical Trials. Available: http://www.who.int/medicinedocs/en/d/Js4926e/#Js4926e. Accessed 2012 Aug 29.
5. US National Center for Complementary and Alternative Medicine (2006) Acupuncture. Available: http://nccam.nih.gov/health/acupuncture/. Accessed 2012 Nov 7.
6. National Health Service (2012) Acupuncture: Evidence for its effectiveness. Available: http://www.nhs.uk/Conditions/Acupuncture/Pages/Evidence.aspx. Accessed 2012 Aug 14.
7. Sun Yong (2011) Analysis of clinical studies of acupuncture. CJCM 3: 69–70.
8. Xu L, Li J, Zhang M, Ai C, Wang L (2008) Chinese authors do need CONSORT: reporting quality assessment for five leading Chinese medical journals. Contemp Clin Trials 29: 727–731.
9. Geng LL, Lin RS, Sun XY, Wu L, Zhong MM, et al. (2008) Critical appraisal of randomized clinical trials in Chinese Acupuncture and Moxibustion from 2000 to 2006. Zhongguo Zhen Jiu 28: 439–43.
10. Vickers A, Goyal N, Harland R, Rees R (1998) Do certain countries produce only positive results? A systematic review of controlled trials. Controll Clin Trials 19: 159–166.
11. Lao LX (2008) Acupuncture clinical studies and evidence-based medicine–an update. Zhen Ci Yan Jiu 33: 53–61.
12. WHO International Clinical Trials Registry Platform (ICTRP). Available: http://apps.who.int/trialsearch/Default.aspx. Accessed 2012 Jul 23.
13. Viergever RF, Ghersi D (2011) The quality of registration of clinical trials. PLoS One 6: 1–8.
14. Liu X, Li Y, Yu X, Feng J, Zhong X, et al. (2009) Assessment of registration quality of trials sponsored by China. J Evid Based Med 2: 8–18.
15. Sekeres M, Gold JL, Chan AW, Lexchin J, Moher D, et al. (2008) Poor reporting of scientific leadership information in clinical trial registers. PLoS One 3: e1610.
16. WHO Trial Registration Data Set (TRDS). Available: http://www.who.int/ictrp/network/trds/en/index.html. Accessed 2012 Jul 28.
17. Yang DQ, Tu Y (2008) Investigation of registration of international acupuncture clinical trials. Available: http://www.cnki.net/kcms/detail/Detail.aspx?dbname=CDMDTOTAL&filename=2008113899.nh&filetitle. Accessed 2012 Jul 29.
18. Li ZJ, Liu ML, Wang JN, Liang FR (2012) Method and current situations on acupuncture clinical trial registration in the world. Zhen Ci Yan Jiu 37: 86–7.

19. Reveiz L, Krleza-Jerić K, Chan AW, de Aguiar S (2007) Do trialists endorse clinical trial registration? Survey of a Pubmed sample. Trials 8: 30.
20. Wu B, Liu Y, He J (2002) (Evidence based medicine and the present situation and enlightenment of acupuncture clinical research. Journal of Clinical Acupuncture and Moxibustion 18: 1–2.
21. De Angelis CD, Drazen JM, Frizelle FA, Haug C, Hoey J, et al. (2005) Is this clinical trial fully registered? A statement from the international committee of medical journal editors. Croat Med J 46: 499–501.
22. MacPherson H, Altman DG, Hammerschlag R, Youping L, Taixiang W, et al. (2010) Revised Standards for Reporting Interventions in Clinical Trials of Acupuncture (STRICTA): extending the CONSORT statement. PLoS Med 7(6): e1000261.
23. International Committee of Medical Journal (2004) Clinical Trial Registration: A statement from the International Committee of Medical Journal Editors. Available: http://www.icmje.org/clin_trial.pdf. Accessed 2012 Jun 28.
24. Krleza-Jeric K, Chan AW, Dickersin K, Sim I, Grimshaw J, et al. (2005) Principles for international registration of protocol information and results from human trials of health related interventions: Ottawa statement (part 1). BMJ 330(7497): 956–958.
25. World Medical Association (2008) Declaration of Helsinki. Available: http://www.wma.net/en/30publications/10policies/b3/index.html. Accessed 2012 Jun 28.
26. Wang L, Jiang J, Li X (2007) Promote the whole level of Chinese medical journals through the mechanism of registry and publicity of clinical experiment. Xian Dai Qing Bao 27: 221–22.
27. Ghersi D, Pang T (2009) From Mexico to Mail: four years in the history of clinical trial registration. J Evid Based Med 2(1): 1–7.
28. Dwan K, Altman DG, Arnaiz JA, Bloom J, Chan AW, et al. (2008) Systematic review of the empirical evidence of study publication bias and outcome reporting bias. PLoS One 3(8): e3081.
29. Scherer RW, Langenberg P, von Elm E (2007) Full publication of results initially presented in abstracts. Cochrane Database Syst Rev 18(2): MR000005.
30. Chalmers I, Glasziou P (2009) Avoidable waste in the production and reporting of research evidence. Lancet 374(9683): 86–9.
31. Begg C, Cho M, Eastwood S, Horton R, Moher D, et al. (1996) Improving the quality of reporting of randomized controlled trials. The CONSORT statement. JAMA 276(8): 637–9.

19

Electroacupuncture Decreases Excessive Alcohol Consumption Involving Reduction of FosB/ΔFosB Levels in Reward-Related Brain Regions

Jing Li[1⑨], Yanan Sun[2⑨], Jiang-Hong Ye[1]*

1 Department of Anesthesiology, Pharmacology and Physiology, University of Medicine and Dentistry of New Jersey, New Jersey Medical School, Newark, New Jersey, United States of America, 2 Department of Neurology, Dong-Zhi-Men Hospital, Beijing University of Chinese Medicine, Key Laboratory for Internal Chinese Medicine of Ministry of Education, Beijing, China

Abstract

New therapies are needed for alcohol abuse, a major public health problem in the U.S. and worldwide. There are only three FDA-approved drugs for treatment of alcohol abuse (naltrexone, acamprosate and disulfuram). On average these drugs yield only moderate success in reducing long-term alcohol consumption. Electroacupuncture has been shown to alleviate various drugs of abuse, including alcohol. Although previous studies have shown that electroacupuncture reduced alcohol consumption, the underlying mechanisms have not been fully elucidated. ΔFosB and FosB are members of the Fos family of transcription factors implicated in neural plasticity in drug addiction; a connection between electroacupuncture's treatment of alcohol abuse and the Fos family has not been established. In this study, we trained rats to drink large quantities of ethanol in a modified intermittent access two-bottle choice drinking procedure. When rats achieved a stable baseline of ethanol consumption, electroacupuncture (100 Hz or 2 Hz, 30 min each day) was administered at Zusanli (ST36) for 6 consecutive days. The level of FosB/ΔFosB in reward-related brain regions was assessed by immunohistochemistry. We found that the intake of and preference for ethanol in rats under 100 Hz, but not 2 Hz electroacupuncture regiment were sharply reduced. The reduction was maintained for at least 72 hours after the termination of electroacupuncture treatment. Conversely, 100 Hz electroacupuncture did not alter the intake of and preference for the natural rewarding agent sucrose. Additionally, FosB/ΔFosB levels in the prefrontal cortex, striatal region and the posterior region of ventral tegmental area were increased following excessive ethanol consumption, but were reduced after six-day 100 Hz electroacupuncture. Thus, this study demonstrates that six-day 100 Hz electroacupuncture treatment effectively reduces ethanol consumption and preference in rats that chronically drink excessive amount of ethanol. This effect of electroacupuncture may be mediated by down-regulation of FosB/ΔFosB in reward-related brain regions.

Editor: Lisa Carlson Lyons, Florida State University, United States of America

Funding: This work was supported by National Institutes of Health – National Institute on Alcohol Abuse and Alcoholism [Grants AA016964 and AA016618]. The funders had no role in study design, data collection and analysis, decision to publish, or preparation of the manuscript.

Competing Interests: The authors have declared that no competing interests exist.

* E-mail: ye@umdnj.edu

⑨ These authors contributed equally to this work.

Introduction

Alcohol abuse is a major public health problem in the U.S. and worldwide. To date, there are only three FDA-approved drugs for treatment of alcohol abuse (naltrexone, acamprosate and disulfuram). On average these drugs yield only moderate success in reducing long-term alcohol consumption [1,2,3]. Therefore, new therapies are needed. Acupuncture, consisting of stimulating certain points on the body by means of needles, has been used in China for thousand years. Although it is still not completely clear how the acupuncture signals from the acupoint, such as Zusanli (ST36) are transmitted to the central nervous system, it has been characterized that the afferent impulses induced by acupuncture are mainly transmitted by Aβ and AΔ fibers [4]. Acupuncture activates small myelinated nerve fibers in the muscle, which send impulses to the spinal cord, and then activates three centers (spinal cord, midbrain and pituitary-hypothalamus) and the release of three endorphins (enkephalin, beta endorphin and dynorphin) and other monoamines, eliciting profound physiological effects and self-healing mechanisms [5]. Thus, acupuncture has been regarded widely as an effective mean for some medical conditions, including nausea, pain [6] and drug abuse [7]. Compared with the currently available pharmacological interventions, a clear advantage of acupuncture therapy is that it has the potential to help drug abusers stay away from drugs without major adverse side effects. Previous clinical and preclinical studies have shown that acupuncture or acupuncture combined with electrical stimulation (electroacupuncture, EA) is an effective treatment for alcohol withdrawal syndrome and alcohol abuse [8,9,10,11,12,13]. Recently, we have shown that EA of 2 Hz reduced voluntary alcohol intake in rats [14]. However, many questions regarding the basic mechanisms of acupuncture in general and of alcohol abuse in particular have not been well addressed.

Investigations of long-term changes in brain structure and function that accompany chronic exposure to drugs of abuse suggest that alterations in gene regulation contribute substantially to the addictive phenotype [15]. In particular, two transcription factors – ΔFosB and CREB (cAMP responsive element binding protein) have been implicated in addiction-related neural plasticity [15]. The transcription factor Δ FosB, an unusually stable, C-terminally truncated variant of the immediate early gene product FosB, accumulates in the addiction circuitry after most drugs of abuse, including cocaine, morphine, Δ^9-tetrahydrocannabinol and ethanol [16]. Once expressed, it is relatively stable and can persist in the brain for weeks after the last drug exposure. By regulating numerous genes that are related to dendritic spine architecture and synaptic function and plas-ticity, such as cyclin-dependent kinase 5 and dynorphin [17,18], ΔFosB mediates the synaptic plasticity which contributes to various behavioural phenotypes in response to drug exposure. Previous studies from our and the other laboratories have shown that chronic alcohol exposures induce the accumulation of ΔFosB within the subregions of the striatum and the prefrontal cortex (PFC) [16,19], which involves activation of endogenous opioid systems [19]. Given that existing evidence indicates that EA alleviated alcohol consumption and morphine dependence via interacting with opioid receptors [12,20,21]; and that acupuncture attenuates stress-induced cocaine relapse by suppressing Fos expression and CREB activation within the subregions of the striatum [22], we hypothesized that EA suppression on alcohol consumption may be mediated by transcription factors, such as FosB/ΔFosB protein in reward-related brain regions. To test this possibility, multiple sessions of EA were administered at the bilateral acupoint ST36 of rats that chronically drink large quantities of ethanol under a modified intermittent access two-bottle choice drinking procedure (IE). The expression of FosB/ΔFosB in several reward-related brain regions was assessed using immunohistochemistry, which has higher sensitivity than Western blotting and provides greater anatomical details [23].

Methods

All experiments were performed in accordance with the guidelines of the National Institutes of Health for the Care and Use of Laboratory Animals, and were approved by the Institutional Animal Care and Use Committee of the University of Medicine and Dentistry of New Jersey, Newark, New Jersey.

Animals and housing

Adult Sprague-Dawley (S-D) rats (250–350 g, at the start of the experiments, Taconic Farm, NY) were individually housed in ventilated cages, in a climate-controlled room (20–22°C), kept on a 12-h light/dark cycle (lights off at 6 p.m.). Food and water were available ad libitum.

Alcohol drinking procedure

The animals were first acclimatized to the homecage environment for one week, and were trained to voluntarily drink ethanol under the intermittent access two-bottle choice drinking procedure as described previously [14,19,24,25,26]. Briefly, animals were given 24-h concurrent access to one bottle of 20% (v/v) ethanol in water and one bottle of water, starting at 6:00 p.m. on Monday. After 24 h, the ethanol bottle was replaced with a second water bottle that was available for the next 24 h. This pattern was repeated on Wednesdays and Fridays. The other days of the week the rats had unlimited access to two bottles of water. The days when ethanol was assessable to the rats, the placement of the ethanol bottle was alternated to control for side preferences. In this study, we modified the procedure by adding 5% sucrose to the

20% ethanol solution in the first three ethanol sessions. This modification rapidly and sharply accelerated ethanol intake (Fig. 1). The amount of ethanol or water consumed was determined by weighing the bottles before access and after 24 h of access. The weight of each rat was measured daily Monday through Friday to monitor health and calculate the grams of ethanol intake per kilogram of body weight. Ethanol consumption was determined by calculating grams of alcohol consumed per kilogram of body weight. The preference ratio of ethanol intake was calculated by the following formula: Preference ratio (%) = Ethanol solution intake (ml/24 h)/total fluid intake (ml/24 h ethanol solution + ml/24 h water). Rats were maintained on 20% ethanol intermittent access two-bottle choice procedure for 4 weeks (12 ethanol-access sessions). A bottle containing water in a cage without rats was used to evaluate the spillage due to the experimental manipulations during the test sessions. The spillage was always <1.0 ml (<2.5% of the total fluid intake).

Blood Ethanol Concentrations (BEC)

On the 13th ethanol drinking session, blood samples were collected from the lateral tail vein of rats (n = 11) following 30 min access to 20% ethanol and water. The samples were centrifuged at 4°C for 15 min at 8000 rpm, and 10 μl plasma from each blood sample was analyzed using nicotinamide adenine dinucleotide-alcohol dehydrogenase (NAD-ADH) enzyme spectrophotometric method [27].

Sucrose self-administration

To determine whether EA-induced reduction in drinking was selective to alcohol, a separate group (n = 8) of rats were trained to drink 5% sucrose solution under intermittent-access two-bottle choice drinking procedure, similar to that for alcohol drinking. 5% sucrose was selected according to our previous studies [25,26] and a recent rodent study on the effect of the opioid receptor antagonists, SoRI-9409 on alcohol intake [28]. When SD rats had reached a consistent baseline level after 12 drinking sessions of access to sucrose and water, 100 Hz EA or sham procedures were performed as described below.

EA treatments

To test the effect of EA on ethanol intake in rats that chronically consumed high amounts of ethanol, 100 Hz EA was administered at bilateral ST36, located near the knee joint of the hind limb, 2 mm lateral to the anterior tubercle of the tibia; EA was applied 30 min each day, 30 min prior to the access to ethanol, for 6 consecutive days (Wednesday through Monday, three consecutive drinking sessions).

All rats were prehandled for 2 min/day for 3 consecutive days prior to EA treatments to reduce stress and facilitate handling. On the test day, under light anesthesia with isoflurane, the rats of both EA and sham groups were lightly restrained, which involved being fixed on a rack with a towel covering their eyes, as described in our recent report [14]. Under these conditions, rats were calm and their limbs and tails could be freely extruded. Two stainless-steel needles with diameter of 0.35 mm and length of 13 mm were inserted about 2–3 mm into ST36 of both legs (for EA group). After the animals woke up from anesthesia, 10 min EA (or sham) was administered. A constant current with square-wave stimulation produced by a programmed pulse generator (Han Actens WQ 1002F, Aeron Optoelectronic Technology Corp., Beijing, China) was given via the two needles for the EA group. The EA frequency was 100 Hz, and the intensity was adjusted to provoke light trembling of muscles (about 0.2–0.3 mA). For the sham group, needles were placed

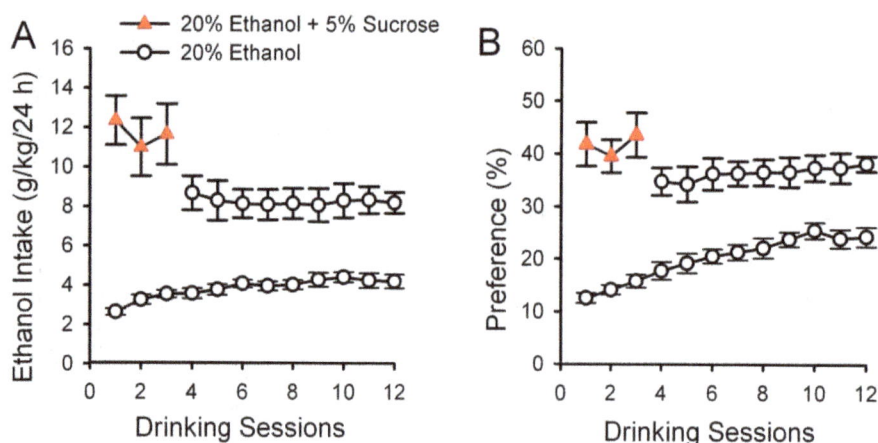

Figure 1. Sucrose induction induced excessive ethanol consumption and high preference in male Sprague-Dawley (SD) rats. The mean (± S.E.M) of ethanol intake (g/kg/24 h) (**A**) and of ethanol preference (**B**) in rats under the intermittent access drinking procedure with 5% sucrose in the first three drinking sessions were much higher than those in rats under the same drinking procedure without sucrose induction (all $p<0.001$). Two-way RM ANOVA followed by Tukey *post hoc* analysis, n = 11 animals for 20% +5% sucrose; n = 22 animals for 20% ethanol.

into non-acupoints of the tail, (1/5 tail length from the proximal region of the tail [13,29]) and no current stimulation was applied. Ethanol (or sucrose) and water intakes were then recorded at 24 h after the onset of drinking. During the 6 treatment days, rats had three ethanol-drinking sessions (day 1, Wednesday; day 3, Friday; and day 6, Monday). Ethanol intake during the drinking session immediately before EA administration and after the last EA administration was recorded respectively as the baseline or post-treatment baseline drinking level. The effects of multiple sessions of low (2 Hz) frequency EA on ethanol intake in rats that chronically consumed high amounts of ethanol was checked in a separate group of rats, in which 2 Hz EA was administered at bilateral ST36 (30 min each day) for six consecutive days. Ethanol and water intakes were recorded as in the above experiment.

Immunohistochemistry

We have recently reported that chronic ethanol intake induces the accumulation of FosB/ΔFosB in a sub region-specific manner [19]. To determine whether EA-induced reduction in ethanol intake was associated with changes in FosB/ΔFosB expression, we analyzed FosB/ΔFosB immunoreactivity (IR) in reward-related areas of the mesocorticolimbic dopamine system. A group of rats (n = 12) were first trained to drink ethanol using the modified intermittent access two-bottle choice drinking paradigm as described above. When rats voluntarily consumed high amounts of ethanol, they were divided into two subgroups: one (n = 6) received 100 Hz EA at bilateral ST36, the other sham treatment at the tail (n = 6) for 6 consecutive days. During the 6 treatment days, rats had three ethanol-drinking sessions (day 1, Wednesday; day 3, Friday; and day 6, Monday). Rats in the control group (ethanol naïve control, n = 5) were allowed to access to water and food without limitation. There were no significant differences in body weight between the ethanol naïve and ethanol-drinking rats at the end of the experiments.

Ethanol drinking rats treated with EA or sham were sacrificed immediately after the last session of 24 h ethanol access. Ethanol naïve rats were also sacrificed at the same time point. Rats were overdosed with ketamine/xylazine (80 mg/10 mg/kg, i.p.) and transcardially perfused with cold saline followed by 4% paraformaldehyde in 0.1 M sodium phosphate buffer (pH 7.4).

Brains were removed, postfixed (2 hours, at 4°C) in the same fixative solution and cryoprotected (overnight at 4°C, 20% sucrose in 0.1 M phosphate buffer, pH 7.4). Serial 30-μm coronal sections of the forebrain were cut on a freezing microtome (Microm HM550, Walldorf, and German), and a 1-in-4 series of brain sections was processed for immunohisto-chemical detection of FosB/ΔFosB-protein. Sections were incubated in the following series of antibodies: pan-FosB antibody (1:2000, #sc-48; Santa Cruz Biotechnology, Santa Cruz, California) overnight, at 4°C, biotinylated anti-rabbit IgG (2 hours, 1:200) (Vector Laboratories, Burlingame, CA). Sections were then incubated in an avidin-biotin-horseradish peroxidase complex solution (45 min) (Vector Elite Kit, Vector Labs, Burlingame, California). Horseradish peroxidase activity was visualized with nickel-diaminobenzidine (Vector Laboratories, Burlingame, CA). Sections from each experimental group were processed simultaneously. Omission of the primary antisera on a subset of sections resulted in a loss of immunoreactivity. Sections were mounted onto chrome-alum slides, dehydrated, and cover slipped.

Quantization of FosB/ΔFosB immunoreactivity

Changes in FosB/ΔFosB immunoreactivity were measured in sections from prefrontal cortices (PrL, IL and orbitofrontal cortex (OFC)), NAc (core and shell) and dorsolateral striatum (DLS) and dorsomedial striatum (DMS). These brain regions were identified based on the Atlas of Paxinos and Watson [30]. Quantitative measurement was performed using an assisted image analysis system, consisting of an Nikon Eclipse 80i bright field microscope (Micron Optics, Cedar Knoll, NJ) interfaced with a color digital camera Nikon DS-Ri1 (Micron Optics, Cedar Knoll, NJ), and a computer with a NIS-Elements BR 3.0 software (Micron Optics, Cedar Knoll, NJ). Images were obtained at 20×magnification and were averaged from right and left hemispheres in each subject. Two dimensional counts of labeled nuclei from each image [200×images (0.1 mm^2 area) of FosB/ΔFosB-like immunoreactive nuclei within brain regions of interest] were determined without knowledge of treatment conditions from three separate sections per animal using NIS-Elements BR 3.0 software.

Statistical Analysis

All data are expressed as mean ± S.E.M. (standard error of the mean). Behavioral data were analyzed with two-way repeated measure ANOVA (RM ANOVA) with the main factors of treatment (EA or sham) and days [baseline (0 day), day 1, 3, 5, postbasline (7 day)]. Tukey *post hoc* analysis was conducted using contrast analysis when day × treatment interaction was $p<0.05$. Immunohistochemical results were analyzed with one-way ANOVA followed by Tukey test.

Results

Intermittent access to 20% ethanol (IE) with sucrose added in the first three drinking sessions induces excessive consumption and high preference for ethanol in male SD rats

We previously showed that the IE procedure led the majority of the SD rats to drink moderate levels of ethanol [14]. In this study, we added 5% sucrose in the first three drinking sessions, which greatly increased the amount of ethanol consumed by SD rats that lasted for >3 weeks after sucrose withdrawal (Fig. 1A). Under these conditions, at the 4th to 12th drinking sessions, SD rats consumed 8.2 ± 0.1 g/kg/24 h, which were substantially greater than 4.1 ± 0.1 g/kg/24 h, consumed by rats under the identical procedure but without sucrose induction. Two-way RM ANOVA revealed significant main effects for treatment ($F_{1,\,337}=269.63$, $p<0.001$), day ($F_{11,\,337}=2.09$, $p<0.05$), and treatment × day interaction ($F_{11,\,337}=6.51$, $p<0.001$). Post-hoc analysis of the mean amount of ethanol consumed by rats at 4th to 12th drinking sessions showed significant difference between groups with and without sucrose induction.

The preference for ethanol in rats with sucrose induction was also greater than that in those rats without sucrose induction (Fig. 1B). During the 4th to 12th sessions, the mean preference for ethanol was $36.4\pm0.4\%$ and $22.0\pm0.8\%$, respectively for rats with and without sucrose induction. Two-way RM ANOVA revealed significant main effects for treatment ($F_{1,\,337}=125.73$, $p<0.001$) and treatment × time interaction ($F_{11,\,337}=5.08$, $p<0.001$) with strong tendency of time ($F_{11,\,337}=1.79$, $p=0.05$). Post-hoc analysis of the preference for ethanol at 4th to 12th drinking sessions was significantly higher in rats with sucrose than that in rats not given sucrose (all $p<0.001$, Fig. 1B).

We measured BEC of rats from the sucrose induction drinking group described above at the 13th drinking session immediately after the 30-min period of access to ethanol. The BEC ranged from 26.8 to 136.0 mg% with an average of 60.5 ± 10.4 mg%. There was a significant positive correlation between BEC and g/kg ethanol consumed ($r^2=0.75$, $n=11$, $p<0.001$; data not illustrated).

Multiple sessions of high (100 Hz), but not low frequency (2 Hz) EA treatment reduces excessive consumption of and preference for ethanol, but not sucrose

A recent rat study found that multiple sessions of high frequency (100 Hz) EA was more effective than the single session of high frequency (100 Hz) in alleviating morphine withdrawal syndrome. Furthermore, the after-effect of multiple sessions EA lasted for at least 7 days [31]. We sought to determine whether multiple sessions of 100 Hz EA treatment can alter ethanol consumption in rats that chronically drink excessive amounts of ethanol. We applied multiple sessions of 100 Hz EA at ST36 or sham to rats when they had reached stable baseline levels of ethanol consumption (see Fig. 1). As shown in Fig. 2A, consecutive 6-day 100 Hz EA, 30 min each day, but not the sham treatment significantly reduced ethanol consumption over the 24-h access period. Two-way RM ANOVA revealed significant main effects of treatment ($F_{1,\,51}=18.59$, $p<0.001$), day ($F_{4,51}=9.81$, $p<0.001$) and treatment × day interaction ($F_{4,51}=5.31$, $p=0.001$). Post hoc analysis revealed that ethanol intake over the 24-h access on day 3 and 6 was clearly decreased in the EA treatment group compared with that of sham (all $p<0.001$, Fig. 2A). Remarkably, when EA treatments were terminated on day 6, the reduction was maintained at the 48-72 h drinking session after the last EA administration ($p<0.01$, EA *vs.* sham, Fig. 2A). There was no overall main effect of sham treatment on ethanol intake on all test days compared with baseline drinking levels.

Although the preference ratio for ethanol at 24-h time point examined was not significantly different among groups during the EA-free baseline period, this ratio was significantly reduced after multiple administration of 100 Hz EA. Two-way RM ANOVA revealed significant main effects of treatment ($F_{1,51}=11.22$, $p=0.004$), day ($F_{4,51}=5.49$, $p<0.001$, and the interaction term ($F_{1,51}=5.66$, $p<0.001$). Post hoc analysis revealed that the preference for ethanol at 24-h time point on day 3 and 6 in the multiple sessions of 100 Hz EA treated group was lower than that of sham (all $p<0.001$, Fig. 2B). Furthermore, EA-induced reduction in preference ratio was maintained at the 48–72 h drinking session when EA administrations were terminated ($p<0.05$, EA *vs.* sham, Fig. 2B). There was no overall main effect of sham treatment on the preference for ethanol on test days compared with baseline preference for ethanol (Fig. 2B). Interestingly, consecutive 6-day 100 Hz EA treatment also produced significant effects on water intake (main effect of treatment [$F_{1,51}=5.21$, $p<0.05$] and day [$F_{4,51}=2.97$, $p<0.05$], with no effect of treatment × time interaction [$F_{4,51}=1.23$, $p=0.31$]) (Fig. 2C). Water intake at 24-h time point on day 5 and 7 was significantly increased in EA treated rats compared with sham ($p<0.05$). On all test days, total fluid intake was not affected by consecutive 6-day 100 Hz EA compared with sham treatment (Fig. 2D).

We previously showed that single low but not high frequency EA reduced moderate ethanol consumption [14]. To determine whether the effect of multiple sessions of EA also depends on its frequency, multiple sessions of low frequency (2 Hz) EA at ST36 was administered to rats that chronically consumed large quantities of ethanol under the IE procedure with sucrose induction as described above. As illustrated in Fig. 3A, under these experimental conditions, multiple sessions of 2 Hz EA did not alter ethanol intake over the 24-h access period on all test days (Fig. 3A). Two-way RM ANOVA for ethanol consumption failed to reveal main effects of treatment ($F_{1,\,37}=1.43$, $p>0.05$), day ($F_{3,37}=1.15$, $p>0.05$) and treatment × time interaction ($F_{3,37}=0.25$, $p>0.05$). Accordingly, multiple sessions of 2 Hz EA did not change the preference ratio for ethanol at the 24-h time point on all test days [no main effects of treatment ($F_{1,\,37}=0.003$, $p=0.95$), day ($F_{3,37}=0.54$, $p=0.65$) or treatment × time interaction ($F_{3,37}=0.30$, $p=0.82$, Fig. 3B]; or water intake and total fluid (data not shown).

To determine whether the reduction in ethanol consumption induced by multiple sessions of 100 Hz EA is specific to ethanol, we measured the intake of preferred substance sucrose using an intermittent access to 5% sucrose in a two-bottle choice drinking procedure. As shown in Fig. 4, neither sucrose intake nor preference for sucrose at 24-h time point was altered by multiple sessions of 100 Hz EA at ST36. Two-way RM ANOVA for sucrose consumption failed to reveal main effects of treatment (F_1,

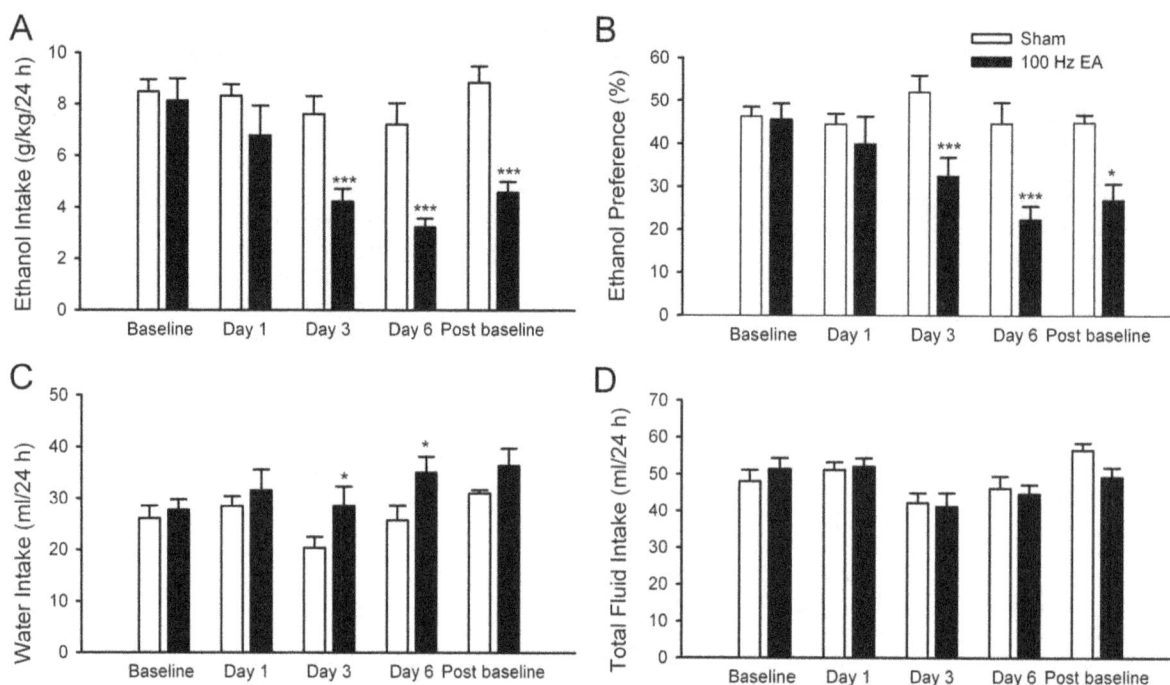

Figure 2. Multiple sessions of high frequency (100 Hz) EA sharply decreased excessive consumption of and preference for ethanol. 100 Hz EA or sham was administered to two different groups of rats for 6 consecutive days, 10 min before the start of ethanol- or water-drinking session. The effect was measured on day 1, 3, and 6. There was no significant difference regarding the baseline drinking levels between the EA and the sham group. Rats in EA group (filled bars) but not in sham group (blank bars) sharply reduced ethanol intake (g/kg/24 h) (**A**) and preference (**B**) for ethanol at the 24 h after the onset of drinking. EA treatment also increased water intake (**C**). Total fluid intake was not affected by multiple EA treatment at 24-h time point on all test days (**D**). The values are expressed as mean ± SEM. *$p<0.05$, ***$p<0.001$ compared with sham (two-way RM ANOVA followed by Tukey *post hoc* analysis), n = 8 animals in each group.

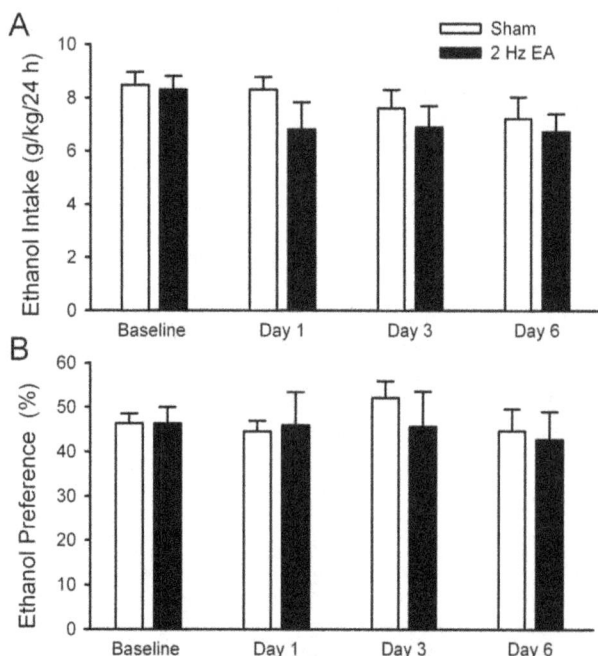

Figure 3. Multiple sessions of low frequency (2 Hz) EA did not alter the excessive intake of and preference for ethanol. EA at low frequency (2 Hz) or sham were administered to rats for 6 consecutive days 10 min before the start of ethanol- or water-drinking session. The effect was measured on day 1, 3, and 6. The values are expressed as mean ± SEM. n = 8 animals in each group.

$_{18} = 0.23$, $p = 0.65$), day ($F_{3,18} = 1.39$, $p = 0.27$) or treatment × time interaction ($F_{3,18} = 0.19$, $p = 0.90$). Furthermore, no significant difference was found between EA and sham for either water consumption or total fluid (data not shown).

Multiple sessions of 100 Hz EA decreases excessive ethanol consumption-induced accumulation of FosB/ΔFosB in specific reward-related brain regions

The results described above showed that consecutive 6-day 100 Hz EA selectively lowered the intake of and preference for ethanol in rats that chronically drink excessive amounts of ethanol. Many studies have proposed that the persistent activation of ΔFosB may be a common pathway for addictive disorders [32]. We previously reported that chronic ethanol consumption induces ΔFosB accumulation selectively in the prefrontal cortex and striatal region [19]; dysfunction of these brain reward-related brain regions is associated with ethanol craving and impairment of new learning processes in abstinent alcoholics [33]. Therefore, we assessed FosB/ΔFosB IR in the following reward-related brain regions of the mesocorticolimbic dopamine system (Fig. 5).

Striatal region. FosB/ΔFosB expression was regulated differentially within the striatal region as a function of both ethanol and EA treatment. In keeping with our recent report [19], FosB/ΔFosB IR increased robustly within the core of the nucleus accumbens (NAc-Core) and dorsolateral striatum (DLS) (Fig. 6), but not within the dorsal shell (NAc-Shell) and dorsomedial striatum (DMS) in animals that chronically consumed large amounts of ethanol with sham treatment, compared with ethanol naïve controls. Multiple sessions of 100 Hz EA significantly decreased the FosB/ΔFosB IR within the DLS and NAc-Core

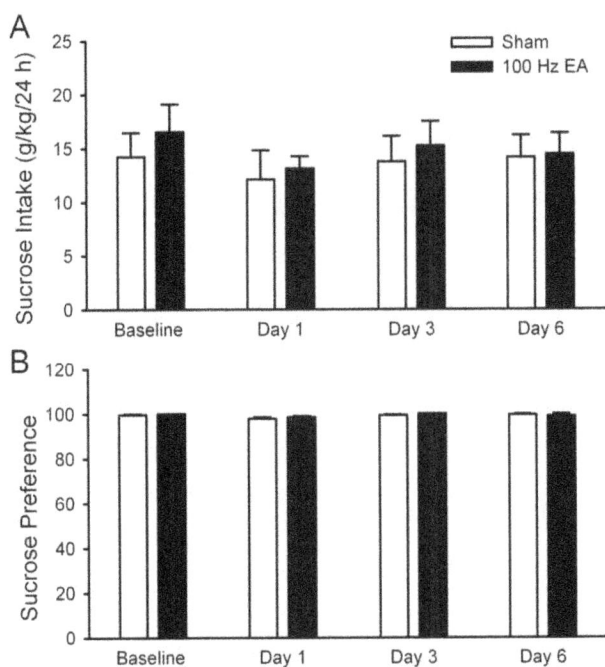

Figure 4. Multiple sessions of 100 Hz EA did not alter the intake of and preference for sucrose. Rats were trained to drink 5% sucrose solution under the intermittent access drinking procedure, similar to that for ethanol drinking. When rats had achieved a consistent baseline level, 100 Hz EA or sham were administered to rats for 6 consecutive days, 10 min before the start of sucrose- or water-drinking session. The effect was measured on day 1, 3, and 6. The values are expressed as mean ± S.E.M. n = 4 animals in each group.

induced by long-term excessive ethanol consumption (Fig. 6). These observations are supported by one-way ANOVA which revealed a significant main effect of treatment in NAc-Core ($F_{2, 33} = 6.27$, $p = 0.005$) and DLS ($F_{2, 33} = 28.54$, $p<0.001$), but not in NAc-shell ($F_{2, 33} = 1.36$, $p>0.05$) and DMS ($F_{2,33} = 2.47$, $p>0.05$).

Prefrontal cortex. We recently reported that chronic ethanol exposure robustly increases FosB/ΔFosB IR in orbitofrontal cortex (OFC), but not the medial prefrontal cortex [19]. However, in the current study, FosB/ΔFosB IR was significantly increased in both of the prelimbic area of the prefrontal cortex (PrL) and OFC in animals that chronically consumed large amounts of ethanol with sham treatment (Fig. 7, $p<0.001$ sham vs. ethanol naïve). No statistical differences in FosB/ΔFosB-positive nuclei counts were found between the sham group and ethanol naïve control group in the infralimbic area of the prefrontal cortex (IL). Multiple sessions of 100 Hz EA significantly decreased FosB/ΔFosB IR in the PrL, the OFC and the IL (all $p<0.01$ EA group vs. sham). Accordingly, one-way ANOVA yielded a significant main effect of treatment in IL ($F_{2, 33} = 7.06$, $p = 0.003$), PrL ($F_{2, 33} = 18.61$, $p<0.001$) and OFC ($F_{2, 33} = 13.23$, $p<0.001$).

The ventral tegmental area (VTA). VTA is believed to be a critical brain region of reward. A recent study showed that chronic psychostimulant administration induces the accumulation of ΔFosB, specifically in the posterior tail of the VTA [23,34]. As illustrated in Fig. 8, FosB/ΔFosB IR in the posterior region of the VTA (Bregma − 5.20 mm to Bregma −6.8 mm) was robustly increased in rats that chronically consumed large amounts of ethanol compared to that in ethanol naïve group ($p<0.001$), and was substantially reduced after multiple sessions of EA ($p<0.001$, EA group vs. sham) but not after sham treatment. There was an

overall main effect of treatment on FosB/ΔFosB IR in the posterior VTA ($F_{2,33} = 12.04$, $p<0.001$, Fig. 8).

Discussion

We reported here that six-day 100 Hz EA (30 min each day) at the bilateral acupoint ST36 selectively reduced excessive consumption of and preference for ethanol over 24 h access period. The reduction maintained for at least 72 h after the termination of EA treatment. Furthermore, this EA regiment decreased FosB/ΔFosB expression induced by chronic ethanol exposure in the reward-related brain regions.

We have recently reported that a single 20 min low (2 Hz), but not high (100 Hz) frequency EA at ST36 lowered the moderate intake of ethanol in SD rats [14]. There is recent evidence that multiple sessions of high frequency EA are more effective than the single session of high frequency EA in alleviating morphine withdrawal syndrome [31]. In this study we investigated whether 100 Hz EA was effective in reducing excessive ethanol consumption in rats under a modified IE drinking procedure, in which all rats consumed high amounts of ethanol (8.2±0.1 g/kg) with high preference ratio for ethanol (36.4±0.4%). Although we did not monitor withdrawal signs in the current study, we have previously reported that rats under the similar drinking program did show mild withdrawal signs [14,25]. The BEC of rats in the current study was 60.5±10.4 mg%, which was almost two times higher than that of SD rats [14] and similar to that of Long-Evans rats [25] which showed withdrawal signs. Thus, it is highly possible that rats under the current experimental conditions may develop ethanol dependence and have signs of withdrawal. Remarkably, consecutive six-day 100 Hz EA reduced free ethanol intake by almost half over the 24-h access period. Intriguingly, this EA regiment also significantly enhanced water intake, suggesting that these animals were going to the direction opposite to ethanol drinking. Importantly, the reduction on ethanol intake was maintained for >72 h after the termination of EA treatments. Conversely, multiple sessions of 100 Hz EA did not change the intake of and preference for the natural reward substance sucrose. Our current finding is in line with a recent study showing that multiple sessions of EA suppressed the morphine withdrawal syndrome, which was maintained for at least 7 days in a treatment-free period. This long-lasting effect of EA may be attributable to the increased dynorphin, since multiple sessions of 100 Hz EA is very efficient in accelerating the biosynthesis of dynorphin, as reflected by the prompt up-regulation of preprodynorphin mRNA, which was maintained for at least 7 days in the brain [31].

Previous evidence indicates that dynorphin released in CNS, via interacting with κ-opioid receptor (KOR) plays an important role in 100 Hz EA-induced suppression of morphine withdrawal syndrome [20,35,36]. Furthermore, multiple sessions of 100 Hz EA were shown to be more effective than single EA in blocking the down-regulation of preprodynorphin mRNA induced by chronic morphine exposure [31]. It has been demonstrated that dynorphin-κ opioid systems may have an important role in driving compulsive drug intake [37]. The expression of dynorphin and KORs were lower in rodents who consumed high levels of ethanol than their low drinking counterparts [38,39,40]. Furthermore, systemic administration of the KOR agonist U50,488H in rats significantly reduces ethanol intake [41], whereas administration of the KOR antagonist increases ethanol intake [42]. Importantly, polymorphisms in dynorphin and the KOR have been associated with increased risk of alcoholism in humans [43]. Taken together, these data suggest a modulatory role of dynorphin over ethanol

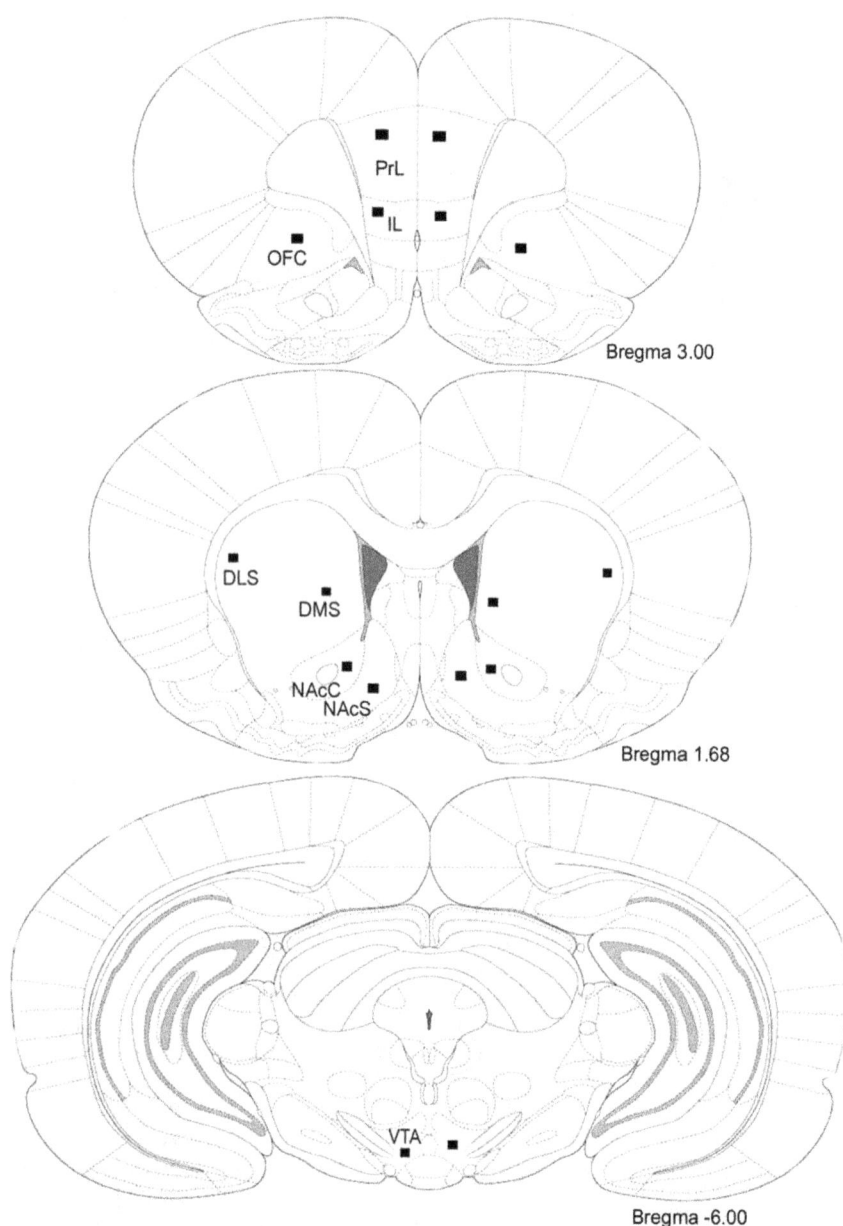

Figure 5. Schematic diagrams of coronal sections of rat brain. The locations that FosB/ΔFosB immunoreactivity was quantified in the following regions: prelimbic cortex (PrL), infralimbic cortex (IL), orbitofrontal cortex (OFC), nucleus accumbens core (NAcC), nucleus accumbens shell (NAcS), dorsolateral striatum (DLS), dorsomedial striatum (DMS), and the ventral tegmental area (VTA). The black squares correspond to a fixed area 200 μm×200 μm in size.

drinking, in which the dynorphin/KOR system functions to reduce ethanol drinking. Since 100 Hz EA can specifically facilitate dynorphin release [44], we hypothesized that dynorphin mediates at least in part of the reduction in ethanol consumption induced by 100 Hz EA observed in the current study. However, the mechanism underlying the dynorphin mediated reduction in ethanol consumption is not completely clear. A reduction in ethanol consumption induced by the increase of dynorphin was also observed in previous studies [45,46]. These authors interpreted their data to indicate that dynorphin may provide postingestive feedback to regulate subsequent ethanol consumption bouts.

Predynorphin gene is one of the transcriptional targets for ΔFosB [18,32]. Over-expression of ΔFosB in the NAc and the dorsal striatum increased locomotor activity and rewarding responses to morphine partly through the suppression of dynorphin expression [18]. Since 100 Hz EA accelerated the release of dynorphin in the spinal cord, and restored the expression of prodynorphin gene in the brain in morphine dependent animal [31,36], we propose that 100 Hz EA may alter the function of ΔFosB in the brain.

This study shows that ΔFosB transcription factors in the prefrontal cortex, the striatal region and the posterior VTA may play an important role in 100 Hz EA-induced reduction of excessive ethanol intake. It highlights that EA-induced reduction

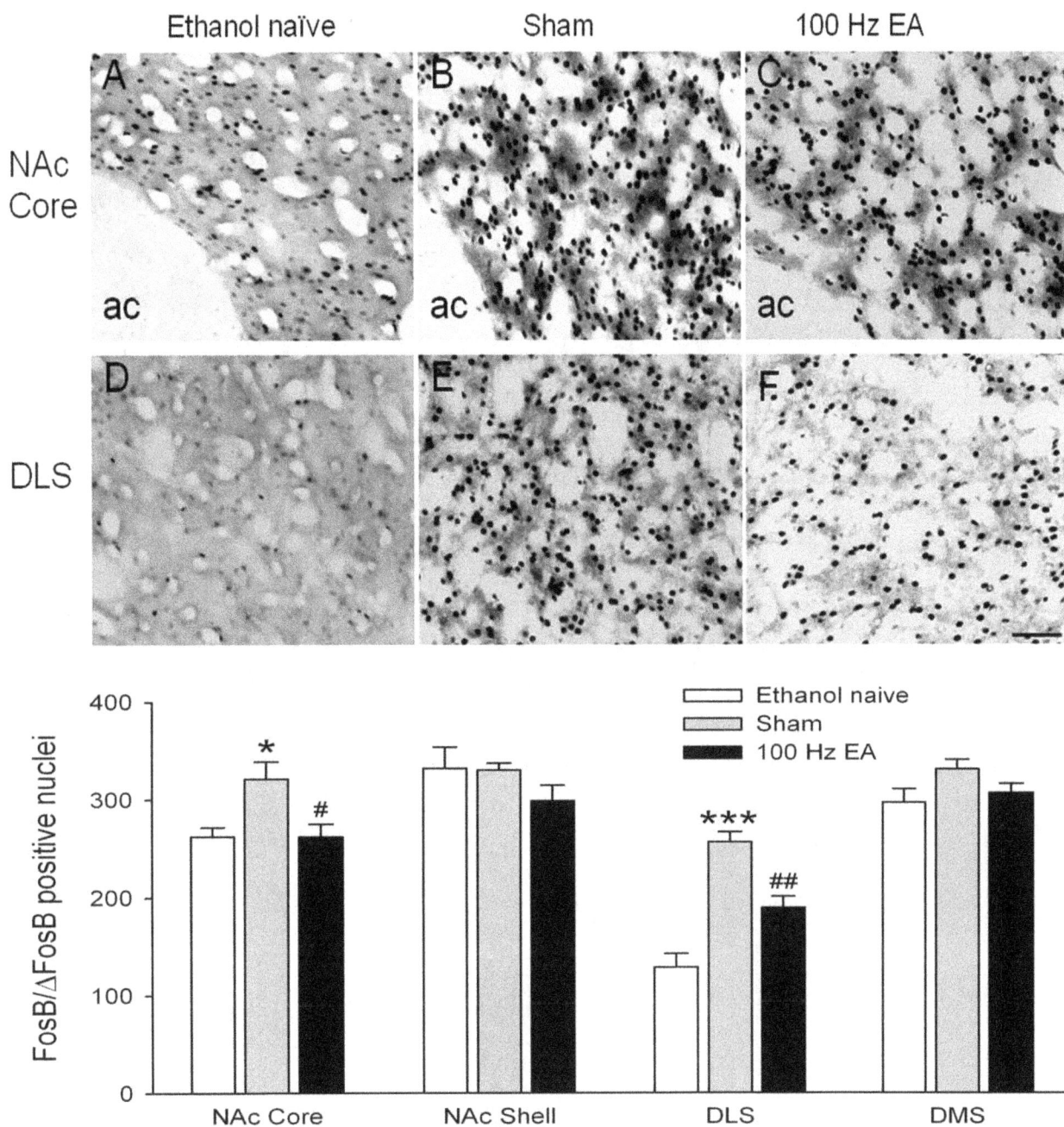

Figure 6. Photomicrographs depicting typical regions of analysis for the NAc core, shell, dorsolateral striatum (DLS) and dorsomedial striatum (DMS). Panels indicate FosB/ΔFosB-positive cells in animals that were drinking water (ethanol naïve, **A, D**), drinking large amounts of ethanol treated with sham (**B, E**), and drinking large amounts of ethanol treated with multiple sessions of 100 Hz EA (**C, F**). Increased numbers of FosB/ΔFosB-positive cells were observed in the NAc core and DLS, but not in the NAc shell and DMS in rats that chronically consumed large amounts of ethanol with sham treatment, as compared with ethanol naive animals. Multiple sessions of 100 Hz EA decreased the accumulation of FosB/ΔFosB in the NAc core and DLS induced by excessive ethanol consumption. Data are expressed as mean ± S.E.M. * $p < 0.05$, *** $p < 0.001$ indicates a significant difference from ethanol naïve; # $p < 0.05$, ## $p < 0.01$ indicates a significant difference from sham. Scale bar = 200 μm. ac: anterior commissure.

of ethanol consumption may involve diverse pathways that contribute to ethanol drinking, including cognitive, motivational and motor neural circuits. The NAc core may contribute to conditioned stimulus-supported drug-seeking behavior [47]. Likewise, dorsal striatum may contribute to the compulsive or habit-like nature of drug consumption [48]. The lateral (DLS) and medial (DMS) parts of dorsal striatum have distinct anatomical

inputs and outputs and therefore different functions [49]. For instance, endogenous brain-derived neurotrophic factor in the DLS but not in the DMS controls voluntary ethanol intake [50]. In line with these findings, we showed that chronic ethanol self-administration induced pronounced accumulation of ΔFosB in the NAc core and the DLS, but not in the NAc shell and the DMS. Importantly, we further showed that multiple sessions of 100 Hz

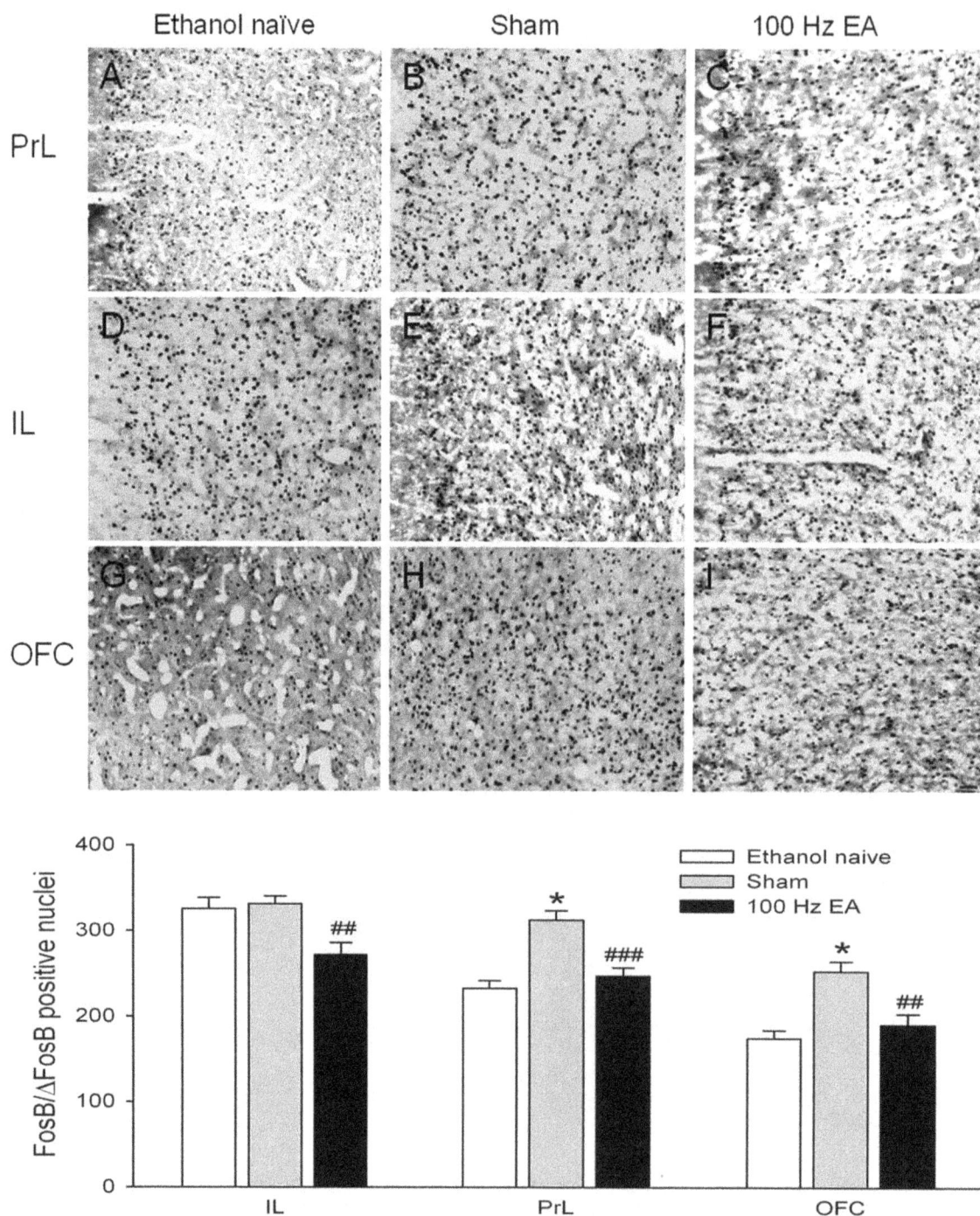

Figure 7. Photomicrographs depicting typical brain regions of analysis for the prelimbic (PrL), infralimbic (IL) and the orbitofrontal cortex (OFC) divisions of the prefrontal cortex. Panels indicate FosB/ΔFosB-positive cells in animals that were drinking water (ethanol naïve, **A**, **D** and **G**), drinking large amounts of ethanol treated with sham (**B**, **E** and **H**), and drinking large amounts of ethanol treated with multiple high frequency EA (**C**, **F** and **I**). Increased numbers of FosB/ΔFosB-positive cells were observed in the PrL and OFC, but not in the IL in rats that chronically consumed large amounts of ethanol with sham treatment, as compared with ethanol naive animals. Multiple sessions of 100 Hz EA significantly decreased the numbers of FosB/ΔFosB positive nuclei in the IL, PrL and OFC in rats that consumed large amounts of ethanol. Data are expressed as mean ± S.E.M. * indicates significant difference from ethanol naïve ($p < 0.001$); ## $p < 0.01$, ### $p < 0.001$ indicates a significant difference from sham. Scale bar = 100 μm.

EA significantly attenuated the accumulation of FosB/ΔFosB IR in the NAc core and the DLS induced by excessive ethanol consumption, and the attenuation was more significant in DLS than in NAc core.

The PFC is responsible for executive function, decision-making, and the implementation of goal-directed actions. Subregions of the PFC include the PrL that guides response initiation and the IL that mediates response inhibition; both

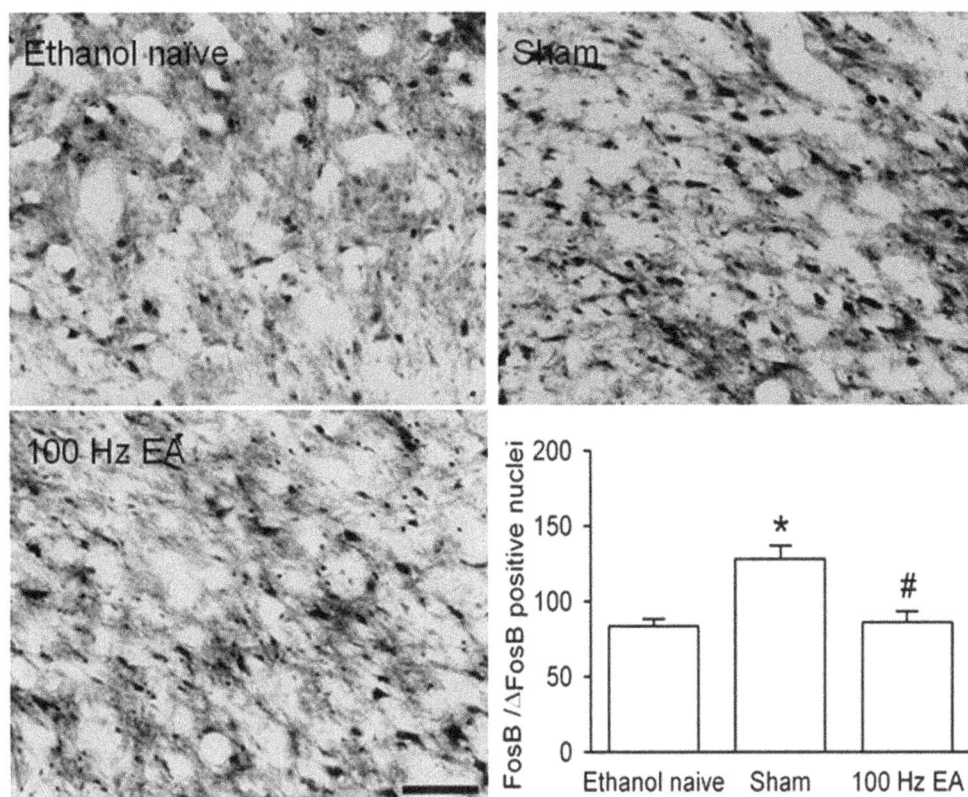

Figure 8. Photomicrographs depicting typical brain regions of analysis for the posterior VTA. Panels indicate FosB/ΔFosB-positive cells in animals that were drinking water (ethanol naïve), drinking large amounts of ethanol treated with sham (Sham), and drinking large amounts of ethanol treated with multiple sessions of 100 Hz EA (100 Hz EA). Increased numbers of FosB/ΔFosB-positive nuclei were observed in the posterior VTA in rats that chronically consumed large amounts of ethanol with sham treatment, as compared with ethanol naive animals. Multiple sessions of 100 Hz EA decreased the accumulation of FosB/ΔFosB in the VTA induced by excessive ethanol consumption. Data are expressed as mean ± S.E.M. * indicates significant difference from ethanol naïve ($p<0.001$), #, a significant difference from sham ($p<0.001$). Scale bar = 200 μm.

regions guide actions and outcomes. The PrL and IL may serve as on-off mechanisms in both conditioned drug and fear responses. Furthermore, the subregion of OFC is a key brain region implicated in regulating goal-directed behavior and impulsivity [51]. Accumulation of ΔFosB in the PFC is thought to be directly involved in addiction maintenance by producing tolerance to the cognitive disrupting effects of drugs via its actions in the PFC [52]. During drug withdrawal, overexpression of ΔFosB enhances impulsivity, which further promotes drug self-administration [53,54]. Importantly, genetic or viral overexpression of ΔJunD -a dominant negative mutant of JunD that antagonizes ΔFosB and other AP1-mediated transcriptional activity – in the OFC blocks these key effects of drug exposure [53]. The current study showed that excessive ethanol intake induced high levels of ΔFosB in PrL and OFC, which were blocked by multiple sessions of 100 Hz EA; furthermore, although FosB/ΔFosB IR in the IL was not altered by excessive ethanol consumption, it was reduced by multiple sessions of 100 Hz EA.

The VTA, the origin of mesolimbic dopamine system, is critical for motivated behaviors of abused drugs, including ethanol. Previously Perrotti and colleagues have provided evidence that following acute or chronic exposure to several psychostimulant such as cocaine and amphetamine, the expression of FosB/ΔFosB in the posterior/tail VTA was increased. Importantly, the expression is essentially presented in the GABAergic neurons, with no detectable expression in the DA

neurons [23,55]. In keeping with Perrotti's finding, we found that following chronic ethanol exposure, the expression of FosB/ΔFosB in the posterior/tail VTA was increased. Although we did not identify the cell types where FosB/ΔFosB was expressed in the present study, based on Perrotti's finding described above, we speculate that FosB/ΔFosB may be expressed in the GABAergic neurons; although the mechanism of ΔFosB induction solely in the subset of GABA neurons of posterior VTA is still unclear. Given that repeated administration of a dopamine uptake inhibitor induced FosB/ΔFosB in the VTA [23], it has been suggested that dopamine system mediates ΔFosB induction. Interestingly, six-day 100 Hz EA significantly decreased FosB/ΔFosB IR in the posterior/tail VTA. Given that activation of KORs in the VTA can hyperpolarize DA neurons and suppress dopamine release by direct actions at the release site [56], we propose that by the activation of KORs, multiple sessions of 100 Hz EA might suppress dopamine release, which leads to the inhibition of FosB/ΔFosB expression in the VTA GABA neurons [23], although the consequence of GABA neuron inhibition requires further investigation. Furthermore, recent studies have demonstrated that KORs are functionally expressed on the PFC- and amygdala- but not NAc-projecting DA neurons in the VTA [57,58]; thus, the inhibition of alcohol intake induced by multiple sessions of 100 Hz EA could be due to selective inhibition of the VTA-PFC or VTA-amygdala DA circuits or both via selective activation of KORs in the VTA.

In summary, this study shows that multiple sessions of EA at high frequency (100 Hz) at acupoint ST36 are effective in reducing (1) ethanol consumption and preference in rats that chronically consumed high amounts of ethanol, and (2) FosB/ΔFosB IR in reward-related brain regions. Given that the ΔFosB and FosB are important members of the Fos family of transcription factors implicated in neural plasticity in drug addiction, it appears that ΔFosB and FosB in the reward-related brain regions are key players of EA action in reducing excessive alcohol consumption.

Author Contributions

Conceived and designed the experiments: JHY JL YS. Performed the experiments: JL YS. Analyzed the data: JL YS. Wrote the paper: JHY JL.

References

1. Anton RF, O'Malley SS, Ciraulo DA, Cisler RA, Couper D, et al. (2006) Combined pharmacotherapies and behavioral interventions for alcohol dependence: the COMBINE study: a randomized controlled trial. JAMA 295: 2003–2017.
2. Mann K, Lehert P, Morgan MY (2004) The efficacy of acamprosate in the maintenance of abstinence in alcohol-dependent individuals: results of a meta-analysis. Alcohol Clin Exp Res 28: 51–63.
3. Meyers RJ, Smith JE, Lash DN (2003) The Community Reinforcement Approach. Recent Dev Alcohol 16: 183–195.
4. Lu GW (1983) Characteristics of afferent fiber innervation on acupuncture points zusanli. Am J Physiol 245: R606–612.
5. Stux G (1987) Acupuncture text book and atlas. Berlin: Springer-Verlag.
6. Jindal V, Ge A, Mansky PJ (2008) Safety and efficacy of acupuncture in children: a review of the evidence. J Pediatr Hematol Oncol 30: 431–442.
7. Han J, Cui C, Wu L (2011) Acupuncture-related techniques for the treatment of opiate addiction: a case of translational medicine. Front Med 5: 141–150.
8. Yoshimoto K, Kato B, Sakai K, Shibata M, Yano, et al. (2001) Electro-acupuncture stimulation suppresses the increase in alcohol-drinking behavior in restricted rats. Alcohol Clin Exp Res 25: 63S–68S.
9. Karst M, Passie T, Friedrich S, Wiese B, Schneider U (2002) Acupuncture in the treatment of alcohol withdrawal symptoms: a randomized, placebo-controlled inpatient study. Addict Biol 7: 415–419.
10. Kim YH, Schiff E, Waalen J, Hovell M (2005) Efficacy of acupuncture for treating cocaine addiction: a review paper. J Addict Dis 24: 115–132.
11. Kunz S, Schulz M, Lewitzky M, Driessen M, Rau H (2007) Ear acupuncture for alcohol withdrawal in comparison with aromatherapy: a randomized-controlled trial. Alcohol Clin Exp Res 31: 436–442.
12. Overstreet DH, Cui CL, Ma YY, Guo CY, Han JS, et al. (2008) Electroacupuncture reduces voluntary alcohol intake in alcohol-preferring rats via an opiate-sensitive mechanism. Neurochem Res 33: 2166–2170.
13. Yang CH, Lee BB, Jung HS, Shim I, Roh PU, et al. (2002) Effect of electroacupuncture on response to immobilization stress. Pharmacol Biochem Behav 72: 847–855.
14. Li J, Zou Y, Ye JH (2011) Low frequency electroacupuncture selectively decreases voluntarily ethanol intake in rats. Brain Res Bull 86:428–434.
15. Robison AJ, Nestler EJ (2011) Transcriptional and epigenetic mechanisms of addiction. Nat Rev Neurosci 12: 623–637.
16. Perrotti LI, Weaver RR, Robison B, Renthal W, Maze I, et al. (2008) Distinct patterns of DeltaFosB induction in brain by drugs of abuse. Synapse 62: 358–369.
17. Bibb JA, Chen J, Taylor JR, Svenningsson P, Nishi A, et al. (2001) Effects of chronic exposure to cocaine are regulated by the neuronal protein Cdk5. Nature 410: 376–380.
18. Zachariou V, Bolanos CA, Selley DE, Theobald D, Cassidy MP, et al. (2006) An essential role for DeltaFosB in the nucleus accumbens in morphine action. Nat Neurosci 9: 205–211.
19. Li J, Cheng Y, Bian WL, Liu X, Zhang C, et al. (2010) Region-specific induction of FosB/deltaFosB by voluntary alcohol intkae: effects of naltrexone. Alcohol Clin Exp Res 34.
20. Cui CL, Wu LZ, Luo F (2008) Acupuncture for the treatment of drug addiction. Neurochem Res 33: 2013–2022.
21. Yang CH, Yoon SS, Hansen DM, Wilcox JD, Blumell BR, et al. (2010) Acupuncture inhibits GABA neuron activity in the ventral tegmental area and reduces ethanol self-administration. Alcohol Clin Exp Res 34: 2137–2146.
22. Yoon SS, Yang EJ, Lee BH, Jang EY, Kim HY, et al. (2012) Effects of acupuncture on stress-induced relapse to cocaine-seeking in rats. Psychopharmacology (Berl).
23. Perrotti LI, Bolanos CA, Choi KH, Russo SJ, Edwards S, et al. (2005) DeltaFosB accumulates in a GABAergic cell population in the posterior tail of the ventral tegmental area after psychostimulant treatment. Eur J Neurosci 21: 2817–2824.
24. Simms JA, Steensland P, Medina B, Abernathy KE, Chandler LJ, et al. (2008) Intermittent access to 20% ethanol induces high ethanol consumption in Long-Evans and Wistar rats. Alcohol Clin Exp Res 32: 1816–1823.
25. Li J, Bian W, Dave V, Ye JH (2011) Blockade of GABA(A) receptors in the paraventricular nucleus of the hypothalamus attenuates voluntary ethanol intake and activates the hypothalamic-pituitary-adrenocortical axis. Addict Biol.16:600–614.
26. Li J, Nie H, Bian W, Dave V, Janak PH, et al. (2012) Microinjection of Glycine into the Ventral Tegmental Area Selectively Decreases Ethanol Consumption. J Pharmacol Exp Ther.341:196–204.

27. Poklis A, Mackell MA (1982) Evaluation of a modified alcohol dehydrogenase assay for the determination of ethanol in blood. Clin Chem 28: 2125–2127.
28. Nielsen CK, Simms JA, Pierson HB, Li R, Saini SK, et al. (2008) A novel delta opioid receptor antagonist, SoRI-9409, produces a selective and long-lasting decrease in ethanol consumption in heavy-drinking rats. Biol Psychiatry 64: 974–981.
29. Zhao RJ, Yoon SS, Lee BH, Kwon YK, Kim KJ, et al. (2006) Acupuncture normalizes the release of accumbal dopamine during the withdrawal period and after the ethanol challenge in chronic ethanol-treated rats. Neurosci Lett 395: 28–32.
30. Paxinos G, Watson C (2007) The Rat brain in stereotaxic coordinates 6th edition, Academic press.
31. Wang GB, Wu LZ, Yu P, Li YJ, Ping XJ, et al. (2011) Multiple 100 Hz electroacupuncture treatments produced cumulative effect on the suppression of morphine withdrawal syndrome: Central preprodynorphin mRNA and p-CREB implicated. Peptides 32: 713–721.
32. Nestler EJ (2005) Is there a common molecular pathway for addiction? Nat Neurosci 8: 1445–1449.
33. Chen G, Cuzon Carlson VC, Wang J, Beck A, Heinz A, et al. (2011) Striatal involvement in human alcoholism and alcohol consumption, and withdrawal in animal models. Alcohol Clin Exp Res 35: 1739–1748.
34. Kaufling J, Veinante P, Pawlowski SA, Freund-Mercier MJ, Barrot M (2009) Afferents to the GABAergic tail of the ventral tegmental area in the rat. J Comp Neurol 513: 597–621.
35. Shi XD, Wang GB, Ma YY, Ren W, Luo F, et al. (2004) Repeated peripheral electrical stimulations suppress both morphine-induced CPP and reinstatement of extinguished CPP in rats: accelerated expression of PPE and PPD mRNA in NAc implicated. Brain Res Mol Brain Res 130: 124–133.
36. Wu LZ, Cui CL, Tian JB, Ji D, Han JS (1999) Suppression of morphine withdrawal by electroacupuncture in rats: dynorphin and kappa-opioid receptor implicated. Brain Res 851: 290–296.
37. Wee S, Koob GF (2010) The role of the dynorphin-kappa opioid system in the reinforcing effects of drugs of abuse. Psychopharmacology (Berl) 210: 121–135.
38. Fadda P, Tronci S, Colombo G, Fratta W (1999) Differences in the opioid system in selected brain regions of alcohol-preferring and alcohol-nonpreferring rats. Alcohol Clin Exp Res 23: 1296–1305.
39. Marinelli PW, Kiianmaa K, Gianoulakis C (2000) Opioid propeptide mRNA content and receptor density in the brains of AA and ANA rats. Life Sci 66: 1915–1927.
40. Winkler A, Spanagel R (1998) Differences in the kappa opioid receptor mRNA content in distinct brain regions of two inbred mice strains. Neuroreport 9: 1459–1464.
41. Lindholm S, Werme M, Brene S, Franck J (2001) The selective kappa-opioid receptor agonist U50,488H attenuates voluntary ethanol intake in the rat. Behav Brain Res 120: 137–146.
42. Mitchell JM, Liang MT, Fields HL (2005) A single injection of the kappa opioid antagonist norbinaltorphimine increases ethanol consumption in rats. Psychopharmacology (Berl) 182: 384–392.
43. Xuei X, Dick D, Flury-Wetherill L, Tian HJ, Agrawal A, et al. (2006) Association of the kappa-opioid system with alcohol dependence. Mol Psychiatry 11: 1016–1024.
44. Han JS (2003) Acupuncture: neuropeptide release produced by electrical stimulation of different frequencies. Trends Neurosci 26: 17–22.
45. Logrip ML, Janak PH, Ron D (2008) Dynorphin is a downstream effector of striatal BDNF regulation of ethanol intake. FASEB J 22: 2393–2404.
46. Logrip ML, Janak PH, Ron D (2009) Blockade of ethanol reward by the kappa opioid receptor agonist U50,488H. Alcohol 43: 359–365.
47. Everitt BJ, Robbins TW (2005) Neural systems of reinforcement for drug addiction: from actions to habits to compulsion. Nat Neurosci 8: 1481–1489.
48. Vanderschuren LJ, Di Ciano P, Everitt BJ (2005) Involvement of the dorsal striatum in cue-controlled cocaine seeking. J Neurosci 25: 8665–8670.
49. Voorn P, Vanderschuren LJ, Groenewegen HJ, Robbins TW, Pennartz CM (2004) Putting a spin on the dorsal-ventral divide of the striatum. Trends Neurosci 27: 468–474.
50. Jeanblanc J, He DY, Carnicella S, Kharazia V, Janak PH, et al. (2009) Endogenous BDNF in the dorsolateral striatum gates alcohol drinking. J Neurosci 29: 13494–13502.
51. Krawczyk DC (2002) Contributions of the prefrontal cortex to the neural basis of human decision making. Neurosci Biobehav Rev 26: 631–664.

52. Nestler EJ (2008) Review. Transcriptional mechanisms of addiction: role of DeltaFosB. Philos Trans R Soc Lond B Biol Sci 363: 3245–3255.

53. Winstanley CA, LaPlant Q, Theobald DE, Green TA, Bachtell RK, et al. (2007) DeltaFosB induction in orbitofrontal cortex mediates tolerance to cocaine-induced cognitive dysfunction. J Neurosci 27: 10497–10507.

54. Winstanley CA, Green TA, Theobald DE, Renthal W, LaPlant Q, et al. (2009) DeltaFosB induction in orbitofrontal cortex potentiates locomotor sensitization despite attenuating the cognitive dysfunction caused by cocaine. Pharmacol Biochem Behav 93: 278–284.

55. Kaufling J, Waltisperger E, Bourdy R, Valera A, Veinante P, et al. (2010) Pharmacological recruitment of the GABAergic tail of the ventral tegmental area by acute drug exposure. Br J Pharmacol 161: 1677–1691.

56. Ford CP, Beckstead MJ, Williams JT (2007) Kappa opioid inhibition of somatodendritic dopamine inhibitory postsynaptic currents. J Neurophysiol 97: 883–891.

57. Margolis EB, Lock H, Chefer VI, Shippenberg TS, Hjelmstad GO, et al. (2006) Kappa opioids selectively control dopaminergic neurons projecting to the prefrontal cortex. Proc Natl Acad Sci U S A 103: 2938–2942.

58. Margolis EB, Mitchell JM, Ishikawa J, Hjelmstad GO, Fields HL (2008) Midbrain dopamine neurons: projection target determines action potential duration and dopamine D(2) receptor inhibition. J Neurosci 28: 8908–8913.

20

Electrical vs Manual Acupuncture Stimulation in a Rat Model of Polycystic Ovary Syndrome: Different Effects on Muscle and Fat Tissue Insulin Signaling

Julia Johansson[1], Louise Mannerås-Holm[1], Ruijin Shao[1], AnneLiese Olsson[1], Malin Lönn[2], Håkan Billig[1], Elisabet Stener-Victorin[1,3]*

1 Institute of Neuroscience and Physiology, Department of Physiology, Sahlgrenska Academy, University of Gothenburg, Gothenburg, Sweden, 2 Institute of Biomedicine, Department of Clinical Chemistry and Transfusion Medicine, Sahlgrenska Academy, University of Gothenburg, Gothenburg, Sweden, 3 Department of Obstetrics and Gynecology, First Affiliated Hospital, Heilongjiang University of Chinese Medicine, Harbin, China

Abstract

In rats with dihydrotestosterone (DHT)-induced polycystic ovary syndrome (PCOS), repeated low-frequency electrical stimulation of acupuncture needles restores whole-body insulin sensitivity measured by euglycemic hyperinsulinemic clamp. We hypothesized that electrical stimulation causing muscle contractions and manual stimulation causing needle sensation have different effects on insulin sensitivity and related signaling pathways in skeletal muscle and adipose tissue, with electrical stimulation being more effective in DHT-induced PCOS rats. From age 70 days, rats received manual or low-frequency electrical stimulation of needles in abdominal and hind limb muscle five times/wk for 4–5 wks; controls were handled but untreated rats. Low-frequency electrical stimulation modified gene expression (decreased *Tbc1d1* in soleus, increased *Nr4a3* in mesenteric fat) and protein expression (increased pAS160/AS160, Nr4a3 and decreased GLUT4) by western blot and increased GLUT4 expression by immunohistochemistry in soleus muscle; glucose clearance during oral glucose tolerance tests was unaffected. Manual stimulation led to faster glucose clearance and modified mainly gene expression in mesenteric adipose tissue (increased *Nr4a3, Mapk3/Erk, Adcy3, Gsk3b*), but not protein expression to the same extent; however, Nr4a3 was reduced in soleus muscle. The novel finding is that electrical and manual muscle stimulation affect glucose homeostasis in DHT-induced PCOS rats through different mechanisms. Repeated electrical stimulation regulated key functional molecular pathways important for insulin sensitivity in soleus muscle and mesenteric adipose tissue to a larger extent than manual stimulation. Manual stimulation improved whole-body glucose tolerance, an effect not observed after electrical stimulation, but did not affect molecular signaling pathways to the same extent as electrical stimulation. Although more functional signaling pathways related to insulin sensitivity were affected by electrical stimulation, our findings suggest that manual stimulation of acupuncture needles has a greater effect on glucose tolerance. The underlying mechanism of the differential effects of the intermittent manual and the continuous electrical stimulation remains to be elucidated.

Editor: Cornelis B. Lambalk, VU University Medical Center, The Netherlands

Funding: For the use of technical equipment and support we thank the Genomics Core Facility at the Sahlgrenska Academy, University of Gothenburg, which was funded by a grant from the Knut and Alice Wallenberg Foundation. The funders had no role in study design, data collection and analysis, decision to publish, or preparation of the manuscript.

Competing Interests: The authors have declared that no competing interests exist.

* E-mail: elisabet.stener-victorin@neuro.gu.se

Introduction

Polycystic ovary syndrome (PCOS), a complex female endocrine disorder, is associated with hyperinsulinemia, insulin resistance, dyslipidemia, obesity, and other metabolic derangements [1]. Insulin resistance in PCOS is ascribed to defects in insulin signaling in adipocytes and skeletal muscle [2,3,4,5]. Insulin action through intracellular GLUT4 translocation depends on insulin-dependent pathways involving insulin receptors, insulin receptor substrates, phosphatidylinositol 3-kinase, protein kinase B (Akt), and Akt substrate of 160 kDa (AS160), as well as insulin-independent mechanisms such as muscle contraction/exercise [6,7]. Insulin-stimulated glucose transport, mediated by glucose transporter 4 (GLUT-4), is reduced in adipocytes of women with PCOS, especially those who are lean [8]. Women with PCOS also

have reduced GLUT4 mRNA expression [9] and reduced GLUT4 protein content in whole-cell lysates and membrane preparations of adipose tissue [8,10].

In clinical studies, low-frequency (2-Hz) electrical stimulation of acupuncture needles placed in skeletal muscles, so-called electroacupuncture (EA), in combination with manual stimulation of the needles improves endocrine disturbances in women with PCOS [11,12,13]. In obese women with PCOS, acupuncture without electrical stimulation is superior to metformin for improving endocrine disturbances, while both treatments improve insulin sensitivity and lipid profile [14]. In experimental studies, muscle contractions elicited by electrical stimulation induce changes in skeletal muscle signaling pathways similar to changes induced by exercise [15,16,17,18]. But when the afferent nerves in the treated hind limb were cut, the increased insulin responsiveness after electrical stimulation was lost, indicating that the response is mediated by activation of afferent nerves rather than by the contractions *per se* [19].

In rats with DHT-induced PCOS, which have insulin resistance, obesity, and a PCOS phenotype including estrous cycle irregularities and ovaries with multiple large atretic antral follicles, low-frequency EA 3 times weekly for 4–5 wks increases insulin sensitivity (euglycemic hyperinsulinemic clamp) and modulates expression of genes related to insulin resistance, obesity and sympathetic activity in adipose tissue [20,21,22]. Recently, we demonstrated that intense (5 days/wk) low-frequency EA for 4–5 wks completely restores insulin sensitivity and improves skeletal muscle signaling defects in this model [18]. Moreover, GLUT4 protein expression increased in all compartments of soleus muscle, including the plasma membrane, suggesting an increase in glucose transport capacity. The improved insulin sensitivity after EA in DHT-treated PCOS rats might due in part due to increased expression of GLUT4, which may increase the translocation capability from intracellular compartments to the plasma membrane [18]. Similar results have been demonstrated in Goto-Kakizaki rats and db/db mice, in which low-frequency EA increased insulin sensitivity [16,23]. Although these initial experimental findings show that electrical stimulation of needles in the muscle can reduce insulin resistance, the underlying signaling mechanism is not identified. Also, it is not known whether manual stimulation of needles in skeletal muscle improves insulin sensitivity to the same extent as electrical stimulation or whether the two types of stimulation have similar effects on regulatory mechanisms in skeletal muscle and adipose tissue.

We hypothesized that repeated acupuncture (5 d per wk for 4–5 wks) with electrical or manual muscle stimulation improves whole-body insulin sensitivity in rats with DHT-induced PCOS, with electrical stimulation being more effective. We also hypothesized that the two stimulation methods have different effects on insulin sensitivity–related signaling pathways in skeletal muscle and visceral adipose tissue. To test these hypotheses, we performed oral glucose tolerance tests (OGTTs), assessed the morphology of pancreatic islets of Langerhans, measured glycogen content in skeletal muscle, adipose tissue, and liver, and analyzed gene and protein expression of molecules related to androgen secretion, glucose transport, MAPK, lipid metabolism, and sympathetic/adrenergic activation in skeletal muscle and adipose tissue.

Materials and Methods

Animals, Ethics and Study Procedure

Three Wistar dams, each with 10 female pups (not their biological offspring) were purchased from Charles River (Sulzfeld, Germany). Pups stayed with their lactating dam until 21 d of age and were then housed five per cage under controlled conditions (21–22°C, 55–65% humidity, 12-h light/12-h dark cycle). All rats had free access to tap water and commercial chow (Harlan Teklad Global Diet, 16% protein rodent diet; Harlan Winkelmann, Harlan, Germany). Animal care was based on the principles of the Guide to the Care and Use of Experimental Animals (www.sjv.se). The study was approved by the Animal Ethics Committee of the University of Gothenburg.

At 21 d of age, rats were randomly assigned to three groups: low-frequency EA, manual stimulation, and control (n = 10 per group). Ninety-day continuous-release pellets containing 7.5 mg of DHT (daily dose, 83 μg) (Innovative Research of America, Sarasota, FL) were implanted subcutaneously in the neck to induce PCOS phenotypic characteristics, including metabolic disturbances (insulin resistance and obesity), at adult age [22].

Microchips (AVID, Norco, CA) for numbering and identification were inserted along with the pellets. From 21 d of age throughout the study, body weight was monitored weekly. Acupuncture treatments started at 70 d of age, 7 wks after the start of DHT exposure. The study was concluded after 11–12 wks of DHT exposure, including 4–5 wks of treatment.

Treatment

Rats were treated daily from Monday to Friday for 4–5 wks (20–25 treatments in total). The duration of treatment was 15 min in week 1, 20 min in wks 2 and 3, and 25 min wks 4 and 5. PCOS rats in the control group were handled in the same way as rats in the electrical and manual muscle stimulation groups except for needle insertion and electrical or manual stimulation. Two acupuncture needles (HEGU Svenska, Landsbro, Sweden) were inserted to a depth of 0.5–0.8 cm in the rectus abdominis and one in each triceps surae muscles bilaterally as described [18,24,25]. After insertion, needles in the electrical stimulation group were attached to an electrical stimulator (CEFAR ACU II; Cefar-Compex Scandinavia, Malmo, Sweden) and continuously stimulated at 2 Hz (so-called low-frequency EA) during each treatment session. For manual stimulation, after insertion the needles were rotated back and forth five times every fifth minute during the treatment [26].

Vaginal Smears

Vaginal smears were obtained daily during the final 2 wks of the experiment, and the stage of cyclicity was determined by microscopic analysis of the predominant cell type [27]. Female rats exposed to DHT are acyclic. During the treatment period, rats were sacrificed in the estrus phase if they showed signs of estrous cycle change.

Oral Glucose Tolerance Test

Blood glucose was measured at baseline after a 5-h fast (Accu-Chek Compact Plus Glucometer, Roche Diagnostics, Indianapolis, IN). A physiological dose of glucose (0.5 g/ml; total 2 g/kg) (G5146, Sigma-Aldrich, Stockholm, Sweden) was given orally by gavage, and glucose levels were measured 15, 30, 60, and 120 min later. At 0, 15, and 30 min, 10 μl of blood was collected from the tail for ELISA analysis of insulin (90060 Ultra Sensitive Rat Insulin ELISA Kit, Crystal Chem, Downers Grove, IL) and proinsulin (10-1232-01 Rat/Mouse Proinsulin ELISA, Mercodia, Uppsala, Sweden), as recommended by the manufacturer. Glucose tolerance was calculated from the area under the curve, the slope of glucose concentration curve (0–15 min and 15–30 min), and the insulin sensitivity index [28]. Intra- and inter-assay coefficients of variation and sensitivity were (<2%, <2% and 10 mg/dl for glucose, ≤10%, ≤10%, and 0.1 ng/ml for insulin, and 2.5%, 6.3%, and 3 pmol/l for proinsulin.

Tissue Collection

One hour after the last acupuncture treatment, rats were sedated with isoflurane (2% in a 1:1 mixture of oxygen and air; Isoba Vet; Schering-Plough, Stockholm, Sweden) and decapitated. The hind limb muscles, soleus, gastrocnemius, and extensor digitorum longus (EDL) were dissected, as were the subcutaneous, inguinal, and visceral fat depots (parametrial, retroperitoneal, and mesenteric), the pancreas, and part of the liver. The tissues were weighed, snap frozen in liquid nitrogen, and stored at –80°C. Portions of the tissue samples were fixed in Histofix containing 6% formaldehyde (Histolab, Göteborg, Sweden) and stored in 70% EtOH.

Table 1. Total selection of putative reference genes, genes related to the androgen and insulin receptor pathway, MAPK activators/inactivators, lipid metabolism, sympathetic/adrenergic pathway and adipokines on the TaqMan low-density arrays including TaqMan gene expression assay number, and GenBank accession number.

Gene Symbol	Gene Description	TaqMan Gene Expression Assay Number	GenBank Accession Number
Putative reference genes			
Gapdh	Glyceraldehyde-3-phosphate dehydrogenase	Rn99999916_s1	NM_017008.3
Ppia	Peptidylprolyl isomerase A	Rn00690933_m1	NM_017101.1
Actb	Beta-actin	Rn00667869_m1	NM_031144.2
Hprt1	Hypoanthine guanine phosphoribosyl transferas	Rn01527840_m1	NM_012583.2
Target genes			
Androgen signaling			
Cyp17a1	Cytochrome P450, family 17, subfamily a, polypeptide 1	Rn00562601_m1	NM_012753.1
Cyp19a1	Cytochrome P450, family 19, subfamily a, polypeptide 1	Rn01422547_m1	NM_017085.2
Ar	Androgen receptor	Rn00560747_m1	NM_012502.1
Insulin signaling			
Insr	Insulin receptor	Rn00567070_m1	M29014.1
Irs1	Insulin receptor substrate 1	Rn02132493_s1	NM_012969.1
Pik3r1	Phosphoinositide-3-kinase, regulatory subunit 1 (alpha)	Rn00564547_m1	NM_013005.1
Pik3cb	Phosphoinositide-3-kinase, catalytic, beta polypeptide	Rn00585107_m1	NM_053481.1
Prkaa2	5-activated protein kinase	Rn00576935_m1	NM_023991.1
Tbc1d1	TBC1 domain family, member 1	Rn01413271_m1	XM_341215.4
Akt2	Protein kinase B, beta, thymoma viral oncogene homolog 2	Rn00690901_m1	NM_017093.1
Pdk4	Pyruvate dehydrogenase kinase isoenzyme 4	Rn00585577_m1	NM_053551.1
Gsk3b	Glycogen synthase kinase 3 beta	Rn00583429_m1	NM_032080.1
Gsk3a	Glycogen synthase kinase 3 alpha	Rn00569232_m1	NM_017344.1
Nuak2	NUAK family, SNF1-like kinase, 2	Rn01759072_m1	NM_001007617.1
Slc2a4	Glucose transporter 4	Rn00562597_m1	NM_012751.1
Mtor	Mammalian target of rapamycin	Rn00571541_m1	NM_019906.1
Rps6kb1	Ribosomal protein S6 kinase, 70kDa, polypeptide 1	Rn00583148_m1	NM_031985.1
Nr4a1/Nur77	Orphan nuclear receptor	Rn00577766_m1	NM_024388.1
Nr4a3	Orphan nuclear receptor	Rn00581189_m1	NM_031628.1
MAPK activators/inactivators			
Mapk1/ERK2	Mitogen-activated protein kinase 1	Rn00671828_m1	NM_053842.1
Mapk3/ERK1	Mitogen-activated protein kinase 3	Rn00820922_g1	NM_017347.2
Mapk14/p38 MAPK	Mitogen-activated protein kinase 14	Rn00578842_m1	NM_031020.2
Mapk8/JNK	Mitogen-activated protein kinase 8	Rn01218952_m1	XM_341399.5
Dusp1	Mitogen-activating protein kinase phosphatase 1	Rn00678341_g1	NM_053769.3
Dusp4	Mitogen-activated protein kinase phosphatase 4	Rn00573501_m1	NM_022199.1
Ppargc1a	Peroxisome proliferator–activated receptor γ coactivator-1 α	Rn01453111_m1	NM_031347.1
Sirt1	Sirtuin (silent mating type information regulation 2 homolog) 1 (S. cerevisiae)	Rn01428093_m1	NM_001107627.1
Lipid metabolism			
Fasn	Fatty acid synthase	Rn01463550_m1	NM_017332.1
G6pc	Glucose-6-phosphatase	Rn00565347_m1	NM_013098.2
Pparg	PPAR gamma	Rn00440945_m1	NM_001145366.1/NM_013124.3
Fabp4	Adipocyte fatty acid binding protein, aP2	Rn00670361_m1	NM_053365.1
Lpl	Lipoprotein lipase	Rn00561482_m1	NM_012598.2
Lipe	Lipase, hormone sensitive	Rn00689222_m1	NM_012859.1
Sympathetic/adrenergic pathway			
Atf2	Activating transcription factor 2	Rn01276559_m1	NM_031018.1
Adcy3	Adenylate cyclase 3	Rn00590729_m1	NM_130779.2

Table 1. Cont.

Gene Symbol	Gene Description	TaqMan Gene Expression Assay Number	GenBank Accession Number
Adcy4	Adenylate cyclase 4	Rn00570644_m1	NM_019285.2
Adrb1	Adrenergic receptor, beta 1	Rn00824536_s1	NM_012701.1
Adrb2	Adrenergic receptor, beta 2	Rn00560650s1	NM_012492.2
Adrb3	Adrenergic receptor, beta 3	Rn00565393_m1	NM_013108.1
Adipokines			
Rbp4	Retinol binding protein 4	Rn01451318_m1	NM_013162.1
Adipoq	adiponectin	Rn00595250_m1	NM_144744.2
Adipor1	Adiponectin receptor 1	Rn01483784_m1	NM_207587.1
Adipor2	Adiponectin receptor 2	Rn01463177_m1	NM_001037979.1

Glycogen Content

Glycogen content was measured in skeletal muscle (soleus and EDL) and liver. Snap-frozen tissue was placed in 200 µl of distilled water on ice, homogenized with a pestle, boiled for 5 min, and centrifuged for 5 min at 13,000 rpm. Glycogen levels in the supernatant were analyzed with a colorimetric assay (Glycogen Assay Kit, BioVision, Mountain View, CA).

Immunohistochemistry of Pancreas

Two paraffin sections, a couple of sections apart, from each animal were placed on Superfrost glass slides, deparaffinized in xylene, rinsed in ethanol, and rehydrated in decreasing concen-trations of ethanol. For antigen retrieval, the sections were boiled with an antigen-unmasking solution (Vector Laboratories, Burlingame, CA) for 4 min, heated in a microwave oven for 10 min at 170 W, cooled, rinsed in PBS, and placed in 3% H_2O_2 to quench endogenous peroxidase activity. Nonspecific binding was blocked with Background Sniper (Biocare Medical, Concord, CA) for 10 min at room temperature. The sections were incubated in a humidified chamber at room temperature for 1 h with the primary antibody against insulin (A0564 polyclonal guinea-pig; Dako, Glostrup, Denmark; 1:300). The sections rinsed with PBS and incubated with horseradish peroxidase–conjugated rabbit anti-guinea pig immunoglobulin (P0141, Dako; 1:50). Immunostaining

Table 2. Weight of dissected individual fat depots and skeletal muscles.

	Control (n = 8)	Manual (n = 9)	Electrical (n = 9)	Control vs. Manual	Control vs. Electrical	Electrical vs. Manual
Body weight, 70 d (g)	252.8±12.9	256.4±15.8	252.3±23.7	0.441	0.847	0.556
Body weight, EP (g)	304.6±5.0	307.0±5.9	295.0±10.2	0.700	0.290	0.270
Fat depots (g)						
Inguinal	1.57±0.11	1.49±0.11	1.27±0.05	0.847	**0.021**	**0.015**
Parametrial	2.98±0.29	2.98±0.43	2.95±0.43	0.773	0.441	0.566
Retroperitoneal	2.33±0.28	2.21±0.24	2.08±0.34	0.773	0.208	0.441
Mesenteric	1.66±0.14	1.72±0.11	1.60±0.17	0.501	0.336	0.310
Fat depots (g/kg body weight)						
Inguinal	5.15±0.35	4.83±0.32	4.33±0.22	1.000	**0.043**	0.058
Parametrial	9.77±0.89	9.64±1.36	9.81±1.20	0.700	0.700	0.895
Retroperitoneal	7.63±0.84	7.15±0.74	6.69±0.46	1.000	0.178	0.310
Mesenteric	5.43±0.39	5.59±0.32	5.38±0.41	0.700	0.923	0.627
Muscles (g)						
EDL	0.14±0.004	0.15±0.004	0.13±0.003	0.923	0.102	**0.047**
Soleus	0.12±0.005	0.13±0.004	0.13±0.003	0.290	0.211	0.627
Tibialis	0.61±0.012	0.63±0.018	0.59±0.019	0.248	0.248	0.093
Muscles (g/kg body weight)						
EDL	0.47±0.011	0.48±0.014	0.46±0.006	0.773	0.336	0.402
Soleus	0.40±0.014	0.42±0.014	0.45±0.013	0.083	**0.007**	0.508
Tibialis	2.02±0.044	2.07±0.07	2.01±0.05	0.923	0.923	0.093

Values are mean ± SEM. EDL, extensor digitorum longus; EP, end point. *P* values were determined with the Mann-Whitney U-test.

A

B

C

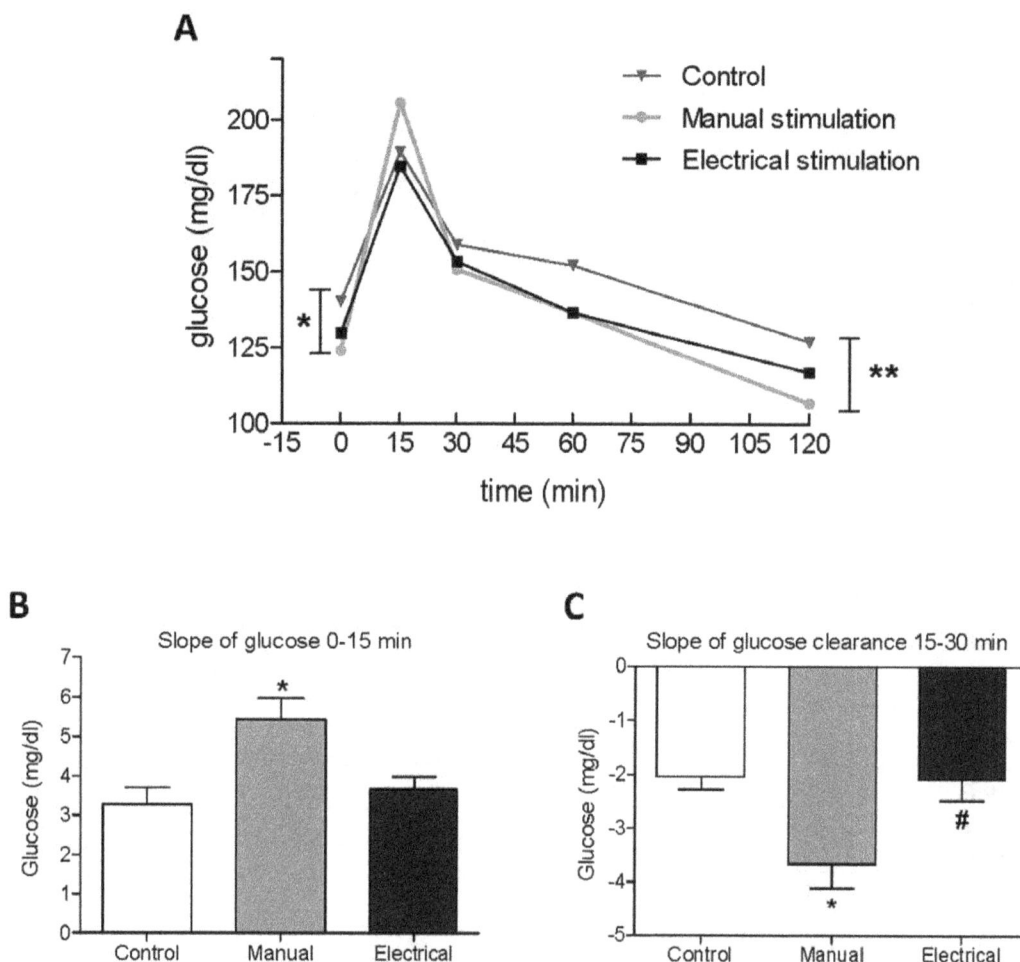

Figure 1. Results of OGTT in rats with DHT-induced PCOS after 4–5 wks of treatment. (A) Glucose concentration in plasma at 0, 15, 30, 60 and 120 min. (B, C) Slope of glucose clearance at 15 min (B) and 30 min (C). Values are mean ± SEM, *P<0.05 manual stimulation vs. controls, **P<0.01 manual stimulation vs. controls. #P<0.05 electrical vs. manual stimulation.

was visualized with DAB (Vector Laboratories). Sections were counterstained with hematoxylin, dehydrated in increasing concentrations of xylene, and placed on coverslips. Islet area, total section area, and the ratio of islet area to total area were determined with a light microscope (Leica DM 6000B, Leica Microsystems, Wetszlar, Germany) and StereoInvestigator Software V.7 (MBF Bioscience, Williston, VT). The virtual drawing tool was used to manually trace the perimeter of the section/islet, and the area was calculated by the program. Mean values of the two sections were used for statistical analyses.

RNA Isolation, cDNA Synthesis, and Real-time RT-PCR

Total RNA was extracted from mesenteric adipose tissue and soleus muscle with RNeasy Lipid Tissue Mini Kits and RNeasy Fibrous Tissue Mini Kits (Qiagen, Hilden, Germany) in a QIAcube according to the manufacturer's protocol. RNA concentrations were determined with a spectrophotometer (ND1000, NanoDrop Technologies, Wilmington, DE). First-strand cDNA in a total volume of 20 μl was synthesized from 1 μg of total RNA using random hexamers (Applied Biosystems, Warrington, UK) and Superscript III reverse transcriptase (Invitrogen Life Technologies, Paisley, UK), all according to the manufacturer's instructions. To prevent RNase-mediated degradation, RNaseout Recombinant Ribonuclease Inhibitor (Invitro-

gen) was added to each reaction. For each rat, cDNA reactions were done in triplicate and then pooled to assure good quality. mRNA expression was quantified by real-time RT-PCR and custom TaqMan low-density arrays (Applied Biosystems, Foster City, CA) with primers and probes for 48 selected genes. These genes and the corresponding TaqMan gene expression assay numbers and GenBank accession numbers are listed in Table 1.

The low-density arrays were run according to the manufacturer's protocol. Samples were run in singletons, and each loading port contained 100 ng of total RNA converted to cDNA. The stability of expression of reference genes (*18S; Actb, Gapdh, Hprt1, Ppia*) was assessed by using the NormFinder algorithm (http://www.mdl.dk/publicationsnormfinder.htm) to determine the lowest intra- and intergroup variability. The most stable gene combinations were *Gapdh* and *Ppia* (mesenteric adipose tissue) and *Actb* and *Hprt1* (soleus). These combinations served as endogenous controls. Gene expression values were calculated by the $2^{-\Delta\Delta Ct}$ method [29]. The ΔCycle threshold value (ΔCt) was calculated by subtracting the average Ct value of the reference genes from the average Ct value of the target gene. $2^{-\Delta\Delta Ct}$ was estimated as the resulting target gene expression level relative to the expression of the control group. ΔCt values were used for statistical analysis.

A

B

C

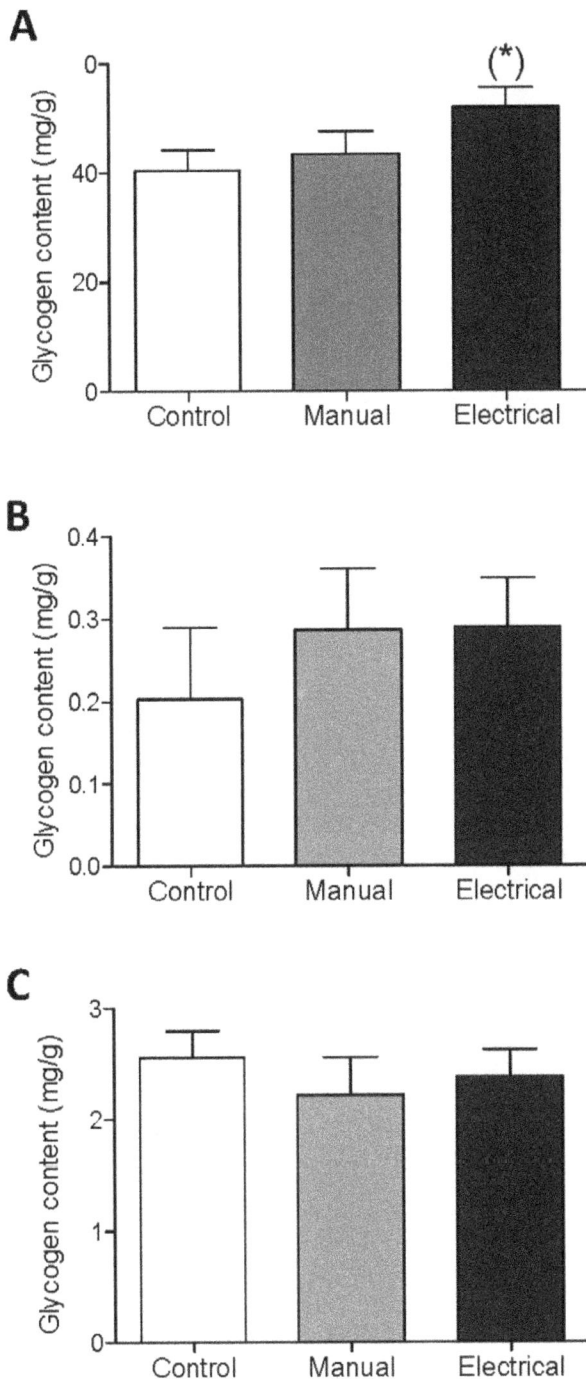

Figure 2. Glycogen content in rats with DHT-induced PCOS after 4–5 wks of treatment. Glycogen content in (A) liver, (B) EDL, and (C) soleus determined with a colorimetric assay. Values are mean ± SEM. (*)P = 0.074 (Mann-Whitney U test).

Protein Preparation and Western Blot Analysis

Frozen tissue (soleus muscle and mesenteric adipose tissue) was homogenized with a pellet pestle mixer (Merck, Darmstadt, Germany) in ice-cold buffer (25 mM Tris-HCl, 0.15 M NaCl, 1% Triton-X, 1 mM dithiothreitol, 5 mM EDTA, 0.5 mM phenyl-methylsufonyl fluoride, 1% sodium dodecyl sulfate, 200 µM sodium deoxycholate, 10 mM N-ethylmaleimide, 10 mM iodoacetamide) containing 1× complete protease inhibitor cocktail

(Roche Diagnostics, Basel, Switzerland). Samples were centrifuged for 30 min at 16.1 x g at 4°C, and supernatants were collected. A portion of the supernatant was used for analysis of protein concentration with the BCA protein assay kit (Pierce Biotechnology, Rockford, IL); bovine serum albumin served as the standard. The rest of the supernatant was stored at −80°C.

Aliquots of protein were pretreated with NuPAGE LDS Sample Buffer (Invitrogen, Carlsbad, CA), heated to 70°C for 10 min, and separated on NuPAGE Novex 3–8% Tris-acetate gels (Invitrogen) under reducing conditions with a Tris-acetate buffer system. Proteins were transferred to nitrocellulose membranes (Invitrogen), which were rinsed in Tris-buffered saline containing 0.1% Tween-20 (TBS-T), blocked in 3% albumin fraction V (BSA) (Merck, Darmstadt, Germany) in TBS-T for 1 h at room temperature, and incubated with primary antibody overnight at 4°C. The following antibodies were used: AS160, P-AS160[thr642], Tbc1D1, horseradish peroxidase–conjugated anti-mouse IgGs (#2670S, #4288S, #4629S, #7076; Cell Signaling Technology, Danvers, MA), GLUT-4 (ab33780, Abcam, Cambridge, UK), Nr4a3 (#pp H7833-00, Perseus Proteomics, Tokyo, Japan), β-actin (A1978, St. Louis, USA), and horseradish peroxidase-conjugated anti-rabbit IgGs (PI-1000, Vector Laboratories, Burlingame, CA). The next day, membranes were rinsed in TBS-T, incubated with the secondary antibodies [α-mouse IgG (#7076, Cell Signaling Technology) or α-rabbit IgG (PI-1000, Vector Laboratories)] for 1 h at room temperature, and rinsed in TBS-T. Protein bands were detected with SuperSignal West Dura Extended Duration Substrate (Pierce Biotechnology) and photographed with the LAS-1000 camera system (Fujifilm, Tokyo, Japan). The intensity of protein signals was quantified by densitometry with MultiGauge software Ver. 3.0; β-actin was used as a loading control and for normalization. Values are expressed in arbitrary densitometric units of relative abundance. Nr4a3 membranes were stripped (30 min, 50°C) in Restore PLUS stripping buffer (Thermo Scientific, Rockford, IL), reblocked with 3% BSA, and reprobed with β-actin.

Immunofluorescence Staining

The level and location of GLUT4 expression in paraffin-embedded sections of soleus muscle and mesenteric fat were determined by immunofluorescence staining with GLUT4 antibody (ab33780, Abcam) as described [30]. Nuclei were identified by staining with 4′,6-diamidino-2-phenylindole (DAPI). Slides were examined on an Axiovert 200 confocal microscope (Zeiss, Jena, Germany) equipped with the laser-scanning confocal imaging LSM 510 META system (Carl Zeiss) and photomicrographed. Negative control sections were used to adjust background settings. Images of GLUT4 immunoreactivity were adjusted to make optimal use of the dynamic range of detection.

Statistical Analysis

Values are reported as mean ± SEM or mean ± SD. Body weight gain was analyzed with a mixed between-within subjects ANOVA. The Mann-Whitney U test was used for comparisons of the electrical stimulation, manual stimulation, and control groups. Secondary comparisons were between the two treatment groups (electric vs. manual stimulation). SPSS software (version 17.0, SPSS, Chicago, IL) was used for all statistical analyses. $P<0.05$ was considered significant.

Results

Four rats, two in the PCOS group and one in each treatment group, were excluded from analysis because they did not have the

Table 3. Relative gene expression in soleus muscle and mesenteric adipose tissue depot.

Gene	Control (n =8)	Manual(n =9)	Electrical(n =9)	Control vs. Manual	Control vs. Electrical	Electrical vs. Manual
Soleus muscle						
Tbc1d1	1±0.28	0.67±0.13	0.54±0.06	0.068	0.016	0.354
Nr4a3	1±0.23	1.38±0.64	0.4±0.07	0.630	0.054	0.200
Mapk1/Erk2	1±0.06	1.18±0.24	0.82±0.05	0.962	0.054	0.031
Mesenteric adipose tissue						
Nr4a3	1±0.12	3.36±1.79	1.57±0.27	0.027	0.046	0.923
Mapk3/Erk1	1±0.15	2.03±0.32	1.14±0.14	0.006	0.401	0.021
Adcy3	1±0.11	1.75±0.3	1.09±0.16	0.012	0.916	0.054
Gsk3b	1±0.13	1.6±0.23	1.25±0.14	0.043	0.115	0.312

Presented values are $2^{-\Delta\Delta Ct}$ (mean ± SEM) relative control group. P values were determined with the Mann-Whitney U-test. The mean cycle threshold (Ct) value for all genes was 26.84±4.03 (range 8.88–37.45) in soleus muscle and 26.65±3.76 (range 9.81–37.15) in mesenteric adipose tissue.

PCOS phenotype (e.g., had regular cycles, normal ovarian morphology, no obesity, and no insulin resistance). We suspect that the DHT pellets in those rats were faulty.

Body and Tissue Weight

To assess the effects of manual and electrical stimulation of acupuncture needles on weight gain during treatment in DHT-induced PCOS rats, we used a mixed between-within subjects analysis of variance across the 11-week study period and during 4 wks of treatment. The main effect comparing weight gain in each group was not significant. Body weight at 70 d (before the start of treatment) or at the end point did not differ between the groups (Table 2). The inguinal fat depot weighed less in the electric stimulation group than in the controls (Table 2). In relation to total body weight, the inguinal fat depot weighed less and the soleus muscle weighed more in the low-frequency EA group than in the controls (Table 2).

Oral Glucose Tolerance Test

The levels of insulin and pro-insulin and the pro-insulin/insulin ratio did not differ between groups at baseline or during the OGTT (data not shown). However, after 4–5 wks of treatment glucose levels were lower in the manual stimulation group than in controls at time point 0 (124.2±1.9 mg/dl vs. 140.4±4.7 mg/dl, P =0.017) and at 120 minutes (106.8±2.0 mg/dl vs. 127.1±3.3 mg/dl, P =0.001) in the OGTT (Fig. 1A).

There were no differences in the area under curve of glucose or insulin or in the insulin sensitivity index between groups (data not shown). The glucose increase and clearance rate was determined by calculating the slope of glucose concentration from 0–15 and 15–30 minutes of the OGTT. Electrical stimulation did not affect any outcome of the OGTT (Fig. 1B, C). In the manual stimulation group, glucose clearance rate was higher than in controls (Fig. 1B, C).

Glycogen Content

There were no significant intergroup differences in glycogen content in liver, soleus, or EDL after treatment. However, there was a trend toward a higher glycogen content in liver in the electrical stimulation group than in controls (P =0.074) (Fig. 2).

Pancreas and Islets of Langerhans

There were no differences in the mean size of pancreatic islets or the ratio of the insulin-positive area to pancreatic area (control

vs. manual stimulation P =0.386 and P =0.211, control vs. electrical stimulation P =0.564 and P =0.773, manual stimulation vs. electrical stimulation P =0.122 and P =0.270, respectively).

Electrical and Manual Stimulation Differentially Regulate Gene Expression in Soleus and Mesenteric Fat

mRNA expression of 43 target genes related to androgen secretion, glucose transport, MAPK, lipid metabolism, adipokines, and sympathetic/adrenergic activation and five putative endogenous control genes were measured in soleus muscle and mesenteric adipose tissue (Table 1). Expression of nine genes in soleus and five in mesenteric fat were not detected at levels sufficient for statistical analysis (Ct>30).

In soleus muscle, the expression of Tbc1d1 mRNA was lower in the electrical stimulation group than in controls (Table 3). Although none of the stimulation groups differed from control, mRNA expression of Mapk1 was lower after electrical stimulation than after manual stimulation. Expression of Nr4a3 (P =0.054) tended to be lower in the electrical stimulation group than in controls, although non-significant.

In mesenteric adipose tissue, the expression of Nr4a3 mRNA was higher in the electrical stimulation group than in controls, and Nr4a3, Mapk3, Adcy3, and Gsk3b mRNA was higher in the manual stimulation group than in controls (Table 3).

Electrical and Manual Stimulation Differentially Regulate the Expression of Proteins in Soleus Muscle and Mesenteric Adipose Tissue

Next, we determined whether changes in insulin sensitivity and gene expression in soleus muscle and mesenteric adipose tissue after electrical and manual stimulation are reflected by alterations in protein expression. Analyses of protein content were limited to GLUT4, AS160, Tbc1d1 and Nr4a3.

In soleus muscle, total GLUT4 content in soleus muscle measured by western blot was significantly lower in the electrical stimulation group than in controls (P =0.012) or in the manual stimulation group (P =0.019) (Fig. 3A). However, both electrical and manual stimulation increased GLUT4 expression in soleus muscle (Fig. 4C1–C3), as confirmed by immunofluorescence staining. Both stimulations increased immunoreactivity in the nucleus, cell membrane, and cytosolic fraction (Fig. 4C2, C3), but the staining was notably more intense after electrical stimulation.

Soleus muscle

Mesenteric fat

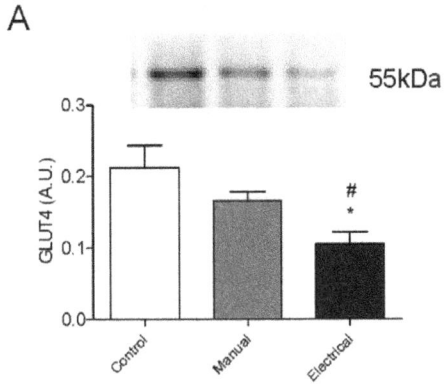

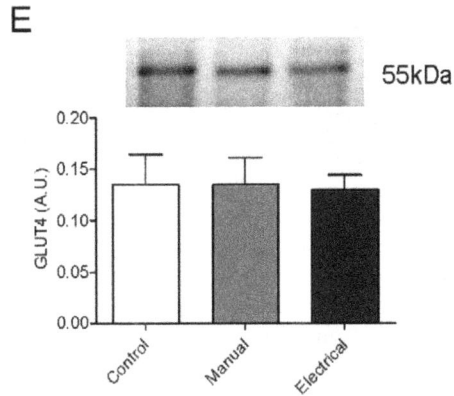

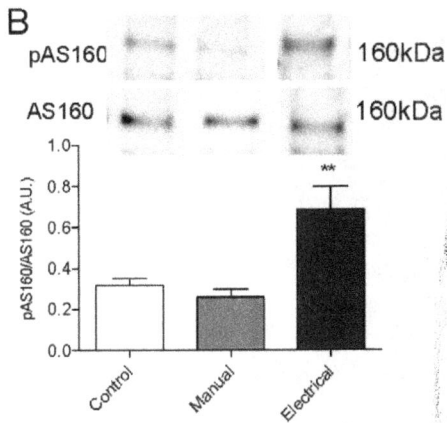

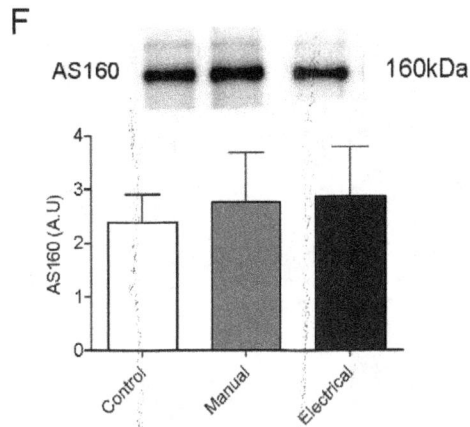

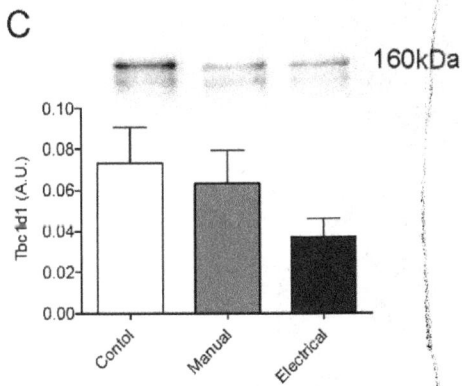

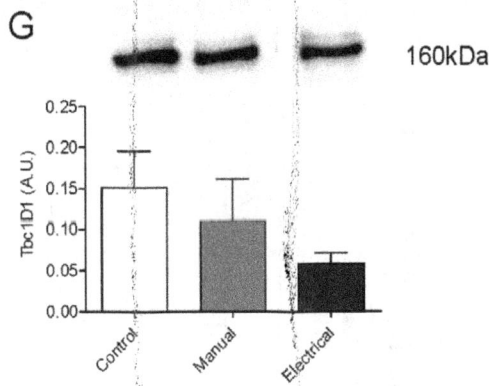

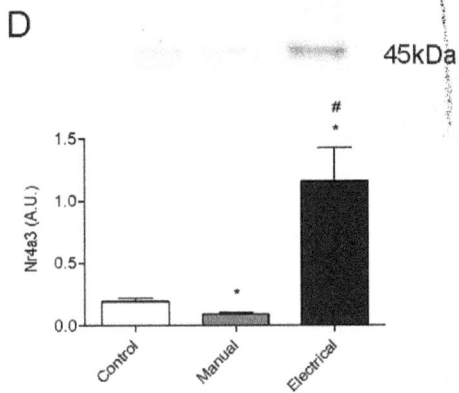

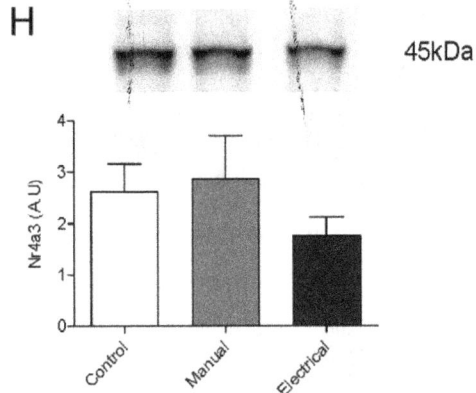

Figure 3. Protein levels in soleus muscle and mesenteric adipose tissue detected by western blot after 4–5 wks of treatment in rats with DHT-induced PCOS. GLUT4 (A, E), pAS160/AS160 ratio (B), AS160 (F), TBC1D1 (C, G), and Nr4a3 (D, H). Representative immunoblots of each protein are shown. Values were normalized to β-actin and are expressed in arbitrary units (A.U.) (mean ± SEM). *$P<0.05$ vs. controls, **$P<0.01$ vs. controls, #$P<0.05$ vs. manual stimulation (Mann-Whitney U test).

The ratio of phosphorylated to nonphosphorylated AS160 in soleus muscle was almost three times higher in the electrical stimulation group than in the manual stimulation group ($P = 0.004$) and controls ($P = 0.005$) (Fig. 3B). Nonphosphorylated AS160 in soleus muscle did not differ between groups (Fig. 3B). Protein expression of TBC1D1 in soleus muscle was almost 50% lower in the electrical stimulation group than in controls ($P = 0.054$) (Fig. 3C). Expression of Nr4a3 in soleus muscle was six times higher in the electrical stimulation group than in the manual stimulation group ($P = 0.004$) and controls ($P = 0.034$),

while manual stimulation downregulated Nr4a3 ($P = 0.012$) in soleus muscle compared with controls (Fig. 3D).

In mesenteric adipose tissue, neither electrical nor manual stimulation affected the protein expression (Fig. 3E–H).

Discussion

The novel finding of this study is that repeated electrical and manual muscle stimulation of acupuncture needles has different effects on insulin sensitivity and signaling mechanisms in an

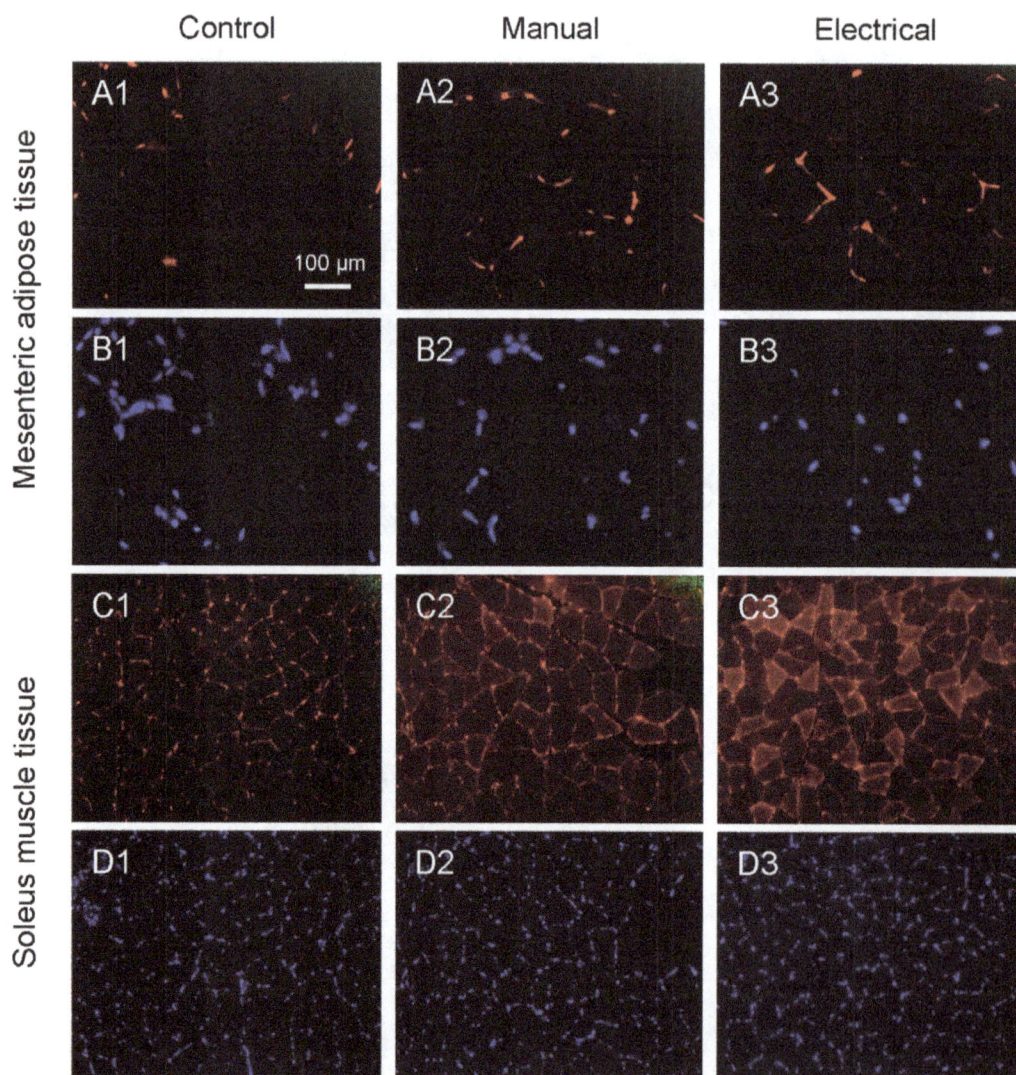

Figure 4. Distribution and expression of GLUT4, determined by immunofluorescence staining, in soleus muscle and mesenteric adipose tissue of rats with DHT-induced PCOS. No visual difference in immunoreactivity is observed in the mesenteric adipose tissue depot (A1–A3). In soleus muscle of control rats, GLUT4 is predominantly localized in the nucleus and cell membrane (C1). Both manual and electrical stimulation increased immunoreactivity in the nucleus, cell membrane, and cytosolic fraction (C2, C3). Staining was notably more intense after electrical stimulation than manual stimulation. Similar results were obtained when the staining was repeated in 3 rats/group for mesenteric adipose tissue and 4 rats/group for soleus muscle. The selected immunofluorescence images are representative of those in randomly selected section from multiple animals. B1–B3 and D1–D3: DAPI staining for nuclei in corresponding rat (A1–A3 and C1–C3). All photographs were taken with a ×20 objective.

insulin-resistant, obese rat PCOS model. Electrical stimulation decreased the weight of the subcutaneous fat depot, increased the weight of the soleus muscle, and affected the expression of genes and proteins related to insulin signaling pathways in soleus skeletal muscle. In contrast, manual stimulation of needles improved whole-body glucose tolerance and affected gene expression in mesenteric adipose tissue but had no major effect on protein expression.

Improved Glucose Tolerance Only after Manual Stimulation in DHT-induced PCOS

One of the main characteristics of rats with DHT-induced PCOS is decreased whole-body insulin sensitivity measured by euglycemic hyperinsulinemic clamp [18,20,22]. Repeated electrical stimulation of the needles, 3 or 5 times weekly for 4–5 wks, restores insulin sensitivity as measured by the clamp [18,20]. To avoid influence of an insulin load by the clamp on gene and protein expression, we measured glucose tolerance and insulin secretion (beta-cell function) with an OGTT the week before tissues were collected.

The lack of response on the OGTT in the electrical stimulation group is interesting, as we have repeatedly shown a positive effect on glucose disposal rate measured by the clamp [18,20]. One may argue that the results of the gold standard clamp method and the OGTT cannot be completely correlated, as the OGTT is less sensitive and provides somewhat different information [31]. In a previous study, we attributed the increased insulin sensitivity after electrical muscle stimulation to an increase in soleus muscle mass, suggesting that muscle twitches evoked have local effects in the muscle [20]. In the present study, we found a similar increase in soleus muscle mass only in the electrical stimulation group. Moreover, only electrical stimulation reduced the weight of the subcutaneous (inguinal) adipose tissue depot. Thus, electrical stimulation has a positive effect on body composition that may affect insulin sensitivity although not reflected by the OGTT in this study, although it was in previous euglycemic clamp experiments. Other potential explanations for the differences in response after electrical stimulation in the OGTT and the clamp include small sample sizes or that the effect of treatment involves increased responsiveness to high insulin levels rather than sensitivity.

Although the area under the curve did not differ between the groups, the glucose concentration at 0 min (fasting) and at 120 min of the OGTT was lower in the manual stimulation group than in controls with no differences in concurrent insulin levels. This could represent improved hepatic insulin sensitivity or decreased pancreatic glucagon release with lowering of high endogenous fasting glucose production, as in type 2 diabetes [32]. Because the sample volume was limited, we could not measure circulating glucagon. The increased glucose clearance rate after manual stimulation, together with lower glucose level at 2 h indicates improved glucose tolerance and possibly increased peripheral insulin sensitivity after manual stimulation, with no effect on pancreatic insulin function.

Next we aimed to elucidate the molecular mechanisms of action of the improved insulin sensitivity after 4–5 wks of manual stimulation in this study and after electrical stimulation in previous studies [18,20,22]. Muscle contractions during electrical stimulation of needles may stimulate glucose uptake by an insulin-independent pathway, as occurs after exercise [16,18,20,33,34]. Whether manual stimulation also activates insulin-independent pathways in skeletal muscle or adipose tissue has not previously been investigated.

First, we performed a more extensive screening by analyzing the expression of genes related to androgen secretion, glucose transport, MAPK, lipid metabolism, and sympathetic/adrenergic activation in soleus skeletal muscle and mesenteric adipose tissue (Table 1). Since the assessed gene expression revealed changes in several genes associated with insulin signaling, we analyzed expression of GLUT4 and its most proximal effectors (AS160, TBC1D1, and Nr4a3) by western blot. This was based on the changes in gene expression of Tbc1d1 and Nr4a3 with an addition of AS160, the homologue of Tbc1d1.

Molecular Effects of Electrical and Manual Stimulation in Soleus Skeletal Muscle

Immunofluorescence staining of GLUT4 in soleus muscle was increased after electrical stimulation and, to a lesser extent, after manual stimulation. These results are consistent with our previous finding that electrical muscle stimulation increases GLUT4 protein expression after insulin stimulation (clamp) [18]. Staining was stronger in cytosolic compartments, cell membranes, and nucleus after both stimulation techniques than in controls, which at least in part reflect increased protein expression as well as translocation. However, in contrast to our previous findings, neither gene nor protein expression of GLUT4/Slc2a4 aligned with immunofluorescense staining, indicating a stronger effect on translocation than expression. Data from membrane fractionation experiments are needed to elucidate this effect. One plausible explanation for the discrepancy in GLUT4 protein expression in soleus muscle in the present and previous study may be the absence of high insulin levels during the clamp, driving GLUT4 expression and translocation. The inconsistency between western blot and immunofluorescence might therefore reflect differences in experimental conditions or the fact that more GLUT4 in the electrical stimulation group is membrane bound as a consequence of translocation.

Two of the most distal proteins in the insulin signaling cascade closely linked to GLUT4 are AS160 and the related homologue TBC1D1, both downstream of Akt (protein kinase B). Non-phosphorylated AS160 functions as a brake on GLUT4 translocation. Phosphorylation in response to insulin, AMP-activated protein kinase (AMPK) activator 5-aminoimidazole-4-carboxamide-1-β-D-ribofluranotide (AICAR), or exercise-associated contraction inactivates this brake to allow glucose transport [35,36,37]. In support of this hypothesis, electrical muscle stimulation increased the ratio of pAS160/AS160 in the soleus muscle, indicating reduced functional activity, increased GLUT4 translocation, and possibly increased insulin sensitivity. Unphosphorylated TBC1D1 may have a role in GLUT4 traffic [36], and reduced expression of TBC1D1 in skeletal muscle increases glucose uptake and oxidation of fatty acids [38]. TBC1D1 protein expression is several times more abundant in skeletal muscles than in fat and, like AS160, insulin, muscle contraction, and AICAR increase phosphorylation (inactivation of brake) in vivo [39]. Here, electrical stimulation significantly lowered expression of Tbc1d1 mRNA in soleus muscle, and manual stimulation tended to lower it. The reduced Tbc1d1 mRNA expression in soleus muscle is supported by the reduction in protein expression ($P = 0.054$). The lack of change in Slc2a4 (GLUT4) mRNA expression suggests a potential role for TBC1D1 in the posttranscriptional modifications of GLUT4 translocation. Consistent with our hypothesis, these results also indicate that low-frequency electrical stimulation causing muscle contractions improves glucose uptake and oxidation of fatty acids in muscle.

Lastly, NR4A3, a member of the NR4A family of orphan nuclear receptors, is widely expressed in different cell types and mediates diverse biological processes [40,41]. *Nr4a3* expression is reduced in skeletal muscle and adipose tissue in multiple rodent models of insulin resistance, while increased expression of *Nr4a3* increases insulin responsiveness and GLUT4 translocation [41]. At the protein level, electrical but not manual stimulation dramatically increased Nr4a3 expression in soleus muscle. This finding is consistent with previous studies of electrical stimulation causing muscle contractions and exercise and might indicate increased insulin sensitivity [42,43].

Molecular Effects of Electrical and Manual Stimulation in Mesenteric Adipose Tissue

Although the molecular effects of electrical and manual stimulation were less pronounced in the mesenteric adipose tissue than in soleus muscle, manual stimulation had the strongest effect on gene expression in mesenteric adipose tissue. mRNA expression of *Adcy3* and *Erk1* increased in adipose tissue by manual stimulation, indicating that the effects after manual acupuncture stimulation may involve modulation of autonomic activity and MAPK signaling. Also, expression of *Nr4a3* mRNA in mesenteric adipose tissue was increased by both manual and electrical stimulation, indicating increased insulin responsiveness and GLUT4 translocation by both methods [41]. However, protein expression was not changed in mesenteric adipose tissue.

Acupuncture Mechanism

Both manual and electrical stimulation cause afferent activity in Aα, β, δ, and unmyelinated C-fibers [44,45], similar to some of the effects of exercise [46]. Both stimulations may, via supraspinal pathways, directly or indirectly modulate the sympathetic output to target organs [47,48,49]. Electrical stimulation of the needles enhances insulin sensitivity in rats, probably through mechanisms related to activation of afferent sensory nerve fibers and modulation of efferent sympathetic nerve activity [19,21,50]. In addition, acupuncture with combined electrical and manual stimulation decreases high sympathetic nerve activity in women with PCOS [51]. This effect may be related, at least in part, to the release of β-endorphin [52,53].

The differential effects of manual and electrical acupuncture stimulation in this study could reflect differences in stimulation duration, given that needles were manually stimulated every 5 min

by compared with continuous low-frequency electrical stimulation. For further understanding, the acute effects of the two stimulation modalities with similar duration should be explored. It is also necessary to evaluate the experimental findings in a clinical setting. Although acupuncture would never be a complete alternative to exercise as a first-line therapy, some patients cannot exercise vigorously enough to improve their insulin sensitivity. Also, we have reason to believe that acupuncture enhances the beneficial effects of exercise. Thus, the combination of these treatments may be optimal [54].

Conclusion

Electrical and manual muscle stimulation affect glucose homeostasis through different mechanisms in rats with DHT-induced PCOS. Repeated electrical stimulation of acupuncture needles regulated key functional molecular pathways related to insulin sensitivity in soleus muscle and mesenteric adipose tissue to a larger extent than manual stimulation. Manual stimulation improved whole-body glucose tolerance as measured by OGTT, an effect that was not observed after electrical stimulation, but did not affect molecular signaling pathways to the same extent as electrical stimulation. Although more functional signaling pathways related to insulin sensitivity were affected by electrical stimulation, our findings suggest that manual stimulation of acupuncture needles has a greater effect on glucose tolerance. The underlying mechanism of the differential effects of the intermittent manual and the continuous electrical stimulation remains to be elucidated.

Acknowledgments

For support and the use of technical equipment, we thank the Genomics Core Facility at the Sahlgrenska Academy, University of Gothenburg, which was funded by a grant from the Knut and Alice Wallenberg Foundation. We also thank the Center for Mouse Physiology and Bio-Imaging, University of Gothenburg and Anders Odén for statistical assistance.

Author Contributions

Conceived and designed the experiments: JJ ESV. Performed the experiments: JJ LMH RS ALO. Analyzed the data: JJ ESV. Contributed reagents/materials/analysis tools: ML. Wrote the paper: JJ ESV ML HB.

References

1. Teede HJ, Hutchison S, Zoungas S, Meyer C (2006) Insulin resistance, the metabolic syndrome, diabetes, and cardiovascular disease risk in women with PCOS. Endocrine 30: 45–53.
2. Dunaif A, Segal KR, Shelley DR, Green G, Dobrjansky A, et al. (1992) Evidence for distinctive and intrinsic defects in insulin action in polycystic ovary syndrome. Diabetes 41: 1257–1266.
3. Dunaif A, Wu X, Lee A, Diamanti-Kandarakis E (2001) Defects in insulin receptor signaling in vivo in the polycystic ovary syndrome (PCOS). Am J Physiol Endocrinol Metab 281: E392–E399.
4. Ciaraldi TP, el-Roeiy A, Madar Z, Reichart D, Olefsky JM, et al. (1992) Cellular mechanisms of insulin resistance in polycystic ovarian syndrome. J Clin Endocrinol Metab 75: 577–583.
5. Ciaraldi TP, Aroda V, Mudaliar S, Chang RJ, Henry RR (2009) Polycystic ovary syndrome is associated with tissue-specific differences in insulin resistance. J Clin Endocrinol Metab 94: 157–163.
6. Zierath JR, Krook A, Wallberg-Henriksson H (2000) Insulin action and insulin resistance in human skeletal muscle. Diabetologia 43: 821–835.
7. Krook A, Wallberg-Henriksson H, Zierath JR (2004) Sending the signal: molecular mechanisms regulating glucose uptake. Med Sci Sports Exerc 36: 1212–1217.
8. Rosenbaum D, Haber RS, Dunaif A (1993) Insulin resistance in polycystic ovary syndrome: decreased expression of GLUT-4 glucose transporters in adipocytes. Am J Physiol Endocrinol Metab 264: E197–202.
9. Jensterle M, Janez A, Mlinar B, Marc J, Prezelj J, et al. (2008) Impact of metformin and rosiglitazone treatment on glucose transporter 4 mRNA

expression in women with polycystic ovary syndrome. Eur J Endocrinol 158: 793–801.
10. Seow K-M, Juan C-C, Hsu Y-P, Hwang J-L, Huang L-W, et al. (2007) Amelioration of insulin resistance in women with PCOS via reduced insulin receptor substrate-1 Ser312 phosphorylation following laparoscopic ovarian electrocautery. Hum Reprod 22: 1003–1010.
11. Jedel E, Labrie F, Oden A, Holm G, Nilsson L, et al. (2011) Impact of electro-acupuncture and physical exercise on hyperandrogenism and oligo/amenorrhea in women with polycystic ovary syndrome: a randomized controlled trial. Am J Physiol Endocrinol Metab 300: E37–E45.
12. Pastore LM, Williams CD, Jenkins J, Patrie JT (2011) True and sham acupuncture produced similar frequency of ovulation and improved LH to FSH ratios in women with Polycystic Ovary Syndrome. J Clin Endocrinol Metab 96: 3143–3150.
13. Stener-Victorin E, Baghaei F, Holm G, Janson PO, Olivecrona G, et al. (2012) Effects of acupuncture and exercise on insulin sensitivity, adipose tissue characteristics, and markers of coagulation and fibrinolysis in women with polycystic ovary syndrome: secondary analyses of a randomized controlled trial. Fertility and Sterility 97: 501–508.
14. Lai MH, Ma HX, Yao H, Liu H, Song XH, et al. (2010) [Effect of abdominal acupuncture therapy on the endocrine and metabolism in obesity-type polycystic ovarian syndrome patients]. Zhen Ci Yan Jiu 35: 298–302.
15. Atherton PJ, Babraj JA, Smith K, Singh J, Rennie MJ, et al. (2005) Selective activation of AMPK-PGC-1alpha or PKB-TSC2-mTOR signaling can explain specific adaptive responses to endurance or resistance training-like electrical muscle stimulation. FASEB J: 786–788.

16. Liang F, Chen R, Nakagawa A, Nishizawa M, Tsuda S, et al. (2011) Low-frequency electroacupuncture improves insulin sensitivity in obese diabetic mice through activation of SIRT1/PGC-1alpha in skeletal muscle. Evid Based Complement Alternat Med 2011: 735297.

17. Suwa M, Nakano H, Radak Z, Kumagai S (2008) Endurance exercise increases the SIRT1 and peroxisome proliferator-activated receptor gamma coactivator-1alpha protein expressions in rat skeletal muscle. Metabolism 57: 986–998.

18. Johansson J, Yi F, Shao R, Lonn M, Billig H, et al. (2010) Intense acupuncture normalizes insulin sensitivity, increases muscle GLUT4 content, and improves lipid profile in a rat model of Polycystic ovary syndrome. Am J Physiol Endocrinol Metab: E:551–E559.

19. Higashimura Y, Shimoju R, Maruyama H, Kurosawa M (2009) Electro-acupuncture improves responsiveness to insulin via excitation of somatic afferent fibers in diabetic rats. Auton Neurosci 150: 100–103.

20. Manneras L, Jonsdottir IH, Holmang A, Lonn M, Stener-Victorin E (2008) Low-Frequency Electro-Acupuncture and Physical Exercise Improve Metabolic Disturbances and Modulate Gene Expression in Adipose Tissue in Rats with Dihydrotestosterone-Induced Polycystic Ovary Syndrome. Endocrinology 149: 3559–3568.

21. Manneras L, Cajander S, Lonn M, Stener-Victorin E (2009) Acupuncture and exercise restore adipose tissue expression of sympathetic markers and improve ovarian morphology in rats with dihydrotestosterone-induced PCOS. Am J Physiol Regul Integr Comp Physiol 296: R1124–1131.

22. Manneras L, Cajander S, Holmang A, Seleskovic Z, Lystig T, et al. (2007) A new rat model exhibiting both ovarian and metabolic characteristics of polycystic ovary syndrome. Endocrinology 148: 3781–3791.

23. Ishizaki N, Okushi N, Yano T, Yamamura Y (2009) Improvement in glucose tolerance as a result of enhanced insulin sensitivity during electroacupuncture in spontaneously diabetic Goto-Kakizaki rats. Metabolism 58: 1372–1378.

24. Feng Y, Johansson J, Shao R, Manneras Holm L, Billig H, et al. (2012) Electrical and manual acupuncture stimulation affects estrous cyclicity and neuroendocrine function in a DHT-induced rat polycystic ovary syndrome model. Exp physiol.

25. Feng Y, Johansson J, Shao R, Manneras L, Fernandez-Rodriguez J, et al. (2009) Hypothalamic neuroendocrine functions in rats with dihydrotestosterone-induced polycystic ovary syndrome: effects of low-frequency electro-acupuncture. PLoS One 4: e6638.

26. Feng Y, Johansson J, Shao RJ, Manneras-Holm L, Billig H, et al. (2012) Electrical and manual acupuncture stimulation affect oestrous cyclicity and neuroendocrine function in an 5a-dihydrotestosterone-induced rat polycystic ovary syndrome model. Experimental Physiology 97: 651–662.

27. Marcondes FK, Bianchi FJ, Tanno AP (2002) Determination of the estrous cycle phases of rats: some helpful considerations. Braz J Biol 62: 609–614.

28. Matsuda M, DeFronzo RA (1999) Insulin sensitivity indices obtained from oral glucose tolerance testing: comparison with the euglycemic insulin clamp. Diabetes Care 22: 1462–1470.

29. Livak KJ, Schmittgen TD (2001) Analysis of relative gene expression data using real-time quantitative PCR and the 2-ΔΔCT method. Methods 25: 402–408.

30. Shao R, Weijdegard B, Fernandez-Rodriguez J, Egecioglu E, Zhu C, et al. (2007) Ciliated epithelial-specific and regional-specific expression and regulation of the estrogen receptor-beta2 in the fallopian tubes of immature rats: a possible mechanism for estrogen-mediated transport process in vivo. Am J Physiol Endocrinol Metab 293: E147–E158.

31. Cederholm J, Wibell L (1990) Insulin release and peripheral sensitivity at the oral glucose tolerance test. Diabetes Res Clin Pract 10: 167–175.

32. Rizza RA (2010) Pathogenesis of fasting and postprandial hyperglycemia in type 2 diabetes: implications for therapy. Diabetes 59: 2697–2707.

33. Goodyear LJ, Kahn BB (1998) Exercise, glucose transport, and insulin sensitivity. Annu Rev Med 49: 235–261.

34. Deshmukh AS, Hawley JA, Zierath JR (2008) Exercise-induced phospho-proteins in skeletal muscle. Int J Obes (Lond) 32 Suppl 4: S18–S23.

35. Frosig C, Richter EA (2009) Improved insulin sensitivity after exercise: focus on insulin signaling. Obesity 17 Suppl 3: S15–20.

36. Sakamoto K, Holman GD (2008) Emerging role for AS160/TBC1D4 and TBC1D1 in the regulation of GLUT4 traffic. Am J Physiol Endocrinol Metab 295: E29–E37.

37. Bruss MD, Arias EB, Lienhard GE, Cartee GD (2005) Increased phosphory-lation of Akt substrate of 160 kDa (AS160) in rat skeletal muscle in response to insulin or contractile activity. diabetes 54: 41–50.

38. Chadt A, Leicht K, Deshmukh A, Jiang LQ, Scherneck S, et al. (2008) Tbc1d1 mutation in lean mouse strain confers leanness and protects from diet-induced obesity. Nat genet 40: 1354–1359.

39. Taylor EB, An D, Kramer HF, Yu H, Fujii NL, et al. (2008) Discovery of TBC1D1 as an insulin-, AICAR-, and contraction-stimulated signaling nexus in mouse skeletal muscle. J Biol Chem 283: 9787–9796.

40. Ohkura N, Ito M, Tsukada T, Sasaki K, Yamaguchi K, et al. (1996) Structure, mapping and expression of a human NOR-1 gene, the third member of the Nur77/NGFI-B family. Biochim Biophys Acta 1308: 205–214.

41. Fu Y, Luo L, Luo N, Zhu X, Garvey WT (2007) NR4A orphan nuclear receptors modulate insulin action and the glucose transport system: potential role in insulin resistance. J Biol Chem 282: 31525–31533.

42. Mahoney DJ, Parise G, Melov S, Safdar A, Tarnopolsky MA (2005) Analysis of global mRNA expression in human skeletal muscle during recovery from endurance exercise. FASEB J 19: 1498–1500.

43. Kawasaki E, Hokari F, Sasaki M, Sakai A, Koshinaka K, et al. (2009) Role of local muscle contractile activity in the exercise-induced increase in NR4A receptor mRNA expression. J Appl Physiol 106: 1826–1831.

44. Han JS (1997) Physiology of acupuncture: review of thirty years of research. J Alt Comp Med 3: 101–108.

45. Kagitani F, Uchida S, Hotta H, Aikawa Y (2005) Manual acupuncture needle stimulation of the rat hindlimb activates groups I, II, III and IV single afferent nerve fibers in the dorsal spinal roots. Jpn J Physiol 55: 149–155.

46. Kaufman MP, Waldrop TG, Rybicki KJ, Ordway GA, Mitchell JH (1984) Effects of static and rythmic twitch contractions on the discharge of group III and IV muscle afferents. Cardiovasc Rec 18: 663–668.

47. Stener-Victorin E, Kobayashi R, Kurosawa M (2003) Ovarian blood flow responses to electro-acupuncture stimulation at different frequencies and intensities in anaesthetized rats. Auton Neurosci 108: 50–56.

48. Stener-Victorin E, Fujisawa S, Kurosawa M (2006) Ovarian blood flow responses to electroacupuncture stimulation depend on estrous cycle and on site and frequency of stimulation in anesthetized rats. J Appl Physiol 101: 84–91.

49. Sato A, Sato Y, Uchida S (2002) Reflex modulation of visceral functions by acupuncture-like stimulation in anesthetized rats. International Congress Series 1238: 111–123.

50. Chang S-L, Lin K-J, Lin R-T, Hung P-H, Lin J-G, et al. (2006) Enhanced insulin sensitivity using electroacupuncture on bilateral Zusanli acupoints (ST 36) in rats. Life Sciences 79: 967–971.

51. Stener-Victorin E, Jedel E, Janson PO, Sverrisdottir YB (2009) Low-frequency electroacupuncture and physical exercise decrease high muscle sympathetic nerve activity in polycystic ovary syndrome. Am J Physiol Regul Integr Comp Physiol 297: R387–395.

52. Han J-S (2003) Acupuncture: neuropeptide release produced by electrical stimulation of different frequencies. Trends in Neurosciences 26: 17–22.

53. Ahmed MI, Duleba AJ, El Shahat O, Ibrahim ME, Salem A (2008) Naltrexone treatment in clomiphene resistant women with polycystic ovary syndrome. Hum Reprod 23: 2564–2569.

54. Padmanabhan V, Veiga-Lopez A (2011) Developmental origin of reproductive and metabolic dysfunctions: androgenic versus estrogenic reprogramming. Semin Reprod Med 29: 173–186.

21

The Acceptability of Acupuncture for Low Back Pain: A Qualitative Study of Patient's Experiences Nested within a Randomised Controlled Trial

Ann Hopton[1]*, Kate Thomas[2], Hugh MacPherson[1]

1 Department of Health Sciences, University of York, York, North Yorkshire, United Kingdom, **2** Health Services Research Unit, University of Sheffield, Sheffield, South Yorkshire, United Kingdom

Abstract

Introduction: The National Institute for Health and Clinical Excellence guidelines recommend acupuncture as a clinically effective treatment for chronic back pain. However, there is insufficient knowledge of what factors contribute to patients' positive and negative experiences of acupuncture, and how those factors interact in terms of the acceptability of treatment. This study used patient interviews following acupuncture treatment for back pain to identify, understand and describe the elements that contribute or detract from acceptability of treatment.

Methods: The study used semi-structured interviews. Twelve patients were interviewed using an interview schedule as a sub-study nested within a randomised controlled trial of acupuncture for chronic back pain. The interviews were analysed using thematic analysis.

Results and Discussion: Three over-arching themes emerged from the analysis. The first entitled facilitators of acceptability contained five subthemes; experience of pain relief, improvements in physical activity, relaxation, psychological benefit, reduced reliance on medication. The second over-arching theme identified barriers to acceptability, which included needle-related discomfort and temporary worsening of symptoms, pressure to continue treatment and financial cost. The third over-arching theme comprised mediators of acceptability, which included pre-treatment mediators such as expectation and previous experience, and treatment-related mediators of time, therapeutic alliance, lifestyle advice and the patient's active involvement in recovery. These themes inform our understanding of the acceptability of acupuncture to patients with low back pain.

Conclusion: The acceptability of acupuncture treatment for low back pain is complex and multifaceted. The therapeutic relationship between the practitioner and patient emerged as a strong driver for acceptability, and as a useful vehicle to develop the patients' self-efficacy in pain management in the longer term. Unpleasant treatment related effects do not necessarily detract from patients' overall perception of acceptability.

Editor: John E. Mendelson, California Pacific Medical Center Research Institute, United States of America

Funding: This research was supported by the National Institute for Health Research (NIHR) Health Technology Assessment programme and in part by a NIHR Career Scientist Award, grant number PAS/03/07/CSA/008 awarded to HM. The funders had no role in study design, data collection and analysis, decision to publish, or preparation of the manuscript.

Competing Interests: The authors have declared that no competing interests exist.

* E-mail: ann.hopton@york.ac.uk

Introduction

Chronic low back pain is a problem in the UK. [1] Pain-related anxieties and fearful avoidance of movement are influential psychological factors from pain inception to its chronic stage. [2;3] Concerns about back pain raised through misinformation, learned pain, or distorted significance of the pain are associated with increased disability. [4] Tension between General Practitioners' recommendation to stay active, versus the patients' expectation of prescribed rest can lead to discord in the doctor-patient relationship. [5] Constraints on time and resources have led patients and doctors to feelings of frustration in the management of back pain in primary care [6;7].

The results of the York Acupuncture for Back Pain trial(YACBAC) [8] showed that a short course of acupuncture compared to usual care for chronic low back pain conferred a clinically significant reduction in low back pain for minor extra cost to the NHS. [9] Within the YACBAC trial, 241 participants, aged 18–65 with a history of non-specific low back pain for a period of 4 to 52 weeks were recruited by general practitioners at GP primary care practices in York. Participants were randomly assigned to receive a course of up to 10 acupuncture sessions over three months as an adjunct to usual care, or to receive usual care alone. Six acupuncturists with a minimum of three years' experience and registered with the British Acupuncture Council delivered up to ten treatments, usually weekly, tailored to individual patients' needs. Additional care such as brief massage and acupuncture-specific advice was provided if considered appropriate by the acupuncturists [10].

Evidence from a trialists' collaboration which conducted a meta-analysis of nearly 18,000 cases of acupuncture for chronic pain conditions including non-specific back pain indicated that acupuncture for low back pain is more than a placebo, although the difference between true acupuncture and sham acupuncture is relatively modest. [11] This study suggested that factors in addition to the specific effect of needling are important contributors to therapeutic effects. Based on the growing evidence of clinical effectiveness and cost effectiveness, the National Institute for Health and Clinical Excellence guidelines recommend acupuncture as a referral option for patients with low back pain [12].

According to the MRC guidelines for the evaluation of complex interventions, an important part of an evaluation process is an exploration of the way in which the intervention under study is implemented, because it can provide valuable insight into why an intervention fails or has unexpected consequences, or why a successful intervention works and how it can be optimised. [13] Given the combination of physical, psychological and social components associated with chronic back pain, it remains unclear as to what additional factors contribute to patients' positive and negative experiences of acupuncture and how these factors interact to influence the patients' perception of the treatment. Understanding why a treatment is acceptable to some patients and not others is important because acceptability may influence the patients' rating of clinical benefit. Quantitative data from the YACBAC trial shows on average that there is a reduction in the intensity of back pain [8], but we know little about the factors at an individual level that might influence a patients' recovery and their subsequent decision to try acupuncture again. These qualitative data will help clinicians to be better informed about who might benefit from referral to acupuncture.

To extend our understanding of acceptability, we have used qualitative methods, based on in-depth interviews with patients who received acupuncture for chronic low back pain nested within a randomised controlled trial. Our aim has been to capture patients' reports on their thoughts, attitudes and experiences of treatment and to understand and describe the elements that they ascribe to the acceptability, or not, of acupuncture.

Methods

Setting and Ethics Statement

This research was a qualitative sub-study nested within the York Acupuncture for Back Pain Trial (YACBAC)(ISRCTN80764175) [14] funded by the Health Technology Assessment programme. The trial was conducted collaboratively by researchers at the University of Sheffield and the Foundation for Research into Traditional Chinese Medicine in York, and approved by York's NHS Local Research Ethics Committee. Written consent was obtained from all participants using a consent document and procedure approved by the ethics committee.

In a postal questionnaire at three months after randomisation, 133 participants reported on treatment effects of acupuncture. Of those, twelve interview participants were drawn as a purposive sample, designed to include a range of known patient characteristics: age and gender, previous experience of acupuncture treatment, and both good and less favourable treatment outcomes. All 12 participants approached agreed to participate in the study and consented to a one to one, face-to-face, audio-recorded, semi-structured interview in their own home, and were considered suitable to represent the diversity of known patient characteristics.

Lucy Thorpe, a research associate experienced in investigating acupuncture for back pain and depression and trained in conducting qualitative research recruited and interviewed all 12 participants, and Mike Fitter, a research consultant provided additional supervision.

The interview opened with an introduction designed to draw out the participants' account of treatment received as part of the trial, followed by prompts from a prepared topic guide (Appendix S1) to elicit the participants' expectations of treatment before receiving acupuncture, therapeutic aspects of the consultation and their experiences of the treatment received. Interviews typically lasted for approximately 30–60 minutes; audiotaped recordings were transcribed verbatim and checked for accuracy. The interviews were conducted according to the topic guide and provided rich detail without further need to re-interview the selected sample. Iterative questioning was used within the interview to establish credibility and trustworthiness of the interviewees. Statements regarding the reduction in back pain experienced, the degree of function regained, and aspects of satisfaction with the time, attention, information and explanations given by the acupuncturist about treatment were crosschecked with quantitative data recorded as part of the trial.

Analytical Methods

An inductive thematic analysis following the methods of Braun & Clarke 2006 [15] was used to search across the dataset of the 12 transcribed interviews, to organise and describe the data in detail, and to actively identify, analyze and report over-arching themes and subthemes. Thematic analysis was selected as a flexible research method with the potential to allow the data to speak for itself and to provide a rich and detailed account of the data. The data was analysed initially by AH by reading each transcript several times to become immersed in the data, and identifying interesting features within individual data sets that might form the foundation of repeated patterns. All data sets were coded manually by annotating notes within the text, and using colour coding to highlight potential patterns. The inductive codes developed from the dataset captured and summarised the participants' experiences. As codes were identified, recorded and organised on an Excel spread sheet, sections of text that demonstrated that code were then added and collated. Coding progressed by moving back and forth across the data set in an iterative process where comparisons were made between codes and phrases. Those with similar context or concepts were grouped together. Identified codes were then matched to data extracts that demonstrated the code and collated together by copying extracts from individual transcripts and inserting them into an Excel spread sheet. This coding was performed sequentially on individual transcripts without software, working systematically throughout the entire dataset. This process was conducted within each interview and across interviews resulting in a codebook of 43 codes and 21 subthemes. Data saturation occurred early with all the codes appearing within the first six interviews. Ongoing analysis refined the specific content of each theme, and the position of codes and themes on the thematic map.

Three over-arching themes were identified and developed from the codes, Figure 1.

The data was checked independently by co-author HM, and the coding and identification of subthemes were discussed and developed collaboratively between AH and HM throughout. The subthemes are illustrated with quotes that embody the participants' experiences embedded within the analytical narrative, as suggested by Braun and Clarke (2006). Additional quotes that support each subtheme within the over-arching themes are set

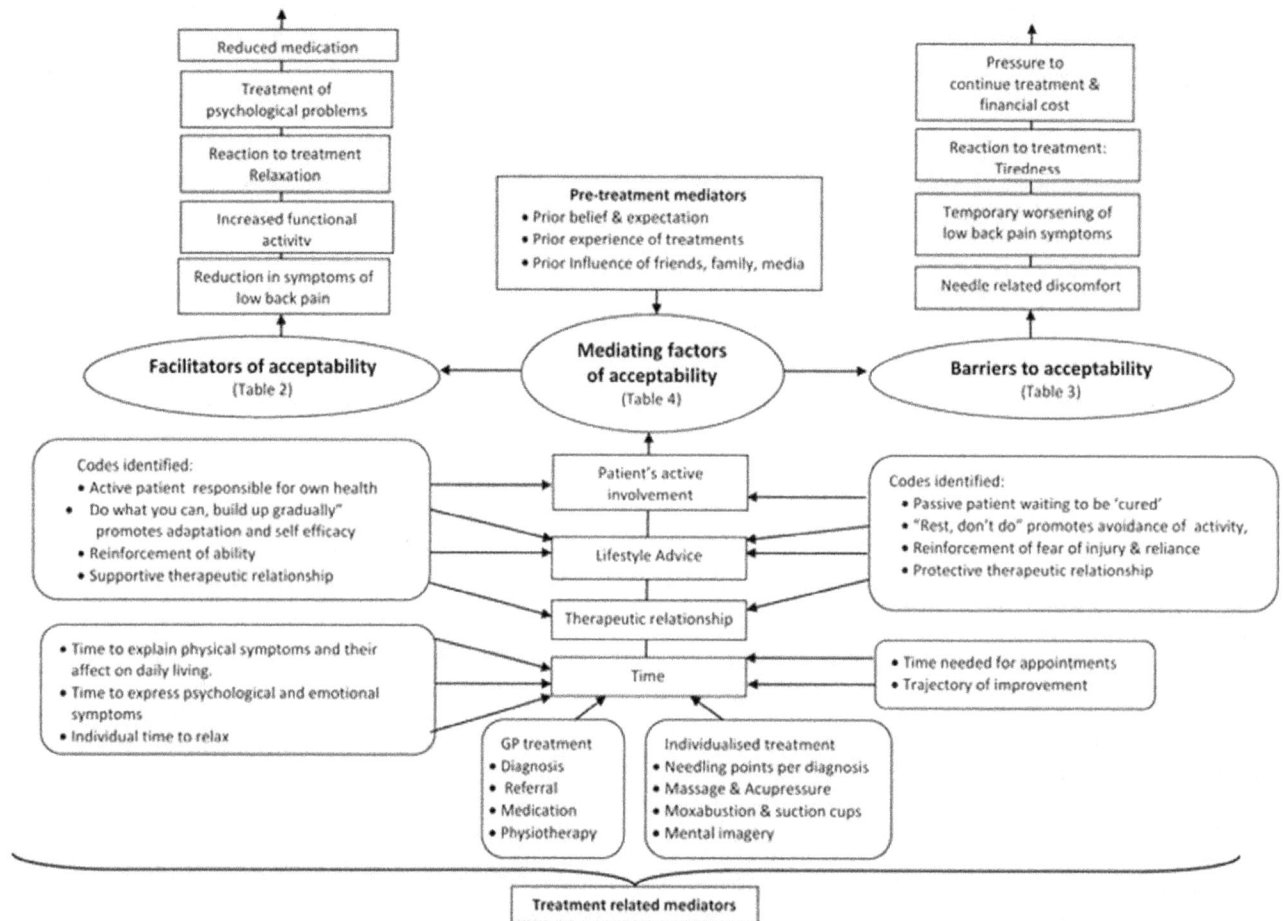

Figure 1. Initial thematic map showing three over-arching themes and related subthemes.

out in Tables 1, 2, 3. To maintain anonymity each participant was numbered. Coding and extractions were checked to verify that the patient's experiences were reflected and summarised accurately. The consolidated criteria for reporting qualitative studies (COREQ): 32-item checklist is available as (Appendix S2).

Results

Participants

The patients interviewed were 2 men and 10 women, purposively sampled to reflect the diversity of known characteristics across all participants in the trial. In the three-month questionnaires, which were completed at around the same time of the interviews, all study participants reported their health as fair to excellent, and the majority reported satisfaction with the acupuncture they had received. Only half of the patients who were interviewed reported satisfaction with the level of their back pain at three months.

Themes

Three over-arching themes pertaining to the acceptability of acupuncture treatment were identified. The first over-arching theme entitled "Facilitators of acceptability" contained five subthemes; reduction in symptoms, improved physical activity, relaxation, reduction of psychological symptoms and reduced reliance on medication (Table1). The second over-arching theme entitled "Barriers to acceptability" encompassed four subthemes:

needle-related discomfort, temporary worsening of symptoms, and tiredness, and the pressure to continue treatment with its' potential financial cost (Table2). The third over-arching theme entitled "Mediating factors" comprised pre-treatment mediators (Table 3), and treatment related mediators with four separate subthemes; time, therapeutic alliance, lifestyle advice, and patient's active involvement, each with the potential to induce positive or negative influences on the patients' perception of the treatment.

Facilitators of Acceptability

Reduction in symptoms. The first facilitator of acceptability of treatment to be identified from the coding was the subtheme "reduction in symptoms of low back pain"(Table1). Two patients reported experiencing a reduction in pain symptoms from the first treatment session. More commonly, the pain relief became apparent gradually, following a trajectory over a period of several weeks. For example, several patients reported that they noticed a reduction in symptoms of low back pain about 4–6 weeks into treatment.

"I had gone at first where it ached for two or three sessions, and I thought, this is not going to work, and then on the fourth session it was a lot easier. It was either the fifth or the sixth session when it was severe, and after that great. Each time I went then I got better and better. It got to the last one and I thought well really I don't need it". (p10)

Table 1. Over-arching theme 1: Benefits of acupuncture.

Reduction of symptoms of low back pain

I am not going though as much of the aches and pains that I was. It has... it's done some good. I still have the odd twinge and it was only the other day I felt like a tug but it seemed to stop quite quickly....I'd probably say I felt about 70% better. I've not felt 100% better. Before the acupuncture my back felt really weak, and since the acupuncture its felt stronger.(P2)

I've had no feeling at all down my calf and my ankle and my instep, and she's even got rid of that....As each week goes by it gets better and there are some days when I just don't feel it. I can forget about it now which is marvellous.(P7)

For me it was quite immediate...it was almost immediately I felt benefits. I felt that my foot had become alienated from my body because of the surgery... It was like a strange feeling that I had this foot but it was just like a lump, I didn't have a bodily association with it... and then I did feel that because of the treatment the warmth and everything else and the way she sort of channelled everything I did feel that I had actually had again an association with my foot... its like she brought it back to me...(P9)

For the first couple of weeks I didn't feel any difference and long term I did, as I say in the beginning, nothing,. Then it did start after a month then it started getting better and better every time I went, it was easier and easier..I didn't seem to get sciatica as often... I must be honest when I bend over it still hurts, it still hurts when I wash my hair in the shower and I bend forward, ... My pain is so much less than ever before over these years, so its been really great. I had a problem with my right shoulder as well. The muscle right inside your bone, that was really sore and I could hardly move, lift my arm and when It told the ladies about it at acupuncture, they were happy to work on it for me, ... now I can lift my shoulder (P12)

Improved physical activity

I hadn't walked for 2–3 months, you know pain does that to anybody I am sure...but I would have no qualms of setting out to do, well... ten mile walks., you know, with a 20 pound ruck sack on your back, so I guess I was back to normal... I still wash the car... bending down, and cleaning that will give me problems but its not giving me problems at the minute.(P1)

I'm much more mobile, I'm standing better, I can tolerate standing and sitting for slightly longer periods of time, and I can walk further. I'm sleeping better. I'm gradually doing a bit more.(P5)

The main thing was going back to work, the other thing was doing household chores. When I had my bad back I was trying to do the ironing, but I was doing like a shirt at a time and then lying down for five minutes and then doing another shirt.... It was horrendous trying to do anything... trying to do anything below waist level was virtually impossible. And I mean now, now I can do anything.(P7)

I think I've been able to focus more on what I can do, and not worry about that I can't do... now I swim more because I can do that and I enjoy it and its good for you(P9)

Relaxation

You can generally feel something happening, its quite strange because you feel all tingly, you feel a bit warm, you feel tired... it does help relax you...The best part of it is just laying out and letting it be done to you.(P3)

I felt more relaxed in my back... that sort of feeling of well being and positive thoughts. That can change you physically at least for a while. I did actually find it relaxing lying on that couch thing with the needles in my back... conked out for a while... I'm more relaxed because I'm sleeping better as well.(P4)

I did feel extremely relaxed when I had treatment...she did actually give me a lot of energy... She did seem to channel quite a lot of energy and I felt that I had... after treatment I felt quite revitalized. It was really positive for me. I used to feel the next day that I had a lot, like a wham of energy and that she'd channelled through me, so it was really good.(P9)

I fell asleep; it was so relaxing, brilliant... I just used to lie there and relax and think oh I've got some freedom, some time to myself and I loved that..., it helps me clear my mind it gets me out, everything into one and of course its painless and its relaxing and it works.(P12)

Psychological benefit

Personally it did more for me head than it actually did for me back. you get a load of stress in your head and your body doesn't work properly, you know that stress is transmitted into your posture and everything else. Some weeks she'd say right we'll just completely forget about your back and just treat you for your emotional problems... (the acupuncturist) influenced that in making me feel better, giving me the ability to feel more positive about myself through going to see her. (P3)

Oh my God, my life is just going, where's it going, suddenly days go into months and you just become aware of all sorts of things, time a, age, and everything. I haven't been able to work... I'm getting worried about how I will ever get another job it's a nightmare. I'm getting sick pay, it's just above the line to be able to claim for income support, I'm building up enormous debt, I can't pay the mortgage, I can't pay it....... what can I do? when I am able I'll man a reception, anything really, collating stuff, anything that's within my ability... I feel I've been treated incredibly well. I feel I've been listened to... I felt supported, I felt listened to really. (P5)

Through the patients' descriptions of pain relief, different types of pain were identified; commonly, severe pain was referred to in threatening terms such as sharp, stabbing, burning, whilst dull and aching pain was considered more tolerable. Two patients reported a reduction in their severe pain, to leave a dull aching, which they considered a good outcome. The relief from constant pain was reported in some cases, whereas for others, the specific types of pain changed in nature. Several patients reported a reduction in the frequency of radiating nerve pain or sciatic pain, bodily dissociation and numbness associated with back pain. One patient graphically described improvement as a sensation of energy flowing, warmth generated, and *"the nerves have come back to life"* (p7). Most patients still experienced a degree of pain during specific household or work related tasks.

"I don't have constant pain like I did before, I know when I do certain things I'm going to get pain, but I don't have it constantly which is a big difference to me in my life" (p12)

The reduction in painful symptoms was not limited to low back pain; two patients reported that their chronic knee pain had been relieved, and another patient was pleased that her shoulder pain was treated during the course of treatment. In summary, the perceived reduction in the symptoms of back pain appeared to facilitate the acceptability of acupuncture.

Improved physical activity. A second subtheme to facilitate acceptability of treatment was the improvement in energy levels and physical functioning. For the majority of patients the awareness of the reduction in daily pain became apparent through their ability to increase physical activity. Several patients

Table 2. Over-arching theme 2: Barriers to acceptability.

Needle-related discomfort

One of the things about acupuncture is when you first start, you go the first one or two times and come out feeling slightly sore, not so much sore from the needles but just slightly worse in general. There seems to be a bit of an adverse effect and this has always happened. But as the success builds up then of course that doesn't happen… it's a dull sore ache but this was only for the first one or two times. My very last session… she really hit the bad spots with the needles and I asked her to take the needle out. It's the first time in all my acupuncture that I've had real pain not needle pain, you know, the needle going in sharp, but the actual spot being hurt …(P1)

I got a twitching finger for four days, it was on the pressure point here, she'd hit a nerve. I had a very bad week with everything on the left hand side of my spine was agony every needle… she could scrape me off the ceiling with pain it was like a sword and I said you're going to have to take it out and so she took it out and I could still feel the pain. (P6)

You'd be lying there waiting for it and it would be like an electric shock when she eventually got there, and my leg would react sort of jerk and it was Hush. Most sessions were quite painful, the actual insertion of the needles.(P7)

I had some needles in my hand for some reason… she had to take them out because my fingers just were numb, I got pins and needles so she said I'll take them straight out. So she'd obviously hit a point where, probably a nerve or something. (P8)

Temporary worsening of symptoms

Sometimes when I got back I would feel, you know, a bit worse for wear. … one or two occasions it felt worse actually, but I'm not sure how much that's then what I have gone on to do…. generally it only lasted a day and a night… I might not sleep so well that night, occasionally its gone on till I've had the next acupuncture, or almost… it's just been wearing off when I've gone back for more torture.(P5)

The treatment did knock me about a bit to begin with, you know I felt worse to be honest. I'd got aches and pains all over my body and I was really, really, stiff.. I'd start to feel it within a couple of hours or so and then you start to feel all achey and thinking 'oh golly'… is this really working, I feel worse now than I did before I went. (P8)

Five or six into the sessions when she nearly killed me… It just started really aching. Ached and ached and I got no sleep that night… It was really very, very, bad and it lasted the following day and the day after…it was just so severe, all the burning came back, I felt shattered the following day, no sleep (P10)

I had all that treatment yesterday and it hasn't done any good for me, in fact I'm worse… I haven't done anything since yesterday to make it worse… So why should I be so bad this morning? I mean it could be a positive thing I suppose.(P11)

Tiredness

I'm always glad I've been, and I always feel better after it, although it does tend to tire you out, but that's ok, that doesn't matter, you know it means you feel relaxed, very relaxed. I'd yawn a lot, yawn like the devil all the way home. I did it for the first three treatments. You know you feel a bit spaced out, you feel warm and a bit tingly/ I had this tremendous yawning and desire to lay down, you know, which I do, I'd come back and lay down or just relax.(P3)

The first 2 or 3 sessions she said I'd be tired but I was literally yawning at the bus stop. It lasted for a couple of hours in the morning I think, Yeah, I found myself incredibly tired, Yawning away. Suddenly it seemed to come on, it was incredible. It didn't happen every one, but I noticed it the first 2 or 3, you know I don't normally stand yawning in the middle of the day (P4)

I used to feel very tired… It was just a progression maybe of just your body saying you know you needed time to heal, and I would just go with it and not want anything else from myself, just have the treatment and set that time aside just to go through."(P9)

Pressure to continue

She talked about, well look, ten is not really enough, I think we should consider more…(P1)

I don't think it is doing me any good you know, and yet I keep going and paying them money.. their care of you and their courtesy is you know second to none they are so nice, and the privacy and everything… that's very special, and you don't get that from your GP do you?(P11)

Financial cost

I felt she was trying to sell me things which I don't think should have been part of the trial… I felt if I hadn't thought about it, it could have been a bit of pressure on people… there is the potential for not so much being ripped off, but being misused. (P1)

I'd always longed to try acupuncture but couldn't afford it because they won't put it on the NHS….If my back plays up I will go for a session of acupuncture and I will get rid of it instead of moaning about it…as long as I can afford it. (P6)

She suggested some tablets so I said well I'll give them a try, so I bought them off her and I got home and they were twelve months out of date, so I had to ring her up and say are they going to do me any harm? and she says well the strength will have gone out of them, so we left it alone and the problem cleared up on its own eventually. (P8)

---

compared their levels of activity before and after acupuncture. Their descriptions allude to the debilitating nature of chronic pain and illustrate how pain regularly interrupted everyday tasks, whereby short periods of rest were necessary in order to complete the task in hand. Over the course of treatment, several patients noticed an increase in their level of energy, which enabled them to complete daily chores more easily.

> "My energy level has increased. I can now cook a meal without having to lie down every couple of minutes in between doing something, which is better". (p5)

The salience of improved physical function differed; for one patient the ability to conduct self-care and simple activities of daily living were a very positive aspect. For several others the improvement in energy levels meant they could engage in beneficial exercise, an aspect that helped to focus the patient on their abilities rather than disability. This served to reduce frustration and, for some, led to being able to engage in gentle exercise activities to help regain strength and fitness. These positive outcomes in functioning were a welcome effect of the treatment.

> "You can get about; you can do things you're not just kind of stuck to a chair or confined to the house… I like to go swimming which you know I couldn't do and I've done it since the treatment. I've been back swimming I do that, and I hoover up now, which I didn't do before and I've done a lot of walking" (p8).

Table 3. Over-arching theme 3; Mediating factors.

Pre-treatment mediators

Expectation

I know it works, ... I am expecting a very high success rate from this trial.(P1)

It was something I had experienced before so I had no fear of it...I thought it will help.(P3)

My friends sister and her partner are both acupuncturists and they gave me some acupuncture and particularly (name) just literally used about four needles ad it helped tremendously, almost immediately. So therefore, I felt this was going to help.(P4)

I'm sure it (acupuncture) still does work for people. I'm sure that another form of acupuncture for me you know would work(P5)

I had to believe you see, you've got to believe in it, you've got to persevere...How on earth do you expect to get better if you don't believe in it...I expected it to work more quickly.(P7)

I didn't really know what I was hoping for I just wanted to get rid of this pain...I know of an instance second-hand where someone else has had treatment and it hasn't done anything for them. (P8)

Prior I was always positive about going and my expectations were unknown because I didn't know what to expect...I welcomed it really to give me the opportunity to try something that was away from trying drugs(p9)

I was a bit doubtful whether this would work... but quite willing to try it because I was in such a lot of pain.... (P11)

I was very excited, because anything to help my back problem I was prepared to try, anything...nothing else has helped... I couldn't expect a complete cure for it (P12)

Treatment related mediators

Time

One of the interesting things is that they were 45 minute sessions and I had the needles in for say 35 minutes. Compared with when I am having it for my knee, it is no more than 10 minutes.... I know with Doc X if he carries on the treatment if I have any more back problems he will just do the 10 minute sessions.(P1)

I wasn't benefiting (from acupuncture) and I found it interfered. If I was benefitting then I would have taken time aside, but I had started getting busy with work.(P4)

Generally speaking the impression you get at the doctors' is that you're one of hundreds of thousands, they want to get you in and out as quickly as possible. It's not their fault that they haven't got time.(P7)

She made me feel that when I went it was my time, that she was totally focussed on what she was doing for me and you know the continuity of the treatment... there was an hour set aside for me, instead of going to the Drs surgery and feeling that you know you had to remember everything you wanted to say, instead of doing that you were going to somebody you knew, you know you'd gone through the back ground they know what they were looking for, they knew what they were going to work on, and when you went they were prepared for you to continue treatment.(P9)

Blow the GP, because you wait to get in to see your GP, you can be waiting months and months to go for an appointment elsewhere, whereas all you've got to do is phone and say can I see so- an-so. (P10)

Part of it is slightly that Acupuncturist is busy going from room to room. There is little problem about that I think that you know that she is not with you all the time and she's moving off to somebody else and then coming back and so she must be distracted, it's quite difficult when she knows people are waiting for her, so she's trying to give you the time, and yet she, so it's the same system as in the Health Service, in the one sense in that yes there are always time constraints.(P11)

The therapeutic relationship

I don't tend to go to the Drs for any treatment for it, cos they don't seem to know much about backs...It's a different sort of thing isn't it the way the Dr treats you.... Uhm they just diagnose things don't they... I find my Dr a very sympathetic Dr, so I can easily you know, if I have problems I tell him. He's a really good Dr, he's lovely... he's really sort of enthusiastic. So he's nice, he's a good doctor.(P4)

She was very very good... very involved, and I felt that she knew me as a person, that when I was going I was actually getting really good one to one treatment... I felt she cared about what she was doing and that was really important to me. I felt I had a really good rapport with her. I felt that she had a sensitivity to how I was feeling and she gave me great consideration, and she empathised and awful lot with what I'd been through and the problems that I'd had. I built a very big sort of bond with her because I trusted her and what she was doing, and that to me was a big issue, that I actually trusted somebody to give me the treatment after having really problems before... that was really important (P9).

But I think with backs GPs just don't know what they are talking about. They just don't know. You have to go to someone that is a specialist.... if I do need to go back then I shan't go to my GP. When I went I didn't actually see my GP, I saw a locum and she laid me on the bed and out me through some exercises, my leg this way, that way, examine my back and she said I really can't I do anything for you... She gave me a couple of sheets to do some exercises. I only did them for one day, it nearly killed me. I was in total agony, so I thought this is a waste of time (P10)

I don't think it is doing me any good you know and yet I keep going and paying them money.. their care of you and their courtesy is you know second to none, I mean you just can't fault it, its absolutely superb you know its absolutely superb.... they are so nice, and their care of you and their concern for you and the privacy and everything. That's very special, and you don't get that from your GP do you? They are so patient with you, so kind and so non-judgemental. (P11)

Lifestyle advice

I've got a good strong back, I could lift you up; like that but it wouldn't do my back any good. You can actually do it, you can use all you muscles, physically and sometimes it'll be perfectly alright and other times all you have to do is go like that and it goes you know. (P3)

She asked me once if I felt the weight had anything to do with it... I can remember we talked about something to do with that,...they only tell you to lose weight if you go to the Dr, and I said I've tried and tried over years and years losing weight and I didn't want to be told again, you know. So it wasn't like an option to help me... The things is, things are easing, but it's nothing to do with the acupuncture, it's because I'm losing some weight (P4)

I do my yoga, I can't do the full lotus, I can't do the splits yet, I'm not happy with my neck because I can't do the plough. I can't switch over and put my knees there. I'm not happy. Yesterday I got off the floor in a full crab... going backwards is hard tilting backwards is painful, it doesn't hurt until I try to bend backwards to do a full crab. I'm doing my exercises every morning... I've been to the gym and there are special exercises I can do to build up my back.(P6)

We looked at diet which is quite important... At foods that were cold, foods that were hot, foods that would benefit me because my body had gone cold with the anaesthetic. (P9)

Don't do anything you shouldn't do. Don't go lifting heavy weights... Just take it easy, don't do things... She said no I don't want you to go to the gym... take it easy... she did give good advice, which all except once when I was doing the gardening I followed. I wouldn't say it learned me an awful lot.(sic) (P10)

Table 3. Continued.

She said I should try some yoga exercises and she showed me a couple of exercises how to stretch from my ankle right up through my hip and how to stretch over to one side and then you turn over and do the other side...the recommendations were yoga exercise and that and to go to yoga generally, that would help me relax.(P12)

Patients involvement in recovery

Like any acupuncture session, there was a good question and answer session beforehand and she summed up well saying to me you eat well, walk well, act well, and here is nothing really to change in your lifestyle. I am certainly overweight with lack of walking but that will come down this year (P1)

I stand over this table which is probably not high enough for doing the job. I can tell when I've been doing a job like that because later on in the day I get back pain.(P4)

I have to take responsibility for getting into this mess. It's a hard lesson isn't it, We are in charge of what we do. I will have to make certain changes. I've got to get fitter, I've got to be more disciplined in doing exercise to strengthen my back and this whole area so it won't happen again, I have to really think about my posture 100% of the time, when I am standing, when I'm sitting .... Be aware and perhaps things then become second nature. (P5)

It makes you take control of your life because you have to make a decision to go to acupuncture in the first place, so you've got to a point where you need to do something... It's like a first step, now I've sorted my back out, now I can start living.(P6)

Relaxation. A third facilitator of acceptability of treatment was a positive, and for some unexpected, side effect of treatment, namely relaxation. Within this subtheme, several patients reported feeling very relaxed whilst the acupuncture needles were in situ, although the interpretation of relaxation differed between individuals.

"While I was there having the treatment I felt relaxed…it was just nice to be peace and quiet and just lay there… It's a relaxant, it just levels you, it levels you an talking relaxes you so that you've got time…you walk home floating" (p6)

One patient cited a feeling of well-being, another reported being able to clear their mind during treatment. Two others actually fell asleep during treatment, with one person reporting feeling revitalised afterwards, an effect that continued into the following day.

In summary, independent of whether there was a reduction in symptoms of pain, the feeling of wellbeing and relaxation during the treatment enhanced acceptability of the treatment.

Psychological symptoms reduced. The fourth subtheme of facilitators of acceptability was the psychological change experienced by some patients. Three patients linked the psychological components and physical components of chronic pain from different perspectives. One patient was clear in saying that the *"awful"* pain experienced from neural symptoms was the cause of their low mood and tearful state (p11). Another acknowledged that stress was a major contributor to poor posture and other physical problems.

"You get a load of stress in your head and your body doesn't work properly, you know that stress is transmitted into your posture and everything else". (p3)

This patient explicitly acknowledged the benefit of a holistic approach, where the acupuncturist was able to prioritise the treatment of his psychological symptoms. Unfortunately, for one patient the lack of ability to find suitable work due to chronic pain and the worry of the subsequent financial difficulty created extreme anxiety. Despite these worries the patient said, *"I've been listened to… I felt supported".* (p5) The ability to share the emotional or psychological aspects of chronic pain with a supportive practitioner, who could include these aspects in the treatment, was an important element of acceptability.

Reduced medication. The fifth subtheme identified as a facilitator of acceptability was the reduced use of medication. Several patients reported reliance on a combination of over the counter anti-inflammatory medication and prescribed analgesics. One patient recounted how he took analgesics as a prophylactic measure before engaging in exercise. Another used analgesics as an aid to sleep.

"Prior to the acupuncture I was taking pain killers for my back to get to sleep at night, and then as the acupuncture progressed I didn't take any for my back… I don't like taking pills because of their effects on the body." (p1)

Most patients disliked being dependent on medication, citing unpleasant side effects, fear of addiction and ineffectiveness of commonly used analgesics as major drawbacks. Once acupuncture treatment had started, one patient stopped taking medication as a means of testing the efficacy of acupuncture. Several patients reported a reduction in the dosage and frequency of usage over the course of the treatment. Overall, reduced reliance on medication, along with reduced concern about unwanted side effects was a further contributor to the acceptability of acupuncture.

Barriers to Acceptability

The over-arching theme of barriers to acceptability comprised three subthemes related to treatment - needle-related discomfort, temporary worsening of symptoms, and tiredness - and a further subtheme on the pressure to continue with treatment with its potential financial cost (Table 2).

Needle related discomfort. The first barrier was associated with needling discomfort. Discomfort due to needling varied across several patients; in most cases the type of treatment reactions reported were transient and mild.

"Sometimes the needles themselves, when they put them in a certain point, they twist them and you get a sharp pain, and they do it again till it's a kind of achy pain" (p5)

One patient described a possible needling injury; one of her fingers twitched for four days after treatment and she/he was concerned that a needle had hit a nerve (p6).

Another patient reported finding the treatment somewhat painful at times, but acknowledged that subsequent physical activity may have contributed to their discomfort.

Reactions to treatment: Temporary worsening of symptoms. Two patients reported an unpleasant worsening of back pain symptoms after treatment, which lasted into the following day, and was relieved by taking paracetomol. One patient had been warned of the possibility of a reaction. The warning helped to reduce the patient's concern and enabled them to view the reaction as an acceptable temporary discomfort with potential for overall improvement (p11). In contrast, warning of a possible reaction led the other patient to assume that the discomfort they experienced was entirely due to the treatment. They did not link the worsening of their symptoms to the effects of an extended car journey taken immediately after treatment.

"I got the most awful back-ache in the car...really really bad backache. I ended up taking paracetomol that night. I think it was a temporary thing, a reaction to the acupuncture 'cos in fact she warned me I may get an adverse effect to it to start with and of course I did", (p4)

Reactions to treatment: Tiredness. Three patients felt extremely tired during the earlier sessions of the course of treatment. For one this was quite unexpected and inconvenient when lasting into the following day. In contrast, the second patient found the tiredness difficult to cope with initially, but later construed this reaction as an acceptable part of the healing process. The third patient successfully managed the situation by carefully planning appointment times. In doing so, the tiredness they experienced became part of their relaxation routine, and was viewed as recovery time.

"I used to feel very tired... It was just a progression maybe of just your body saying you know you needed time to heal...I intentionally used to make my appointments later on in the day so I could come home and relax." (p9)

Several patients had previous experience of acupuncture and expected minor discomfort as an acceptable risk as part of the treatment. Although some patients continued to experience unpleasant reactions in later sessions, they had also experienced some benefit and persevered with the course of treatment. For a minority, these reactions detracted from the overall acceptability of the treatment, particularly where any overall benefit from treatment was less than expected.

Pressure to continue treatment and potential financial cost. The fourth barrier to acceptability was the pressure to continue with treatment after the course of treatment paid for by the YACBAC trial had ended. None of the twelve people interviewed reported 100% pain relief without later recurrence of some of the back pain symptoms. Several patients were still in pain at the end of the 10 session course and reported that their acupuncturist had suggested one or two (or more) treatments as a private patient. Two patients welcomed the opportunity to continue. Another, who had not experienced pain relief felt unsure, but had appreciated the care and concern they had received and agreed to pay for additional sessions in the hope that it would work eventually.

"She suggested it; it was her who suggested five more because she thought... she was hoping we would have cracked it really in five more sessions. I mean that must have been at the time when we were still feeling there was some improvement being maintained". (p12)

Two more patients would have liked to continued treatment, or would have considered treatment in the future, but were constrained by the financial cost of each session. Another patient tried to have the treatment continued via the GP but was told that funds were not available. In summary, patients found the cost of treatment more acceptable if they were experiencing some benefits, however, where the benefit was in question, or if they felt pressured to pay or could not pay, then the pressure to continue treatment and the potential financial cost of ongoing treatment were not acceptable.

Mediating Factors

The third over-arching theme is that of mediating factors, which could potentially influence a patient's behaviour, experience and perception of treatment in either positive or negative ways. Pre-treatment mediating factors related to aspects of expectation and previous experience (Table 3). Two treatments related mediating factors, that of time and the therapeutic alliance highlighted contrasts between the consultations with their acupuncturist and their General Practitioner. Two further treatments related mediating factors were life style advice designed to promote and sustain a reduction in back pain and the patient's active involvement, both of which were influenced by the type of advice offered to patients, and the willingness to act on the advice.

Pre-treatment Mediators

Expectation and experience. Expectation of efficacy varied; six patients with previous experience of acupuncture felt that it might be helpful. For those without previous experience, two patients expressed doubt, and were influenced by the attitudes and experiences of others, one had read extensively and was very positive. Another felt excited at the prospect, but realised that the effect may be limited; one was convinced that belief was the key to efficacy. Most patients welcomed the opportunity to try acupuncture because their pain was severe, and they disliked taking medication. Only one patient, based on previous experience, offered an explanation of how he expected acupuncture to work:

"with acupuncture it tends to keep the energy flowing through everything so it can obviously work better...if you've got energy going through properly which is what acupuncture does really, it controls these hidden energy lines which goes through and activates or deactivates muscles really or invigours(sic) them, so if you can organise that and get that kind of thing balanced then your back's going to be straight and that's how I think it works for me anyway" (p3).

Treatment Related Mediators

Time. Time, the first mediating subtheme, represented a component of treatment that had a multifaceted impact that underpinned all aspects of the treatment process. The majority of patients interviewed enjoyed the time spent within an acupuncture consultation and contrasted it with that of a GP consultation. The acupuncture consultation was found to be more acceptable by several patients because it allowed them time to fully explain their experience of pain, receive individualised treatment for their back pain and other concurrent physical and psychological symptoms within the same consultation.

"It's totally for you, not for anybody else, totally for you and its lovely to have the attention instead of being on this five minutes list at a doctors

and they don't listen. They've got to listen to you and she's interested".
(p6)

One patient reported her enjoyment of the acupuncture session as a personal time to relax and reflect. In contrast, another patient who had a pressing workload found the treatment too time consuming for the pain relief gained and resented setting time aside to attend sessions. Even where GPs had given a diagnosis, prescribed several medications and made a referral to a physiotherapist, the brevity of the GP consultation was the overriding memory for most patients. For most people interviewed, the disparity in the time allowed for the GP consultation enhanced the perceived acceptability of the acupuncturists' consultation.

> *It's a very nice sort of atmosphere there all friendly there and very relaxed. It's not like sitting in the doctor's waiting room you know pretending not to look at each other and waiting... You know it's completely different ... well it's holistic compared to hustle-istic in the doctors. (p3)*

The therapeutic alliance.   Underpinned by the subtheme of time, the second mediating factor was the subtheme of the therapeutic alliance. On a superficial level, three patients reported that their acupuncturist was kind, considerate and friendly. For two patients the development of good rapport and a trusting bond were key components of the therapeutic alliance and instilled faith in the acupuncturist's abilities.

> *"She's well trained to do things, she'd know what she was doing... they are more thorough in examining you and ironing out your problems"* (p5)

For one patient, the level of courtesy and privacy was a special feature of the acupuncturist's care. Two patients also comment on the acupuncturist's care, concern and understanding of their condition compared to a perceived lack of sympathy from their doctor. Although one patient considered their doctor enthusiastic and sympathetic, the patient still lacked confidence in the doctor's knowledge of treatment for back pain.

> *"I think, with backs, GPs just don't know what they are talking about. They just don't know. You have to go to someone that is a specialist... if I do need to go back then I shan't go to my GP"* (p10)

In contrast, where an acupuncturist was working in a multi-bed setting in a college clinic and moving between several patients at a time, the attention was not as personal, and the patient was left to glean information from passing acupuncture students.

In summary, for most patients the provision of sufficient time and one-to-one attention clearly facilitated the development of the therapeutic relationship and contributed to the acceptability of the treatment.

Lifestyle advice.   The third component within the theme of mediating factors was the provision of appropriate lifestyle advice. For the majority of patients, lifestyle advice was a common feature in consultations within both acupuncture and GP care. Patients were offered lifestyle advice related to their acupuncture diagnosis over the course of treatment. For several patients, the supportive encouragement from the acupuncturist helped them to engage in gentle exercise and regular activity according to their individual ability and with realistic expectations. In contrast, one patient

seemed to be irritated with advice on exercise as at the time they regularly engaged in exercise that they considered appropriate to help them regain function and mobility. Three patients received dietary advice to lose weight, whereas another was offered individualised dietary advice to help them understand the importance of warm and cold foods in relation to their traditional Chinese diagnosis. Several patients received advice from the acupuncturist about their posture when walking:

> *"She did give me two exercises to do with my hips which I have tried to do. She also talked to me about trying to look at myself in the mirror and see, try to be aware of my posture and also try to walk... keep my hips mobile and keep them moving in the right way really. So it's been more to do with physical posture and things like that"* (p11)

Two patients were advised to take more rest. One of these was specifically asked to do exercise to strengthen their back muscles but very clearly not to go beyond the point where the pain would get worse. The second was advised not to do anything, and to take it easy, and the patient summed up that "I wouldn't say they *learned me an awful lot*" (p10).

Overall, lifestyle advice was reported to be more acceptable when the acupuncturist provided it gradually, over the course of treatment.

Patients' active involvement.   The fourth mediating factor was the subtheme of the patients' personal involvement in their own recovery. Three people reported that the treatment had brought them to an acceptance of their back pain. Two of those accepted that there was always going to be a certain amount of pain, but they could live with that. Another two patients became more aware of their fragility, but managed their back pain by maintaining personal vigilance of their posture and engaging in specific strengthening exercises.

Two patients reported regaining a strong sense of control of their life and cited taking personal control as a key feature of their ongoing recovery, and the importance of setting time aside for themselves. Although acupuncture was not particularly effective for another person, they felt better placed to seek other treatment rather than putting up with back pain. In contrast, two people knew what steps to take in order to manage their back pain, but were unwilling to make changes. One other patient felt that he had taken all lifestyle steps possible to ensure a good recovery, and though capable of lifting heavy objects, he remained fearful of taking a labouring job that might lead to re-injury. In summary, for most patients, the taking of responsibility and being supported to gain control were potential facilitators of acceptability.

> *"The start of curing yourself is to take steps to do something about it. That's an acceptance, you know something's wrong with you and you've got to get it sorted out. It does help to create a positive attitude. I deliberately altered me posture, trying to get it back over a year or two".*
> (p3)

Discussion

Key Findings

The results of this study show that acceptability of acupuncture for patients is based on a complex and multifaceted appraisal of the treatment, which incorporates potentially positive and negative experiences and perceptions. The therapeutic relationship between the practitioner and patient appears to be a strong driver of acceptability, but not the only reason. In addition to offering care and compassion, the supportive therapeutic alliance is a useful vehicle to promote learning, and to develop the patient's self-efficacy in pain management, two aspects that might contribute towards a beneficial outcome and its maintenance. In this study, patients reported a range of beneficial outcomes and drawbacks of treatment. However, the judgment on how each of the benefits and drawbacks contributed to acceptability varied with the patients' individual experience. These qualitative findings should be considered in the context that the quantitative data showed acupuncture had a clinically and statistically significant effect in reducing chronic pain. An understanding of the underlying mechanisms of effectiveness was not considered important by patients in their reports on efficacy or acceptability of treatment.

Strengths and Limitations

Qualitative studies nested within randomised controlled trials are particularly suited to exploring in depth the reasons why an intervention might be successful or not. Our use of in-depth interviews provided a deep understanding of what acceptability means to patients receiving acupuncture for low back pain and presented rich detail of how they interpret their experience of treatment. The bottom-up process of thematic analysis was conducted following the steps recommended by Braun and Clarke. [15] This method allowed the themes to develop directly from the patients' own voices, and enabled a more accurate representation of their experiences without the constraint of preconceived ideas.

Our findings provide insight into a key factor related to effectiveness, namely acceptability of treatment. Acceptability is an important factor because it will impact on the take-up of the treatment offered and the compliance or willingness to see the course of treatment through. We have reported on patients' experiences of acceptability, whether the outcomes from acupuncture were beneficial or not. A strength of our study is that we have been able to qualify the quantitative results on effectiveness with our data on acceptability. A better understanding of the underlying factors that impact on acceptability and effectiveness enhances our understanding of the potential transferability of the intervention to practitioners of acupuncture across the UK. For example, our study adds to the quantitative data by providing an understanding on the impact of the patient-practitioner relationship on the acceptability of acupuncture treatment, and what steps the practitioner and patient might take to maximise the likelihood of acceptability for the patient.

A limitation of the study was the small number of interviews, however, the coding for each theme was congruent across the majority of the sample and data saturation occurred within six interviews. Individual differences were included in the results to illustrate contrasts where they occurred, and to avoid bias in representation. The researchers AK and HM were in accordance with each other on the data extracted and their interpretation; however lack of wider consultation may be a potential source of bias. A further limitation was the minimal integration with the quantitative data available from the YACBAC trial. [16] Although the qualitative data presented here support the quantitative findings that the majority of patients were satisfied with the treatment received in terms of time and attention and were willing to try acupuncture again, the quantitative data provided insufficient depth of detail to crosscheck and integrate with the components of acceptability reported in this study.

Comparison with Other Studies

Willingness to have acupuncture again has been found to be a quantitative indicator of acceptability among patients with low back pain. [16] Our previous paper on the willingness to have acupuncture after experiencing a reaction to treatment reported that the benefit of reduced back pain over the course of treatment outweighed negative experiences associated with treatment reactions. [17] The qualitative analysis conducted in the current study is consistent with these previous findings and complements them by identifying the therapeutic alliance and the active engagement of the patient in their own recovery as a driving force for beneficial change.

The expectation of pain relief is reported to have a significant impact on outcomes in patients with chronic pain. [18;19] However, in this study, although expectation was a pre-treatment mediator of acceptability of treatment, the patients with no experience of acupuncture had a higher expectation of pain relief and reported less benefit than anticipated. In contrast, those who had previous experience of acupuncture were more realistic in their expectation of efficacy. This finding is consistent with the quantitative data from the YACBAC trial population that reported weak evidence of an interaction effect whereby positive belief of those receiving acupuncture was associated with less benefit [16]. The finding is also consistent with research which suggests that perceived outcomes are related to patient-practitioner relationship factors [20;21].

An awareness of gaining greater control over back pain enhanced the acceptability of the treatment for some patients. Within the therapeutic alliance, the development of the learning processes appeared to engender greater efficacy in the patients' personal management of back pain. These findings are consistent with practitioner reports from two other qualitative studies[22;23]. In contrast, acceptability diminished in patients who reported a reluctance or inability to put self-care into practice or make adaptive changes to working practices. This was more apparent where patients continued to expect the acupuncturist to provide an immediate and long lasting cure, and supports Foster's [24] finding that the lack of belief in a personal ability to manage back pain and the assumption of the inevitability of a future with pain, are major psychological obstacles to recovery.

Acceptability of acupuncture treatment appears to increase when the combined processes of care lead the patient to accept responsibility for their ongoing back care, and helps to shift their focus from pain elimination to the restoration of function. This shift in focus creates of an opening for a transition from the biomedical model which focuses on healing through techniques, toward the 'healing through adaptation,' based on a biopsycho-social explanatory model of back pain [7].

Implications for Practice and Future Research

The time allowed for each acupuncture session was an important contributor to acceptability, however, the time-frame needed for the processes of treatment to occur is not possible within the consultation time available within the GP surgery. [6] The partnership developed between the therapist and patient was a key factor of acceptability, this opened up the potential for learning processes to be utilised as a means of increasing patient's self-efficacy in pain management. Our research has reinforced the value of improving patient's perceptions of their personal control over pain and of reducing the expectation of the inevitability of an ongoing back problem and passive progression to disability. Looking at acceptability in this way has opened up the possibility of investigating the mechanisms of action from the patients' perspective, and generates the hypothesis that increased self-efficacy is one such mechanism that may underpin the long-term effects of acupuncture. These qualitative data suggest that the inclusion of a self-efficacy measure [25] in a randomised controlled trial could identify whether those patients who may be already predisposed to improve irrespective of treatment do better, and determine whether or not other patients can gain efficacy in pain management through the processes of acupuncture treatment. Secondly, the optimum time after the onset of back pain for acupuncture treatment to reduce pain and prevent chronicity and disability is unknown.

Conclusions

Acceptability of acupuncture treatment for low back pain is associated with a complex appraisal of the treatment processes and outcomes, and reflects the quality of the care received. Acceptability is enhanced by beneficial physiological and psychological outcomes, and the development of learning processes that engender personal responsibility and increased self-efficacy in the management of low back pain. Dissatisfaction with the amount of pain relief received, and unpleasant treatment effects do not necessarily detract from the patients' overall perception of acceptability of the treatment.

References

1. Webb R, Brammah T, Lunt M, Urwin M, Allison T, et al. (2003) Prevalence and Predictors of Intense, Chronic, and Disabling Neck and Back Pain in the UK General Population. Spine 28.
2. Cedraschi C, Allaz AF (2005) How to identify patients with a poor prognosis in daily clinical practice. Best Prac Res Cl Rh 19: 577–591.
3. Newcomer KL, Shelerud RA, Vickers Douglas KS, Larson DR, et al.(2010) Anxiety Levels, Fear-avoidance Beliefs, and Disability Levels at Baseline and at 1 Year among Subjects with Acute and Chronic Low Back Pain. AAPM&R 2: 514–520.
4. Rainville J, Smeets RJEM, Bendix T, Tveito TH, Poiraudeau S, et al.(2011) Fear-avoidance beliefs and pain avoidance in low back pain translating research into clinical practice. J Spine 11: 895–903.
5. Corbett M, Foster N, Ong BN (2009) GP attitudes and self-reported behaviour in primary care consultations for low back pain. Fam Pract 26: 359–364.
6. Breen A, Austin H, Campion-Smith C, Carr E, Mann E (2007) You feel so hopeless: A qualitative study of GP management of acute back pain. Eur J Pain 11: 21–29.
7. Toye F, Barker K. (2012) Persistent non-specific low back pain and patients' experience of general practice: a qualitative study. Prim Health Care Res Dev13: 72–84. Cambridge University Press. Ref Type: Electronic Citation.
8. Thomas KJ, MacPherson H, Thorpe L, Brazier J, Fitter M, et al. (2006) Randomised controlled trial of a short course of traditional acupuncture compared with usual care for persistent non-specific low back pain. BMJ 333: 623–626.
9. Ratcliffe J, Thomas KJ, MacPherson H, Brazier J (2006) A randomised controlled trial of acupuncture care for persistent low back pain: cost effectiveness analysis. BMJ 333: 626–628.
10. Macpherson H (2004) Pragmatic clinical trials. Complement Ther Med 12: 136–140.
11. Vickers A, Cronin A, Maschino A, Lewith G, MacPherson H, et al. (2012) Acupuncture for chronic pain: an individual patient data meta-analysis of randomized trials. Arch Int Med 172: 14444–53.
12. NICE guideline 88 (2009) Low back pain. Early management of persistent non-specific low back pain. London, UK, National Institute for Health and Clinical Excellence.1: 6.1 Available: http://www.nice.org.uk/nicemedia/live/11887/44343/44343.pdf. Accessed 23 January 2013.
13. Craig P, Dieppe P, MacIntyre S, Mitchie S, Nazareth I, (2008) Developing and evaluating complex interventions: the new Medical Research Council guidance. BMJ 337: 979–983.

Supporting Information

Appendix S1   TOPIC GUIDE.
(DOC)

Appendix S2   COREQ 32-ITEM CHECKLIST.
(DOC)

Acknowledgments

Our thanks are due to Research Fellow, Lucy Thorpe (MSc) of the Medical Care Unit, University of Sheffield, who conducted the interviews, and Mike Fitter(PhD), independent research consultant, Sheffield, for advice on planning and conduct of the study.

Author Contributions

Conceived and designed the experiments: HM KT. Performed the experiments: HM KT. Analyzed the data: AH HM. Contributed reagents/materials/analysis tools: AH. Wrote the paper: AH HM. Revised critically important intellectual content: KT.

14. Thomas KJ, MacPherson H, Thorpe L, Brazier J, Fitter M, Campbell MJ, et al. (2006) Randomised controlled trial of a short course of traditional acupuncture compared with usual care for persistent non-specific low back pain. BMJ 333: 623–626.
15. Braun V, Clarke V (2006) Using thematic analysis in psychology. Qual Res Psych 3: 77–101.
16. Thomas KJ, MacPherson H, Ratcliffe J, Thorpe L, Brazier J, et al (2005) Longer term clinical and economic benefits of offering acupuncture care to patients with chronic low back pain. Health Technol Assess 9: 1–126.
17. Hopton AK, Thomas KJ, MacPherson H (2010) Willingness to try acupuncture again: reports from patients on their treatment reactions in a low back pain trial. Acupunct Med 28: 185–188.
18. Wasan AD, Kong J, Pham LD, Kaptchuk TJ, Edwards R, et al. (2010) The Impact of Placebo, Psychopathology, and Expectations on the Response to Acupuncture Needling in Patients With Chronic Low Back Pain. J Pain 11: 555–563.
19. Linde K, Witt CM, Streng A, Weidenhammer W, Wagenpfeil S, et al. (2007) The impact of patient expectations on outcomes in four randomized controlled trials of acupuncture in patients with chronic pain. Pain 128: 264–271.
20. So DW (2002) Acupuncture outcomes, expectations, patient-provider relationship, and the placebo effect: implications for health promotion. Am J Public Health 92: 1662–1667.
21. White P, Bishop FL, Prescott P, Scott C, Little P, et al. (2012) Practice, practitioner, or placebo? A multifactorial, mixed-methods randomized controlled trial of acupuncture. Pain 153: 455–462.
22. MacPherson H, Thorpe L, Thomas KJ (2006) Beyond needling - therapeutic processes in acupuncture care: a qualitative study nested within a low-back pain trial. J Altern Complement Med 12: 873–880.
23. Evans M, Patterson C, Wrye L, Chapman R, Robinson J et al. (2012) Lifestyle and Self-Care Advice Within Traditional Acupuncture Consultations: A Qualitative Observational Study Nested in a Co-Operative Inquiry. J Altern Complement Med 17: 519–529.
24. Foster NE, Thomas E, Bishop A, Dunn KM, Main CJ (2010) Distinctiveness of psychological obstacles to recovery in low back pain patients in primary care. Pain 148: 398–406.
25. Nicholas MK (2007) The pain self-efficacy questionnaire: Taking pain into account. Eur J Pain 11: 153–163.

22

Altered Small-World Efficiency of Brain Functional Networks in Acupuncture at ST36: A Functional MRI Study

Bo Liu[1,9]*, **Jun Chen**[1,9], **Jinhui Wang**[2,9], **Xian Liu**[1] , **Xiaohui Duan**[1], **Xiaojing Shang**[1], **Yu Long**[1], **Zhiguang Chen**[1], **Xiaofang Li**[1], **Yan Huang**[1], **Yong He**[2]

1 Department of Radiology, Guangdong Provincial Hospital of Traditional Chinese Medicine, Guangdong, China, **2** State Key Laboratory of Cognitive Neuroscience and Learning, Beijing Normal University, Beijing, China

Abstract

Background: Acupuncture in humans can produce clinical effects via the central nervous system. However, the neural substrates of acupuncture's effects remain largely unknown.

Results: We utilized functional MRI to investigate the topological efficiency of brain functional networks in eighteen healthy young adults who were scanned before and after acupuncture at the ST36 acupoints (ACUP) and its sham point (SHAM). Whole-brain functional networks were constructed by thresholding temporal correlations matrices of ninety brain regions, followed by a graph theory-based analysis. We showed that brain functional networks exhibited small-world attributes (high local and global efficiency) regardless of the order of acupuncture and stimulus points, a finding compatible with previous studies of brain functional networks. Furthermore, the brain networks had increased local efficiency after ACUP stimulation but there were no significant differences after SHAM, indicating a specificity of acupuncture point in coordinating local information flow over the whole brain. Moreover, significant ($P<0.05$, corrected by false discovery rate approach) effects of only acupuncture point were detected on nodal degree of the left hippocampus (higher nodal degree at ACUP as compared to SHAM). Using an uncorrected $P<0.05$, point-related effects were also observed in the anterior cingulate cortex, frontal and occipital regions while stimulation-related effects in various brain regions of frontal, parietal and occipital cortex regions. In addition, we found that several limbic and subcortical brain regions exhibited point- and stimulation-related alterations in their regional homogeneity ($P<0.05$, uncorrected).

Conclusions: Our results suggest that acupuncture modulates topological organization of whole-brain functional brain networks and the modulation has point specificity. These findings provide new insights into neuronal mechanism of acupuncture from the perspective of functional integration. Further studies would be interesting to apply network analysis approaches to study the effects of acupuncture treatments on brain disorders.

Editor: Mark W. Greenlee, University of Regensburg, Germany

Funding: This work was partly supported by the Guangdong Science and Technology Department (No. 2008B080703041 and 2010B080701025), the Natural Science Foundation of China (Grant Nos. 81030028 and 30870667), the Beijing Natural Science Foundation (Grant No. 7102090) and the Scientific Research Foundation for the Returned Overseas Chinese Scholars (State Education Ministry, YH). The funders had no role in study design, data collection and analysis, decision to publish, or preparation of the manuscript.

Competing Interests: The authors have declared that no competing interests exist.

* E-mail: lbgdhtcm@163.com

⑨ These authors contributed equally to this work.

Introduction

Acupuncture, which utilizes fine needles to pierce through specific anatomical points (called "acupoints"), has been extensively used in traditional Chinese medicine and has emerged as an important modality of complementary and alternative therapy to Western medicine [1,2]. Many studies have demonstrated that acupuncture plays an important role in relieving pain and anesthetizing patients for surgery [3,4,5]. Therefore, it is vital and necessary to explore the underlying biological mechanisms of acupuncture.

Recently, researchers have begun to utilize blood oxygenation level-dependent functional MRI (fMRI), a non-invasive imaging technique mapping brain function, to investigate biological mechanisms underlying the acupuncture therapy. Several fMRI studies have shown that acupuncture stimulation is associated with extensive alterations of brain activity [6,7,8,9,10,11]. In particular, research has shown that acupuncture stimulation produces brain activation in several regions of the limbic system, such as the cingulate cortex and insula [6,7,8,9,10,11]. However, other fMRI studies showed deactivation in these regions [7,9,10,12,13,14,15,16]. The results of these studies are inconsistent in regards to the responses of the limbic system to acupuncture stimulation.

Traditional Chinese medicine training on the acupuncture practice supports the concept of acupoint specificity, which typically states that a particular acupuncture point has specific functional effects on the target organ systems. Several previous fMRI studies have indicated that acupuncture at specific acupoints can modulate the brain activity of disease-related neuromatrix [17,18,19]. For example, Li et al. [19] showed that acupuncture at traditional "vision-related" acupoints elicited neuronal activity predominantly in the visual cortex. However, other fMRI studies reported that multiple brain regions were activated by such a stimulus [20,21,22]. The specificity of acupuncture stimulation remains to be further elucidated.

Despite extensive research on acupuncture-related changes in regional brain activities, very few studies have yet investigated the functional architecture of whole-brain connectivity networks in acupuncture. Currently, there are several different connectivity approaches in studying functional brain networks, such as regional homogeneity (ReHo) [23], seed-based connectivity analysis [24] and independent component analysis (ICA) [25]. Although these connectivity methodologies have been successfully applied to map brain networks from different perspectives and revealed disease-related alterations, they can not capture the topological architecture of brain's functional connectivity networks (i.e., connectome) (we will return this issue in the discussion). By contrast, graph theoretical approaches allow us to map functional connections among all the brain units simultaneously and to study the underlying topologically organizational principles (e.g., network efficiency and hubs) governing the connectivity networks. Specially, graph theoretical approaches enable us to explore how the entire assemblages of the connectivity networks respond to different external stimulations such as acupuncture. Given that acupuncture is typically thought to modulate and balance the brain activity from global rather than local levels [26,27], the current study therefore exclusively employed graph theoretical approaches to study how acupuncture affects the topological architecture of whole-brain functional brain networks. Specifically, we focused on small-world organization [28], a consistently observed organizational principle in functional brain networks [29,30,31,32,33,34]. The small-wordness is attractive for the characterization of brain function because it not only supports both segregated and integrated information processing but also maximizes the efficiency while minimizing wiring costs [35]. However, no studies reported acupuncture-related changes in small-world properties of whole-brain functional networks.

Given that functional connectivity between different brain areas could be modulated by acupuncture [6,36], we hypothesize that the small-world properties of brain functional networks would be altered after acupuncture. To test this hypothesis, we used fMRI data to construct brain functional networks of ninety brain regions (Table 1) in acupuncture and examined their topological properties such as small-world attributes and hub regions, followed by group comparisons between the acupuncture at acupoints and sham points, and before and after acupuncture. In this study, we selected the acupuncture point Zusanli (ST 36, ACUP) (Fig. 1) because it is the most frequently used acupuncture point in Chinese acupuncture, especially for treating pain, hypertension, gastrointestinal and other physiological dysfunctions [37,38]. Sham point (SHAM) stimulation was devised with needling at nonmeridian points (2–3cm away from ST36) with the same acupuncture method used in the acupoints.

Results

Acupuncture Sensation

None of the subjects experienced sharp pain after acupuncture. The prevalence of various acupuncture sensations was expressed as the percentage of individuals in the group that reported the given sensations. The statistical analysis revealed no difference between the ACUP and the SHAM groups in regards to the prevalence of acupuncture sensations ($P>0.05$). There was no significant difference in the pain intensity measured by the VAS between ACUP and SHAM groups ($P>0.05$).

Global Properties of Functional Brain Networks

Small-worldness. In the present study, we constructed four brain networks for each participant under each of the four conditions: before stimulation at SHAM (BE-SHAM), after stimulation at SHAM (AF-SHAM), before stimulation at ACUP (BE-ACUP), and after stimulation at ACUP (AF-ACUP). We found that the local efficiency was higher in the regular networks than that in the corresponding random graphs (Fig. 2A), but the global efficiency was higher in the random graphs than that in the corresponding regular networks (Fig. 2B). Furthermore, we found that the efficiency curves of actual brain networks located between the curves of the random and regular graphs in a wide range of cost under each condition, suggesting small-world architectures in the brain functional networks. In addition, all the networks exhibited an economical behavior since both local and global efficiency rose much faster than the required wiring cost (Fig. 2). For example, at approximately 15% wiring cost, the functional brain networks reached local and global efficiency of approximately 50%. These findings were in accordance with previous human brain structural and functional networks studies [39].

Point and stimulation effects. To determine point- and stimulation-related differences, we performed two-way repeated-measures ANOVA using integrated measures (i.e., AUCs). Neither the point effect nor the stimulation effect was significant on any of the five global network parameters (all $P>0.05$). However, we observed a significant point–stimulation interaction on local efficiency ($F(1,17) = 5.66$, $P = 0.03$, Fig. 3). Further paired t-test analysis indicated that this interaction resulted from significantly larger local efficiency ($t(17) = 2.76$, $P = 0.01$) at AF-ACUP when compared to BE-ACUP, but non-significant differences between AF-SHAM and BE-SHAM ($t(17) = -0.75$, $P = 0.46$).

Regional Nodal Degree

Network hubs. In the current study, hubs were defined as those regions with one standard deviation larger than the mean of nodal degree over all regions. The hubs identified under each condition were listed in Table 2 and mapped onto brain surface for visualization (Fig. 4). With the exception of AF-ACUP, we found that the hubs were predominately located in the occipital, parietal and temporal lobes, such as the bilateral lingual gyrus (LING), right angular gyrus (ANG) and left superior temporal gyrus (STG). Moreover, we found that the spatial distributions of hub regions were similar among conditions of BE-SHAM, AF-SHAM and BE-ACUP, but changed a lot under AF-ACUP condition. Several frontal regions (e.g., bilateral superior frontal gyrus, medial [SFGmed], right superior frontal gyrus, medial orbital [ORBsupmed], left middle frontal gyrus [MFG] and right gyrus rectus [REC]) became hubs and several occipital regions (e.g., bilateral LING and left STG) no longer served as hubs at AF-ACUP.

Table 1. Regions of interest (ROIs).

Index	Regions	Abbr.	Index	Regions	Abbr.
1,2	Superior frontal gyrus, dorsolateral	SFGdor	47,48	Middle frontal gyrus, orbital part	ORBmid
3,4	Middle frontal gyrus	MFG	49,50	Inferior frontal gyrus, orbital part	ORBinf
5,6	Inferior frontal gyrus, opercular part	IFGoperc	51,52	Superior frontal gyrus, medial orbital	ORBsupmed
7,8	Inferior frontal gyrus, triangular part	IFGtriang	53,54	Gyrus rectus	REC
9, 10	Rolandic operculum	ROL	55,56	Insula	INS
11,12	Supplementary motor area	SMA	57,58	Anterior cingulate and paracingulate gyri	ACG
13,14	Superior frontal gyrus, medial	SFGmed	59,60	Median cingulate and paracingulate gyri	DCG
15,16	Cuneus	CUN	61,62	Posterior cingulate gyrus	PCG
17,18	Lingual gyrus	LING	63,64	Parahippocampal gyrus	PHG
19,20	Superior occipital gyrus	SOG	65,66	Temporal pole: superior temporal gyrus	TPOsup
21,22	Middle occipital gyrus	MOG	67,68	Temporal pole: middle temporal gyrus	TPOmid
23,24	Inferior occipital gyrus	IOG	69,70	Olfactory cortex	OLF
25,26	Fusiform gyrus	FFG	71,72	Hippocampus	HIP
27,28	Superior parietal gyrus	SPG	73,74	Amygdala	AMYG
29,30	Inferior parietal, but supramarginal and angular gyri	IPL	75,76	Caudate nucleus	CAU
31,32	Supramarginal gyrus	SMG	77,78	Lenticular nucleus, putamen	PUT
33,34	Angular gyrus	ANG	79,80	Lenticular nucleus, pallidum	PAL
35,36	Precuneus	PCUN	81,82	Thalamus	THA
37,38	Paracentral lobule	PCL	83,84	Precental gyrus	PreCG
39,40	Superior temporal gyrus	STG	85,86	Calcarine fissure and surrounding cortex	CAL
41,42	Middle temporal gyrus	MTG	87,88	Postcentral gyrus	PoCG
43,44	Inferior temporal gyrus	ITG	89,90	Heschl gyrus	HES
45,46	Superior frontal gyrus, orbital part	ORBsup			

The regions are listed in terms of a prior template of Anatomical Automatic Labeling atlas (57). Regions in the left and right hemispheres are indexed by odd and even numbers, respectively.

Point and stimulation effects. Two-way repeated-measures ANOVA revealed that only the left hippocampus (HIP) exhibited significant ($P<0.05$, false discovery rate [FDR] corrected) point main effect. No regions showed significant stimulation main effect and interaction under this significance level. Post-hoc paired t-tests indicated higher nodal degree of the left HIP at ACUP as compared to SHAM. To further illustrate relatively subtle effects of point and stimulation on nodal centrality, we listed and mapped those brain regions reaching a less rigorous significance level of $P<0.05$ (uncorrected) (Table 3 and Fig. 5). Another 10 brain regions showed point main effects, including 5 regions with increased nodal degree (right REC, right anterior cingulate and paracingulate gyri [ACG], left olfactory cortex [OLF] and left superior frontal gyrus, dorsolateral [SFGdor]) and 6 regions with decreased nodal degree (bilateral calcarine fissure and surrounding cortex [CAL], right STG, left caudate [CAU], right LING and right superior occipital gyrus [SOG]) at ACUP as compared to SHAM. As for stimulation main effects, 4 regions showed increased nodal degree (left superior frontal gyrus, orbital part [ORBsup], right supplemental motor area [SMA], left inferior frontal gyrus, orbital part [ORBinf] and right superior parietal gyrus [SPG]) and 5 regions showed decreased nodal degree (bilateral cuneus [CUN], right CAL and bilateral LING) after the stimulation. Interestingly, all the decreased regions of nodal degree after acupuncture stimulation were located in occipital lobe and were identified as hubs in the brain network (Table 3).

Regional Nodal Homogeneity

In addition to the abovementioned network metrics based on interregional functional connectivity, we also calculated intraregional homogeneity for each brain area [40]. No brain regions exhibited significant ($P<0.05$, FDR corrected) point and stimulation effects. Under an uncorrected $P<0.05$, several limbic and subcortical brain regions were found to be relatively sensitive to acupuncture point (increased nodal homogeneity in the left HIP, left posterior cingulate gyrus [PCG] and left thalamus [THA] at ACUP as compared to SHAM) and simulation (decreased nodal degree in the right parahippocampal [PHG], right amygdala [AMYG] and right THA after the stimulation) (Table 4 and Fig. 6).

Discussion

This is the first study to investigate the small-world properties of brain functional networks in acupuncture at ACUP and SHAM and between states before and after acupuncture. We found that brain functional networks exhibited efficient small-world topology under each condition. However, increased local efficiency in brain functional networks was demonstrated only after stimulating acupuncture point ST36. Furthermore, our study revealed that nodal degree was profoundly affected. at several regions of the limbic system, prefrontal, parietal, temporal and occipital cortices, a finding that is compatible with previous studies in acupuncture. Our results suggested that the topological organization of functional brain networks is altered after acupuncture and the

(A)

(B)

(C)

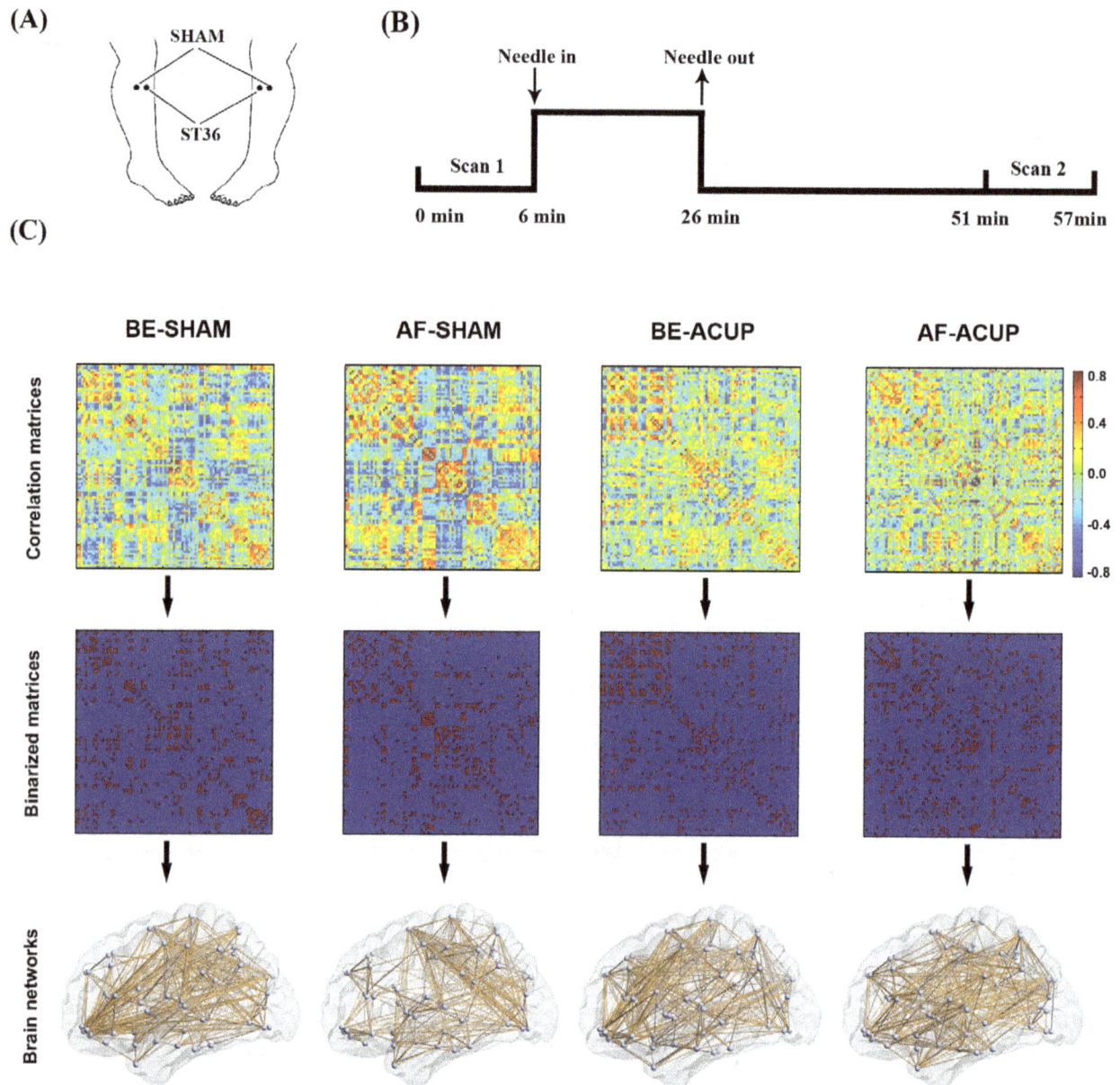

Figure 1. A schematic illustration of the design paradigm and brain network construction. (A), The points of stimulation used in the present study: verum acupuncture at ST36 (ACUP) and sham points (SHAM); (B), Two scans were performed before and after the stimulation at both ACUP and SHAM, which were used to construct brain networks, respectively. (C) Top, under each condition, a correlation matrix was obtained for each subject by calculating inter-regional Pearson correlation coefficient of mean time series among 90 regions; Middle, these correlation matrices were further converted into binary versions (i.e., adjacency matrices) by applying a thresholding procedure such that the elements were set to 1 if their absolute correlation coefficients were larger than a predefined threshold and 0 otherwise; Bottom, the obtained binary matrices could be finally represented as networks or graphs that were composed of brain nodes and edges.

alterations have point specificity, thus providing further evidence for brain modulation associated with point and stimulation.

In the current study, we utilized a specific connectivity analysis method, graph-based network analysis, to explore the acupuncture mechanism. Currently, several connectivity approaches exist, including ReHo (23), seed-based connectivity analysis (24) and ICA (25). ReHo quantifies the similarity of the time series of a given voxel to those of its nearest neighbors, thus only measuring the relationships between the given voxel and those spatially adjacent voxels without taking into account long-range connections. Seed-based approach measures functional connectivity

between a specific region of interest (ROI) and all the other voxels in the brain and thus it only takes into account of the connectivity relevant to the ROI without taking into account of the relationships among other regions. ICA attempts to identify sets of brain regions that are separable on the basis of statistical patterns in their dynamic time series, thus providing information about how regions may be related within subnetworks (i.e., components) but not capturing the connectivity information between these components. Although these connectivity methodologies have been successfully applied to map brain connectivity networks from different perspectives and revealed disease-related

(A)

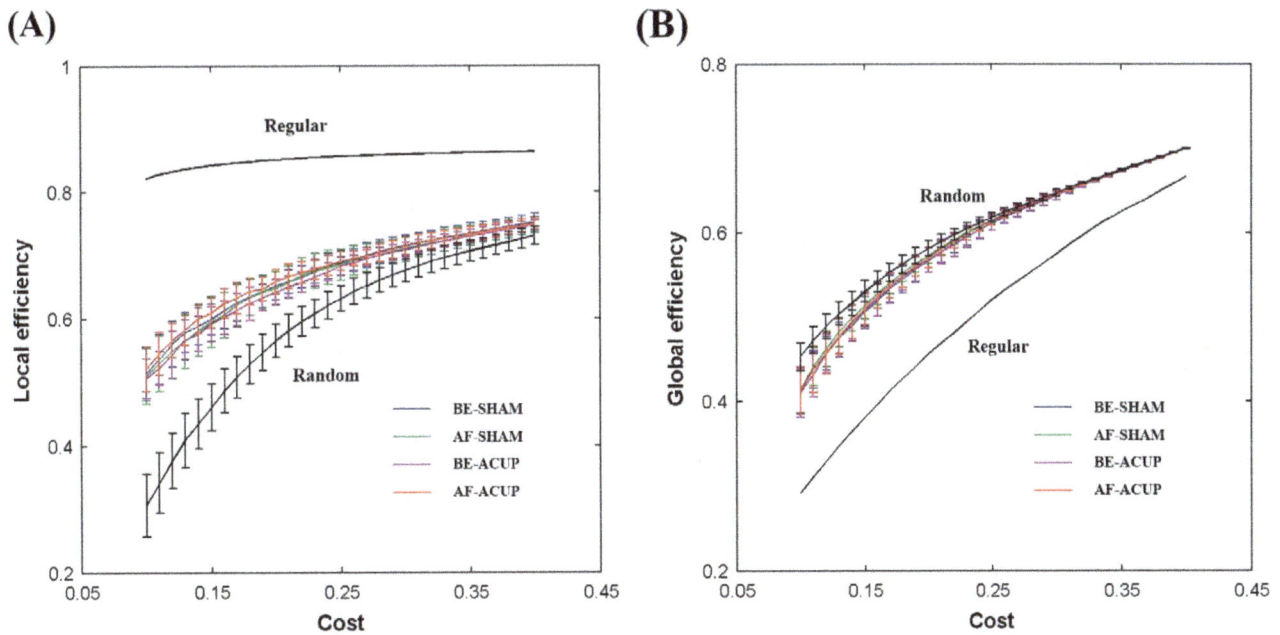

(B)

Figure 2. The local and global efficiency of random, regular and actual functional brain networks as a function of cost. The brain networks under each condition showed higher local efficiency than the matched random networks (A) and higher global efficiency than the matched regular networks (B) at the whole cost range between 0.1 and 0.4 used in the present study. Thus, the brain networks under each condition exhibited small-world properties. The brain networks were also found to be economical because both the local and global efficiency were much higher than the required cost.

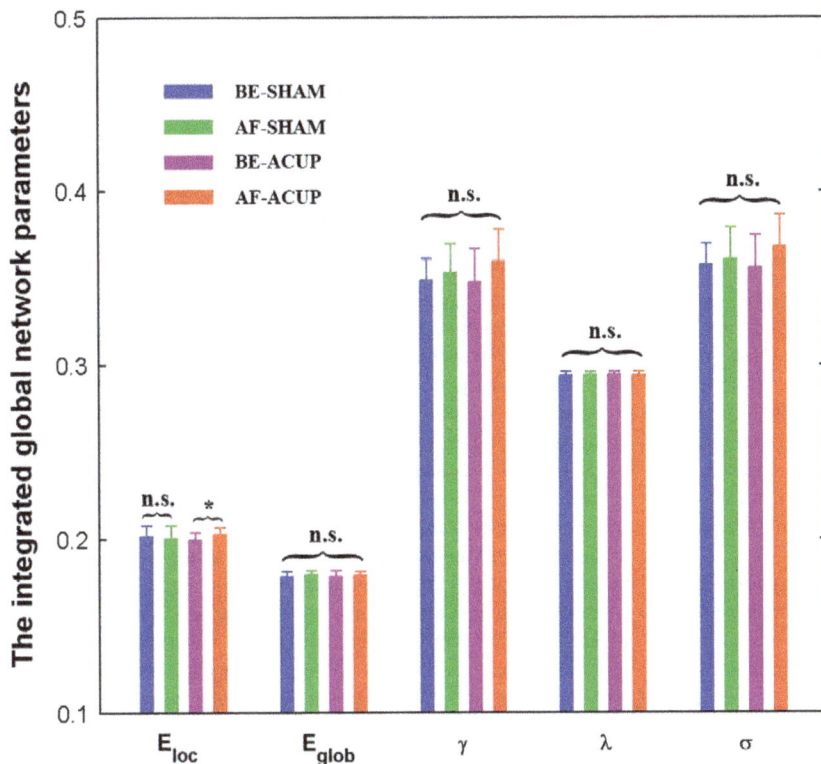

Figure 3. Between-condition differences in the integrated global network parameters. E_{loc}, E_{glob}, γ, λ and σ denote the local efficiency, global efficiency, normalized local efficiency, normalized global efficiency, and efficiency-based small-worldness, respectively. Note that the local efficiency (E_{loc}) was greater after acupuncturing ST36, but not in the case of SHAM. n.s., non-significant, *, $P<0.05$.

Table 2. The hubs in the brain functional networks.

Region	Classification	Nodal degree	Region	Classification	Nodal degree
BE-SHAM			**BE-ACUP**		
LING.R	Occipital	1.47	LING.L	Occipital	1.36
LING.L	Occipital	1.43	PoCG.R	Parietal	1.27
CAL.R	Occipital	1.39	STG.L	Temporal	1.27
SOG.R	Occipital	1.37	INS.R	Insula	1.26
SOG.L	Occipital	1.36	LING.R	Occipital	1.25
STG.L	Temporal	1.32	CUN.R	Occipital	1.24
CAL.L	Occipital	1.31	SOG.L	Occipital	1.23
STG.R	Temporal	1.30	SMG.R	Parietal	1.22
ANG.R	Parietal	1.26	TPOsup.R	Limbic	1.22
PoCG.R	Parietal	1.25	PCUN.R	Parietal	1.22
MFG.R	Frontal	1.23	ANG.R	Parietal	1.21
CUN.L	Occipital	1.23	ACG.R	Limbic	1.21
CUN.R	Occipital	1.22	ACG.L	Limbic	1.19
			PoCG.L	Parietal	1.19
			SOG.R	Occipital	1.19
AF-SHAM			**AF-ACUP**		
STG.R	Temporal	1.44	SFGmed.L	Frontal	1.34
STG.L	Temporal	1.32	MFG.L	Frontal	1.33
LING.R	Occipital	1.31	SOG.L	Occipital	1.26
LING.L	Occipital	1.26	SPG.L	Parietal	1.23
CAL.R	Occipital	1.22	ORBsupmed.R	Frontal	1.23
SOG.R	Occipital	1.20	REC.R	Frontal	1.22
CUN.R	Occipital	1.20	SPG.R	Parietal	1.22
ANG.R	Parietal	1.20	IPL.L	Parietal	1.21
SPG.R	Parietal	1.19	SFGmed.R	Frontal	1.21
MTG.R	Temporal	1.18	TPOmid.R	Limbic	1.21
CAL.L	Occipital	1.18	INS.R	Insula	1.20
SOG.L	Occipital	1.18			

Regions were considered hubs if their normalized nodal degree was at least one standard deviation greater than the average across all regions. For the abbreviation of brain regions, see Table 1.

alterations in these networks, none of them can capture the topological structure of these brain networks. In contrast, graph theoretical approaches allow us to map the entire functional connectivity pattern among all the brain units simultaneously and to explore how the layout is organized and modulated in response to external stimulus, such as acupuncture. Moreover, studying the full connectivity network at a system level conforms to conditional view that acupuncture modulates and balances the brain activity from global rather than local levels [26,27].

Previous researches have shown that human brain functional networks follow a small-world configuration [30,33]. In agreement with the previous findings, in the present study, we also observed the features of small-world architecture in the functional brain networks during acupuncture at ACUP and SHAM between before and after acupuncture. Moreover, the functional networks showed economical properties, which was in accordance with previous human brain structural and functional networks studies [41,42,43].

The topology of after acupuncture signal was altered as compared to the before acupuncture signal. The result showed

an after-larger-than-before local efficiency at ACUP but non-significant differences at SHAM. The local efficiency is a measure of local network connectivity. Previous studies have shown that the connectivity of distinct brain regions can be modulated by acupuncture. For example, Qin et al. [6] indicated that acupuncture can increase connectivity between amygdala with other brain regions including the medial prefrontal cortex, postcentral gyrus, insula and periaqueductal gray. Dhond et al. [36] reported that acupuncture increased not only the default mode network (DMN) connectivity with pain, affective and memory related brain regions, but also the sensorimotor network (SMN) connectivity with pain-related brain regions. These alterations may contribute to the increasing tendency of local efficiency in the brain network after acupuncture. We thus suspected that the higher value of local efficiency after acupuncture observed here might suggest a kind of regional reorganization mechanism in response to an external stimulus.

The regional nodal degree measures the extent to which a given node connects all other nodes of a network and indicates the importance or centrality of the node in the whole-brain network.

(A) BE-SHAM

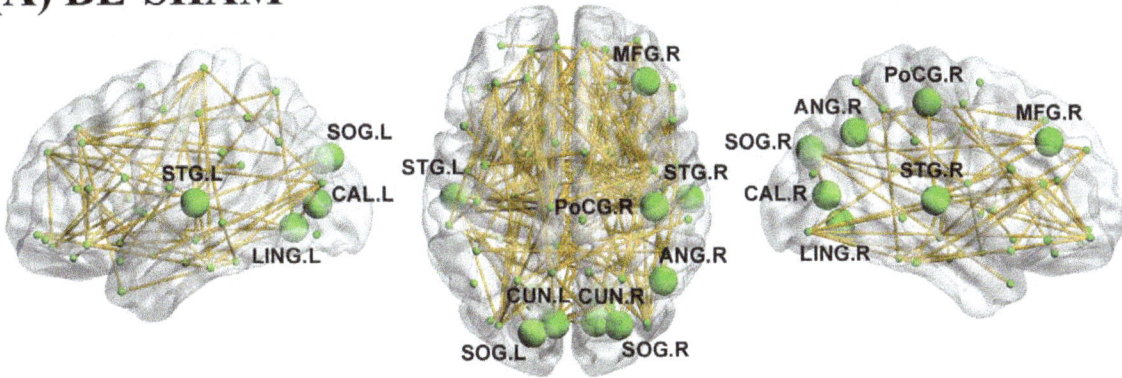

(B) AF-SHAM

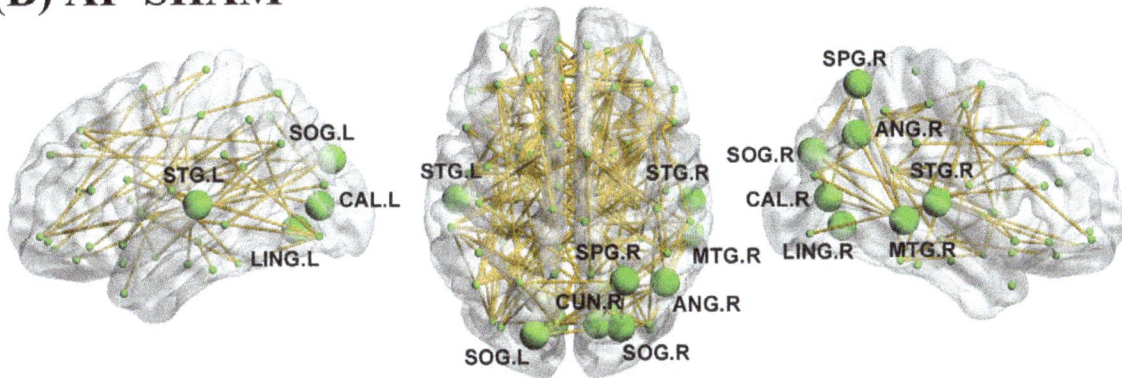

(C) BE-ACUP

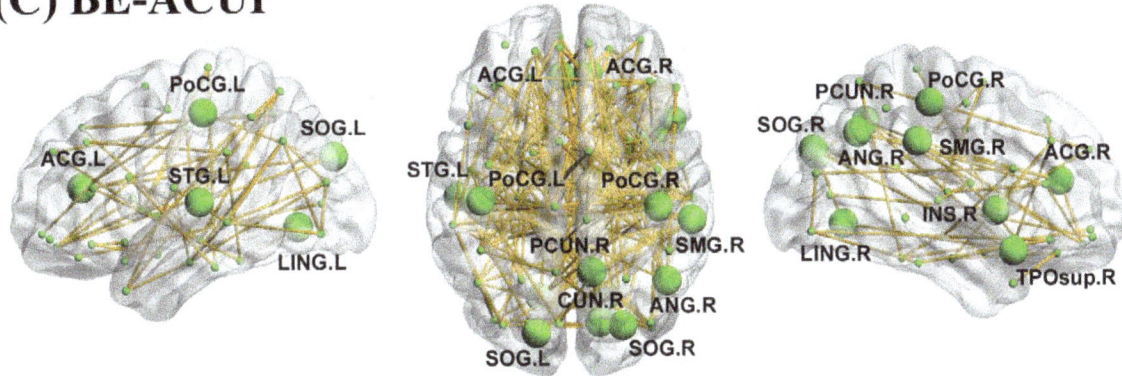

(D) AF-ACUP

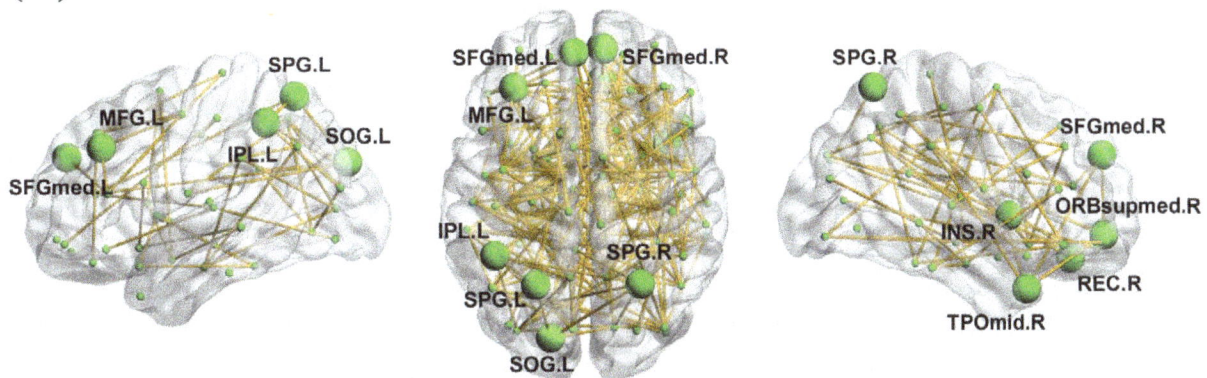

Figure 4. The hubs of functional brain networks. The nodal sizes indicate their relative nodal degree within each condition. Regions with normalized nodal degree greater than mean + SD were identified as hubs. Note that the connectivity backbone (sparsity = 5%) was obtained by thresholding the mean correlation matrix under each condition. For more details, see Table 2. L, left; R, right.

Using this measure, we found several occipital (e.g., the LING, CUN and SOG), temporal (e.g., the STG) and parietal (e.g., the PCUN, ANG and PoCG) regions exhibited high nodal degree and therefore were considered hubs. These hubs were highly consistent among conditions of BE-SHAM, BE-ACUP and AF-SHAM and many of them were identified as functional and/or structural core regions in previous studies [29,32,44,45,46,47,48,49]. Nonetheless, we noted that there were still several regions that were detected as hubs previously but not in the current study, such as medial prefrontal cortex [45]. These discrepancies could be due to different preprocessing strategies, sample characteristics and nodal metrics employed by these studies. As for AF-ACUP, hubs regions were predominantly located in frontal and parietal lobes, suggesting a redistribution of hubs regions, which presumably is due to the modulation of ACUP.

Further statistical analysis revealed altered regional nodal degree centrality associated with point-related effects in several regions, involving the limbic system (e.g., right ACG and left HIP), temporal (right STG), occipital (bilateral CAL, right LING and

Table 3. Effects of interest on regional nodal degree.

Regions	Classification	F(1,17)	Effect	Hub
Main effect of point				
HIP.L	Limbic	6.66	ACUP>SHAM	No
REC.R	Frontal	13.24	ACUP>SHAM	Yes
ACG.R	Limbic	9.27	ACUP>SHAM	Yes
OLF.L	Frontal	8.00	ACUP>SHAM	No
SFGdor.L	Frontal	4.75	ACUP>SHAM	No
CAL.L	Occipital	12.85	SHAM>ACUP	Yes
CAL.R	Occipital	12.56	SHAM>ACUP	Yes
STG.R	Temporal	11.97	SHAM>ACUP	Yes
CAU.L	Subcortical	6.45	SHAM>ACUP	No
LING.R	Occipital	6.17	SHAM>ACUP	Yes
SOG.R	Occipital	4.94	SHAM>ACUP	Yes
Main effect of stimulation				
ORBsup.L	Frontal	14.61	AFTER>BEFORE	No
SMA.R	Frontal	6.56	AFTER>BEFORE	No
ORBinf.L	Frontal	6.42	AFTER>BEFORE	No
SPG.R	Parietal	4.78	AFTER>BEFORE	Yes
CUN.R	Occipital	10.84	BEFORE>AFTER	Yes
CAL.R	Occipital	10.76	BEFORE>AFTER	Yes
LING.R	Occipital	8.23	BEFORE>AFTER	Yes
CUN.L	Occipital	8.09	BEFORE>AFTER	Yes
LING.L	Occipital	5.13	BEFORE>AFTER	Yes

R, right hemisphere; L, left hemisphere. The effects of points and stimulation were determined by two-way repeated-measures ANOVA. The directions of the effect of interest were determined by post-hoc paired t-tests. The threshold was $P<0.05$ (uncorrected). Only the HIP.L survives after the multiple comparison correction ($P<0.05$, FDR corrected). "Yes" indicates that the region was identified as a "hub" of any of the four conditions of networks and "No" indicates that the region was not a hub. For the abbreviation of brain regions, see Table 1.

right SOG) and frontal (left SFGdor, left OLF and right REC) regions. Compared with SHAM, ACUP induced increased regional nodal degree in the ACG, HIP and frontal regions, and decreased nodal centrality in the temporal and occipital cortices. These findings are compatible with previous functional imaging studies [7,12,13,16] and suggest distinct modulation mechanisms recruited by ACUP and SHAM in regulating nodal centrality. According to traditional Chinese medicine, ACUP point is a specific anatomical position of the human body, but SHAM point is not. Subjects receiving stimulations at ACUP point usually generate sensations of DeQi (a series of unique sensations of numbness, tingling, fullness, and dull ache that develop at the site of acupuncture). Although the sensations of DeQi could also appear at SHAM point, there are more varied and stronger sensations evoked by needling at ACUP as compared to SHAM points [30]. Previous functional MRI studies have showed point-related differences in the neural activities induced by acupuncture between at ACUP and at SHAM points [10,13,30]. Our findings of point-related effects on regional nodal centrality reported here indicate that the nodal centralities in brain functional networks are profoundly affected by different points, therefore providing further evidence of acupoint specificity. However, it is worth noting that we did not find significant between-group differences in DeQi for the samples employed in the current study, which could be due to the relatively small sample size. Further large sample studies are needed to provide more insights into this issue.

In this study, we also showed altered regional nodal degree centrality associated with stimulation-related effects in several regions, including the frontal (left ORBsup, right SMA and left ORBinf), parietal (right SPG) and occipital (right CAL, bilateral LING and CUN) regions. The left ORBsup, left ORBinf and right SPG are located in the frontal-partial circuit, which is associated with the attention and executive function network [50]. Increased nodal centrality in the frontal and parietal cortex after needle stimulation was consistent with several functional imaging studies that have found activation in these regions [51,52], which might suggest the enhancement of attention and executive function after needle stimulation. In contrast, several regions belonging to occipital cortices were also found to exhibit decreased nodal centrality. Evidence shows that stimulation of human frontal [53] and parietal [54] regions can affect visual cortical activity. When increasing load of attention and executive function, visual cortical activity became attenuated [55]. Our results showed increased nodal centrality in frontal and parietal regions and decreased nodal centrality in occipital regions, which are compatible with a previous study showing acupuncture-related functional alteration in these regions [56]. Together, the findings of stimulation-related changes in the regional nodal centrality reported here suggest that the nodal roles in brain functional networks are profoundly affected by needle stimulation. Further, we suspect that the cooperation among frontal, parietal and occipital cortex regions could contribute to the effect of acupuncture.

In addition to stimulation- and point-related alterations on nodal degree that measures the extent to which a given node connects to other nodes in a network, we also found that several limbic and subcortical brain regions were modulated with respect to their local homogeneity. It should be noted that after multiple comparison correction, significant modulation was observed only

(A) Effects of point

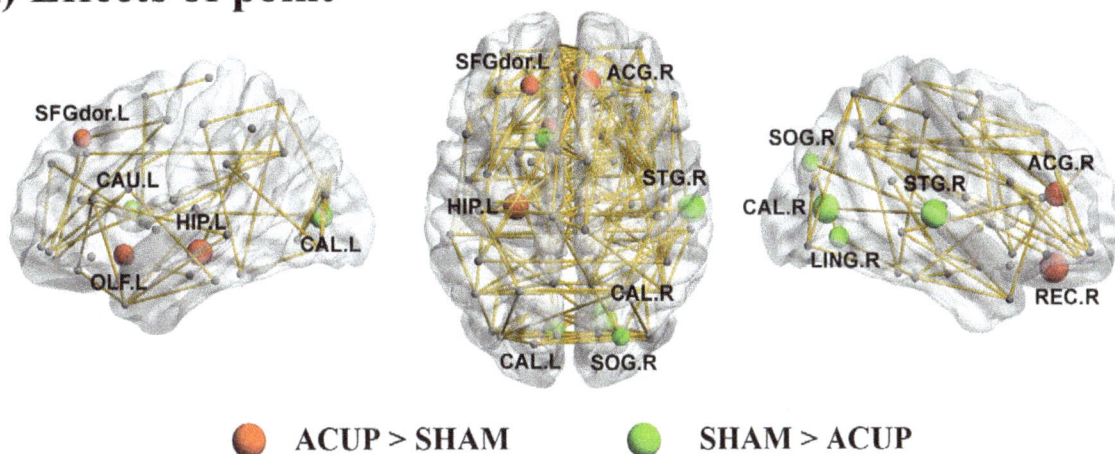

● **ACUP > SHAM**   ● **SHAM > ACUP**

(B) Effects of stimulation

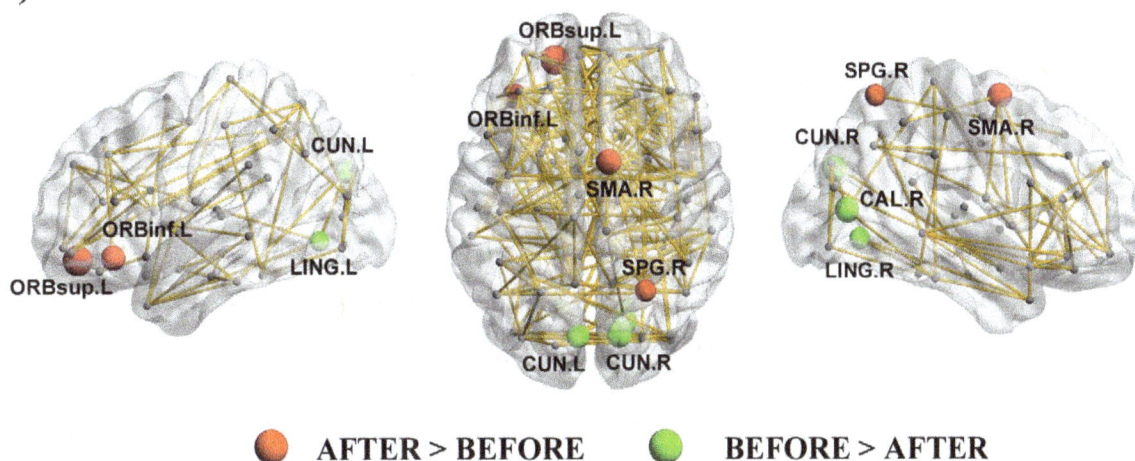

● **AFTER > BEFORE**   ● **BEFORE > AFTER**

Figure 5. Regions showing significant point- (A) and stimulation- (B) related differences in regional nodal degree. The node sizes indicate the effects (i.e., t values) of interest on nodal degree. The threshold was $P < 0.05$ (uncorrected). Note that the connectivity backbone (sparsity = 5%) was obtained by thresholding the mean correlation matrix across all subjects and conditions. For more details, see Table 3. ACUP, acupuncture at ST36; SHAM, acupuncture at sham point; Before, before stimulation; After, after stimulation; L, left; R, right.

for nodal degree, implying the regulation of acupuncture mainly on interregional connectivity.

Several issues need to be further addressed. First, the subjects in our study were healthy individuals, but previous studies found that acupuncture was an effective treatment for pathological conditions (e.g., Parkinson's disease). Thus, studying the effects of acupuncture under different conditions of clinical diseases would be an interesting subject for future studies. Second, we constructed whole-brain functional networks and investigated their topological attributes in responding to acupuncture. Several previous studies suggest that the topological behavior of specific brain subsystems or functional modules is different from that of the whole network [29,57]. Consequently, the investigation of specific sub-networks associated with acupuncture (e.g., pain-related networks) would provide further insights into the mechanism of acupuncture. Finally, the nodal centrality results reported in the current study were not corrected by multiple comparisons, meaning this finding needs to be considered an exploratory analysis. Future studies

using a large sample of participants or selecting a limited number of ROIs can increase the statistical power.

To summarize, we evaluated the stimulation- and point-related differences in human brain functional networks based on fMRI. Our results indicate that the topological organization of human brain functional networks can be modulated by different acupuncture points and stimulations. Together, our results indicate that graph theoretical network analysis could provide an important tool to explore the mechanism of acupuncture.

Methods

Subjects

The experiment was performed on 18 healthy, right-handed Chinese college students (9 males and 9 females; aged $= 23{\sim}27$ years, mean age $= 25.1$ years, SD $= 2.83$ years; mean education level $= 15.28$ years, SD $= 2.19$ years). Subjects with a medical history of any neurological or psychiatric conditions were excluded

216

Table 4. Effects of interest on regional nodal homogeneity.

Regions	Classification	F(1,17)	Effect	Hub
Main effect of point				
HIP.L	Limbic	6.66	ACUP>SHAM	No
PCG.R	Limbic	5.68	ACUP>SHAM	No
THA.L	Subcortical	4.65	ACUP>SHAM	No
Main effect of stimulation				
PHG.R	Limbic	8.04	BEFORE>AFTER	No
AMYG.R	Subcortical	6.20	BEFORE>AFTER	No
THA.R	Subcortical	4.58	BEFORE>AFTER	No

R, right hemisphere; L, left hemisphere. The effects of points and stimulation were determined by two-way repeated-measures ANOVA. The directions of the effect of interest were determined by post-hoc paired t-tests. The threshold was $P<0.05$ (uncorrected). No regions survive after the multiple comparison correction ($P<0.05$, FDR corrected). "Yes" indicates that the region was identified as a "hub" of any of the four conditions of networks and "No" indicates that the region was not a hub. For the abbreviation of brain regions, see Table 1.

from the study. All subjects were naïve to acupuncture and had not been previously exposed to a high magnetic field. Written informed consent was obtained from each participant, and the study was approved by the ethics committee of the Second Affiliated Hospital, Guangzhou University of Traditional Chinese Medicine.

Experimental Design

The experiment lasted a total of 57 minutes and was composed of an initial rest scan of 6 minutes, 20 minutes of acupuncture treatment (actual or sham), a 25-minute resting period after the needle was removed, and a 6-minute post-acupuncture scan (Fig. 1).

Acupuncture was performed at the acupoint ST36 (zusanli, located four finger width below the lower margin of the patella and one finger width laterally from the anterior crest of the tibia) using disposable sterile needles (40 mm long ×0.30 mm diameter supplied by Huatuo, Suzhou Medical Application Company). The needle was inserted perpendicularly to the skin surface to a depth of 15 mm. In the ACUP, the needle was manipulated rotationally with a flipping range of ±180° at a frequency of 120 flips/min for 1 min at 0 minutes, 7 minutes and 14 minutes. The total needle retention time was twenty minutes per run. In the SHAM, acupuncture was carried out with needling at non-meridian points (2–3 cm away from ST36) with needle depth, stimulation intensity, and manipulation identical to that of ACUP group. The procedure was performed by the same experienced and licensed acupuncturist on all subjects.

Most of the acupuncture studies use unilateral acupoint only with a short needle retention time (a few minutes) without any needle rotation. In the actual clinical practice of acupuncture, it is usually performed on both limbs with needle retention time ranging from 20 to 30 minutes along with needle rotation at specified time intervals. In this study we have emulated the clinical practice of acupuncture in its entirety and we thus presume that the results would truly reflect the clinical effects of acupuncture.

All 18 subjects were divided into two groups, each with 9 subjects: one group received ACUP, whereas the other received SHAM, and the groups were alternated each week. To eliminate the anticipatory effects of the acupuncture, the presentation sequence of these two runs (SHAM and ACUP) was randomized

and each participant was subjected only once each week. The subjects were not informed of the order in which the two runs would be carried out, and they were instructed to remain tranquil without engaging in any mental task. To facilitate blinding, the subjects were also asked to keep their eyes closed to prevent them from actually observing the procedures. At the end of each scan, all subjects were questioned to confirm that they had stayed awake during the entire process.

Image Acquisitions and Data Preprocessing

The fMRI data were obtained using a 1.5 T Siemens scanner at the department of radiology of the Second Affiliated Hospital of Guangzhou University of Traditional Chinese Medicine. A total of 180 volumes of EPI images were obtained axially (repetition time, 2000 ms; echo time, 30 ms; slices, 30; thickness, 4 mm; gap, 1 mm; field of view, 240×240 mm^2; matrix, 64×64; flip angle, 90°). Prior to preprocessing, the first 5 volumes were discarded to allow for scanner stabilization and the subjects' adaptation to the environment. Data preprocessing was then conducted by SPM5 (http://www.fil.ion.ucl.ac.uk/spm/). Briefly, the remaining functional scans were first corrected for within-scan acquisition time differences between slices, and they were then realigned to the first volume to correct for inter-scan head motions. This realigning step provided a record of head motions within each fMRI run. One subject was found to have excessive head motion (larger than 2 mm and/or 2 degree in any direction) and was therefore excluded from further analysis. Subsequently, the functional scans were spatially normalized to a standard Montreal Neurological Institute space with the EPI image provided by SPM5 as a reference template and resampled to 3×3×3 mm^3 resolution. Finally, the waveform of each voxel was passed through a band-pass filter (0.01–0.1 Hz) to reduce the effects of low-frequency drift and high-frequency physiological noise.

Construction of Functional Brain Networks

In the current study, functional brain networks were constructed for each participant with nodes denoting brain regions and edges denoting functional connectivity between nodes. To define network nodes, we employed an automated anatomical labeling (AAL) atlas [58] to divide the brain into 90 ROIs (45 in each hemisphere). The names of the ROIs and their corresponding abbreviations are listed in Table 1. The mean time series was then acquired for each ROI by averaging the signals of all voxels within that region. Prior to the interregional functional connectivity estimation, multiple linear regressions were performed to remove several sources of spurious variances arising from estimated head-motion profiles and global activity from each regional mean time course [59]. Pearson correlation coefficients between any pair of regional residual time series were subsequently calculated, thus generating a 90×90 correlation matrix for each subject. Finally, each absolute correlation matrix was thresholded into a binary matrix with a fixed sparsity level, S (defined as the total number of edges in a network divided by the maximum possible number of edges). Setting a sparsity threshold ensured that all the resultant networks had the same number of edges or wiring cost. Given that there is currently no definitive way to determine a single threshold level, we thresholded each absolute correlation matrix repeatedly over a wide range of sparsity levels ($10\% \leq S \leq 40\%$) at an interval of 0.01. This range of sparsity was chosen to allow prominent small-world properties in brain networks to be observed [32,43]. Through this thresholding procedure, a set of unweighted and undirected graphs were obtained for each subject. See Figure 1C for the flowchart of brain network construction.

(A) Effects of point

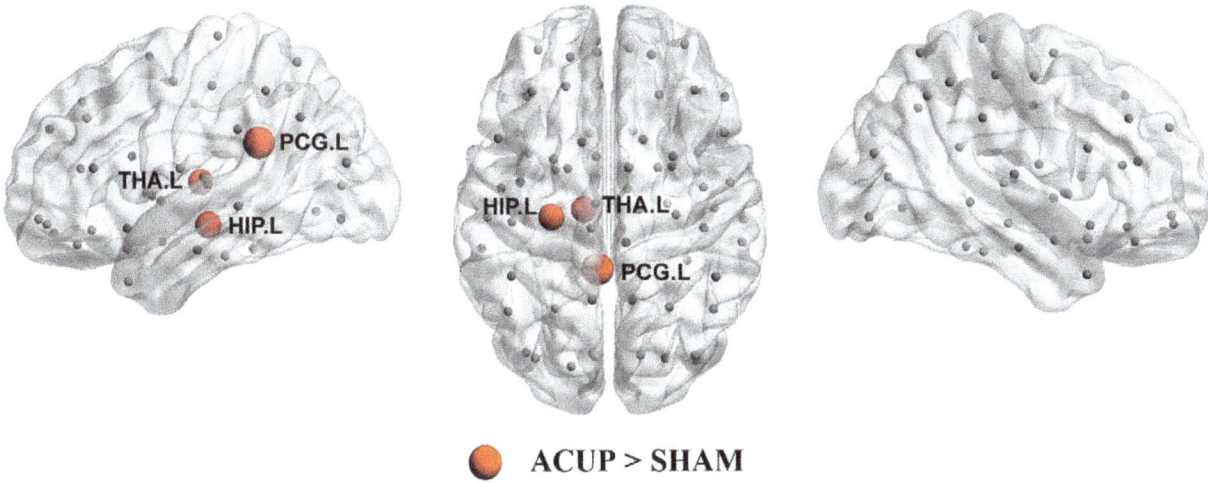

ACUP > SHAM

(B) Effects of stimulation

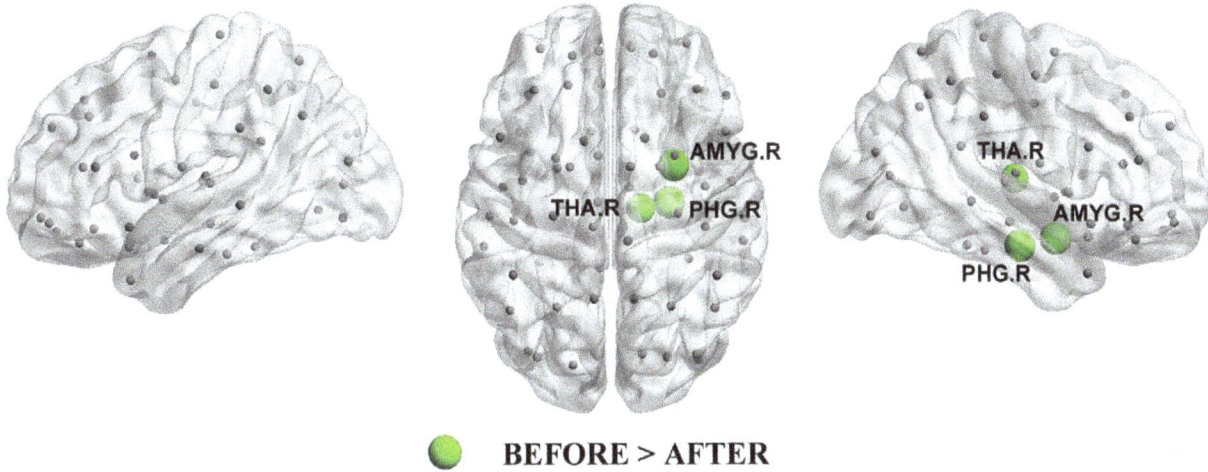

BEFORE > AFTER

Figure 6. Regions showing significant point- (A) and stimulation- (B) related differences in regional nodal homogeneity. The node sizes indicate the effects (i.e., t values) of interest on nodal degree. The threshold was $P<0.05$ (uncorrected). Note that the connectivity backbone (sparsity = 5%) was obtained by thresholding the mean correlation matrix across all subjects and conditions. For more details, see Table 4. ACUP, acupuncture at ST36; SHAM, acupuncture at sham point; Before, before stimulation; After, after stimulation; L, left; R, right.

Network Analysis

Small-world analysis. The small-world model, originally proposed by Watts and Strogatz [60], can be quantified by characteristic path length, L_p and clustering coefficient, C_p. In a small-world network, the shortest path length between any pair of nodes was approximately equivalent to a comparable random network, but the nodes of the network had greater local interconnectivity than a random network [60]. Recently, more biologically relevant measures of network efficiency have been widely used to characterize the capability of parallel information flow in functional brain networks [29,34,41,61]. Network efficiency provides a single measure to capture both the local and the global behavior of a network and can also address either disconnected or non-sparse graphs or both [62]. In this study, we used the efficiency measures to investigate the effects of acupuncture and differences between actual and sham acupoints

in functional brain functional networks. Briefly, for a graph G with N nodes and K edges, the global efficiency was defined as

$$E_{glob}(G) = \frac{1}{N(N-1)} \sum_{i \neq j \in G} \frac{1}{d_{ij}},$$

where d_{ij} is the shortest path length between node i and node j in G. The local efficiency of G was measured as

$$E_{loc}(G) = \frac{1}{N} \sum_{i \in G} E_{glob}(G_i),$$

where $E_{glob}(G_i)$ is the global efficiency of G_i, the sub-graph comprised of the neighbors of node i. Global efficiency and local efficiency measure the ability of a network to transmit information at the global and local level, respectively [62]. In this study, we also investigated the ratios of local efficiency $\left(E_{loc}/E_{loc-s}\right)$ and global efficiency $\left(E_{glob}/E_{glob-s}\right)$ between the real brain functional networks and 100 random networks to assess small-world properties of functional brain networks. The random networks were generated by matching the number of nodes and edges as well as degree distribution with actual brain networks [63,64]. Typically, a small-world network has a higher local efficiency $\left(E_{loc}/E_{loc-s}>1\right)$ and an approximately equivalent global efficiency $\left(E_{glob}/E_{glob-s}\approx1\right)$ as compared to its random counterparts.

Nodal centrality. To examine the regional properties of brain functional networks, we employed nodal degree among numerous nodal metrics because of its high test-retest reliability [65]. For a given node i, the nodal degree k_i measures the connectivity of this node with all the other nodes in a network and is calculated as the number of edges linked to it.

In this study, all the network metrics used (E_{loc}, E_{glob} and k_i) were functions of the sparsity threshold because functional brain networks were constructed over a continuous threshold level (10% $\leq$ S $\leq$40%). To provide a summarized scalar for each metric and simplified subsequent statistical analysis, we calculated the integrated global efficiency, local efficiency and nodal degree as areas under curves (AUCs) for each subject, which has been used in previous brain network studies [29,34,41].

In addition to the abovementioned network metrics based on interregional functional connectivity, we also calculated intraregional homogeneity in the time series fluctuations for each brain area [40]. For a region or node, the intraregional homogeneity is calculated as.

$$W=\frac{\sum(R_i)^2 - n(\bar{R})^2}{\frac{1}{12}K^2(n^3-n)},$$

where R_i is the sum rank of the ith time point; $\bar{R}$ is the mean of R_i;

K is the number of voxels in the region; and n is the length of the time series.

Statistical Analysis

To determine whether there were significant differences in any of the global efficiency, local efficiency, nodal degree and nodal homogeneity, two-way repeated-measures analysis of variance (ANOVA) was performed on the these metrics (AUCs) with points (ACUP and SHAM) and stimulation time (before and after stimulation) as within-subject factors. The ANOVA was performed by (http://www.mathworks.com/matlabcentral/fileexchange/6874-two-way-repeated-measures-anova).

Acupuncture Sensation Analysis

At the end of each fMRI scan, all subjects completed a questionnaire based on a 10-point visual analog scale (VAS) to rate their experience of any pain sensation (sharp, full, dull), soreness, numbness, fullness, heaviness, throbbing, warmth, coolness and any other sensations experienced during the scan [7,66]. The VAS was scaled at 0 = no sensation, 1–3 = mild, 4–6 = moderate, 7–8 = strong, 9 = severe, and 10 = unbearable sensation. Sharp pain was considered to be an inadvertent noxious stimulation [66]. Fisher's exact test and Student's t test were used to compare the frequency and the intensity of sensations between ACUP and SHAM. Subjects who experienced sharp pain (greater than two standard deviations above the mean pain level) were excluded from further analysis.

Acknowledgments

We would like to acknowledge the participants from Guangzhou University of Traditional Chinese Medicine for their time and enthusiastic participation.

Author Contributions

Conceived and designed the experiments: BL. Performed the experiments: BL JC XL XD XS YL ZC XL Y. Huang. Analyzed the data: JW Y. He. Wrote the paper: BL JC JW Y. He.

References

1. Richardson PH, Vincent CA (1986) Acupuncture for the treatment of pain: a review of evaluative research. Pain 24: 15–40.
2. Eisenberg DM, Davis RB, Ettner SL, Appel S, Wilkey S, et al. (1998) Trends in alternative medicine use in the United States, 1990–1997: results of a follow-up national survey. JAMA 280: 1569–1575.
3. Molsberger AF, Mau J, Pawelec DB, Winkler J (2002) Does acupuncture improve the orthopedic management of chronic low back pain–a randomized, blinded, controlled trial with 3 months follow up. Pain 99: 579–587.
4. Witt C, Brinkhaus B, Jena S, Linde K, Streng A, et al. (2005) Acupuncture in patients with osteoarthritis of the knee: a randomised trial. Lancet 366: 136–143.
5. Wang SM, Kain ZN, White PF (2008) Acupuncture analgesia: II. Clinical considerations. Anesth Analg 106: 611–621, table of contents.
6. Qin W, Tian J, Bai L, Pan X, Yang L, et al. (2008) FMRI connectivity analysis of acupuncture effects on an amygdala-associated brain network. Mol Pain 4: 55.
7. Hui KK, Liu J, Marina O, Napadow V, Haselgrove C, et al. (2005) The integrated response of the human cerebro-cerebellar and limbic systems to acupuncture stimulation at ST 36 as evidenced by fMRI. Neuroimage 27: 479–496.
8. Biella G, Sotgiu ML, Pellegata G, Paulesu E, Castiglioni I, et al. (2001) Acupuncture produces central activations in pain regions. Neuroimage 14: 60–66.
9. Wang SM, Constable RT, Tokoglu FS, Weiss DA, Freyle D, et al. (2007) Acupuncture-induced blood oxygenation level-dependent signals in awake and anesthetized volunteers: a pilot study. Anesth Analg 105: 499–506.
10. Wu MT, Hsieh JC, Xiong J, Yang CF, Pan HB, et al. (1999) Central nervous pathway for acupuncture stimulation: localization of processing with functional MR imaging of the brain–preliminary experience. Radiology 212: 133–141.
11. Zhang WT, Jin Z, Cui GH, Zhang KL, Zhang L, et al. (2003) Relations between brain network activation and analgesic effect induced by low vs. high frequency electrical acupoint stimulation in different subjects: a functional magnetic resonance imaging study. Brain Res 982: 168–178.
12. Fang J, Jin Z, Wang Y, Li K, Kong J, et al. (2009) The salient characteristics of the central effects of acupuncture needling: limbic-paralimbic-neocortical network modulation. Hum Brain Mapp 30: 1196–1206.
13. Hui KK, Liu J, Makris N, Gollub RL, Chen AJ, et al. (2000) Acupuncture modulates the limbic system and subcortical gray structures of the human brain: evidence from fMRI studies in normal subjects. Hum Brain Mapp 9: 13–25.
14. Wu MT, Sheen JM, Chuang KH, Yang P, Chin SL, et al. (2002) Neuronal specificity of acupuncture response: a fMRI study with electroacupuncture. Neuroimage 16: 1028–1037.
15. Napadow V, Makris N, Liu J, Kettner NW, Kwong KK, et al. (2005) Effects of electroacupuncture versus manual acupuncture on the human brain as measured by fMRI. Hum Brain Mapp 24: 193–205.
16. Kong J, Ma L, Gollub RL, Wei J, Yang X, et al. (2002) A pilot study of functional magnetic resonance imaging of the brain during manual and electroacupuncture stimulation of acupuncture point (LI-4 Hegu) in normal subjects reveals differential brain activation between methods. J Altern Complement Med 8: 411–419.
17. Cho ZH, Chung SC, Jones JP, Park JB, Park HJ, et al. (1998) New findings of the correlation between acupoints and corresponding brain cortices using functional MRI. Proc Natl Acad Sci U S A 95: 2670–2673.
18. Chung SC, Min BC, Kim CJ, Cho ZH (2000) Total activation change of visual and motor area due to various disturbances. J Physiol Anthropol Appl Human Sci 19: 93–100.
19. Li G, Liu HL, Cheung RT, Hung YC, Wong KK, et al. (2003) An fMRI study comparing brain activation between word generation and electrical stimulation of language-implicated acupoints. Hum Brain Mapp 18: 233–238.
20. Campbell A (2006) Point specificity of acupuncture in the light of recent clinical and imaging studies. Acupunct Med 24: 118–122.

21. Gareus IK, Lacour M, Schulte AC, Hennig J (2002) Is there a BOLD response of the visual cortex on stimulation of the vision-related acupoint GB 37? J Magn Reson Imaging 15: 227–232.

22. Yan B, Li K, Xu J, Wang W, Liu H, et al. (2005) Acupoint-specific fMRI patterns in human brain. Neurosci Lett 383: 236–240.

23. Zang Y, Jiang T, Lu Y, He Y, Tian L (2004) Regional homogeneity approach to fMRI data analysis. Neuroimage 22: 394–400.

24. Biswal B, Yetkin FZ, Haughton VM, Hyde JS (1995) Functional connectivity in the motor cortex of resting human brain using echo-planar MRI. Magn Reson Med 34: 537–541.

25. Beckmann CF, DeLuca M, Devlin JT, Smith SM (2005) Investigations into resting-state connectivity using independent component analysis. Philosophical Transactions of the Royal Society B: Biological Sciences 360: 1001–1013.

26. Mayer DJ (2000) Acupuncture: an evidence-based review of the clinical literature. Annu Rev Med 51: 49–63.

27. Beijing University of Chinese Medicine, Shanghai University of T.C.M, Nanjing University Of Chinese Medicine (2005) Essentials of Chinese Acupuncture. Beijing: Foreign Language Press.

28. Watts DJ, Strogatz SH (1998) Collective dynamics of 'small-world' networks. Nature 393: 440–442.

29. He Y, Wang J, Wang L, Chen ZJ, Yan C, et al. (2009) Uncovering intrinsic modular organization of spontaneous brain activity in humans. PLoS One 4: e5226.

30. Bullmore E, Sporns O (2009) Complex brain networks: graph theoretical analysis of structural and functional systems. Nat Rev Neurosci 10: 186–198.

31. Salvador R, Suckling J, Coleman MR, Pickard JD, Menon D, et al. (2005) Neurophysiological architecture of functional magnetic resonance images of human brain. Cereb Cortex 15: 1332–1342.

32. Achard S, Salvador R, Whitcher B, Suckling J, Bullmore E (2006) A resilient, low-frequency, small-world human brain functional network with highly connected association cortical hubs. J Neurosci 26: 63–72.

33. He Y, Evans A (2010) Graph theoretical modeling of brain connectivity. Curr Opin Neurol 23: 341–350.

34. Wang J, Wang L, Zang Y, Yang H, Tang H, et al. (2009) Parcellation-dependent small-world brain functional networks: a resting-state fMRI study. Hum Brain Mapp 30: 1511–1523.

35. Sporns O, Chialvo DR, Kaiser M, Hilgetag CC (2004) Organization, development and function of complex brain networks. Trends Cogn Sci 8: 418–425.

36. Dhond RP, Yeh C, Park K, Kettner N, Napadow V (2008) Acupuncture modulates resting state connectivity in default and sensorimotor brain networks. Pain 136: 407–418.

37. Chen K (1995) Personal experience with acupuncture therapy. J Tradit Chin Med 15: 203–208.

38. Chen K (1995) Personal experience with acupuncture therapy. J Tradit Chin Med 15: 203–208.

39. Cheng TO (2000) Stamps in cardiology. Acupuncture anaesthesia for open heart surgery. Heart 83: 256.

40. Stam CJ, Reijneveld JC (2007) Graph theoretical analysis of complex networks in the brain. Nonlinear Biomed Phys 1: 3.

41. Zang Y, Jiang T, Lu Y, He Y, Tian L (2004) Regional homogeneity approach to fMRI data analysis. Neuroimage 22: 394–400.

42. Achard S, Bullmore E (2007) Efficiency and cost of economical brain functional networks. PLoS Comput Biol 3: e17.

43. He Y, Chen ZJ, Evans AC (2007) Small-world anatomical networks in the human brain revealed by cortical thickness from MRI. Cereb Cortex 17: 2407–2419.

44. He Y, Chen Z, Evans A (2008) Structural insights into aberrant topological patterns of large-scale cortical networks in Alzheimer's disease. J Neurosci 28: 4756–4766.

45. Hagmann P, Cammoun L, Gigandet X, Meuli R, Honey CJ, et al. (2008) Mapping the Structural Core of Human Cerebral Cortex. PLoS Biol 6: e159.

46. Buckner RL, Sepulcre J, Talukdar T, Krienen FM, Liu H, et al. (2009) Cortical hubs revealed by intrinsic functional connectivity: mapping, assessment of stability, and relation to Alzheimer's disease. J Neurosci 29: 1860–1873.

47. Gong G, He Y, Concha L, Lebel C, Gross DW, et al. (2009) Mapping Anatomical Connectivity Patterns of Human Cerebral Cortex Using In Vivo Diffusion Tensor Imaging Tractography. Cereb Cortex 19: 524–536.

48. Cole MW, Pathak S, Schneider W (2010) Identifying the brain's most globally connected regions. Neuroimage 49: 3132–3148.

49. Tomasi D, Volkow ND (2010) Functional connectivity density mapping. Proc Natl Acad Sci U S A 107: 9885–9890.

50. Zuo XN, Ehmke R, Mennes M, Imperati D, Castellanos FX, et al. (2011) Network Centrality in the Human Functional Connectome. Cereb Cortex. In press.

51. Makris N, Biederman J, Valera EM, Bush G, Kaiser J, et al. (2007) Cortical thinning of the attention and executive function networks in adults with attention-deficit/hyperactivity disorder. Cereb Cortex 17: 1364–1375.

52. Yeo S, Choe IH, van den Noort M, Bosch P, Lim S (2010) Consecutive acupuncture stimulations lead to significantly decreased neural responses. J Altern Complement Med 16: 481–487.

53. Hsieh CW, Wu JH, Hsieh CH, Wang QF, Chen JH (2011) Different brain network activations induced by modulation and nonmodulation laser acupuncture. Evid Based Complement Alternat Med doi:10.1155/2011/951258.

54. Ruff CC, Blankenburg F, Bjoertomt O, Bestmann S, Freeman E, et al. (2006) Concurrent TMS-fMRI and psychophysics reveal frontal influences on human retinotopic visual cortex. Curr Biol 16: 1479–1488.

55. Ruff CC, Bestmann S, Blankenburg F, Bjoertomt O, Josephs O, et al. (2008) Distinct causal influences of parietal versus frontal areas on human visual cortex: evidence from concurrent TMS-fMRI. Cereb Cortex 18: 817–827.

56. Schwartz S, Vuilleumier P, Hutton C, Maravita A, Dolan RJ, et al. (2005) Attentional load and sensory competition in human vision: modulation of fMRI responses by load at fixation during task-irrelevant stimulation in the peripheral visual field. Cereb Cortex 15: 770–786.

57. Luo F, Wang JY (2008) Modulation of central nociceptive coding by acupoint stimulation. Neurochem Res 33: 1950–1955.

58. Zhang T, Wang J, Yang Y, Wu Q, Li B, et al. (2011) Abnormal small-world architecture of top-down control networks in obsessive-compulsive disorder. J Psychiatry Neurosci 36: 23–31.

59. Tzourio-Mazoyer N, Landeau B, Papathanassiou D, Crivello F, Etard O, et al. (2002) Automated anatomical labeling of activations in SPM using a macroscopic anatomical parcellation of the MNI MRI single-subject brain. Neuroimage 15: 273–289.

60. Fox MD, Snyder AZ, Vincent JL, Corbetta M, Van Essen DC, et al. (2005) The human brain is intrinsically organized into dynamic, anticorrelated functional networks. Proc Natl Acad Sci U S A 102: 9673–9678.

61. Watts DJ, Strogatz SH (1998) Collective dynamics of 'small-world' networks. Nature 393: 440–442.

62. Bassett DS, Bullmore ET (2009) Human brain networks in health and disease. Curr Opin Neurol 22: 340–347.

63. Latora V, Marchiori M (2001) Efficient behavior of small-world networks. Phys Rev Lett 87: 198701.

64. Maslov S, Sneppen K (2002) Specificity and stability in topology of protein networks. Science 296: 910–913.

65. Sporns O, Zwi JD (2004) The small world of the cerebral cortex. Neuroinformatics 2: 145–162.

66. Wang J-H, Zuo X-N, Gohel S, Milham MP, Biswal BB, et al. (2011) Graph Theoretical Analysis of Functional Brain Networks: Test-Retest Evaluation on Short- and Long-Term Resting-State Functional MRI Data. PLoS ONE 6: e21976.

67. Kong J, Gollub R, Huang T, Polich G, Napadow V, et al. (2007) Acupuncture de qi, from qualitative history to quantitative measurement. J Altern Complement Med 13: 1059–1070.

23

Favorable Circulatory System Outcomes as Adjuvant Traditional Chinese Medicine (TCM) Treatment for Cerebrovascular Diseases in Taiwan

Hsienhsueh Elley Chiu[1,2,4]*, Yu-Chiang Hong[1,4], Ku-Chou Chang[2,4], Chun-Chuan Shih[5], Jen-Wen Hung[3,4], Chia-Wei Liu[2,4], Teng-Yeow Tan[2,4], Chih-Cheng Huang[1]

1 Department of TCM, Chang Gung University College of Medicine, Kaohsiung, Taiwan, 2 Department of Neurology, Chang Gung University College of Medicine, Kaohsiung, Taiwan, 3 Department of Rehabilitation, Chang Gung University College of Medicine, Kaohsiung, Taiwan, 4 Chang Gung Memorial Hospital, Chang Gung University College of Medicine, Kaohsiung, Taiwan, 5 School of Chinese Medicine for Post-Baccalaureate, I-Shou University, Kaohsiung, Taiwan

Abstract

Background: This study searches the National Health Insurance Research Database (NHIRD) used in a previous project, aiming for reconstructing possible cerebrovascular disease-related groups (DRG),and estimating the costs between cerebrovascular disease and related diseases.

Methods and Materials: We conducted a nationwide retrospective cohort study in stroke inpatients, we examined the overall costs in 3 municipalities in Taiwan, by evaluating the possible costs of the expecting diagnosis related group (DRG) by using the international classification of diseases version-9 (ICD-9) system, and the overall analysis of the re-admission population that received traditional Chinese medicine (TCM) treatment and those who did not.

Results: The trend demonstrated that the non-participant costs were consistent with the ICD-9 categories (430 to 437) because similarities existed between years 2006 to 2007. Among the TCM patients, a wide variation and additional costs were found compared to non-TCM patients during these 2 years. The average re-admission duration was significantly shorter for TCM patients, especially those initially diagnosed with ICD 434 during the first admission. In addition, TCM patients demonstrated more severe general symptoms, which incurred high conventional treatment costs, and could result in re-admission for numerous reasons. However, in Disease 7 of ICD-9 category, representing the circulatory system was most prevalent in non-TCM inpatients, which was the leading cause of re-admission.

Conclusion: We concluded that favorable circulatory system outcomes were in adjuvant TCM treatment inpatients, there were less re-admission for circulatory system events and a two-third reduction of re-admission within ICD-9 code 430 to 437, compared to non-TCM ones. However, there were shorter re-admission duration other than circulatory system events by means of unfavorable baseline condition.

Editor: Jinglu Ai, St Michael's Hospital, University of Toronto, Canada

Funding: This study was supported by the Chung Gung Research Project, CMRPG 890961. The corresponding author and the first author had full access to all data in the study and had final responsibility for the decision to submit the paper for publication. The funders had no role in study design, data collection and analysis, decision to publish, or preparation of the manuscript.

Competing Interests: All authors and contributors declared that no conflict of interest exists.

* E-mail: elleychiu@hotmail.com

Introduction

Cerebrovascular diseases pose a critical threat to human health. The prevalence of cerebrovascular diseases in the study population older than 45 years old was 17.5/1000 (95% confidence interval 17.0–18.0) [1]. Cerebrovascular diseases, such as hemorrhage, thrombosis and necrosis, are malignant and can cause death or disability, which has a detrimental effect on individuals, families, and society [2,3]. According to World Health Organization (WHO) reports, cerebrovascular diseases in high income countries were among the world's top 10 leading causes of death in 2005, and were the second highest cause of death overall. Every year, 770 000 people die from cerebrovascular diseases, and in middle-income countries they are the leading cause of death (3.14 million

deaths per year). [4]. Taiwan's Health Department reported that cerebrovascular disease has been among the top three leading causes of death for 10 consecutive years, and in 2005 and 2006, it was responsible for the second highest number of deaths (malignant tumors were the leading cause of death). Numerous inpatients survive with appropriate stroke management. However, acute stage patients are in a compromised situation that could easily lead to infections, it could result in a sequel of neurological deficits, such as limb, language, bowel control, vision, and emotional dysfunctions. The health burden of cerebrovascular diseases was measured at an annual population prevalence of 11.7/1000 (95% confidence interval of 11.3 to 12.1), and it is estimated that up to 67% of cerebrovascular disease survivors are unable to be self-supporting [1], and 10% of survivors require

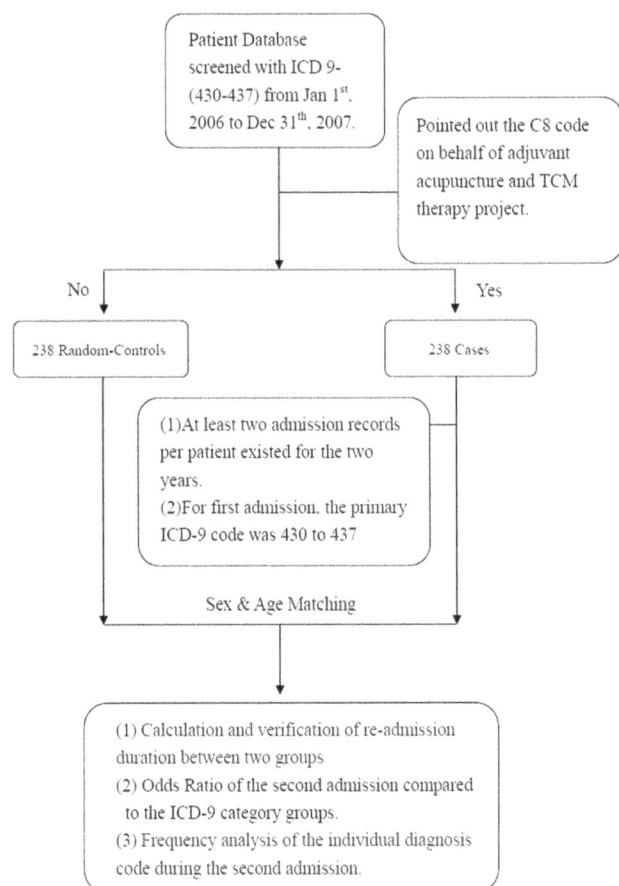

Figure 1. Analysis Strategy (2006–2007).

long-term care in paramedical institutions [5]. Cerebrovascular disease not only causes a great inconvenience for inpatients, but also has a tremendous impact on families. In addition, the cost to the community is high, and effectively managing the medical and social support costs remains a challenge.

Traditional Chinese medicine (TCM) has been used to treat cerebrovascular disease for millenary. Treatments include passive massage and Tai-Chi rehabilitation. Acupuncture and moxibustion have been used for at least two thousand years [6]. Traditional Chinese medicine acupuncturists select specific

acupoints on both the healthy and affected side of the body, based on the Zang-Fu thesis for patients who clinically suffer hemiplegia. Most patients experience functional recovery to varying degrees. Numerous animal and human experiments have indicated that acupuncture can lead to improved blood circulation and induces various biochemical reactions. Acupuncture, moxibustion, and electro-acupuncture could cause localized biological reactions through remote response or systemic reactions. These treatments work mainly through the excitement of the central nervous pathway, and consequently influence more than one physical system, including the central and peripheral nervous systems [10–14]. Recently, acupuncture has become widely used around the world, and according to a statement by the National Institutes of Health in the U.S.A., the application of acupuncture has been recognized for cerebrovascular diseases [7,12]. Studies on acupuncture and moxibustion conducting in China and Europe indicated positive results for treating cerebrovascular disease [8]. A double-blinded study, using computed tomography, found that the severity of neuronal damage of patients who accepted acupuncture treatment was half that of patients who did not accept. In addition, acupuncture reduced the severity of motor paralysis [9].

Since 2006, the Pilot Scheme of National Health Policy in Stroke Adjuvant Acupuncture and Traditional Chinese Medicine (TCM) Therapy has been applied. Our previous reports demonstrated that verum acupuncture, in moderate to severe ischemic stroke patients, might play a protective role against comorbidity and mortality during admission, as well as for 6 months after discharge. However, the studies did not find improvements in neurological deficits [15]. Thus, the severe stroke burden contributed to clinical and economic policies. We therefore conducted a nationwide retrospective cohort analysis in stroke inpatients, aiming for reconstructing possible cerebrovascular disease-related groups (DRG),and estimating the costs between cerebrovascular disease and related diseases. we examined the overall costs in three municipals in Taiwan, and estimated the possible costs for the expecting diagnosis related group (DRG) using the ICD-9 system, and an overall analysis of the re-admission population (including inpatients who did and did not receive TCM treatment).

Methods and Materials

We analyzed inpatient costs using the 2006 to 2007 research database. Ambulatory care costs were analyzed using the profiles international classification of diseases version-9 (ICD-9) code 430 to 437 from the research database of the National Health Insurance (NHIRD) to determine attributes such as in-patient

Table 1 Database of Case Groups.

ICD-9 CM_CODE	Number of Cases (First admission)	Number of Re-admissions	Duration (days)	Age
430	40	20	55.90±60.66	52.85±18.49
431	209	93	67.58±86.15	60.56±12.68
432	0	0	-	-
433	8	6	128.50±109.84	66.83±9.93
434	291	114	67.00±88.55	66.46±12.01
435	1	1	30	58
436	3	1	5	74
437	4	3	58.33±60.75	67.33±2.89

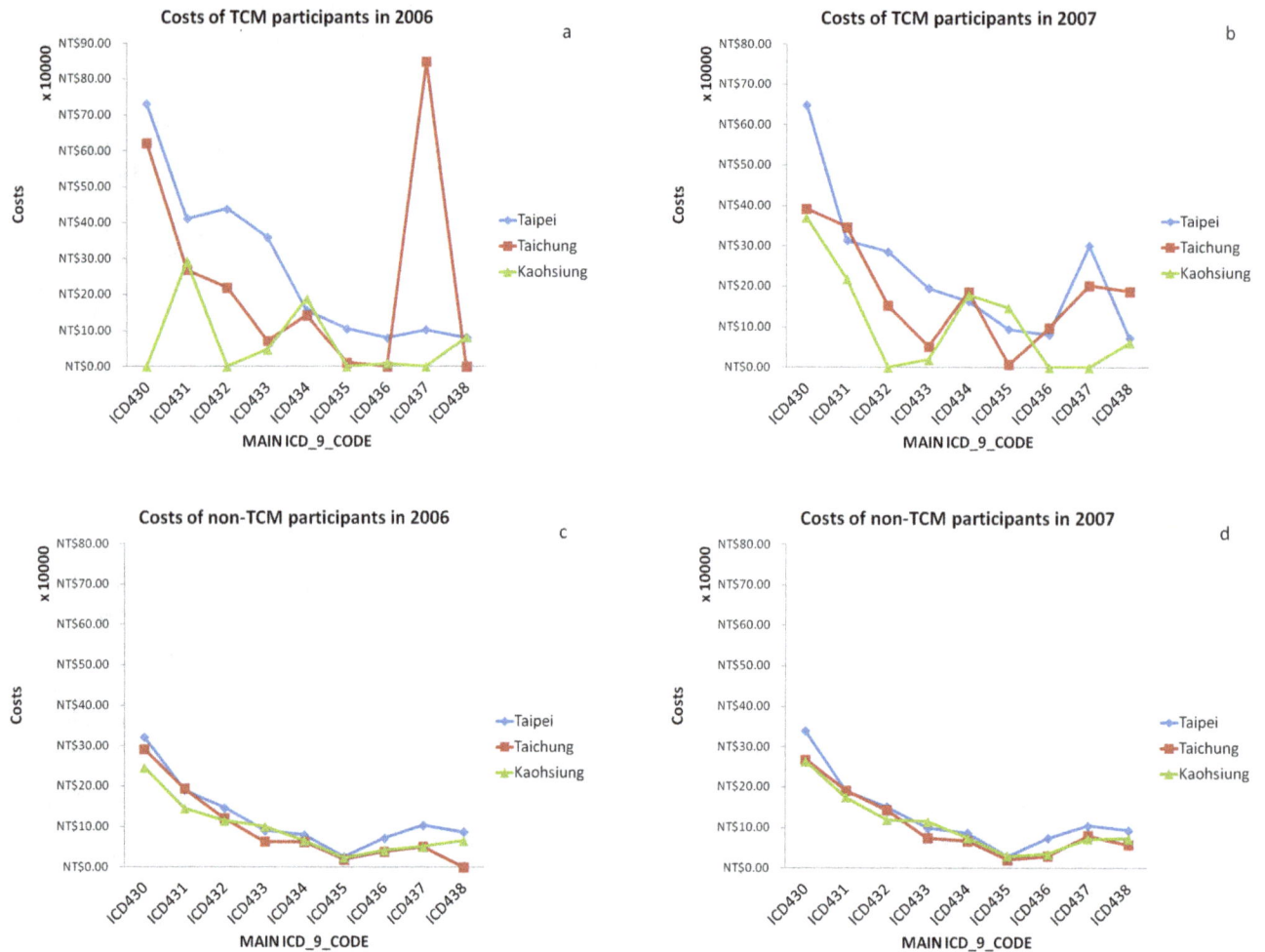

Figure 2. The inpatients expenditures as admission in year 2006 and 2007 (by insurance covered city).

duration-time, age, and sex. The investigation project was approved by the ethical committee of Chang Gung Memorial Hospital (Institution Review Board No.99-1800B). The apriori association rule was used to perform data mining using the primary ICD-9 code to identify cerebrovascular disease-related groups. To analyze expenses, we first combined the identity number (ID) and the first date of admission (IN_DATE) column as an index key to distinguish duplicative data based on a screen of the ICD code (430–437). Second, we classified medical institution types based on column of contract hospital type (HOSP_CONT _TYPE). Third, if the department type for selecting if Chinese Medical Treatment records (FUNC_TYPE) column number 60–69 existed, we considered it as a TCM treatment. In Taiwan, acupuncture and Chinese Traumatology manipulation are classified as one TCM therapeutic method. Finally, to determine whether combined TCM and western medical treatment data existed, we used the ID column to compare the medical records.

Because the detail document (DD document) of the hospital medical costs database is screened under the main diagnosis code bar unit and filtered under a cerebrovascular code from the research database of the Bureau of National Health Insurance, the first time follow-up patient data were analyzed by (1) merging the ID digital number field and the hospital date as the index key, which was differentiated using repeat gender data, (2) distinguishing between medical institution and special category field

outpatient data, (3) regarding the column of interview specialty on medical character, if a TCM code (60 to 69) appeared, we defined it as a rational to distinguish between TCM and western medicine patient treatments, (4) finally, comparing ID digital numbers to identify if any duplications existed in the combination of TCM and western medicine treatments. The analysis of outpatient costs included outpatient visits, and character counting, and was scaled to 100,000 inpatients and the details of the drug and diagnosis and treatments, and pharmacy services costs, as well as information on the amount and average amount of costs related to partial cash payments for treatments. A decomposition analysis of medical cost was conducted to investigate cost trends compared to average medical costs per annum per person. All medical causes of the disease were influenced by age. Therefore, high costs are an accepted factor for aging populations, and result in a rise in total costs. In addition, the average age of the population is growing, which influences average costs. Therefore, the first step of the medical treatment cost analysis was to consider the average age of the population and include an analysis of the population structure. We filtered inpatients out using the ICD-9 code (430 to 437), and included all inpatients that received TCM treatments (case group), and also evaluated the re-admission inpatients database for the 2 years covered by this study. The random-control population was selected from inpatients who did not receive TCM treatments. (Figure 1) The multivariate Cox proportional hazard models by

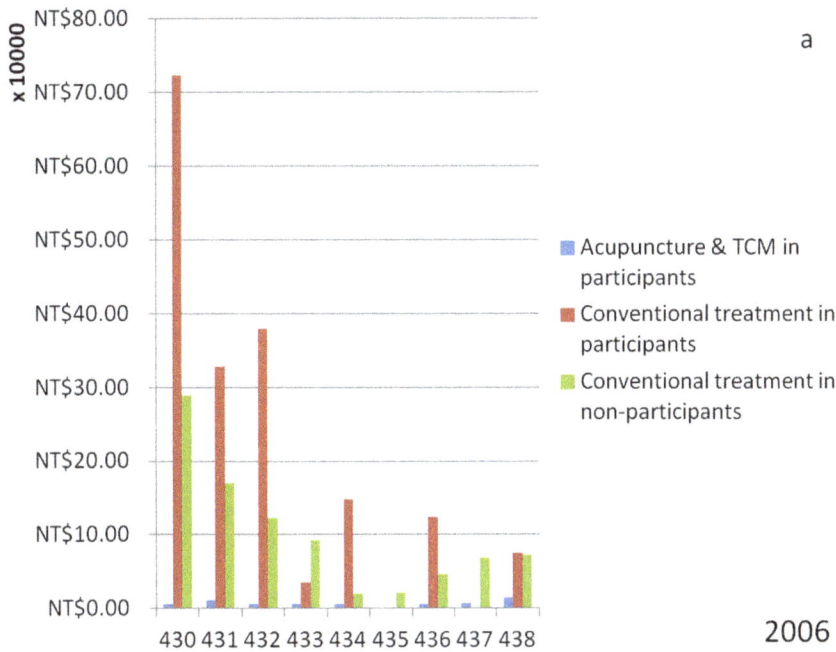

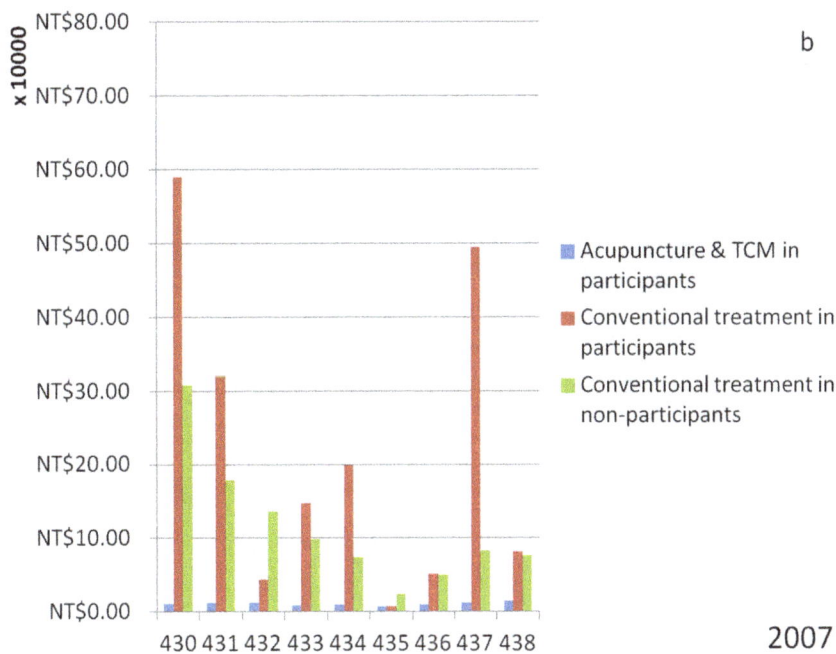

Figure 3. The inpatient expenditures as admissions in each diagnosis related groups (DRG) in year 2006 (3a) and 2007 (3b).

adjusting age, sex, occupation, low income, diabetes, hypertension, hyperlipidemia, mental disorder, anticoagulant medication, anti-platelet medication, and lipid-lowering medication. The odds ratio was calculated by Chi-square test according to 17 disease categories. The 95% confidence interval is analyzed for the significance of OR. Independent T test is used for continuous variable such as age variable. If the sample size violated parametric assumption, we replaced Independent T test with

Mann-Whitney U test. Defied as statistical significance if p value is less than 0.05. The impact of adjuvant TCM therapy on the frequency and expenditure of emergency care and hospitalization after the index stroke admission, were analyzed in the general linear regressions by adjusted for age, sex, occupation, low income, coexisting medical conditions, stroke-related medication, medical center, types of stroke, history of stroke, length of stay, and neurosurgery.

a

b

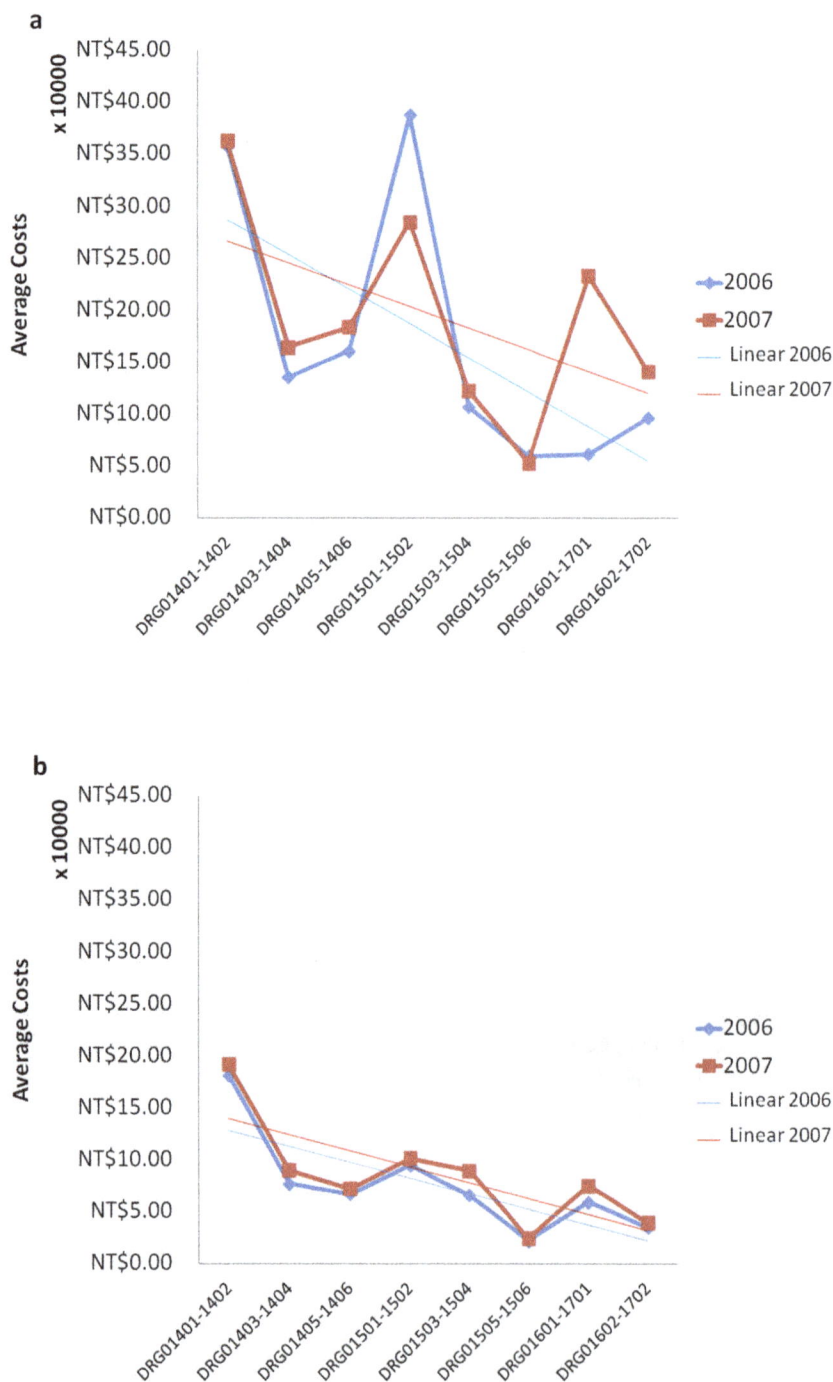

Figure 4. Expected costs of TCM participants (4a) and non-TCM participants (4b) with DRG in year 2006 and 2007.

Results

In 2006, the inpatients' first ICD-9 code between 430–437 as the primary analysis population, random-control group matched for sex, age by propensity score matching procedures. (Table 1) The adjusted hazard ratios (HRs) and 95% confidence intervals (CIs) of post-stroke complications and mortality associated with adjuvant TCM treatments were calculated again in ICD-9 codes. The number of hospitalizations in 2006–2007 was of 3,140,164 people, while the random-control group was 131,789 inpatients (deduction of TCM consultation inpatients within ICD-9 code

430–437). Adjuvant TCM treatment inpatients as the first diagnosis code within 430–437 were 558 inpatients, which including 238 re-admission ones.

Analysis showed that the adjuvant TCM treatment group had less odds (68.4%/31.6% = 2.16) than non-TCM treatment group (87.4%/12.6% = 6.93), favorable odds on non-TCM treatment group by re-admission ICD-9 code 430 ~ 437 (relative risk ratio, 6.93/2.16 = 3.2), 95% confidence interval not containing 1, P<0.01. A two-third reduction of re-admission within ICD-9 code 430 ~ 437 favored the adjuvant TCM treatment group, the difference was statistically significant.

Table 2 Duration of Re-admission Cases and Random-Controls.

ICD-9 CM_CODE	Numbers of Re-admissions	Sex	Age	Control Population	Re-admission Duration (days)		P
					Cases	Controls	
430	20	M: 12	44.17±16.19	3820	66.58±76.09	55.83±61.79	.707
		F: 8	65.88±13.88		39.88±19.99	115.38±173.07	.258
431	93	M: 63	58.32±12.90	21281	63.40±76.77	89.35±142.98	.219
		F: 30	65.27±10.96		76.37±104.04	127.67±170.26	.165
433	6	M: 4	62.00±7.12	4664	143.75±127.23	283.50±232.20	.331
		F: 2	76.50±7.78		98.00±94.75	103.50±126.57	.965
434	114	M:59	62.56±12.38	73784	63.00±78.05	134.21±149.94	.001
		F: 55	70.65±10.14		71.29±99.14	115.77±129.83	.047
435	1	M:1	58	17852	30	167	-
		F: 0	-		-		-
436	1	M: 0	-	6203	-		-
		F: 1	74		5	381	-
437	3	M:1	69	4185	1	222	
		F: 2	66.50±3.54		87.00±49.49	198.00±142.84	.408

We estimated that overall, only 4% of the annual budget was spent on TCM treatments, and the rest was spent on conventional treatments. We investigated three municipals— Kaohsiung, Taichung and Taipei, they are on behalf of the south, the middle and the north part of Taiwan. The medical expenditure trend indicated that the costs for non-TCM treatment inpatients were consistent in the ICD-9 category (430 to 437), and were similar for both years. However, wide variation and more costs were incurred by TCM participants than non-TCM ones during these 2 years.(Figure 2)

The overall secondary costs to western medicine treatment for all inpatients were more in 2006, as indicated by ICD 430, 432, 434, and 436, than in 2007. In 2007, ICD 433 and 437 reported higher costs than in 2006. In 2007, the trend demonstrated that

Table 3 Odds Ratio of Major Disease Re-admission in Cases/ Random –Controls.

Disease Group	OR			Lower 95% CI			Upper 95% CI		
	total	men	women	total	men	women	total	men	women
Disease 1	0.43	0.40	0.48	0.12	0.07	0.04	1.37	1.81	3.45
Disease 2	0.84	1.97	0.19	0.26	0.41	<0.01	2.72	12.39	1.74
Disease 3	0.48	0.96	-	0.08	0.13	-	2.28	7.32	-
Disease 4	1.95	-	-	0.10	-	-	115.49	-	-
Disease 5	0.48	0.96	-	0.01	0.01	-	9.35	76.23	-
Disease 6	1.47	1.72	0.97	0.46	0.43	0.07	5.11	8.21	13.77
Disease 7	0.27[*]	0.20[*]	0.44[*]	0.17	0.10	0.21	0.44	0.37	0.91
Disease 8	0.93	1.07	0.75	0.54	0.52	0.30	1.62	2.24	1.85
Disease 9	1.47	1.17	2.07	0.70	0.45	0.61	3.13	3.15	8.00
Disease 10	1.94	2.00	1.90	0.87	0.60	0.61	4.55	7.65	6.51
Disease 11	-	-	-	-	-	-	-	-	-
Disease 12	1.22	0.48	2.00	0.26	0.01	0.28	6.22	9.31	22.53
Disease 13	0.41	0.64	0.24	0.07	0.05	<0.01	1.82	5.67	2.47
Disease 14	0.48	-	-	0.01	-	-	9.35	-	-
Disease 15	-	-	-	-	-	-	-	-	-
Disease 16	0.86	1.21	0.57	0.28	0.25	0.09	2.56	6.25	3.06
Disease 17	0.50	0.31	0.63	0.18	0.03	0.17	1.29	1.79	2.08

Disease group means ICD-9 category 1 to 17;
OR means odds ratio.
*means $P < .01$, favors random-controls.

a

b

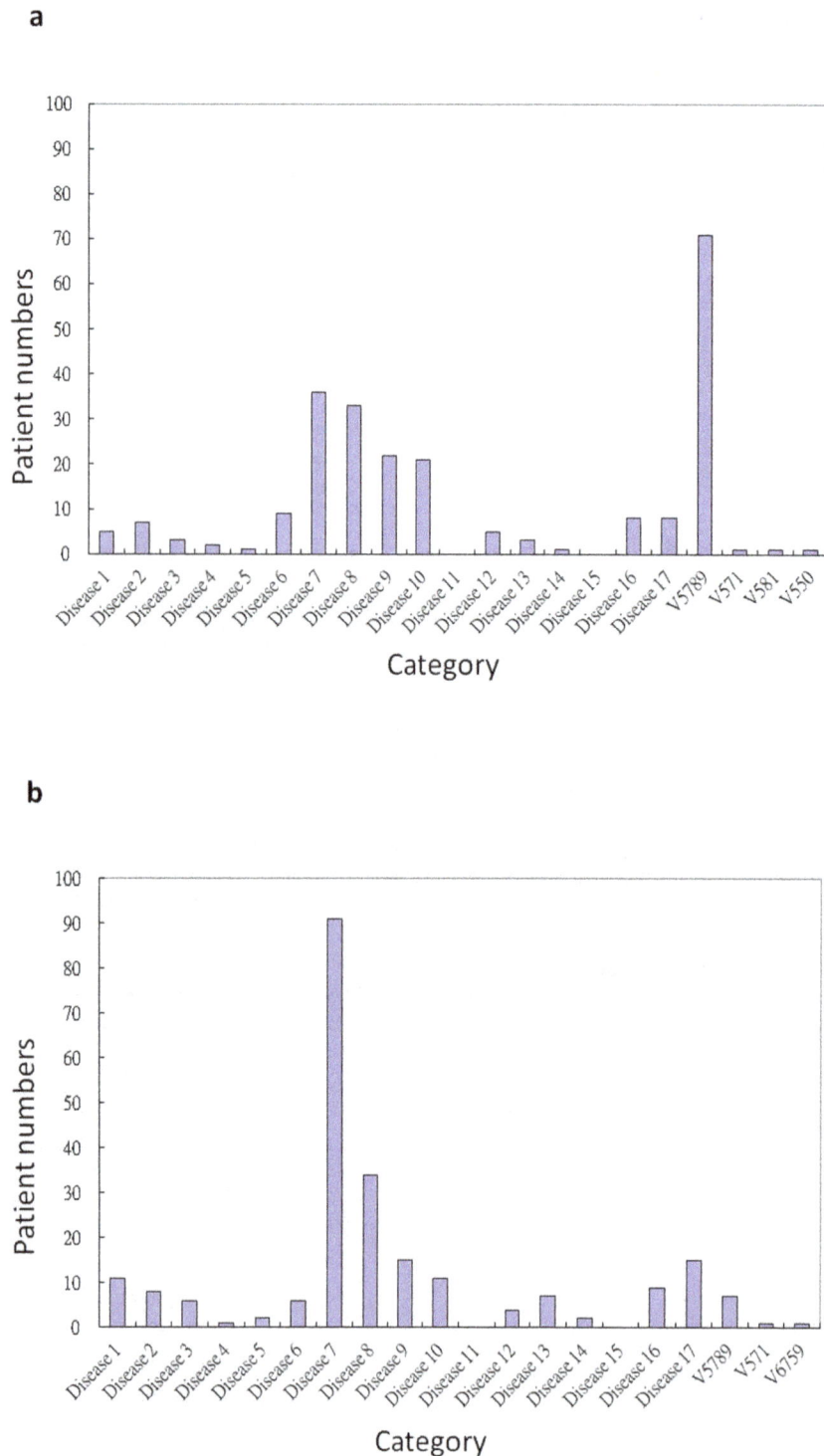

Figure 5. The distribution of ICD-9 category in re-admission of cases (5a) and random-controls (5b) group.

adjuvant TCM treatment inpatients paid less for conventional treatments, with the exception of ICD 437, which appeared to be higher in the first instance.(Figure 3)

This study demonstrated that for inpatients receiving TCM treatments for the DRG1501-02 Project, the annual costs during 2007 were significantly lower than in 2006. By contrast, for DRG1601-1702, if the TCM associated medical costs were

excluded, the medical treatment costs for the 2 years were similar.(Figure 4)

During the first hospitalization, the percentage of adjuvant TCM treatments was 0.82% in 2006 and 1.70% in 2007. In addition, the re-admission rate of TCM inpatients was 17.84% in 2006 and 19.04% in 2007. During the first hospitalization, 99.18% (2006) and 98.3% (2007) of the whole population were non-TCM inpatients, and the re-admission rate was 10.56% in 2006 and 9.43% in 2007. The average re-admission duration was significantly shorter for TCM participants, especially for the initial ICD 434 cases.(Table 2) However, during subsequent re-admission episodes, the odds ratio for Disease 7 of ICD-9 category, representing circulatory system diseases, significantly favored non-TCM participants among all potential causes. (Table 3)(Figure 5)

Discussion

Among inpatients who were diagnosed with ICD-9 code (430 to 437) upon first admission, the average re-admission duration was significantly shorter for TCM inpatients. In addition, the inpatients being introduced to TCM demonstrated more severe general symptoms, which were costly to deal with conventional treatments, and the severity of underline diseases might be causative re-admission. However, adjuvant TCM treatment inpatients appeared to have significantly lower circulatory system events while re-admission. However, there were shorter re-admission duration other than circulatory system events by means of unfavorable baseline condition.

The disease diagnosis related group (DRG) measure enforces equal medical fee payments for diagnosis-related groups and helps to reduce unnecessary medical costs that burden the system. Recently, Taiwan has been planning to implement the DRG. However, after numerous meetings, consultations, commissioning of scholars and experts to lead relevant research projects, some public interest-related support measures have been developed for the short-term, but no guarantee exists that public health interests are not negatively influenced by the waste of additional medical resources. Since 2009, DRG measures have focused on the gradual implementation of health payments with a pilot project. This study's design was based on a previous study focusing on data from 2006 and 2007 Taiwanese National Health Insurance Research Database, and included study participants that were diagnosed under the international standard code for diagnosis of disease (ICD-9) in the cerebrovascular disease Group (430 to 437) for analysis. In April 2006, the National Health Council issued a Pilot Scheme of Health Policy in Stroke Adjuvant Acupuncture

and TCM Therapy [15], and we used this scheme to investigate the statistics on TCM participation per patient per year for all inpatients hospitalized during 2006 and 2007. We then analyzed the overlapping use of integrative Chinese and Western medicine in hospitals to understand regional differences between inpatients that participated in pilot scheme in three municipals by analyzing the costs of admission and number of outpatients. In addition, we partially launched the DRG project in 2011. The 2006 to 2007 database of the NHIRD was used to perform cost predictions for retrospective classifications. However, the national medical institutions failed to timeously implement the pilot scheme in 2006, and ragged data could not be avoided. Therefore, additional research of the health insurance database is needed.

Conclusion

Among inpatients diagnosed with ICD-9 code 430 to 437 upon first admission, the adjuvant TCM treatment patients appeared to be significantly less re-admission for circulatory system events. A two-third reduction of re-admission within ICD-9 code 430 ~ 437 favored the adjuvant TCM treatment patients.

Supporting Information

File S1   Appendix S1.
(DOCX)

Acknowledgments

The authors give thanks to the Taiwan Traditional Chinese Medicine Association for providing information of HPSAAT. We acknowledge the contribution of Hen-Hong Chang MD/PhD and Sheng-Teng Huang MD/PhD in the administration support of this study, and Jer-Ming Sheen MD, Cheng-Nan Lu MD, Guo-Wei Bi MD, and Wu-Long Hu MD in treating the HPSAAT patients in KCGMH.

Author Contributions

Conceived and designed the experiments: HEC. Performed the experiments: HEC KCC JWH CWL TYT. Analyzed the data: HEC CCS JWH. Contributed reagents/materials/analysis tools: HEC YCH. Wrote the paper: HEC. Critical review of Statisitcs: HEC CCH.

References

1. O'Mahony PG, Thomson RG, Dobon R (1999) The prevalence of stroke and associated disability. J Public Health Med 21:1666–1671.
2. Hackett ML, Duncan JR, Anderson CS, Broad JB, Bonita R (2000) Health-related quality of life among long-term survivors of stroke: results from the Auckland Stroke Study, 1991–1992. Stroke 31:440–447.
3. Murry CJ, Lopez AD (1997) Mortality by cause for eight regions of the world: Global Burden of Disease Study. Lancet 349:1269–1276.
4. World Health Organization (2007) The Top Ten Causes of Death. Fact sheet N° 310. February 2007:5.
5. Southampton and South West Hampshire Health Commission (1994). Annual report. Director of Public Health.
6. Wu JN (1996) A short history of acupuncture. J Altern Complement Med 2:19–21.
7. Han JS, Terenius L (1982) Neurochemical basis of acupuncture analgesia. Annu Rev Pharmacol Toxicol 22:193–220.
8. Jansen G, Lundeberg T, Kjartansson S, Samuelson UE (1989) Acupuncture and sensory neuropeptides increase cutaneous blood flow in rats. Neurosci Let 97:305–309.

9. Magnusson M, Johansson K, Johansson BB (1994) Sensory stimulation promotes normalization of postural control after stroke. Stroke 25:1176–1180.
10. Sun HL, Li XM (2001) Clinical study on treatment of cerebral apoplexy with penetration needling of scalp acupoints. Chin Acupunct Moxi 21:275–278.
11. NIH Consensus Conference (1998) Acupuncture. JAMA 280:1518–1524.
12. Chen ZM, Sandcock P, Xie JX, Collins R, Liu LS (1997) Hospital management of acute ischemic stroke in China. J Stroke Cerebrovasc Dis. 6:361–367.
13. Naeser MA, Alexander MP, Stiassny-Eder D, Galler V, Hobbs J, et al (1994) Acupuncture in the treatment of paralysis in chronic and acute stroke patients--improvement correlated with specific CT scan lesion sites. Acupunct Electrother Res 19:227–249. javascript:PopUpMenu2_Set(Menu7625245);
14. Dean RH (2004) Retrospective Studies and Chart Reviews. Respir Care 49:1171–1174.
15. Wei YC, Sun MF, Chang KC, Chang CJ, Hung YC, et al (2011) Pilot scheme of health policy in stroke adjuvant acupuncture therapy for acute and subacute ischemic stroke in Taiwan. eCAM 2011:689813.

PERMISSIONS

The contributors of this book come from diverse backgrounds, making this book a truly international effort. This book will bring forth new frontiers with its revolutionizing research information and detailed analysis of the nascent developments around the world.

We would like to thank all the contributing authors for lending their expertise to make the book truly unique. They have played a crucial role in the development of this book. Without their invaluable contributions this book wouldn't have been possible. They have made vital efforts to compile up to date information on the varied aspects of this subject to make this book a valuable addition to the collection of many professionals and students.

This book was conceptualized with the vision of imparting up-to-date information and advanced data in this field. To ensure the same, a matchless editorial board was set up. Every individual on the board went through rigorous rounds of assessment to prove their worth. After which they invested a large part of their time researching and compiling the most relevant data for our readers.

The editorial board has been involved in producing this book since its inception. They have spent rigorous hours researching and exploring the diverse topics which have resulted in the successful publishing of this book. They have passed on their knowledge of decades through this book. To expedite this challenging task, the publisher supported the team at every step. A small team of assistant editors was also appointed to further simplify the editing procedure and attain best results for the readers.

Apart from the editorial board, the designing team has also invested a significant amount of their time in understanding the subject and creating the most relevant covers. They scrutinized every image to scout for the most suitable representation of the subject and create an appropriate cover for the book.

The publishing team has been an ardent support to the editorial, designing and production team. Their endless efforts to recruit the best for this project, has resulted in the accomplishment of this book. They are a veteran in the field of academics and their pool of knowledge is as vast as their experience in printing. Their expertise and guidance has proved useful at every step. Their uncompromising quality standards have made this book an exceptional effort. Their encouragement from time to time has been an inspiration for everyone.

The publisher and the editorial board hope that this book will prove to be a valuable piece of knowledge for researchers, students, practitioners and scholars across the globe.

LIST OF CONTRIBUTORS

Junqi Chen
Department of Rehabilitation, The Third Affiliated Hospital of Southern Medical University, Guangzhou, China

Jizhou Wang
The First Clinical Medical School, Southern Medical University, Guangzhou, China

Yong Huang and ShanshanQu
School of Traditional Chinese Medicine, Southern Medical University, Guangzhou, China

Xinsheng Lai, Chunzhi Tang and Junjun Yang
School of Acupuncture and Rehabilitation,Guangzhou University of Traditional Chinese Medicine, Guangzhou, China

Junxian Wu
Department of Acupuncture and Moxibustion, Shantou Central Hospital, Shantou, China

TongjunZeng
The First People's Hospital of Shunde, Foshan, China

Myeong Soo Lee
Brain Disease ResearchCenter, Korea Institute of Oriental Medicine, Daejeon, Republic of Korea

Hyun-Woo Cho and Kwang-Ho Heo
Department of Rehabilitation Medicine of Korean Medicine, Spine and Joint Center, Pusan National University Korean Medicine Hospital, Yangsan, Republic of Korea,

Eui-Hyoung Hwang and Byung-Cheul Shin
Department of Rehabilitation Medicine of Korean Medicine, Spine and Joint Center, Pusan National University Korean Medicine Hospital, Yangsan, Republic of Korea
Division of Clinical Medicine, School of Korean Medicine, Pusan National University, Yangsan, Republic of Korea

Byungmook Lim
Division of Humanities and Social Medicine, School ofKorean Medicine, Pusan National University, Yangsan, Republic of Korea

Jian-Ping Liu
Center for Evidence-Based Chinese Medicine, Beijing University of Chinese Medicine, Beijing,China

Kiichiro Tsutani
Department of Drug Policy and Management, Graduate School of Pharmaceutical Sciences, The University of Tokyo, Tokyo, Japan

Xiao Lu and Shang Hongcai
Tianjin University of Traditional Chinese Medicine, Tianjin, China
MOE Virtual Research Center of Evidence-Based Medicine, Chengdu, China

Wang Jiaying
Tianjin University of Traditional Chinese Medicine, Tianjin, China
Evidence BasedMedicine Center in Tianjin, Tianjin, China

Hu Jing
Peking University, Beijing, China

Xiong Jun
Department of Acupuncture, Jiang Xi Hospital of Traditional Chinese Medicine, JiangxiProvince, China

Huijuan Cao
Centre for Complementary Medicine Research, University of Western Sydney, Penrith, Australia
Centre for Evidence-Based Chinese Medicine, Beijing University ofChinese Medicine, Beijing, China

Xun Li and Jianping Liu
Centre for Evidence-Based Chinese Medicine, Beijing University of Chinese Medicine, Beijing, China

Ling Zhao, Xilin Dong, YulinPeng, Fumei Wu, Ying Li and Fanrong Liang
Acupuncture and Tuina School, Chengdu University of Traditional Chinese Medicine, Chengdu, Sichuan, China

Zili Tang
German Cancer Consortium (DKTK),Heidelberg, Germany

Fuwen Zhang
School of Clinical Medicine, Chengdu University of Traditional Chinese Medicine, Chengdu, Sichuan, China

Wei Qin, Kai Yuan, Karen M. von Deneen and Jixin Liu
School of Life Science and Technology, XidianUniversity, Xi'an, Shaanxi, China

Qiyong Gong
Department of Radiology,The Center for Medical Imaging, Huaxi MR Research Center, West China Hospital of Sichuan University, Chengdu, Sichuan, China

Chun-Chuan Shih, Chin-Chuan Tsai and Hsin-Long Lane
School of Chinese Medicine for Post-Baccalaureate, I-Shou University, Kaohsiung, Taiwan

Hwang-Huei Wang
Graduate Institute of Integrated Medicine, College of Chinese Medicine, China Medical University, Taichung, Taiwan

Ta-Liang Chen
Department of Anesthesiology, Taipei Medical University Hospital, Taipei, Taiwan
Health Policy Research Centre, Taipei Medical University Hospital, Taipei, Taiwan
School of Medicine, College of Medicine, Taipei Medical University, Taipei, Taiwan

Chun-ChiehYeh
Graduate Institute of Clinical Medical Science, China Medical University, Taichung, Taiwan

Fung-Chang Sung
Department of Public Health, China Medical University, Taichung, Taiwan

Wen-Ta Chiu
Graduate Institute of Injury Prevention and Control, Taipei Medical University, Taipei,Taiwan

Yih-GiunCherng
Department of Anesthesiology, Shuang Ho Hospital, Taipei Medical University, New Taipei City, Taiwan

Chien-Chang Liao
Department of Anesthesiology, Taipei Medical University Hospital, Taipei, Taiwan
Health Policy Research Centre, Taipei Medical University Hospital, Taipei, Taiwan
School of Medicine, College of Medicine, Taipei Medical University, Taipei, Taiwan
Management Office for Health Data, China MedicalUniversity Hospital, Taichung, Taiwan

Yi-Ting Hsu
Neuroscience Laboratory, Department of Neurology, China Medical University Hospital, Taichung, Taiwan

Claudia M. Witt
University of Maryland School of Medicine, Center for Integrative Medicine, Baltimore, Maryland, United States of America

Charité University Medical Center, Institutefor Social Medicine, Epidemiology and Health Economics, Berlin, Germany

Eric Manheimer, Lixing Lao and Brian M. Berman
University of Maryland School of Medicine, Center for Integrative Medicine, Baltimore, Maryland, United States of America,

Richard Hammerschlag
Research Department, Oregon College of Oriental Medicine, Portland, Oregon, United States of America

Rainer Lüdtke
Carstens Foundation, Essen, Germany

Sean R.Tunis
Center for Medical Technology Policy, Baltimore, Maryland, United States of America

Zhiqun Wang, Zhilian Zhao and Jie Lu
Department of Radiology, Xuanwu Hospital of Capital Medical University, Beijing, China

Peipeng Liang
Department of Radiology, Xuanwu Hospital of Capital Medical University, Beijing, China,

Ying Han and Haiqing Song
Department of Neurology, Xuanwu Hospital of Capital Medical University,Beijing, China

Jianyang Xu
General Hospital of ChinesePeople's Armed Police Forces, Beijing, China

Kuncheng Li
Department of Radiology, Xuanwu Hospital of Capital Medical University, Beijing, China
Key Laboratory for Neurodegenerative Diseases, Ministry of Education, Beijing, China
Beijing Key Laboratory of Magnetic Resonance Imaging and Brain Informatics, Beijing, China

Haomin Wang and Xinhong Wang
Neuroscience Research Institute, Peking University, Beijing, People's Republic of China

Yanli Pan
Science and Education Office, Beijing An Ding Hospital, Beijing, People'sRepublic of China

Bing Xue
Medical Experiment and Test Center, Capital Medical University, Beijing, People's Republic of China

Feng Zhao
School of Public Health and Family Medicine,Capital Medical University, Beijing, People's Republic of China

Jun Jia
Department of Physiology, Capital Medical University, Key Laboratory for Neurodegenerative Disorders ofthe Ministry of Education, Beijing, People's Republic of China

Xibin Liang
Department of Neurology and Neurological Sciences, Stanford University, Stanford, California, UnitedStates of America

XiaominWang
Neuroscience Research Institute, Peking University, Beijing, People's Republic of China
Department of Physiology, Capital Medical University, Key Laboratory for Neurodegenerative Disorders ofthe Ministry of Education, Beijing, People's Republic of China

Zhenyu Liu, Wenjuan Wei, LijunBai, Ruwei Dai and Youbo You
Key Laboratory of Molecular Imaging and Functional Imaging, Institute of Automation, Chinese Academy of Sciences, Beijing, China

Shangjie Chen
Department of Acupuncture andMassage, Bao'an Hospital, Southern Medical University, Shenzhen, China

JieTian
Key Laboratory of Molecular Imaging and Functional Imaging, Institute of Automation, Chinese Academy of Sciences, Beijing, China
Life Sciences Research Center, School of Life Sciences and Technology, Xidian University, Xi'an,Shaanxi, China

Hugh MacPherson
Department of Health Sciences, University of York, York, United Kingdom

Emily Vertosick and Andrew J. Vickers
Memorial Sloan-Kettering Cancer Center, New York, New York, United States of America

George Lewith
Faculty of Medicine, Primary Care and Population Sciences, University of Southampton, Southampton, United Kingdom

Klaus Linde
Institute of General Practice, TechnischeUniversitätMünchen, Munich, Germany

Karen J. Sherman
Group Health Research Institute, Seattle, Washington, United States of America

Claudia M. Witt
Center for Complementary and IntegrativeMedicine, University Hospital Zurich, Zurich, Switzerland
Institute for Social Medicine, Epidemiology and Health Economics, Charité - Universitätsmedizin, Berlin,Germany

Zhang-Jin Zhang, Roger Ng, Sui Cheung Man, Tsui Yin Jade Li, Wendy Wong and HeiKiu Wong
School of Chinese Medicine, LKS Faculty of Medicine, The University of Hong Kong, Hong Kong, China

Qing-Rong Tan
Department of Psychiatry, Fourth Military Medical University, Xi'an, Shaanxi, China

Man-Tak Wong, Wai-KiuAlfert Tsang and Ka-chee Yip
Department of Psychiatry, Kowloon Hospital, Hong Kong, China,

Ka-Fai Chung
Department of Psychiatry, LKS Faculty of Medicine, The University of Hong Kong, Hong Kong, China

Eric Ziea and Vivian TaamWong
Chinese Medicine Section, Hospital Authority, Hong Kong, China

Yangbo Liu, Cailong Liu, Jing Wang, Lei Chen and Jiandong Yuan
Orthopedics, The First Affiliated Hospital of Wenzhou Medical University, Wenzhou, Zhejiang, China

Jingye Pan
Intensive Care Unit, The First Affiliated Hospital of WenzhouMedical University, Wenzhou, Zhejiang, China

Keke Jin
Pathophysiology, Wenzhou Medical University, Wenzhou, Zhejiang, China

Li Chen
Biomedicine, The University of Melbourne,Melbourne, Victoria, Australia

Tae-Hun Kim
Acupuncture, Moxibustion& Meridian Research Centre, Korea Institute of Oriental Medicine, Daejeon, South Korea
Department of Cardiovascular and NeurologicDiseases, College of Oriental Medicine, Graduate School, Kyung Hee University, Seoul, South Korea

Jung Won Kang
Acupuncture, Moxibustion& Meridian Research Centre, Korea Institute of Oriental Medicine, Daejeon, South Korea

Department of Acupuncture and Moxibustion, College of Oriental
Medicine, Kyung Hee University, Seoul, South Korea

Kun Hyung Kim
Acupuncture, Moxibustion& Meridian Research Centre, Korea Institute of Oriental Medicine, Daejeon, South Korea
Division of Clinical Medicine, School of Korean Medicine, Pusan National University, Gyeongsangnam-do, South Korea

Kyung-Won Kang, Mi-Suk Shin, So-Young Jung, Ae-Ran Kim, Hee-Jung Jung and Sun-Mi Choi
Acupuncture, Moxibustion& Meridian Research Centre, Korea Institute of Oriental Medicine, Daejeon, South Korea,

Jin-Bong Choi
Department of Oriental Rehabilitation Medicine, Dongshin University, Gwangju, South Korea

Kwon Eui Hong
Department of Acupuncture and Moxibustion, Daejeon University,
Daejeon, South Korea

Seung-Deok Lee
Department of Acupuncture and Moxibustion, Dongguk University, Goyang, South Korea

Mats Lekander
Departmentof Clinical Neuroscience, Osher Centre for Integrative Medicine, Karolinska Institute, Stockholm, SwedenStress Research Institute, Stockholm University, Stockholm,Sweden

Anna Enblom
Division of Nursing Science, Department of Medical and Health Sciences, Linkö ping University, Linkö ping, Sweden

The Vårdal Institute, Lund, Sweden
Departmentof Clinical Neuroscience, Osher Centre for Integrative Medicine, Karolinska Institute, Stockholm, Sweden

Mats Hammar
Department of Clinical and Experimental Medicine, Obstetrics and Gynecology, Linkö ping University, Linkö ping, Sweden

Anna Johnsson
Division of Physiotherapy,Department of Oncology, University Hospital, Lund, Sweden

Erik Onelöv
Division of Clinical Cancer Epidemiology, Department of Oncology, Karolinska Institute, Stockholm, Sweden

Gunnar Steineck
Division of Clinical Cancer Epidemiology, Department of Oncology, Karolinska Institute, Stockholm, Sweden
Division of Clinical Cancer Epidemiology, Department of Oncology, Sahlgrenska Academy, Gothenburg, Sweden

Martin Ingvar
Departmentof Clinical Neuroscience, Osher Centre for Integrative Medicine, Karolinska Institute, Stockholm, Sweden

SussanneBörjeson
Division of Nursing Science, Department of Medical and Health Sciences, Linkö ping University, Linkö ping, Sweden Centre of Surgery and Oncology, Linkö pingUniversity Hospital, Linkö ping, Sweden

Chen Bo, Zhao Xue, Guo Yi, Chen Zelin, Bai Yang and Wang Zixu
College of Acupuncture and Moxibustion, Tianjin University of Traditional Chinese Medicine, Tianjin, China

Wang Yajun
Department of Acupuncture and Massage, Gansu Collegeof Traditional Chinese Medicine, Gansu Province, China

Jing Gu
Evidence-Based Medicine Center, Institute of Integrated Traditional Chinese and Western Medicine, School of Basic Medical Sciences, Lanzhou University, Lanzhou,Gansu, China
Institute of Integrated Traditional Chinese and Western Medicine, Gansu University of Traditional Chinese Medicine, Lanzhou, Gansu, China

Ye Zhao, Xiaogang Wang, JinhuiTian and Kehu Yang
Evidence-Based Medicine Center, Institute of Integrated Traditional Chinese and Western Medicine, School of Basic Medical Sciences, Lanzhou University, Lanzhou,Gansu, China

Jianjun Jiang
SecondSchool of Clinical Medicine of Lanzhou University, Lanzhou, Gansu, China

Jing Li and Jiang-Hong Ye
Department of Anesthesiology, Pharmacology and Physiology, University of Medicine and Dentistry of New Jersey, New Jersey Medical School, Newark, New Jersey,United States of America

Yanan Sun
Department of Neurology, Dong-Zhi-Men Hospital, Beijing University of Chinese Medicine, Key Laboratory for Internal Chinese Medicine of
Ministry of Education, Beijing, China

Julia Johansson, Louise Mannerås-Holm, Ruijin Shao and AnneLiese Olsson and HåkanBillig
Institute of Neuroscience and Physiology, Department of Physiology, Sahlgrenska Academy, University of Gothenburg, Gothenburg, Sweden,

ElisabetStener-Victorin
Institute of Neuroscience and Physiology, Department of Physiology, Sahlgrenska Academy, University of Gothenburg, Gothenburg, Sweden,
Department of Obstetrics andGynecology, First Affiliated Hospital, Heilongjiang University of Chinese Medicine, Harbin, China

MalinLönn
Institute of Biomedicine,Department of Clinical Chemistry and Transfusion Medicine, Sahlgrenska Academy, University of Gothenburg, Gothenburg, Sweden

Ann Hopton and Hugh MacPherson
Department of Health Sciences, University of York, York, North Yorkshire, United Kingdom

Kate Thomas
Health Services Research Unit, University of Sheffield, Sheffield, South
Yorkshire, United Kingdom

Bo Liu, Jun Chen, Xian Liu, XiaohuiDuan, Xiaojing Shang, Yu Long,Zhiguang Chen, Xiaofang Li and Yan Huang
Department of Radiology, Guangdong Provincial Hospital of Traditional Chinese Medicine, Guangdong, China

Jinhui Wang and Yong He
State Key Laboratory of Cognitive Neuroscience andLearning, Beijing Normal University, Beijing, China

Yu-Chiang Hong
Department of TCM, Chang Gung University College of Medicine, Kaohsiung, Taiwan
Chang Gung Memorial Hospital, Chang GungUniversity College of Medicine, Kaohsiung, Taiwan

Chun-Chuan Shih
School of Chinese Medicine for Post-Baccalaureate, I-Shou University, Kaohsiung, Taiwan

Jen-Wen Hung
Department of Rehabilitation, Chang Gung University College of Medicine, Kaohsiung, Taiwan
Chang Gung Memorial Hospital, Chang GungUniversity College of Medicine, Kaohsiung, Taiwan

Chia-Wei Liu, Teng-Yeow Tan and Ku-Chou Chang
Department of Neurology, Chang Gung University College of Medicine,
Kaohsiung, Taiwan
Chang Gung Memorial Hospital, Chang GungUniversity College of Medicine, Kaohsiung, Taiwan

Chih-Cheng Huang
Department of TCM, Chang Gung University College of Medicine, Kaohsiung, Taiwan

HsienhsuehElley Chiu
Department of TCM, Chang Gung University College of Medicine, Kaohsiung, Taiwan
Department of Neurology, Chang Gung University College of Medicine, Kaohsiung, Taiwan
Chang Gung Memorial Hospital, Chang Gung University College of Medicine, Kaohsiung, Taiwan

Index

www.ingramcontent.com/pod-product-compliance
Lightning Source LLC
Chambersburg PA
CBHW080517200326
41458CB00012B/4239

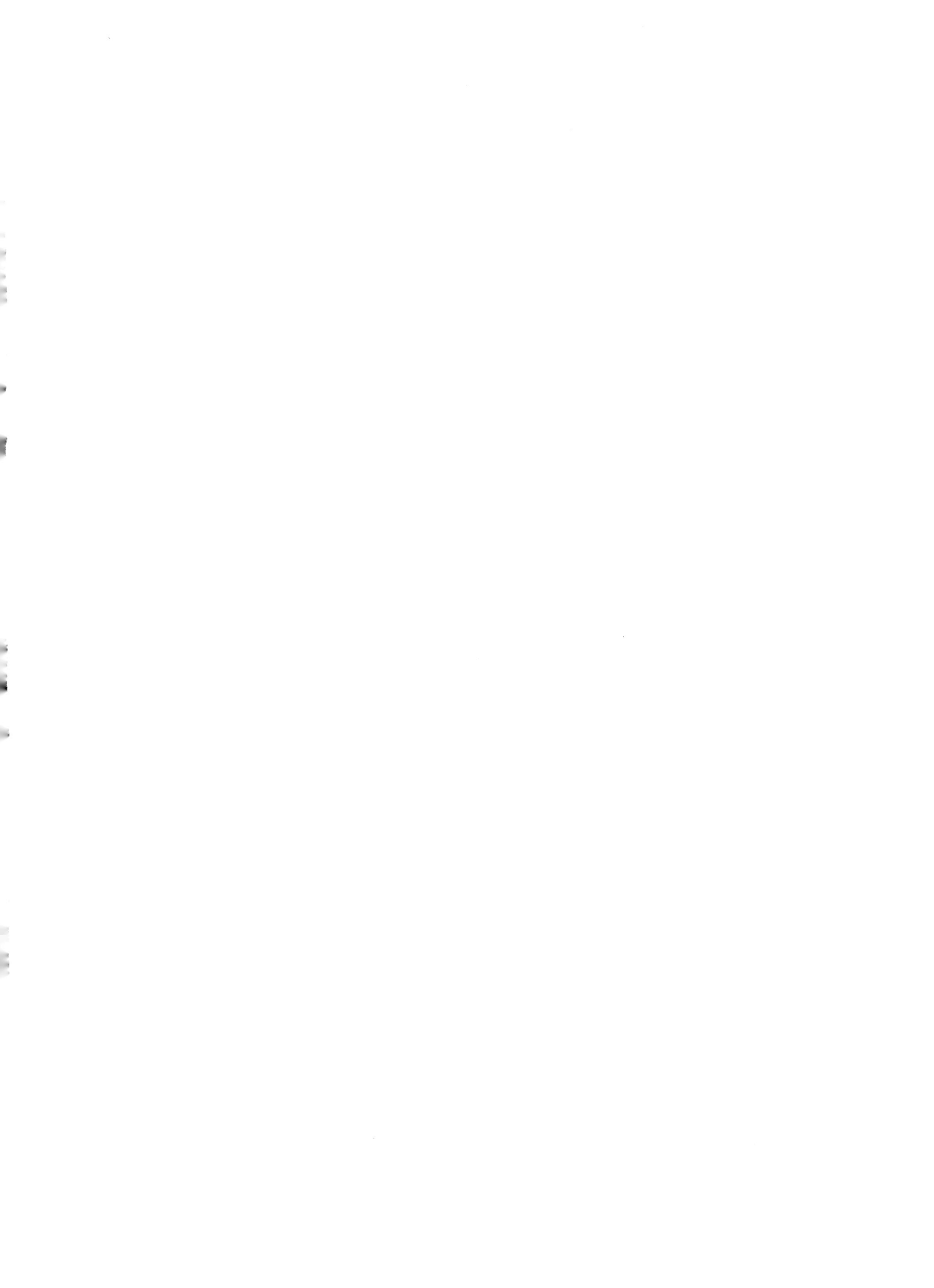

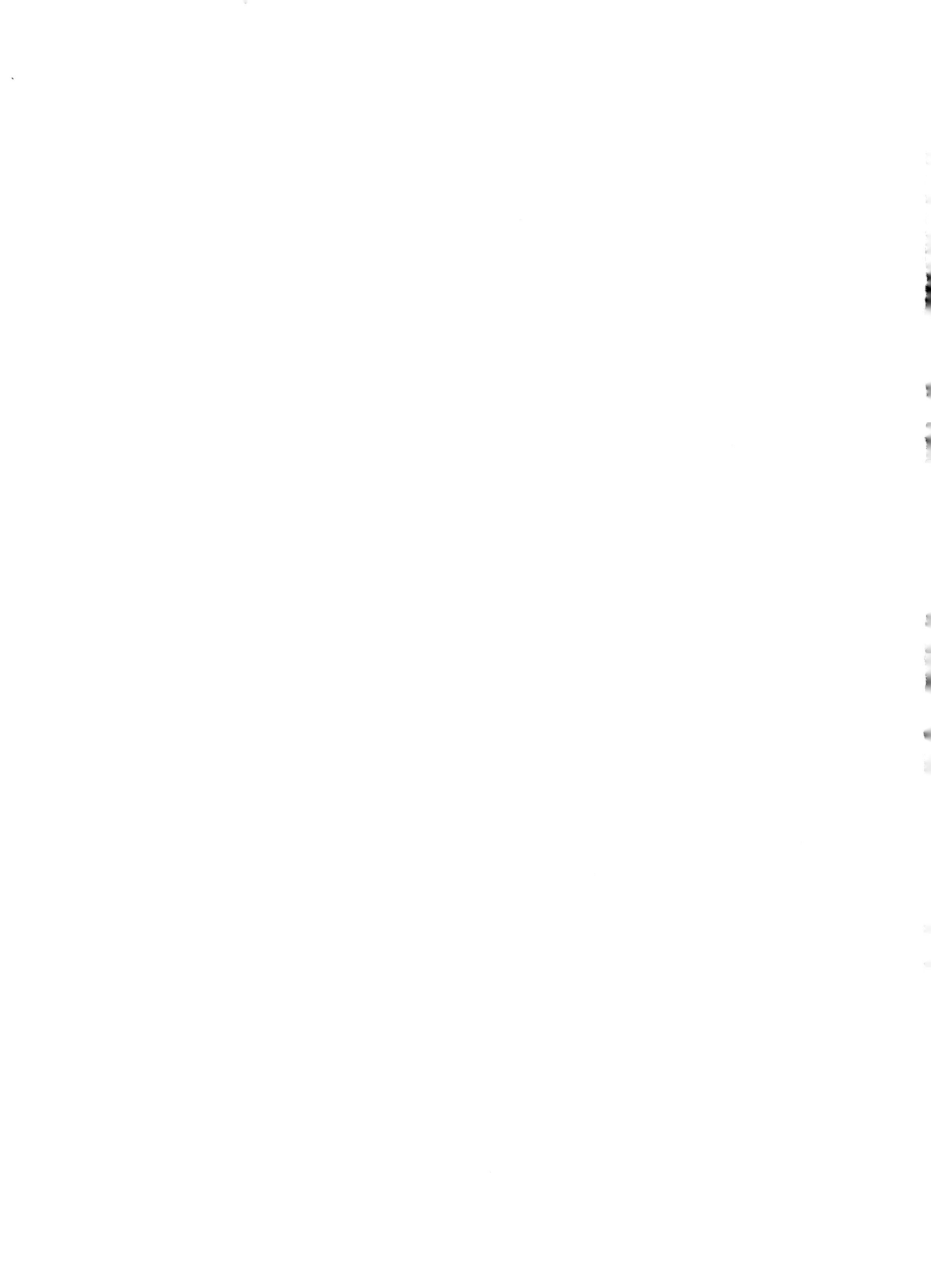